INTERNATIONAL ENCYCLOPEDIA OF
PHARMACOLOGY AND THERAPEUTICS

Executive Editor: A. C. SARTORELLI, *New Haven*

Section 127

ANTIBIOTIC INHIBITORS OF BACTERIAL CELL WALL BIOSYNTHESIS

EDITORIAL BOARD

Some Recent and Forthcoming Volumes

NOTICE TO READERS

Dear Reader

If your library is not already a standing order customer to this series, may we recommend that you place a standing order to receive immediately on publication all new volumes published in this valuable series. Should you find that these volumes no longer serve your needs your order can be cancelled at any time without notice.

The Editors and Publisher will be glad to receive suggestions or outlines of suitable titles for consideration for rapid publication in this series.

ROBERT MAXWELL
Publisher at Pergamon Press

INTERNATIONAL ENCYCLOPEDIA OF
PHARMACOLOGY AND THERAPEUTICS

Section 127

ANTIBIOTIC INHIBITORS OF BACTERIAL CELL WALL BIOSYNTHESIS

SECTION EDITOR

DONALD J. TIPPER

Department of Molecular Genetics and Molecular Biology,
University of Massachusetts Medical School, USA

PERGAMON PRESS

OXFORD · NEW YORK · BEIJING · FRANKFURT
SÃO PAULO · SYDNEY · TOKYO · TORONTO

U.K.	Pergamon Press, Headington Hill Hall, Oxford OX3 0BW, England
U.S.A.	Pergamon Press, Maxwell House, Fairview Park, Elmsford, New York 10523, U.S.A.
PEOPLE'S REPUBLIC OF CHINA	Pergamon Press, Room 4037, Qianmen Hotel, Beijing, People's Republic of China
FEDERAL REPUBLIC OF GERMANY	Pergamon Press, Hammerweg 6, D-6242 Kronberg, Federal Republic of Germany
BRAZIL	Pergamon Editors, Rua Eça de Queiros, 346, CEP 04011, Paraiso, São Paulo, Brazil
AUSTRALIA	Pergamon Press Australia, P.O. Box 544, Potts Point, N.S.W. 2011, Australia
JAPAN	Pergamon Press, 8th Floor, Matsuoka Central Building, 1-7-1 Nishishinjuku, Shinjuku-ku, Tokyo 160, Japan
CANADA	Pergamon Press Canada, Suite No. 271, 253 College Street, Toronto, Ontario, Canada M5T 1R5

Copyright © 1987 Pergamon Books Ltd.

First edition 1987

Library of Congress Cataloging in Publications Data

Antibiotic inhibitors of bacterial cell wall biosynthesis.
(International encyclopedia of pharmacology and therapeutics; section 127)
"Published as Supplement no. 27 (1987) to the review journal Pharmacology and therapeutics"—T.p. verso.
Includes bibliographies and index.
1. Bacterial cell walls—Synthesis—Inhibitors.
2. Beta lactam antibiotics—Structure-activity relationships. I. Tipper, Donald J., 1935– .
II. Pharmacology & therapeutics. III. Series.
[DNLM: 1. Antibiotics—biosynthesis. 2. Bacteria—metabolism.
3. Cell Wall—metabolism 4. Drug Resistance, Microbial. QV 4
158 section 127]
QR77.3.A58   1987   589.9′0875   87-21572

British Library Cataloguing in Publication Data

Antibiotic inhibitors of bacterial cell wall biosynthesis.—(International encyclopedia of pharmacology and therapeutics: section 127).
1. Antibiotics
I. Tipper, Donald J. II. Series
615′.329   RM267
ISBN 0-08-036130-7

Published as Supplement No. 27 (1987) to the review journal *Pharmacology and Therapeutics*.

Printed in Great Britain by A. Wheaton & Co. Ltd., Exeter

DEDICATION

This volume is dedicated to Dr. Jack L. Strominger *whose intelligence, profound biochemical insight, enthusiasm, and unfailing ability to ask the right questions has been largely responsible for the major advances made in understanding the mode of action of inhibitors of bacterial cell wall peptidoglycan biosynthesis over the past twenty-five years.*

PREFACE

Antibiotic Inhibitors of Bacterial Cell Wall Biosynthesis: the present and some thoughts on future trends

Epidemic bacterial infectious diseases, such as cholera and plague, have played such a prominent part in the history of the 'Western' world that their horrors still echo in our memories. Although apparently laid to rest by modern medicine, they are still capable of ravaging less fortunate societies. The spectre stirred again in the United States in 1976 with the recognition of Legionella as a 'new', frequently lethal, bacterial epidemic disease. It now looms menacingly in the form of AIDS, a viral disese whose mechanisms could not have been understood as recently as twenty years ago. Such is the pace of modern biological research, however, that there is hope that this disease, undoubtedly the most serious challenge to preventative medicine and therapy of infectious disease ever recognized by man, can be contained by a massive research effort to pinpoint its mechanisms and weaknesses. Fear is widespread; panic may not be far behind.

Nevertheless, it is undoubtedly true that the development of sanitation and other public health measures, dating back at least to the Minoan civilization, by thwarting the food and water-borne routes of transmission of infectious diseases, did more to improve the longevity of Urban man than all of modern microbiology. Moreover, vaccination, developed out of an intuitive response to scientific observation long before infectious agents were identified, conquered smallpox and still provides the best chance of holding in check the pandemic viral and bacterial infections such as influenza, measles, mumps and TB that debilitate, maim, and sometimes kill. It was the establishment of the science of microbiology in the nineteenth century, however, that was the necessary precursor to one of the major success stories of twentieth century medicine—the development of effective antimicrobial chemotherapy.

From the beginning, this was an enterprise carried on the crest of the wave of developing science—microbiology, genetics, organic chemistry, then biochemistry and, more recently, molecular biology and genetics. Slow to develop, it came of age with the introduction of penicillin during the second World War. This volume represents an overview of the field initiated with that event: The mechanisms of action and some major mechanisms of resistance to chemotherapeutic agents that interfere with bacterial cell wall biosynthesis. These agents, and the β-lactam antibiotics in particular, still provide some of the best weapons for treatment of many bacterial infectious diseases, in spite of the spread of resistance to these agents in many genera as a consequence of selection. Diseases such as pneumococcal pneumonia, whose pathogenic agents remain for the most part susceptible, are no longer feared random killers of the relatively healthy. The major challenges for chemotherapy include the increasing population of individuals with severely impaired immunity, the broad range of pathogens to which they are susceptible, including some which are intrinsically resistant to most chemotherapeutic agents, and the variants of common pathogens which have acquired resistance to the commonly used agents and sometimes even to their latest derivatives.

Ward's chapter on the biosynthesis of peptidoglycan and the points of attack by wall inhibitors sets the stage for this field. The chapters by Neuhaus and Hammes on alanine analogues, by Toscano and Storm on Bacitracin, and by Perkins on Vancomycin and related antibiotics, follow in the sequence of their targets in the pathway of peptidoglycan biosynthesis. My own chapter on the mode of action of β-lactam antibiotics, inhibitors of the final stages of cell wall biosynthesis, provides further background for the final chapters on modern β-lactam antibiotics (Sykes *et al.*), the role of permeability barriers in resistance to these agents (Nikaido), and the role of β-lactamase inhibitors in chemotherapy (Neu).

It is worth noting that the more interesting and valuable recent developments in the chemotherapy of bacterial infectious disease have come from the rational application of the tools of modern organic chemistry to the design and synthesis of new derivatives of natural antibiotics, such as the monobactams and the β-lactam containing β-lactamase inhibitors, and to the production of completely synthetic agents such as alafosfalin. It is quite possible that the next significant advances in this field will come from two directions: First, the developing, detailed insight into the mode of action of known antibiotic inhibitors of transpeptidases andother peptidoglycan biosynthetic enzymes, based on the X-Ray crystallographic structural analysis of these targets, should lead to more rational and less empirical methods for the design of better inhibitors. These may either be variants of known antibiotics or completely new types of compound. Second, the rational design of inhibitors of other potential targets in wall biosynthesis for which no adequate natural or synthetic inhibitor currently exists, remains an open challenge. These targets include muramic acid biosynthesis and the production of D-glutamate. Phosphonomycin is an excellent inhibitor of muramic acid synthesis. Although resistance is easily acquired in the laboratory due to loss of the uptake pathways, this apparently does not impair its clinical utility, as shown by experience in Japan.. D-Glutamate production must be as carefully regulated as D-alanine production, but it has not been extensively studied. The mechanisms controlling cell wall autolysis, if sufficiently general, could also be specific targets for selective disruption. They are now known to be triggered in a species- and inhibitor-specific fashion by many of the agents discussed in this volume. Inhibitors of outer membrane assembly, particularly of lipopolysaccharide biosynthesis, might be effective agents specific for Gram-negative bacteria. At least they might disrupt the outer membrane permeability barrier sufficiently to act synergistically with β-lactam or other antibiotics. The recent reports concerning dipeptide derivatives of inhibitors of keto-deoxyoctanate biosynthesis are encouraging. They are highly effective against Gram-negative organisms *in vitro*, though possibly susceptible to hydrolysis by dipeptidase *in vivo*. It also seems possible that the recent application of the the techniques of modern molecular genetics to investigation of the mechanisms of pathogenesis of faculative intracellular parasites, such as *Salmonella, Yersinia* and *Legionella*, will lead to new strategies for treatment involving a dual attack on the bacteria themselves (conventional antibiotics) and on their mechanisms for avoiding intracellular killing mechanisms and surviving in this antibiotic-protected niche. Any such combined strategy may have to be tailored to specifically diagnosed infections. Analysis of the pathogenic mechanisms of several major extracellular bacterial pathogens, such as *Neisseria, Staphylococci, Campylobacter*, and enteropathogenic *E. coli* is also advancing rapidly, and should yield important clues for improvement in methods of prophylaxis and treatment. One aspect of antibacterial chemotherapy seems predictable: it will evolve and become more complex as our knowledge increases and as the pathogens adapt to our best efforts by mutation and plasmid acquisition.

Many of the recent advances listed and suggested above have been and will be pursued, appropriately, in the laboratories of the pharmaceutical industry. As previously implied, however, this enterprise is built on accumulated knowledge in the fields of organic chemistry, biochemistry, microbial physiology, and molecular biology and genetics. These subdisciplines of biology have named themselves as reflections of the aspirations of their practitioners. In turn, these names reflect the history of increasing sophistication in our drive to understand the life process. This intellectual evolution superbly illustrates the benefits to be derived from basic research, research aimed first at understanding, and only later at practical issues. Such basic research must be publicly funded. Applications come when the utility of tools developed by basic research become obvious. It is easy for the controllers of the public purse to identify the targets for such use. It is far more difficult for them to understand that the vitality and progression of the entire field of medicine is dependent on maintenance of an adequate level of funding for basic research and research training. We must continue to attract our ablest minds to this enterprise by demonstrating a firm political commitment to its support. The only argument should concern the appropriate fraction of our national resources to be devoted to this essential activity.

CONTENTS

6. MODERN β-LACTAM ANTIBIOTICS   171

R. B. Sykes, *Glaxo Group Research Ltd, Greenford, Middlesex, UK*, D. P. Booner & E. A. Swabb, *The Squibb Institute for Medical Research, New Jersey, USA*

7. ROLE OF PERMEABILITY BARRIERS IN RESISTANCE TO β-LACTAM ANTIBIOTICS   203

Hiroshi Nikaido, *University of California, USA*

8. THE ROLE OF β-LACTAMASE INHIBITORS IN CHEMOTHERAPY   241

H. C. Neu, *Columbia University, New York, USA*

LIST OF CONTRIBUTORS

DANIEL P. BONNER
The Squibb Institute for Medical Research
P.O. Box 4000
Princeton, NJ 08540
U.S.A.

WALTER P. HAMMES
Institut für Lebensmittel Teknologie
Universität Hohenheim
Garbenstrasse 25
7000 Stuttgart 70
West Germany

HAROLD C. NEU, M.D.
Departments of Medicine and Pharmacology
College of Physicians and Surgeons
Columbia University
630 West 168th Street
New York, NY 10032
U.S.A.

FRANCIS C. NEUHAUS
Department of Biochemistry and Molecular Biology
Northwestern University
Evanston, IL 60201
U.S.A.

H. NIKAIDO
Department of Microbiology and Immunology
University of California
Berkeley
California 94720
U.S.A.

H. R. PERKINS
Department of Microbiology
University of Liverpool
Liverpool L69 3BX
England

DANIEL R. STORM
Department of Pharmacology
University of Washington School of Medicine
Seattle, WA 98195
U.S.A.

EDWARD A. SWABB
Searle Pharmaceuticals Inc.
5300 Old Orchard Road
Skokie, IL 6007
U.S.A.

RICHARD B. SYKES
Glaxo Group Research Ltd
Greenford
Middlesex
U.K.

DONALD J. TIPPER
Department of Molecular Genetics and
    Microbiology
University of Massachusetts Medical School
Worcester, MA 01605
U.S.A.

WILLIAM A. TOSCANO, JR
Laboratory of Toxicology
School of Public Health
Harvard University
665 Huntington Avenue
Boston, MA 02115
U.S.A.

J. B. WARD
Department of Microbial Biochemistry
GLAXO Group Research Ltd
Greenford
Middlesex UB6 0HE
England

CHAPTER 1

BIOSYNTHESIS OF PEPTIDOGLYCAN: POINTS OF ATTACK BY WALL INHIBITORS

J. B. WARD

Department of Microbial Biochemistry, Glaxo Group Research Ltd.,
Greenford, Middlesex, UB6 0HE, England

1. INTRODUCTION

The bacterial wall is of major importance not only to the organism itself, but to man as the focus of interaction between the host, the bacterium and antimicrobial agents. It is now thirty years since Park (1952a,b,c) reported the isolation of the first nucleotide linked precursor of peptidoglycan from *Staphylococcus aureus* grown in the presence of benzylpenicillin. Since that time studies of the biosynthesis of peptidoglycan have been essential in furthering our knowledge not only of the complexities of the biosynthetic mechanisms but also of the mode of action of inhibitors of this process. These now include a wide range of compounds whose sites of action cover the whole biosynthetic pathway.

2. STRUCTURE OF PEPTIDOGLYCAN

The walls of all bacteria, with the exception of the Archaebacteria, contain peptidoglycan as their main structural component. In Gram-positive organisms this polymer alone may account for as much as 80% of the total weight of the wall, although values of 40–50% are more commonly found. In Gram-negative organisms peptidoglycan represents only a minor fraction of the wall. As its name implies, it consists of glycan chains with peptide substituents that are cross-linked. Thus, the organism is enclosed in a network; the bag-shaped macromolecule of Weidel and Pelzer (1964), which is responsible for the shape of the bacterium.

The glycan chains consist of alternating residues of glucosamine and muramic acid, the 3-*O*-D-lactyl ether derivative of glucosamine. In most bacteria the amino groups of these hexosamines are *N*-acetylated although in certain organisms including Bacilli, Clostridia and Rhodopseudomonads, glucosamine is largely unsubstituted. Other minor modifications have been reported (for review see Rogers *et al.*, 1980). Mycobacteria, *Nocardia kirovani* and Micromonospora contain *N*-glycoyl- and rather than *N*-acetylmuramic acid and *O*-acetylation of *N*-acetylmuramic acid occurs in *Staph. aureus* and *Neisseria gonorrhoea*. The biosynthetic aspects of these modifications are discussed elsewhere in this review.

The glycan chains vary considerably in length from several hundred to ten to twenty disaccharide repeating units (Ward, 1973). They appear to be biosynthesized as extremely long chains which are then subject to cleavage by autolytic glycosidases. Fractionation of the glycans isolated from *Bacillus subtilis* walls revealed a heterogeneous population, the largest size class having an average chain length of 500 disaccharide units. This would be approximately 500 nm long (Fox *et al.*, 1977). Even much shorter chains would be too long to be arranged radially in the peptidoglycan and there is now microscopic and physical evidence that the glycan chains of *Escherichia coli* lie more or less perpendicular to the length of the cell (Verwer *et al.*, 1978, 1980).

The carboxyl groups of the muramic acid residues are, with the exception of some residues in *Micrococcus luteus*, substituted with short peptides, a proportion of which are cross-linked, either directly or through a second short peptide. It is this cross-linkage which joins the glycan chains to form the macromolecular network of high tensile strength and rigidity. The configuration of the amino acids in the primary peptide side chain extending from muramic acid are L (or glycine) D, L, D and D. Linkages are α-peptide bonds except for the one between D-glutamic acid and the third residue which is formed by the γ-carboxyl group of the glutamyl residue. In Gram-negative organisms and Bacillus spp. the majority of cross-links are direct between the penultimate D-alanine residue of one peptide side chain and the free amino group of the meso-diaminopimelic acid residue of a second peptide (Fig. 1).

However, recent studies (Glauner and Schwarz, 1983) using high-pressure liquid chromatography of muramidase-solubilized sacculi of *E. coli* demonstrated that the classical monomers and dimers accounted for only some 70% of the total digest. The remaining 30% was made up of other disaccharide-peptides including dimers in which an additional D,D-diaminopimelic acid residue was present. About 20% of the dimers present had this unusual structure, which was associated with the linkage of lipoprotein to the peptidoglycan. Some 30–40% of the peptidoglycan-bound lipoprotein was attached to the D,D-diaminopimelic acid containing dimers and not to those which had direct cross-linkage.

In other Gram-positive bacteria a great variety of peptides are found although the peptidoglycan from any one species still contains no more than four or five amino acids (Fig. 1). Many of these additional amino acids are present in peptides forming a cross-bridge linking two peptide side chains. One such example, in an organism on which much of the earlier biosynthetic work was carried out, is the pentaglycine cross-bridge in *Staph. aureus*. Two major attempts have been made at clasifying peptidoglycans on the basis of their chemical structures (Ghuysen, 1968; Schleifer and Kandler, 1972). In each the type of cross-linking present was regarded as being of major importance.

The extent to which cross-linkage occurs also varies considerably from one organism to another. In Gram-negative organisms and Bacilli about 30–50% of the peptides are cross-linked as dimers, whereas in *Staph. aureus* cross-linkage is almost complete and a high proportion of the peptides may be isolated as oligomers containing an average of five to eight repeating units (Tipper and Berman, 1969). However, recent observations (discussed in detail in a later section) have shown that *Staph. aureus* can grow apparently normally with much reduced cross-linkage (Wyke *et al.*, 1981).

There is no evidence available which suggests any specific location of uncross-linked peptides and they are probably interspersed throughout peptidoglycan. Peptides which do not become involved in cross-linkage often lose either one or both of their terminal D-alanine residues by the action of carboxypeptidases. Hence, peptidoglycan isolated from walls of many bacteria contained an average one or less D-alanine residue per glutamic acid residue.

3. BIOSYNTHESIS OF PEPTIDOGLYCAN

The synthetic pathway has now been studied in many organisms including *Staph. aureus*, *E. coli*, several Bacilli and *M. luteus*. Despite wide differences in bacterial wall structure, from both a chemical and morphological point of view, peptidoglycan synthesis shows an overall similarity in these organisms which confirms the fundamental nature of the process.

Three stages in the synthetic pathway can be recognized, each occurring at a different cellular site. The first stage, catalyzed by soluble enzymes in the cytoplasm, is the formation of the nucleotide-linked precursors. In the second stage, which is presumed to occur at the interface of the cytoplasm and membrane, the precursor subunits are transferred to a lipophilic carrier, undecaprenyl phosphate, and further modified. These reactions are catalyzed by membrane-bound enzymes while the disaccharide pentapeptide subunit remains attached to the lipid carrier. Modifications including the addition of N-acetyl-glucosamine, amidation and the addition of the cross-bridge amino acids may occur at this

E. coli

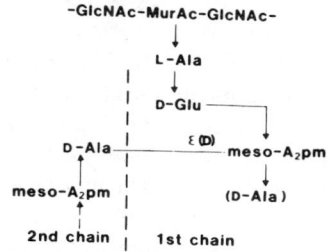

M. luteus

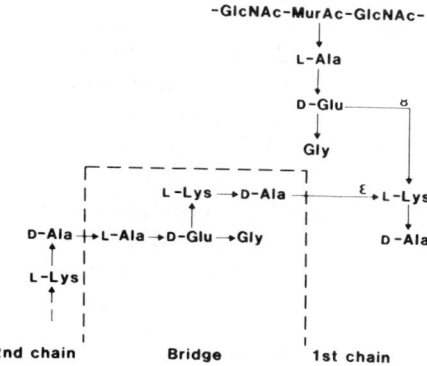

S. aureus Copenhagen

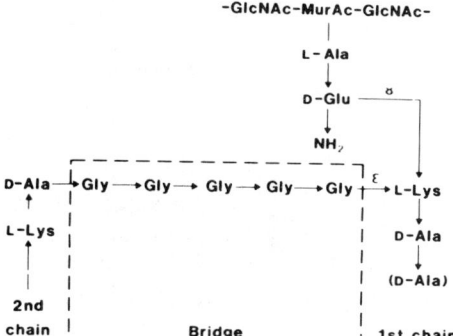

FIG. 1. Examples of peptidoglycan structure.

stage. In addition, recent evidence (discussed in detail below) has suggested that poly-merization of subunits may occur while the growing glycan chain remains linked to the lipid carrier. Stage three of peptidoglycan biosynthesis involves the translocation of the newly-synthesized subunit(s) through the cytoplasmic membrane to the outer surface, where polymerization and transpeptidation occur. In this way the nascent peptidoglycan is incorporated into the pre-existing wall.

Thus peptidoglycan synthesis is a vectorial process leading from intracellular soluble precursors to an extramembranal insoluble cross-linked polymer capable of withstanding a wide range of unfavorable environments. Similar mechanisms are involved in the biosynthesis of other wall polymers in both Gram-positive and Gram-negative bacteria, e.g. lipopolysaccharide and teichoic acids. In this article I will discuss the biosynthesis of peptidoglycan with particular reference to points of attack by cell wall inhibitors. I will briefly mention related aspects of the biosynthesis of other wall polymers.

3.1. SYNTHESIS OF NUCLEOTIDE-LINKED PRECURSORS

The initial reaction of the complex series (Fig. 2) leading to the synthesis of UDP-N-acetylmuramoyl-pentapeptide is the formation of UDP-N-acetylglucosamine from UTP and N-acetylglucosamine-1-phosphate. The pyrophosphorylase catalyzing this reaction is analogous to those involved in the synthesis of UDP-glucose and other sugar nucleotides of this type. Since N-acetylglucosamine is a common constituent of wall polymers in both Gram-positive and Gram-negative bacteria, this reaction is not specific to peptidoglycan synthesis. However, muramic acid is a unique constituent of peptidoglycan. Hence, the following reactions involving the transfer of enolpyruvate to UDP-N-acetylglucosamine and the subsequent reduction of the enolpyruvyl ether to give UDP-N-acetylmuramic acid, are the first specific steps in peptidoglycan biosynthesis.

The two enzymes catalyzing these reactions have been purified from *Enterobacter cloacae* (Zemell and Anwar, 1975) and *E. coli* (Anwar and Vlaovic, 1979) and partially purified from *Staph. epidermidis* (Wickus *et al.*, 1973). The UDP-N-acetylglucosamine:enolpyruvate transferases were found to be subject to feed-back inhibition by either UDP-N-acetylmuramic acid or UDP-N-acetylmuramoyl-peptides (Wickus and Strominger, 1973; Zemell and Anwar, 1975). The possible role of such inhibition in the regulation of peptidoglycan biosynthesis is discussed in a later section.

Phosphoenolpyruvate:UDP-N-acetylglucosamine-3-O-enolpyruvyl transferase is competitively inhibited by phosphonomycin (fosfomycin). This antibiotic acts as an analog of phosphoenolpyruvate and reacts covalently with a cysteine residue in the active site of the

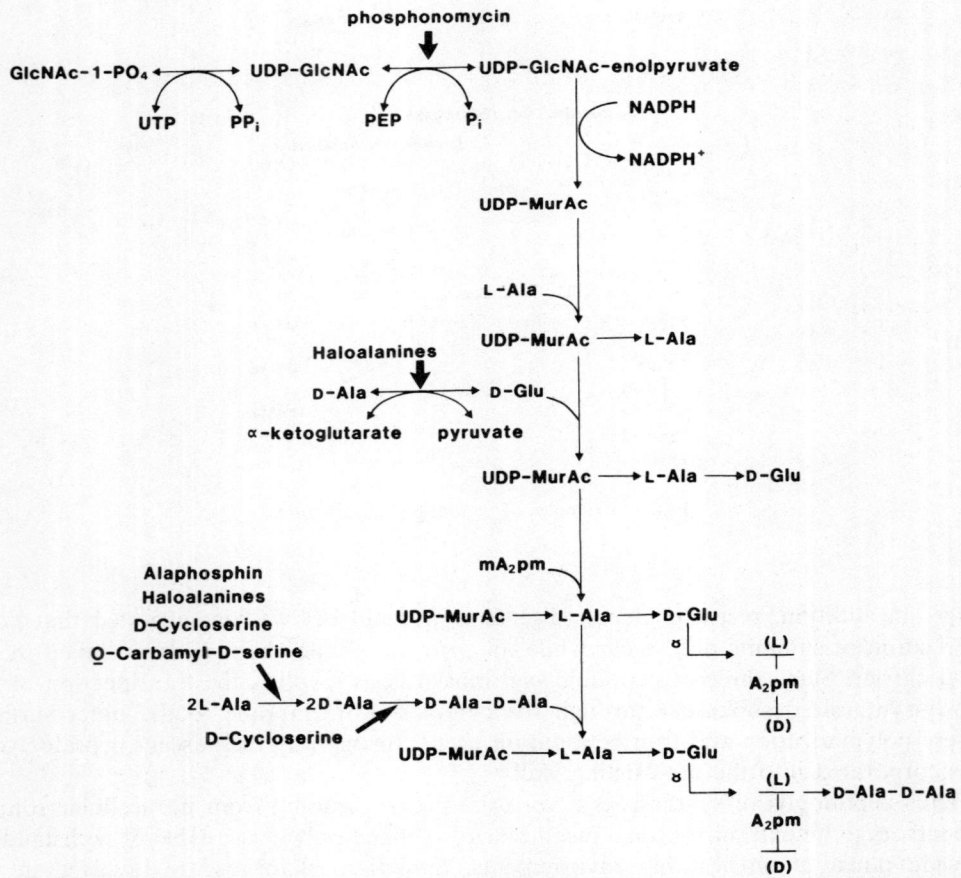

FIG. 2. The reactions involved in the biosynthesis of UDP-N-acetylmuramoyl-pentapeptide and their inhibition by wall antibiotics. The reactions shown are those for the biosynthesis diaminopimelic acid containing UDP-N-acetylmuramoyl-pentapeptide which is present in most Gram-negative bacteria, Bacilli and certain Clostridia. As described in the text, the ligases require either Mn^{2+} or Mg^{2+} for activity and the hydrolysis of ATP.

transferase. Pre-incubation of the enzyme with phosphonomycin leads to irreversible inactivation and 2-S-l-cysteinyl-l-hydroxypropylphosphate has been isolated from proteolytic digests of such inactive enzyme (Kahan et al., 1974). UDP-N-acetylglucosamine is an obligatory cofactor for inhibition.

Since the enolpyruvyl transferase is a cytoplasmic enzyme inhibition by phosphonomycin requires that the antibiotic be transported into the organism. In sensitive bacteria this occurs predominantly via the L-α-glycerophosphate transport system (Hayashi et al., 1964, Kahan et al., 1974). Alternatively, uptake can occur via the inducible hexose monophosphate system (Kadner and Winkler, 1973) and it is the activation of this mechanism that explains the increased sensitivity of several bacteria, including those known to lack the L-α-glycerophosphate transport system, when blood is present in the growth medium. Resistance to phosphonomycin occurs quite readily by loss of either of the above transport systems. In addition, a temperature-sensitive mutant of E. coli has been described in which resistance appears to be associated with decreased affinity of the transferase for both phosphonomycin and the natural substrate, phosphoenolpyruvate (Venkateswaran and Wu, 1972).

Conversion of UDP-N-acetylmuramic acid to form UDP-N-acetylmuramoyl-pentapeptide precursor then occurs by sequential addition of three amino acids and the pre-formed dipeptide, D-alanyl-D-alanine. In each case the addition is catalyzed by a specific ligase which requires a divalent cation (Mg^{2+} or Mn^{2+}) and the hydrolysis of ATP for activity. Unlike protein synthesis where the addition of amino acids is directed by a nucleic acid template, the ordered formation of UDP-N-acetylmuramoyl-pentapeptide is dependent upon the substrate specificities of the ligases. For example the L-lysine ligase of Staph. aureus fails to ligate meso-diaminopimelic acid to UDP-N-acetylmuramoyl-L-alanyl-D-glutamic acid and the converse result has been obtained with m-diaminopimelic acid ligase from E. coli (Ito and Strominger, 1962, 1966, 1973).

D-Glutamic acid, one of the D-amino acids characteristic of peptidoglycan, is produced either by the transamination of D-alanine and α-ketoglutarate (Martinez-Carrion and Jenkins, 1965) or by glutamic acid racemase (Diven, 1969). The transaminase from B. sphaericus is inhibited by β-halo (i.e. chloro- and fluoro-)-D-amino acids and by D-cycloserine (Soper and Manning, 1981). Inhibition by the halo alanines results in inactivation of the enzyme by a β-elimination reaction in which an α-aminoacrylate Schiffs base with pyridoxal phosphate is a key intermediate. Inhibition of the transaminase by D-cycloserine was reversed by dialysis of the inactive enzyme against pyridoxal phosphate at pH 6.5 to 7.0. At higher pHs (8.0 to 8.5) reactivation did not occur. DL-gabaculine (5-amino-1,3-cyclohexyldienyl carboxylic acid) also inhibited the transaminase (Soper and Manning, 1981, 1982). In this case the enzyme was protected from inhibition by D-alanine; α-ketoglutarate was less effective.

As described above the formation of UDP-N-acetylmuramoyl-pentapeptide is completed by the addition of D-alanyl-D-alanine. The synthesis of this dipeptide from L-alanine and its addition to UDP-N-acetylmuramoyl-tripeptide has been studied in detail by Neuhaus and his colleagues. The formation of the dipeptide is unique to prokaryotes and is of particular interest since a number of inhibitors have been described. These aspects are discussed in a recent review (Neuhaus and Hammes, 1981) hence the following description will deal primarily with biosynthesis and addition of the dipeptide. The conversion of L- to D-alanine is catalyzed by alanine racemase. The reaction, which has now been studied in numerous organisms, appears to require pyridoxal phosphate as a cofactor. Alanine racemase is competitively and irreversibly inhibited by cycloserine, the halo alanines and O-carbamyl-D-serine (Wang and Walsh, 1978). In addition L-l-aminoethylphosphonic acid inhibits the racemase of Gram-negative organisms competitively and reversibly and that of Gram-positive bacteria irreversibly in a time-dependent manner (Lambert and Neuhaus, 1972). In recent studies the antibiotic was incorporated into a peptide, L-alanyl-L-l-aminoethylphosphonic acid being most effective. The peptide, after being transported into the bacteria, was hydrolysed intracellularly to yield the antibacterial agent (Allen et al., 1978, 1979; Atherton et al., 1979).

D-alanyl-D-alanine synthetase (D-alanine:D-alanine ligase [ADP]) has been purified from
S. faecalis (Neuhaus, 1962a,b) and Staph. aureus (Ito and Strominger, 1962). Enzyme
activity requires K$^+$, Mg^{2+} (or Mn^{2+}) and the hydrolysis of ATP. In Staph. aureus an
additional unidentified heat-stable cofactor is required. The synthetase has two binding
sites for D-alanine to which residues bind sequentially as the donor (N-terminal) and
acceptor (C-terminal). In S. faecalis K_m values determined for the binding of D-alanine to
the donor and acceptor sites were 0.66 and 10 mM respectively (Neuhaus, 1962b). The
synthetase showed an absolute specificity for D-amino acids or glycine. D-aminobutyric
acid was the only D-alanine analog binding to the donor site. Incorporation of other
D-amino acids at the acceptor site occurred only in the presence of D-alanine to produce
mixed dipeptides with N-terminal D-alanine. Addition of the dipeptide to UDP-N-acetylmuramoyl-tripeptide shows the opposite specificity: i.e. D-alanine is required as the
C-terminal residue with a low specificity for the N-terminal residue. Thus, acting in
concert, the two enzymes ensure that D-alanyl-D-alanine is preferentially synthesized and
added to the tripeptide to form the complete nucleotide precursor, UDP-N-acetylmuramoyl-pentapeptide.

3.1.1. Regulation of UDP-N-Acetylmuramoyl-Pentapeptide Synthesis

The role of feed-back inhibition in the control of UDP-N-acetylmuramoyl-pentapeptide
synthesis remains unclear. As discussed above UDP-N-acetylglucosamine:enolpyruvate
transferases from E. cloacae, B. cereus and E. coli were inhibited by UDP-N-acetylmuramoyl-pentapeptide and -tripeptide (Taku et al., 1970). On the other hand the same
enzyme from Staph. epidermidis was unaffected by these precursors and significant
inhibition was obtained only with UDP-N-acetylmuramic acid (Wickus and Strominger
1973, Wickus et al., 1973). In Staph. aureus UDP-N-acetylmuramoyl-L-alanine and
-L-alanyl-D-glutamic acid both inhibit the L-alanine ligase as does UDP-N-acetylmuramoyl-pentapeptide (Tipper and Wright, 1980). These observations may explain the
accumulation of UDP N-acetylmuramic acid and UDP-N-acetylmuramoyl-L-alanine in
addition to pentapeptide when Staphylococci are treated with β-lactam antibiotics. In
contrast similar antibiotic treatment of E. coli fails to cause the accumulation of either
UDP-N-acetylmuramoyl-pentapeptide or earlier precursors. This finding suggests that in
E. coli UDP-N-acetylmuramoyl-pentapeptide might control its own biosynthesis by
feedback inhibition. Clearly this type of regulation is not apparent in Staph. aureus.
Moreover, treatment of E. coli with D-cycloserine results in significant accumulation of
UDP-N-acetylmuramoyl-tripeptide. Thus regulation by product inhibition in E. coli
appears to be limited to the pentapeptide although, as discussed above, both pentapeptide
and tripeptide precursors inhibit the UDP-N-acetylglucosamine:enolpyruvate transferase.
The amount of D-alanyl-D-alanine synthesized also appears to be carefully regulated.
The synthetase from S. faecalis was inhibited by D-alanyl-D-alanine as well as by
D-cycloserine and certain analogs of the dipeptide (Neuhaus and Lynch, 1964). Since
alanine racemase has an equilibrium constant of approximately one and the synthetase
may be regarded as being physiologically irreversible because of the concomitant hydrolysis of ATP, regulation of the synthetase by product inhibition is necessary to prevent all
the L-alanine pool of the organism being converted to D-alanyl-D-alanine.

3.1.2. Mutants in the Early Stage of Peptidoglycan Synthesis

Osmotically fragile, temperature sensitive mutants of E. coli, Staph. aureus and B.
subtilis, impaired in various steps of UDP-N-acetylmuramoyl-pentapeptide synthesis, have
been isolated and characterized. Selection of these mutants was based on their ability to
grow at the restrictive temperature only in the presence of an osmotic stabilizer such as
sucrose or NaCl. Identification of the temperature-sensitive lesions was, in general, made
by characterization of the nucleotide-linked precursor which accumulated and was
confirmed by assay of the actual enzyme involved. In this way mutants of E. coli with

defects in UDP-N-acetylglucosamine:enolpyruvate reductase (genetic designation *Mur B*) and the L-alanine, meso-diaminopimelic acid and D-alanyl-D-alanine ligases (*Mur C, Mur E* and *Mur F*) were isolated (Matsuzawa *et al.*, 1969; Lugtenberg and de Haan, 1971; Lugtenberg *et al.*, 1972). Additional mutations in alanine racemase (*alr*) (Wijsman, 1972b) and D-alanyl-D-alanine synthetase (*ddl*) (Lugtenberg and van Schijndel van Dam, 1972a,b; 1973) were also obtained. Mapping of the various mutations revealed a clustering of the *mur C, E* and *F* genes together with *ddl* at 1 to 1.5 min on the *E. coli* 100 min genetic map (Wijsman, 1972a). Also located in this region are two temperature-sensitive division loci (*fts A; fts I*) (Fletcher *et al.*, 1978) and a lesion in a D,D-carboxypeptidase (*mra B*) (Miyakawa *et al.*, 1972). A mutation in UDP-N-acetylglucosamine:enolpyruvate transferase (*Mur A*) has been isolated as a phosphonomycin-resistant mutant of *E. coli* (Wu and Venkateswaran, 1974). This gene is located with *Mur B* at 77 min on the *E. coli* map. Several other mutants accumulated UDP-N-acetylmuramoyl-pentapeptide and are probably defective in later stages of peptidoglycan synthesis. These mutations also mapped in the two areas described above, suggesting an organisation of the genes of peptidoglycan synthesis into two loci which would allow coordinate control over their related functions. Only alanine racemase mapped separately at 83 min (Wijsman, 1972b). Similar mutants isolated from *Staph. aureus* were defective in L-alanine, D-glutamic acid and L-lysine ligases and in D-alanine synthetase (Good and Tipper, 1972).

In *B. subtilis* temperature-sensitive mutations in D-alanyl-D-alanine synthetase (*ddl*), N-acetyl-L-diaminopimelic acid deacylase (*dap E*) and at an unidentified late stage in peptidoglycan synthesis were described (Buxton and Ward, 1980). Again the mutations mapped in two regions of the chromosome although in *B. subtilis* both *ddl* and *dal* (alanine racemase) were closely linked.

Nonconditional mutants with defects in peptidoglycan synthesis have been isolated as stable L-forms in *Staph. aureus*, *Streptococcus pyogenes*, *B. subtilis* and *B. licheniformis*, all of which accumulated nucleotide precursors. Lesions in aspartic acid-semialdehyde dehydrogenase, the first enzyme directly involved in diaminopimelic acid biosynthesis, L-alanine ligase and phospho-N-acetylmuramoyl-pentapeptide translocase, the first membrane bound enzyme in peptidoglycan synthesis, were identified in the bacilli (Ward, 1975). Translocase activity was also defective in L-phase variants of *S. pyogenes* (Reusch and Panos, 1976) and *S. faecium* (Gregory and Gooder, 1978).

3.2. THE LIPID CYCLE: MEMBRANE-ASSOCIATED EVENTS

The undecaprenyl phosphate carrier plays a central role in the second stage of peptidoglycan synthesis. The use of such a lipophilic carrier enables the organism to transport the hydrophobic N-acetylmuramoyl-pentapeptide and N-acetylglucosamine precursors from the intracellular sites of synthesis across the hydrophobic environment of the membrane to the membrane exterior surface for polymerization into the growing peptidoglycan (Fig. 3). More or less simultaneously with the first demonstration of their involvement in peptidoglycan synthesis (Higashi *et al.*, 1967), undecaprenyl phosphate linked intermediates were shown to participate in the biosynthesis of the O-side chain of lipopolysaccharide (Wright *et al.*, 1967) and of the lipomannan in *M. luteus* (Scher *et al.*, 1968). Subsequently, isoprenyl-lipid intermediates of this type have been implicated in the biosynthesis of teichoic acid linkage units (for review see Ward, 1981), teichuronic acids of *M. luteus* and *B. licheniformis* (Ward, 1981), several exopolysaccharides (Sutherland, 1977), a neuraminic acid containing polymer in the envelope of *E. coli* (Troy *et al.*, 1975) and the cell wall glycoprotein of *Halobacterium halobium* (Mescher and Strominger, 1976). In eukaryotic cells similar carrier lipids, the dolichols, which differ in that the hydroxy-terminal isoprene unit is saturated, function in the synthesis of glycoproteins (Waechter and Lennarz, 1976). Clearly, the participation of a single carrier lipid in the biosynthesis of wall polymers would provide the organism with a single point of control and perhaps prevent any imbalance occurring in overall wall synthesis.

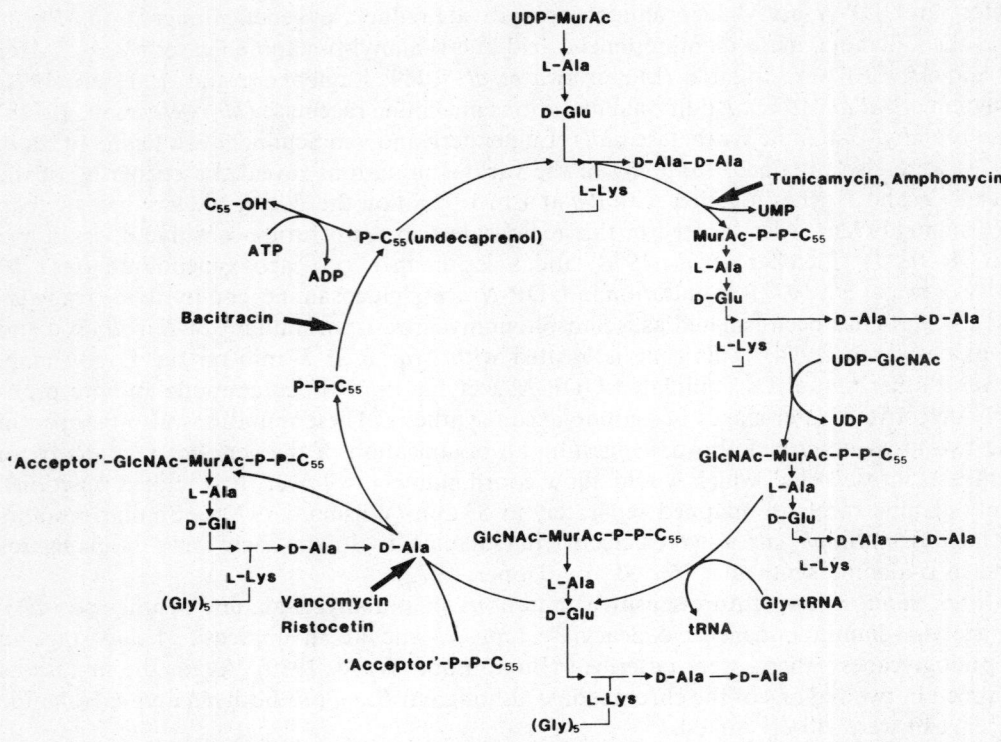

FIG. 3. The biosynthesis of uncross-linked peptidoglycan in *Staph. aureus* and its inhibition by wall antibiotics. Phospho-*N*-acetylmuramoyl-pentapeptide is translocated to the membrane bound lipid carrier, undecaprenyl phosphate (C_{55}-P). The transfer of *N*-acetylglucosamine follows to complete formation of the disaccharide repeating unit. Addition of the five glycyl residues of the cross-bridge and amidation of the α-COOH group of the D-glutamate (not shown) then takes place before polymerization of the newly-synthesized disaccharide-peptide occurs. Covalent linkage to the growing wall requires the formation of cross-links by transpeptidation.

3.2.1. *Biosynthesis of the Carrier Lipids*

Undecaprenol, present either as the free alcohol or in a phosphorylated form, has been isolated from a range of bacteria. In each case it was characterized by mass-spectrometry and various chromatographic techniques as a C_{55}-isoprenoid alcohol with traces of C_{45}, C_{50} and C_{60} homologs.

Undecaprenyl pyrophosphate is synthesized from farnesylpyrophosphate and eight isopentenyl pyrophosphate residues. Soluble and membrane-bound enzymes catalyzing this synthesis have been studied in *Salmonella newington* (Christenson *et al.*, 1969) and *Lactobacillus plantarum* (Keenan and Allen, 1974). The soluble enzymes from *L. plantarum* required either detergent or phospholipid for activity suggesting that this enzyme is also membrane-associated *in vivo* (Keenan and Allen, 1974; Allen *et al.*, 1976, Allen and Muth, 1977).

Undecaprenyl pyrophosphate, the primary biosynthetic product, must be hydrolysed to the monophosphate before it can be used in wall polymer biosynthesis. This reaction also occurs at the end of each cycle of wall polymer biosynthesis where undecaprenyl pyrophosphate is produced. It is this dephosphorylation reaction which is the primary site of action of bacitracin (Siewert and Strominger, 1967, Toscano and Storm, 1982). The reaction is catalyzed by undecaprenyl pyrophosphate phosphatase which has been isolated from *M. luteus* membranes by detergent extraction (Goldman and Strominger, 1972).

Undecaprenyl phosphate can also be dephosphorylated by a membrane-bound phosphatase. This enzyme was detected in *Staph. aureus* but not in membranes of several other bacteria (Willoughby *et al.*, 1972). However, the amount of undecaprenol increases in stationary phase Lactobacilli (Thorne and Kodicek, 1966) suggesting the presence of the undecaprenol phosphatase. At the time that the *Staph. aureus* phosphatase was studied, it was suggested that formation of the free alcohol would allow control over wall polymer biosynthesis by removing undecaprenyl phosphate from the system. Clearly a mechanism of this type would also require a kinase whose activity would serve to increase the proportion of undecaprenyl phosphate present. Such an enzyme, undecaprenyl phosphate phosphokinase, has been studied in a variety of organisms and was purified to homogeneity from butan-1-ol extracts of *Staph. aureus* membranes (Gennis and Strominger, 1976a,b; Gennis *et al.*, 1976, Higashi *et al.*, 1970, Sandermann and Strominger, 1972, Sandermann, 1976a,b). The extracted enzyme was soluble in organic solvents but insoluble in water. Moreover, further purification resulted in the separation of an apoprotein whose activity was restored by a wide range of detergents and phospholipids. Recent results suggest that enzyme activity is dependent on 'lipid hydration' rather than lipid viscosity or the actual chemical structure of the activating lipids polar group (Sandermann, 1976a,b).

Thus the possibility exists that, through the action of these phosphatases and the kinase, undecaprenol may function as a reserve pool of the lipid carrier. Moreover, synthesis of peptidoglycan or other wall polymers could then be controlled by this phosphorylation–dephosphorylation system.

3.2.2. *Phospho*-N-*Acetylmuramoyl*-*Pentapeptide Translocase*

The first membrane-associated reaction in the second stage of peptidoglycan synthesis is the transfer of phospho-N-acetylmuramoyl-pentapeptide from the nucleotide to the lipid carrier, undecaprenyl phosphate. Thus the products of the reaction are undecaprenyl pyrophosphoryl-N-acetylmuramoyl-pentapeptide and UMP. The reaction is called a translocase since it involves an exchange of carriers by the cleavage and synthesis of pyrophosphoryl-bonds of equivalent reactivity (Neuhaus, 1972). As implied by the above statement the reaction is readily reversible and can be assayed either as the transfer of phospho-N-acetylmuramoyl-pentapeptide to a membrane-bound form soluble in certain organic solvents or by a reaction in which free UMP is exchanged with the uridylic acid moiety of UDP-N-acetylmuramoyl-pentapeptide. The equilibrium constant for the reaction is about 0.25. Both transfer and exchange reactions require Mg^{2+} and are stimulated by K^+ and other monovalent cations. The translocase is inhibited by tunicamycin and amphomycin (Tamura *et al.*, 1976; Ward, 1977; Tanaka *et al.*, 1978). Tunicamycin, which contains uracil, N-acetylglucosamine, unsaturated fatty acids and a novel amino sugar, tunicamine (Ito *et al.*, 1977, Takatsuki *et al.*, 1977), inhibits the formation of N-acetylglucosamine-containing lipid intermediates involved in the biosynthesis of teichoic acid linkage units and also similar lipid intermediates used in the glycosylation of proteins in eukaryotic cells (for reviews see Rogers *et al.*, 1980; Yamasaki *et al.*, 1982; Tkacz, 1983).

Phospho-N-acetylmuramoyl-pentapeptide translocase was solubilized, by extraction with Triton X-100, from membranes of *M. luteus* (Umbreit and Strominger, 1972) and *Staph. aureus* (Pless and Neuhaus, 1973). More recently soluble enzyme was obtained from an *E. coli* envelope preparation by repeated cycles of freezing and thawing (Geis and Plapp, 1978). The solubilized enzyme from *M. luteus* had specific lipid requirements for transfer and exchange reactions. Transfer activity was dependent upon undecaprenyl phosphate and was further stimulated by a neutral lipid fraction. In contrast, a phospholipid, possibly phosphatidylglycerol, stimulated the exchange activity. Subsequent detailed studies on the translocase from *Staph. aureus* by Neuhaus and his colleagues suggested that reactivation of the enzyme results from the provision of a lipid microenvironment rather than reflecting a requirement for a specific phospho- or neutral lipid (Lee *et al.*, 1980; Weppner and Neuhaus 1978, 1979). These studies used a variety of physical techniques to investigate the microenvironment in membranes of the fluorescent lipid intermediate undecaprenyl-P-P-N-acetylmuramoyl-(N^c-dansyl) pentapeptide. In addition the physical state of membrane lipids was perturbed by treatment of membranes with butan-1-ol and by change in temperature. The results obtained from both investigations suggest that the lipid intermediate is held in a hydrophobic environment close to the membrane surface. Evidence was also found for strong lipid intermediate–protein interactions which the authors suggest may indicate that the lipid intermediate is held with the translocase in a peptidoglycan synthesizing complex.

Earlier Pless and Neuhaus (1973) proposed a five-step reaction sequence for translocase (Fig. 4). Transfer activity requires reactions (1) to (5) and the presence of a pool of undecaprenyl phosphate whereas the exchange reaction requires reactions (2) to (5) and sufficient undecaprenyl phosphate to form a complex with the translocase. The rate of the transfer reaction is invariably slower than the rate of the exchange reaction. Either reactions (1) or (5), the formation of the enzyme-undecaprenyl phosphate complex or the dissociation of the enzyme-undecaprenyl pyrophosphoryl-N-acetylmuramoyl-penta-peptide complex could be the rate-limiting step for the transfer reaction. In the presence of undecaprenyl phosphate and UDP-N-acetylmuramoyl-pentapeptide a steady-state level of lipid intermediate was formed. However, the exchange reaction continued and after a long period free phospho-N-acetylmuramoyl-pentapeptide was found in the reaction mixtures, presumably arising from dissociation of the enzyme intermediate formed in reaction (3). The transfer reaction can also be uncoupled by treatment of the enzyme preparation with dodecylamine. Under these conditions phospho-N-acetylmuramoyl-pentapeptide is formed and the translocase behaves as though it is depleted of un-decaprenyl phosphate.

The specificity for various nucleotide substrates of the translocases from *Staph. aureus* and *Gaffkya homari* was studied by Hammes and Neuhaus (1974a,b,c) (Table 1). The use of nucleotide precursors modified in amino acid composition of the pentapeptide side chain showed the translocases to have high specificity for L-alanine as residue 1 and D-alanine as residue 4. However, relatively low specificity was found for the D-amino acid in position 3 and the terminal D-alanine residue. Earlier, UDP-N-acetylmuramoyl-L-alanyl-D-isoglut-amyl-L-lysyl-D-alanyl-O-carbamoyl-D-serine and the natural nucleotide-pentapeptide precursor were shown to be equally effective as substrates in the exchange reaction catalyzed by the translocase of *S. faecalis* (Stickgold and Neuhaus, 1967).

Alteration in the length of the peptide side chain has dramatic effects on translocase activity. The staphylococcal enzyme gave 24% activity with UDP N-acetylmuramoyl-tetrapeptide and only 1.3% with the tripeptide (Hammes and Neuhaus (1974c). On the other hand UDP-N-acetylmuramoyl-pentapeptide-pentaglycine was utilized at 70% and 30% of the efficiency of the pentapeptide precursor by membranes of *M. lysodeikticus* (*M. luteus*) and *Staph. aureus* respectively (Matsuhashi *et al.*, 1967). The translocase also has a high specificity for the uracil residue and will not utilize the 5-fluorouracil analog, (Stickgold and Neuhaus, 1967). Since this substituted nucleotide is accepted by the earlier biosynthetic enzymes, FUDP-N-acetylmuramoyl-pentapeptide accumulated in organisms treated with 5-fluorouracil.

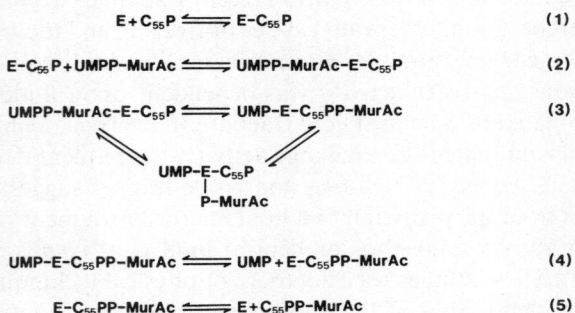

FIG. 4. The proposed reaction sequence for phospho-N-acetylmuramoyl-pentapeptide translocase (Pless and Neuhaus, 1973). E is the enzyme, C_{55} is undecaprenyl, UMPP-MurAc is uridine diphosphate N-acetylmuramoyl-pentapeptide, P is phosphate and PP is pyrophosphate.

TABLE 1. *The Specificity of the Phospho-N-acetylmuramoyl-Pentapeptide Trans-locases from* Gaffkya homari *and* Staphylococcus aureus

Substrate (only the peptide is shown)	Activity (%)		
	G. homari	Staph. aureus	
	Transfer	Transfer	Exchange
-L-Ala-D-Glu-L-Lys-D-Ala-D-Ala	100	100	100
-L-Ala-D-Glu-L-Lys-D-Ala	58	24	40
-L-Ala-D-Glu-L-Lys	0.03	1.3	0.7
-L-Ala-D-Glµ-L-Lys-D-Ala-Gly	65	67	92
-L-Ala-D-Glu-L-Lys-Gly-D-Ala	16	7	8
-Gly-D-Glu-L-Lys-D-Ala-D-Ala	24	11	17
-Gly-D-Glu-L-Lys-D-Ala-Gly	—	—	10
-Gly-D-Glu-L-Lys-Gly-D-Ala	—	—	0.7
-L-Ala-D-Glu-mA$_2$pm-D-Ala-D-Ala	68	57	66
-L-Ala-D-Glu-L-Orn-D-Ala-D-Ala	—	—	100

The effect of modifications to the peptide moiety of UDP-N-acetylmuramoyl peptide on the activity of the enzymes measured in either the transfer or exchange reactions are shown. In each assay the activity of the enzyme with the natural substrate, UDP-N-acetylmuramoyl-L-alanyl-D-isoglutamyl-L-lysyl-D-alanyl-D-alanine, is given as 100%. The data given is taken from Hammes and Neuhaus (1974a,b,c).

Thus the specificity of the translocase together with the specificity of the D-alanyl-D-alanine ligase and the dipeptide:UDP-N-acetylmuramoyl-tripeptide ligase described above ensures that only under exceptional circumstances are unsuitable modifications incorporated into peptidoglycan. Under certain conditions glycine can replace both alanine isomers in UDP-N-acetylmuramoyl-pentapeptide isolated from various organisms. Under these conditions the specificity of the translocase and the two ligases are overridden and the synthesis and incorporation of modified peptidoglycan precursors may explain the inhibitory effects of glycine and certain other D-amino acids on growth of many bacteria (Schleifer *et al.*, 1976).

3.2.3. *Formation of Undecaprenyl-Linked Disaccharide-Pentapeptide*

The second lipid intermediate is synthesized by the transglycosylation of N-acetylglucosamine from UDP-N-acetylglucosamine to undecaprenyl-P-P-N-acetylmuramoyl-pentapeptide with the formation of the disaccharide-pentapeptide lipid intermediate and UDP. The formation of the disaccharide repeating unit prior to polymerization ensures the alternating sequence of N-acetylmuramic acid and N-acetylglucosamine in the completed peptidoglycan.

The enzyme catalyzing this reaction, UDP-N-acetylglucosamine:N-acetylmuramoyl-(pentapeptide)-P-P-undecaprenol N-acetylglucosamine transferase, has been purified from LiCl extracts of toluene-treated *Bacillus megaterium* (Taku and Fan, 1976a,b, Taku *et al.*, 1975). Activity of the purified transferase is also stimulated by the addition of a crude lipid extract to the reaction mixture. The lipid causing this stimulation was not identified. It seems likely that, in common with the translocase, the transferase also requires a lipid microenvironment for optimal activity.

Nisin, a peptide antibiotic produced by *Streptococcus lactis*, was reported to inhibit the transferase by complexing with undecaprenyl-P-P-N-acetylmuramoyl-pentapeptide (Reisinger *et al.*, 1980).

3.2.4. *Modifications of the Pentapeptide Side Chain*

In Gram-negative bacteria, the Bacilli and *G. homari*, the lipid-linked disaccharide pentapeptide units are used without further modification for peptidoglycan synthesis.

However, in other organisms further substitution of the peptide, for example amidation of the D-isoglutamyl residue or addition of other amino acids which will subsequently form cross-bridges in the polymeric peptidoglycan, occurs at the lipid disaccharide stage of the biosynthetic cycle.

3.2.5. *Substitution of the* D-*isoglutamyl Residue*

Amidation of D-isoglutamyl residues was first described in *Staph. aureus* (Tipper *et al.*, 1967) and membrane preparations were subsequently shown to catalyze the amidation reaction utilizing either ammonia or glutamine as the donor of the NH_2-group. Both undecaprenyl-P-P-*N*-acetylmuramoyl-pentapeptide or -disaccharide-pentapeptide were substrates for the reaction which required the concomitant hydrolysis of ATP. UDP-*N*-acetylmuramoyl-pentapeptide was not a substrate. In *M. luteus* the α-carboxyl of the D-isoglutamyl residue is substituted by a glycine residue in a ligation reaction similar to those involved in synthesis of the pentapeptide side chain (Katz *et al.*, 1967). Again both lipid intermediates were substrates and the energy requirements of the reaction were supplied by the concomitant hydrolysis of ATP. It is probable that many other minor differences found in the structure of peptidoglycan such as the addition of single amino acids to the peptide side chain, occur by similar reactions utilizing the lipid intermediates as substrates.

3.2.6. *Formation of Cross-Bridge Peptides*

In bacteria of chemotype subgroup A1 (Schleifer and Kandler, 1972), direct cross-linkage occurs between the penultimate D-alanine residue of one side chain and the free amino group of the diamino acid of a second peptide. In other bacteria additional amino acids, which ultimately form the cross-bridge, are added to the lipid intermediates. Three types of cross-bridge have been distinguished: they contain either (a) single D-amino acids which may be amidated, (b) single L-amino acids, glycine or oligomers of L-amino acids or (c) a mixture of L- and D-amino acids in the same cross-bridge (Table 2). They are synthesized by two distinct methods. Formation of cross-bridge peptides containing glycine or L-amino acids requires the appropriate tRNA whereas D-amino acids are incorporated from activated-derivatives such as D-aspartylphosphate.

3.2.7. *Cross-bridge Formation in Staphylococci*

The involvement of tRNA in the synthesis of the pentaglycine cross-bridge of *Staph. aureus* was first suggested by the finding that *in vitro* incorporation of glycine into staphylococcal peptidoglycan was inhibited by ribonuclease (Chatterjee and Park, 1964). Under identical conditions the incorporation of *N*-acetylmuramoyl-pentapeptide from the

TABLE 2. *Bacteria in which Cross-Bridge Peptide Biosynthesis has been Studied*

Organism	Cross-Bridge Peptide	Intermediates Involved in Biosynthesis
Staph. aureus	Gly-Gly-Gly-Gly-Gly→	Glycyl-tRNA
S. epidermidis T-26	L-Ser-Gly-L-Ser-Gly-Gly→	L-Seryl-tRNA; Glycyl-tRNA
M. roseus	L-Ala-L-Ala-L-Ala-L-Thre→	L-Alanyl-tRNA; L-Threonyl-tRNA
L. viridescens	L-Ser-L-Ala→	L-Seryl-tRNA; L-Alanyl-tRNA
A. crystallopoietes	L-Ala→	L-Alanyl-tRNA
S. faecalis	D-Asp-NH$_2$ β⌐→	β-D-aspartyl phosphate D-Aspartate; ATP; NH_4^+
Sporosarcina ureae	D-Glu γ⌐ Gly→	D-Glutamate; ATP Glycyl-tRNA

nucleotide precursor was unaffected. Subsequent detailed investigation has established the unique way in which bacteria synthesize cross-bridge peptides of this type. In *Staph. aureus*, five glycine residues activated as tRNA derivatives, are added sequentially by membrane-bound enzymes, first to the NH_2-group of the lysyl residue and then to the N-terminus of the growing chain (Matsuhashi *et al.*, 1967, Thorndike and Park, 1969, Kamiryo and Matsuhashi, 1972). This mechanism is in direct contrast to protein synthesis where addition occurs at the carboxy-terminus, and no evidence was obtained for the participation of peptidyl tRNA-intermediates. Three species of glycyl-tRNA were purified from *Staph. aureus* and all would function in peptidoglycan synthesis although only two were active in protein synthesis (Bumsted *et al.*, 1968). Whether the third species alone is used for peptidoglycan synthesis *in vivo* remains unknown.

A more complex situation occurs in *Staph. epidermidis* and four types of cross-bridge have been identified (Petit *et al.*, 1968; Tipper, 1969). Each contains three residues of glycine and two of serine in a characteristic sequence, although glycine is always the substituent of the NH_2 group of lysine. The two amino acids are activated as their tRNA derivatives and incorporation into the cross-bridge peptide involves a membrane bound enzyme system independent of ribosomes and supernatant factors (Petit *et al.*, 1968; Bumsted *et al.*, 1968). In agreement with the chemical structure, incorporation of glycine occurs in the absence of seryl-tRNA whereas maximum serine incorporation requires the simultaneous incorporation of glycine. The ratio of glycine and serine incorporated by the membrane preparations is dependent on the relative concentration of the two charged tRNAs (Matsuhashi *et al.*, 1967, Hilderman and Riggs, 1973). A similar situation may exist *in vivo* where variations in cross-bridge structure can occur in response to medium composition (Schleifer *et al.*, 1976). The peptidoglycan of *Staph. epidermidis* grown in serine-poor medium resembled that of *Staph. aureus* grown in medium enriched with serine (Schleifer *et al.*, 1969).

Four glycyl- and four seryl-tRNAs were found in *Staph. epidermidis* and again, although all would act in peptidoglycan synthesis, one species of each type was inactive in protein synthesis (Petit *et al.*, 1968). Detailed analysis of the peptidoglycan-specific glycyl-tRNA showed it to consist of two distinct iso-accepting species differing in seven bases (Roberts, 1972). They also lacked the GTψc sequence and most minor bases. Since GTψc has previously been implicated in ribosome-tRNA binding the absence of this sequence may explain the inability of these tRNAs to function in protein synthesis. Thus *Staph. epidermidis* and perhaps other organisms utilizing this mechanism of cross-bridge formation, has evolved a means of maintaining the flow of glycine and L-amino acids to peptidoglycan without involving the machinery of protein synthesis. This should ensure that the structural integrity of the wall and hence of the organism, is maintained in those conditions where utilization of the amino acids for protein synthesis would be disadvantageous.

Involvement of aminoacyl tRNAs in the formation of cross-bridges of *Arthrobacter crystallopoietes* (Roberts *et al.*, 1968b), *M. roseus* (Roberts *et al.*, 1968a) and *L. viridescens* (Plapp and Strominger, 1970a,b) was also studied. In *A. crystallopoietes* the membrane-bound ligase which adds a single L-alanyl residue to the lipid-intermediate was also specific for the tRNA. The enzyme was inactive when L-seryl-tRNA, L-cysteinyl-tRNA or L-alanyl-tRNA[cys] prepared by the chemical reduction of L-cysteinyl-tRNA were used as substrates. In contrast the two enzymes involved in the formation of the L-seryl-L-alanine cross-bridge in *L. viridescens* were less specific. The L-alanyl residue was first added by a soluble ligase to the nucleotide pentapeptide precursor to give UDP-*N*-acetylmuramoyl-(L-alanyl-pentapeptide). After translocation of the *N*-acetylmuramoyl-hexapeptide to form a lipid intermediate a membrane-bound enzyme added the L-seryl residue. This enzyme would also transfer residues of L-alanine or L-serine.

3.2.8. *Formation of Cross-Bridges Containing* D-*Amino Acids*

Examples of this type of cross-bridge are the single D-isoasparaginyl residues found in *S. faecalis* (*S. faecium*) and *L. casei* (Schleifer and Kandler, 1972). In this case D-aspartic

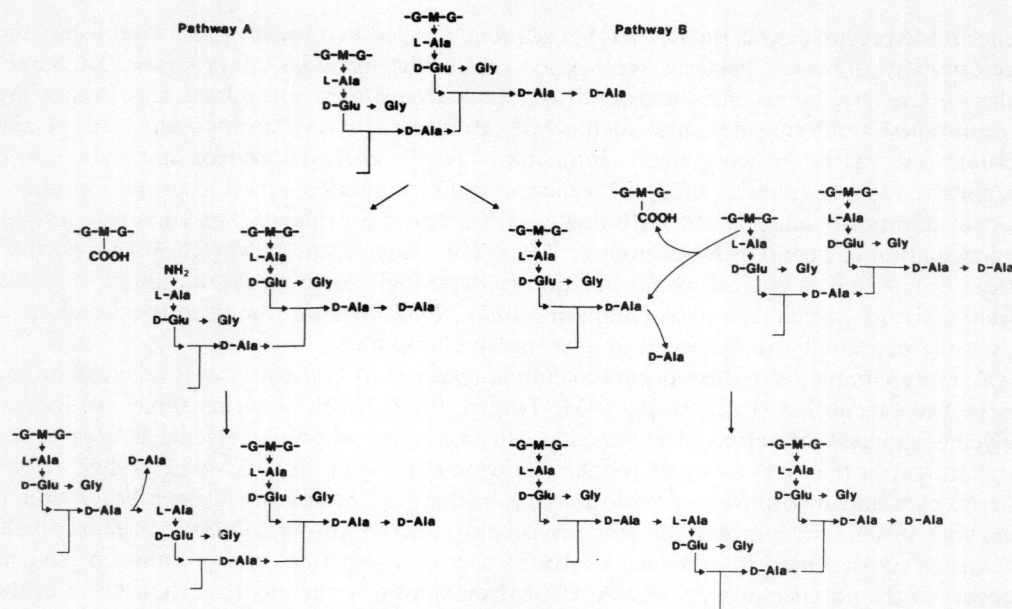

FIG. 5. Suggested mechanisms for the formation of cross-bridge peptides in *M. luteus*. For either mechanism the initial reaction is the formation by transpeptidation of a D-alanyl-N'-L-lysine cross-link. This is followed in pathway A by amidase action to hydrolyse the N-acetylmuramoyl-L-alanine bond of one peptide subunit of the cross-linked dimer. Subsequent transpeptidation to a third peptide, using the released L-alanine residue as the acceptor, would result in the formation of a D-alanyl-L-alanine bond. Alternatively, in pathway B, the terminal D-alanine residue of a third peptide could be removed by a D-alanine carboxypeptidase action. The resulting peptide would then participate as an acceptor in a transamination reaction releasing the N-acetylmuramoyl residue from the N-terminus of the cross-linked dimer with the concomitant formation of the D-alanyl-L-alanine cross-link. Repetition of either series of reactions would result in the synthesis of cross-bridge peptides made up of multiple peptide units in head-to-tail linkage. In the figure ⌐ represents L-lysine.

acid is activated as β-D-aspartylphosphate by a membrane-bound enzyme. This enzyme was partially purified from *S. faecium* membranes by LiCl extraction and would reattach to the membranes on removal of the salt by dialysis (Staudenbauer and Strominger, 1972). This process required the presence of phospholipids but not Mg^{2+}. A second membrane-bound enzyme, which was also released by the above treatment, transferred the aspartyl residue to either UDP-N-acetylmuramoyl pentapeptide or to the lipid intermediate. Amidation of the α-carboxyl group then occurred in a reaction which required NH_4^+ and ATP.

3.2.9. *Formation of 'Hybrid' Cross-Bridges*

The third class of cross-bridge peptides contains both L- and D-amino acids. An example of this group is found in *Sporosarcina ureae* where D-glutamylglycine links the D-alanyl and L-lysyl residues of separate peptide side chains. The synthesis of the cross-bridge is based on the two mechanisms described above (Linnett *et al.*, 1974). The addition of glycine to the ϵ-NH_2 group of lysine requires glycyl-tRNA while D-glutamic acid was activated by a membrane-bound enzyme in the presence of ATP in a reaction presumably analogous to the one described above for D-aspartate.

3.2.10. *Cross-Bridge Formation in M. luteus*

In *M. luteus* and other organisms of sub group A2 the cross-bridge and peptide side chains of peptidoglycan have identical amino acid sequences (Fig. 1). Two possible mechanisms have been suggested which would allow synthesis of this type of structure (Fig. 5). In the first, Ghuysen *et al.* (1968) proposed the sequential action of a transpeptidase and N-acetylmuramoyl-L-alanine amidase. In the first step a conventional cross-bridge is formed between two peptide side chains. One of these is then released from the glycan by action of the amidase (step 2). A second transpeptidation reaction then occurs to form a linkage between the penultimate D-alanyl residue of a third peptide side chain and the free NH_2 group on the L-alanine residue released by amidase action. Repeated cycles of steps 2 and 3, the release of free NH_2-groups of L-alanine and the second transpeptidation reaction would build up cross-bridges of multiple peptide side chains. Evidence for two transpeptidases in $M. luteus$ came from studies on the effect of benzylpenicillin on formation of D-alanyl-L-lysine and D-alanyl-L-alanine bonds in $vivo$ (Mirelman and Bracha, 1974). Formation of D-alanyl-L-lysine bonds was approximately 50-times more sensitive to inhibition (50% inhibition occurred with 0.1 μg benzylpenicillin ml^{-1}) than was the formation of D-alanyl-L-alanine links.

More recently Chatterjee et $al.$ (1977) suggested that synthesis of $M. luteus$ peptidoglycan may involve N-acetylmuramoyl-L-alanine amidase acting as a transaminase. Again the first step would be the formation of a D-alanyl-L-lysine cross-link. A D,D carboxypeptidase would then cleave the terminal D-alanyl residue from a third hexapeptide side chain (step 2). The resultant pentapeptide would participate as an acceptor in a transamination reaction catalyzed by the N-acetyl muramoyl-L-alanine amidase (step 3) to cleave the peptide side chain from the glycan forming a D-alanyl-L-alanine bond in the process. Which, if either of these two mechanisms functions in $M. luteus$, remains unknown.

3.2.11. *Polymerization of Disaccharide Peptide Subunits*

The structure of peptidoglycan shows clearly that two possibilities exist for the incorporation of newly-synthesized subunits into the pre-existing polymer. These require the formation of either glycosyl or peptide bonds. In fact the large disparity between glycan and peptide chain lengths and the independence of glycan polymerization from cross-linkage in many organisms suggest that glycan polymerization precedes transpeptidation. Recent studies concluded that polymeric uncross-linked peptidoglycan is present in some bacteria and have shown that transpeptidation continues to occur after incorporation of newly-synthesized peptidoglycan into the wall. In addition treatment of *Staph. aureus* (Tipper and Strominger, 1968), *M. luteus* (Mirelman *et al.*, 1974) and *B. licheniformis* (Tynecka and Ward, 1975) with β-lactam antibiotics results in the synthesis of soluble uncross-linked peptidoglycan. Glycan polymerization also precedes transpeptidation during the early stages of the reversion of protoplasts and unstable L-forms of *B. licheniformis* (Elliott *et al.*, 1975a,b). Thus polymerization by transglycosylation can occur in the absence of transpeptidation whereas the reverse situation, transpeptidation in the absence of glycan chain elongation, has only been demonstrated with model peptides.

3.2.12. *Elongation of Glycan Chains*

If newly-synthesized disaccharide peptide subunits were added to the non-reducing end of the growing glycan chain then the N-acetylglucosaminyl residue of the disaccharide should be susceptible to periodate oxidation. On the other hand, periodate oxidation would not occur if the units were added to the reducing i.e. N-acetylmuramoyl terminus. In addition units added in this way would undergo a β-elimination reaction to yield lactyl-peptide, providing a free reducing group were present. This proved to be the case in uncross-linked peptidoglycan synthesized by membranes of *B. licheniformis* (Ward and Perkins, 1973) where the newly-incorporated N-acetylglucosamine residues were periodate-resistant and lactyl peptides were obtained after mild acid hydrolysis to yield free reducing groups in the newly-synthesized peptidoglycan. Similar results have since been reported with *B. megaterium* (Fuchs-Cleveland and Gilvarg, 1976) and *M. luteus* (Weston *et al.*, 1977). In each case the reducing termini were blocked by linkages labile to mild acid hydrolysis. Thus in the process of glycan chain elongation the N-acetylmuramoyl terminus

of the growing chain is transfered from its link with the membrane to the nonreducing
N-acetylglucosamine terminus of the newly-synthesized disaccharide peptide subunit
which presumably remains linked to the lipid carrier. This mechanism and the conditions
of mild acid hydrolysis used, suggest that the growing glycan chain also remains attached
to undecaprenyl pyrophosphate, but this has not yet been established. If this were the case,
then the presence of free-reducing groups of muramic acid found in peptidoglycans (Ward,
1973) could result from some mechanism for terminating a particular glycan chain. This
could certainly be the case for organisms lacking endomuramidases e.g. *Staph. aureus* and
certain Bacillus sp. (Rogers, 1979).

Polymerization of uncross-linked peptidoglycan has been studied *in vitro* using reconstituted membranes of *B. megaterium* (Taku and Fan, 1979). A soluble fraction was
isolated by high speed centrifugation after treatment of the membranes with LiCl and
cholate. Removal of the LiCl and detergent by dialysis resulted in the formation of vesicles
which synthesized peptidoglycan from the nucleotide precursors. In addition active vesicles
were also prepared from a fraction of cholate-solubilized membranes designated PG-II,
purified phospho-N-acetylmuramoyl pentapeptide translocase, and N-acetylglucosaminyl
transferase. In the absence of the cholate-soluble fraction, only lipid intermediates were
synthesized by the vesicles, suggesting that PG-II was either peptidoglycan polymerase or,
alternatively, a protein whose presence was necessary for polymerization to occur. More
recently, the polymerase (peptidoglycan transglycosylase) has been purified from membranes of *B. megaterium* (Taku *et al.*, 1982). This protein, which appears to be identical
with PG-II, synthesized lysozyme-sensitive peptidoglycan from the lipid intermediate,
undecaprenyl pyrophosphoryl-disaccharide-pentapeptide. This polymerization was inhibited by vancomycin, but not by benzylpenicillin or tunicamycin. Interestingly, in view
of the results obtained with *E. coli* (described in a later section), the enzyme from *B.
megaterium* bound benzylpenicillin but transpeptidase activity was not detected. SDS-
polyacrylamide gel electrophoresis revealed the transglycosylase to run as a single band
which the authors suggest may correspond to PEP-4 of *B. megaterium* KM.

Moenomycin and related antibiotics were shown to inhibit synthesis of uncross-linked
peptidoglycan in *E. coli* (Van Heijenoort *et al.*, 1978; Van Heijenoort and Van Heijenoort,
1980). Whether this group of antibiotics also interacts with, and inhibits polymerization
by the *B. megaterium* enzyme remains unknown.

3.2.13. *Are There Polymeric Intermediates in Peptidoglycan Biosynthesis?*

Fuchs-Cleveland and Gilvarg (1976) first reported the isolation of soluble peptidoglycan
from *B. megaterium*. This fraction, extracted from whole cells with SDS, was characterized
as uncross-linked peptidoglycan with a glycan chain length of 11 to 13 disaccharide units.
Treatment with lysozyme hydrolysed the oligomeric material into disaccharide pentapeptide subunits and a fragment tentatively identified as undecaprenyl-P-P-disaccharide
peptide. Pulse-chase experiments showed the oligomer to be radioactively labeled and
chased into unknown products with similar kinetics to both the lipid intermediates and
UDP-N-acetylmuramoyl pentapeptide. However, a precursor–product relationship between the oligomeric material and mature peptidoglycan was not established. The
possibility remains that the oligomers may arise by cleavage of nascent uncross-linked
peptidoglycan. A mechanism of this type might explain the puzzling absence of shorter
oligomers i.e. those of glycan chain lengths less than 11 units. It would, however, mean
that polymerization by transglycosylation precedes cross-linking into the wall. Such an
arrangement is supported by the earlier observation that cross-linking in *B. megaterium*
continues for 25 minutes after incorporation of newly-synthesized peptidoglycan into the
wall (Fordham and Gilvarg, 1974). Continued transpeptidation was also reported to occur
in *S. faecalis* (Dezelee and Shockman, 1975).

Mett *et al.* (1980) described the isolation and characterization of detergent-soluble
partially cross-linked peptidoglycan from *E. coli*. This solubilized material was substituted
with lipoprotein and contained more pentapeptide residues than did mature peptidoglycan.

It was proposed to be a synthetic intermediate. In addition, a proportion of lower molecular weight material contained undecaprenyl substituents. However, it should be noted that the conditions of radioactive-labeling used prior to isolation of the soluble polymer were such that the organisms were depleted of diaminopimelic acid for a considerable proportion of the labeling period. The amount of polymer isolated was extremely small, less than 2% of the newly-synthesized peptidoglycan, and might have been released by autolytic activity during this time. Thus the soluble polymer could be mixture of old and new material where lipoprotein was attached to mature peptidoglycan and the pentapeptide residues were newly-synthesized. Pulse-chase experiments showed that during an extended chase of 45 min only half of the detergent soluble polymer became attached to the wall. Clearly, these are not the kinetics we would expect from a true intermediate.

More recently, Goodell et al. (1983) reported that they were unable to detect oligomeric peptidoglycan intermediates in E. coli. Pulse-labeling of growing organisms with [^{3}H]diaminopimelic acid and subsequent fractionation of SDS-soluble material revealed the radioactivity to be present only as UDP-N-acetylmuramoyl-pentapeptide and the lipid-linked intermediates undecaprenyl-pyrophosphoryl-disaccharide-penta-peptide and undecaprenyl-pyrophosphoryl-N-acetylmuramoyl-pentapeptide. Goodell et al. suggested that the oligomeric material seen by others could result from autolytic degradation of newly-synthesized peptidoglycan but this was not established.

Earlier, detergent-soluble oligomeric intermediates were reported to occur during peptidoglycan biosynthesis by deoxycholate-treated M. luteus (Thorpe and Perkins, 1979) and ether-treated P. aeruginosa (Mirelman and Nuchamowitz, 1979a) (Table 3). In M. luteus the addition of small quantities of detergent to wall–membrane preparations led to the accumulation of oligomeric peptidoglycan soluble in hot SDS but not cold SDS. Similar material was also isolated in very small amounts from wall–membrane preparations incubated in the absence of detergent. The average glycan chain length of the oligomer was 40 to 60 disaccharide units and lysozyme treatment gave mainly disaccharide hexapeptides with very small amounts of material having the chromatographic mobility of undecaprenyl-P-P-disaccharide hexapeptide. Covalent linkage of soluble peptidoglycan to the wall (detergent-insoluble fraction) occurred when the deoxycholate was removed and the wall membrane preparations were reincubated with peptidoglycan precursors. This incorporation was inhibited by benzylpenicillin and was therefore dependent upon transpeptidation. However, whether the 'soluble peptidoglycan' represents a true intermediate in the biosynthetic process again remains unclear. From the above results one possible conclusion is that incorporation of nascent glycan into the wall occurs with the normal degree of cross-linkage of its peptides being achieved by delayed transpeptidation. This has not yet been established. An alternative, and perhaps more reasonable possibility is that further disaccharide hexapeptide subunits are added to extend the glycan chain and it is these subunits which become cross-linked into the wall in a reaction coupled to transglycosylation. This mechanism would result in the peptidoglycan which was previously 'soluble' remaining uncross-linked; it would, however, now appear to be trans-

TABLE 3. *Polymeric Intermediates of Peptidoglycan Biosynthesis*

Organism	Size (disaccharide units)	Degree of cross-linkage %	Linkage to undecaprenol	References
B. megaterium	11–13	0	+	Fuchs-Cleveland and Gilvarg (1976)
B. licheniformis protoplasts stage of reversion—early	10	10–15	?	Elliott et al. (1975b)
—late	200	30–35	?	
M. luteus	40–60	?	+	Thorpe and Perkins (1979)
E. coli	'large'	18–26	0–?	Mett et al. (1980)
P. aeruginosa	'large'	'partial'	0	Mirelman and Nuchamowitz (1979a)

peptidated into the wall. Further studies are required to distinguish these possibilities. Evidence for synthesis, by *M. luteus*, of material of a smaller size, soluble in cold SDS, was obtained (Weston *et al.*, 1977) but in this case no evidence for a role as a precursor was obtained. Rather it was concluded that this represented uncross-linked peptidoglycan synthesized by membranes not associated with the wall in the enzyme preparation used.

The oligomeric material isolated from *P. aeruginosa* was a mixture of partially cross-linked peptidoglycan and lower molecular weight material (Mirelam and Nuchamo-witz, 1979a,b). This could be radioactively labeled and was chased into SDS-insoluble peptidoglycan within 20 min of incubation with unlabeled nucleotide precursors. However, although these observations clearly suggest the SDS-soluble material to be a macro-molecular intermediate in peptidoglycan biosynthesis, no blocking of the glycan reducing groups was detected.

As mentioned earlier, relatively uncross-linked peptidoglycan was isolated from revert-ing protoplasts of *B. licheniformis* (Elliott *et al.*, 1975b). In the earliest stages of reversion examined, the peptidoglycan had a glycan chain length of approximately 10 disaccharide units with 20–30% of the diaminopimelyl residues involved in cross-linkage. In mature peptidoglycan obtained from organisms in the final stages of reversion, these values had increased to 200 disaccharide units and 60 to 70% cross-linkage.

These observations suggest that, in all bacteria, the rates of glycan polymerization and transpeptidation may be such that small amounts of uncross-linked peptidoglycan are synthesized prior to cross-linkage. Whether the partially cross-linked peptidoglycan isolated from *E. coli* and *P. aeruginosa* represents an intermediate in peptidoglycan biosynthesis remains questionable.

The mechanism of glycan polymerization described above allows both the synthetic enzymes including penicillin-binding proteins and the growing terminus of the glycan chain to be 'anchored' in the membrane. The formation of cross-links, mediated by membrane-bound transpeptidases, could also occur at this time. Linkage of the nascent peptidoglycan to the lipid carrier might also allow some lateral movement of oligomeric material, provided no linkage to the pre-existing wall took place.

The method of synthesis of the glycan chains of peptidoglycan is analogous to that of lipopolysaccharide O-antigen (Robbins *et al.*, 1967) and teichuronic acid in *B. licheniformis* (Ward and Curtis, 1982). In contrast, the elongation of poly(glycerol phosphate) and poly(ribitol phosphate) teichoic acids occurs in the reverse way (for review see Ward, 1981). The teichoic acids were shown to grow by addition of polyol phosphate units to the terminus of the chain distal to the initial residue, which eventually becomes linked to peptidoglycan.

3.2.14. *Antibiotics Inhibiting Reactions in the Second Stage of Peptidoglycan Synthesis*

The possible inhibition of glycan polymerase by moenomycin and related antibiotics has already been mentioned. The secondary product of the polymerization reaction is undecaprenyl pyrophosphate. This must be dephosphorylated to undecaprenyl mono-phosphate before the carrier can be reutilized in a second cycle of peptidoglycan synthesis, and it is this reaction which is specifically inhibited by bacitracin (Toscano and Storm, 1982). Consequently bacitracin inhibits any biosynthetic reaction in which undecaprenyl pyrophosphate is a product, including formation of the 'O' side chain of lipo-polysaccharide and teichuronic acid biosynthesis (Kanegasaki and Wright, 1970; Ward and Curtis, 1982) and the formation of glycoprotein in the envelope of *Halobacterium halobium* (Mescher and Strominger, 1976). In contrast, polymerizations not involving undecaprenyl derivatives, such as teichoic acid biosynthesis and the formation of the 'core' oligosaccharide of lipopolysaccharide and other reactions involving undecaprenyl-phosphoryl-sugars, in which undecaprenyl phosphate is the product, are not inhibited.

Vancomycin, ristocetin and related antibiotics also inhibit reactions in this second stage of peptidoglycan synthesis. These antibiotics are like bacitracin, extremely effective against many Gram-positive organisms but not against Gram-negative bacteria, apparently because they are excluded by the porins of the outer membrane. The formation of complexes between vancomycin and the acyl-D-alanyl-D-alanine terminus of peptidoglycan precursor is discussed in detail elsewhere (Perkins, 1982). Vancomycin was shown to inhibit synthesis of uncross-linked peptidoglycan by membrane preparation of several bacteria (Anderson *et al.*, 1966, Reynolds, 1971, Ward, 1974). The biosynthetic system of *Gaffkya homari* differs from the others in that synthesis of polymeric material occurs from either UDP-*N*-acetylmuramoyl-pentapeptide, the -tetrapeptide or -tripeptide precursors (Hammes and Neuhaus, 1974b). As expected from the studies of complex formation described above, vancomycin only inhibited synthesis when the pentapeptide substrate was used. Thus the antibiotic does not inhibit the glycan polymerase itself, but rather complexes with the precursor UDP-*N*-acetylmuramoyl-pentapeptide, or the terminal pentapeptide moiety of the growing glycan chain, to exert its inhibitory action. Using membranes of *B. licheniformis*, Ward (1974) found that inhibition of peptidoglycan biosynthesis occurred at much lower concentrations of vancomycin, measured in terms of the ratio of antibiotic to UDP-*N*-acetylmuramoyl-pentapeptide present than did the inhibition of the D,D-carboxypeptidase. Since the carboxypeptidase also interacts with the D-alanyl-D-alanine terminus of the pentapeptide this finding was taken to show that complex formation with the nucleotide precursor was not responsible for antibiotic actions. Johnston and Neuhaus (1975) using *Staph. aureus* membranes were able to demonstrate the formation of a complex between either vancomycin or ristocetin and spin-labeled lipid intermediate. Their results, however, were not able to pinpoint the site of action of these antibiotics.

Newer antibiotics such as diumycin, prasinomycin and other phosphorous-containing glycolipid antibiotics appear to resemble moenomycin as inhibitors of glycan polymerase (Van Heijenoort, *et al.*, 1978; Van Heijenoort and Van Heijenoort, 1980). Whether this is the case with antibiotics such as enduracidin (Matsuhashi *et al.*, 1970), gardimycin (Somma *et al.*, 1977) and janiemycin (Brown *et al.*, 1974) requires further investigation.

3.3. Transpeptidation: the Peptide Cross-Linking System

The importance of cross-linking for the incorporation of newly-synthesized peptidoglycan into the pre-existing wall has been mentioned several times in preceding sections of this chapter. Even when uncross-linked peptidoglycan has glycan chains many disaccharide units in length it remains water soluble. Only when cross-links are formed between peptide side chains does peptidoglycan become an insoluble matrix capable of maintaining the structural integrity of the organism.

By the early 1960's both chemical and biosynthetic studies of peptidoglycan structure had established the reactions leading to formation of uncross-linked polymer. Membrane preparations of *M. luteus* and *Staph. aureus* catalyzed these reactions but in each case the product was uncross-linked (Anderson *et al.*, 1965). Moreover, such peptidoglycan synthesis was not inhibited by β-lactam antibiotics although it was sensitive to other antibiotics known to cause accumulation of peptidoglycan nucleotide precursors in whole organisms. Chemical studies showed that cross-linkage between peptide side chains occurred through the penultimate D-alanine residue which was originally present in the precursor as the D-alanyl-D-alanine terminus of the peptide. Thus, cross-linking appeared to involve a transpeptidation reaction in which the D-alanyl-D-alanine bond in one peptide is cleaved with the concomitant formation of a new peptide bond to a free amino-group of a second peptide (Martin, 1964; Wise and Park, 1965; Tipper and Strominger 1965). The second product of this reaction would be D-alanine. The transpeptidation reaction was proposed as the site of inhibition of peptidoglycan synthesis by β-lactam antibiotics. The obvious attractions of this hypothesis, which we know to be correct, were twofold. It provided an explanation of the apparent universal presence of a D-alanyl-D-alanine terminus in the nucleotide precursor of peptidoglycan although the cross-linked polymer appeared to contain only single D-alanine residues. In addition the total bond energy would change little in transpeptidation allowing the organism to form cross-links to the exterior of the cytoplasmic membrane in the absence of energy sources such as ATP.

Experimental support for the hypothesis soon came from *in vivo* studies on the effects of benzylpenicillin on peptidoglycan synthesis by *Staph. aureus*. Walls prepared from organisms grown in the presence of sublethal concentrations of antibiotic contained a higher ratio of alanine to glycine than did walls from untreated organisms (Wise and Park, 1965). More or less simultaneously, direct chemical analysis of staphylococcal walls, again prepared from organisms grown with sublethal concentrations of benzylpenicillin, showed that the proportion of uncross-linked monomer units increased (Tipper and Strominger, 1965, 1968). These peptide side chains retained the D-alanyl-D-alanine terminus of the nucleotide precursor and were substituted on the ε-amino group of lysine with a pentaglycine cross-bridge peptide. During subsequent growth of the organisms in the absence of benzylpenicillin these uncross-linked monomers did not become cross-linked into the wall. Tipper and Strominger (1968) concluded that the continued formation of polymeric material while cross-linkage was inhibited effectively moved these uncross-linked units outside the reach of transpeptidase molecules held at the wall–membrane interface. In the absence of antibiotic they envisaged that newly-synthesized disaccharide-peptide units were incorporated into the growing wall by almost immediate formation of cross-links to adjacent peptide side chains. A second important hypothesis arising in these studies of cross-linkage was the concept of acyl-intermediates in the transpeptidation reaction. They proposed that the acyl-D-alanyl-D-alanine donor peptide interacted with the enzyme to form an acyl-D-alanyl-enzyme with the immediate release of the terminal D-alanine. In a second stage of the reaction the acyl-D-alanyl-substituent was transferred to the free-amino group of the acceptor. Moreover, it was further hypothesized that β-lactam antibiotics reacted with transpeptidases as analogs of acyl-D-alanyl-D-alanine. The current situation which largely establishes the validity of these hypotheses is discussed in more detail below.

Thus in the late 1960's *in vivo* studies supported the conclusion that cross-linkage of peptidoglycan occurred via transpeptidation in a reaction which was inhibited by β-lactam antibiotics. However, further investigations of the process clearly required the development of suitable *in vitro* systems.

3.3.1. *Transpeptidation* In Vitro

Direct demonstration of transpeptidation *in vitro* was first achieved with particulate membrane preparations from *E. coli* (Araki *et al.*, 1966a,b; Izaki *et al.*, 1966, 1968). Subsequently an increasing number of similar preparations have been isolated from both Gram-positive and Gram-negative bacteria. However, membrane preparations which catalyze transpeptidation have largely been obtained from organisms with type A1 peptidoglycans. Here the cross-linkage occurs directly between peptide side chains without the intervention of cross-bridge amino acids or peptides. In Gram-negative organisms and Bacilli cross-linkage results in the formation of D-alanyl-*meso*-diaminopimelyl bonds (Fig. 6). Among organisms having more complex peptidoglycan structures, membranes of *Sporosarcina ureae* (type A4) and *M. luteus* (type A2) were reported to catalyze cross-linkage (Linnett *et al.*, 1974; Pellon *et al.*, 1976). In *M. luteus* this resulted in the formation of both D-alanyl-L-lysine and D-alanyl-L-alanine bonds, the two types of cross-linkage found in the mature peptidoglycan. Earlier Mirelman and Bracha (1974), studying the formation of these cross-links *in vivo*, found the synthesis of D-alanyl-L-alanine bonds to be some fifty-fold less sensitive to inhibition by benzyl-penicillin than was the synthesis of the D-alanyl-L-lysine cross-link, suggesting that different transpeptidases catalyze these two reactions. Multiple transpeptidases were also suggested by a study of the incorporation of D,D-diaminopimelic acid into peptidoglycan synthesized by membranes from *B. megaterium* (Wickus and Strominger, 1972, 1974).

Although the majority of earlier studies in peptidoglycan biosynthesis utilized sub-cellular fractions from *Staph. aureus* and *M. luteus*, these were membrane preparations

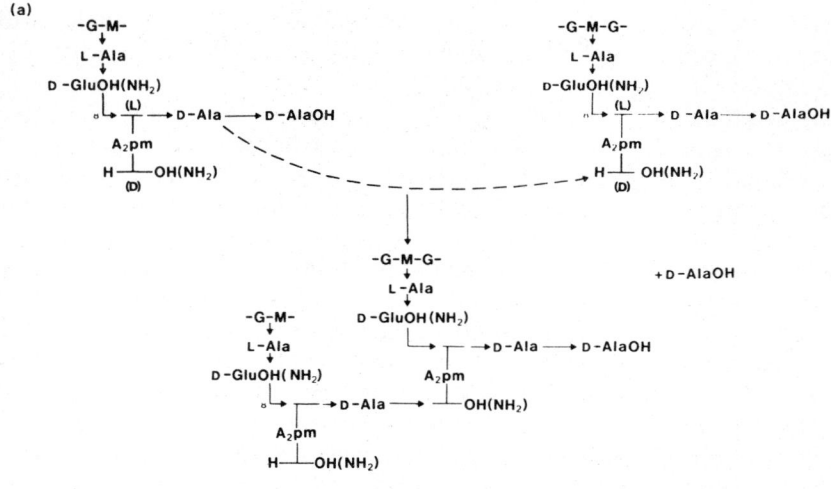

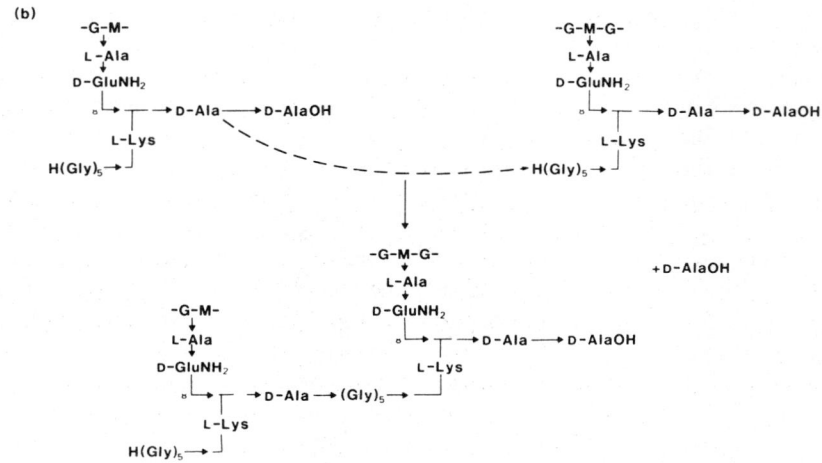

FIG. 6. The transpeptidation reactions occurring in Gram-negative organisms and Bacilli (a) and in *Staph. aureus* (b). The reaction occurs with the release of a terminal D-alanine residue and the cross-linkage of the resulting terminal D-alanine residue of the tetrapeptide with a free-amino group of a second peptide.

which did not catalyze efficient cross linkage. This was finally achieved in *Staph. aureus* with the development of wall–membrane preparations (Mirelman and Sharon, 1972). Subsequently, the major advances in our understanding of the transpeptidation reaction and its role in peptidoglycan synthesis have come through the use of wall–membrane and permeabilized cell preparations (for review see Rogers *et al.*, 1980). A recent exciting development has been the demonstration (Kalomiris *et al.*, 1982) that freeze-thawing of *Gaffkya homari* membranes, in the presence of isolated walls, appears to reactivate transpeptidation. In common with membranes of *M. luteus* and *Staph. aureus*, isolated membranes of *G. homari* only synthesize uncross-linked peptidoglycan. However, after several cycles of freeze-thawing in the presence of *G. homari* walls (walls of *B. megaterium* and cellulose did not substitute), the membranes catalyzed the cross-linkage of newly synthesized peptidoglycan to the walls. The formation of a complex of membranes and walls was demonstrated by density centrifugation but the relationship of this preparation to wall–membrane preparations remains unclear.

In both wall–membrane and permeabilized cell preparations, products of biosynthesis can be easily fractionated by treatment of the preparation with hot detergent. Under these conditions newly-synthesized material cross-linked into the wall remains detergent-insoluble, whereas uncross-linked polymer is solubilized. Recent studies with Gram-negative bacteria, which suggest that a fraction of the detergent-soluble polymer is partially cross-linked, have already been discussed.

In wall-membrane preparations from *Staph. aureus* the synthesis of cross-linked peptidoglycan required, as precursors, UDP-*N*-acetylmuramoyl-pentapeptide, UDP-*N*-acetylglucosamine and glycine (Mirelman and Sharon, 1972). Transpeptidation, determined as the release of D-alanine, was inhibited by low concentrations of benzylpenicillin. Glycine incorporation was sensitive to ribonuclease suggesting the involvement of the glycyl-tRNA intermediate described previously. However, the addition of glycyl-tRNA synthetase and soluble tRNA failed to stimulate synthesis. This may reflect the presence in the membrane of an ordered biosynthetic enzyme complex which did not interact with soluble components. Wall–membrane preparations have now been isolated from *B. licheniformis* (Ward, 1974), *M. luteus* (Mirelman *et al.*, 1972; Weston *et al.*, 1977) and *G. homari* (Hammes and Kandler, 1976). In each case attachment of newly-synthesized peptidoglycan to preexisting wall occurs via a transpeptidation reaction. In *B. licheniformis* this reaction was inhibited by low concentrations of β-lactam antibiotics whereas in *M. luteus* the incorporation of approximately 20–25% of the newly-synthesized material was not inhibited by high concentrations of benzylpenicillin. On the other hand the release of D-alanine was inhibited by as little as $1 \mu g \, ml^{-1}$ of the antibiotic. It appears that in *M. luteus* some extension of glycan chains by a penicillin-insensitive transglycosylation reaction can occur in the absence of transpeptidation. Whether this situation exists *in vivo* remains unclear. The importance of cross-linkage in the attachment of newly-synthesized peptidoglycan to the wall was shown in experiments where cultures of *B. licheniformis* (Tynecka and Ward, 1975), *M. luteus* (Mirelman *et al.*, 1974) and *B. subtilis* (Waxman *et al.*, 1980) were incubated with benzylpenicillin. In all cases linear uncross-linked peptidoglycan was released into the medium. The material from *B. licheniformis* and *B. subtilis* was fully substituted with pentapeptide side chains due to the simultaneous inhibition of the penicillin-sensitive D,D-carboxypeptidases and that from *B. licheniformis* had an average chain length of 44 disaccharide units. Soluble uncross-linked peptidoglycan was also 'secreted' into the medium when *Brevibacterium divaricatum* (Keglevic *et al.*, 1974, Valinger *et al.*, 1982) or 'autoplasts' of *Streptococcus faecium* (Rosenthal and Shockman, 1975a,b; Rosenthal *et al.*, 1975) were incubated in the presence of penicillin.

Schrader and Fan (1974) first used permeabilized bacteria to study peptidoglycan biosynthesis. They showed that toluene-treated *B. megaterium* synthesized cross-linked peptidoglycan when supplied with appropriate precursors. Similar preparations were subsequently obtained from *G. homari* (Giles and Reynolds, 1979), *M. luteus* (S. J. Thorpe and H. R. Perkins, unpublished observations) and *Staph. aureus* (A. W. Wyke and J. B. Ward, unpublished observations). However, it is really with the Gram-negative bacteria that permeabilization has been most widely used. In *E. coli* (Mirelman *et al.*, 1976; Maass and Pelzer, 1981) *P. aeruginosa* (Mirelman and Nuchamowitz, 1979a,b; Moore *et al.*, 1979) and *Neisseria gonorrhoea* (Brown and Perkins, 1979) diethyl-ether treatment of the bacteria yielded preparations catalyzing the synthesis of cross-linked peptidoglycan in which attachment of the newly-synthesized material occurred via a penicillin-sensitive transpeptidation reaction. In *E. coli* and *N. gonorrhoeae* approximately half of the newly-synthesized peptidoglycan was covalently-linked to the sacculus, i.e. insoluble in hot detergent. Suprisingly, in *N. gonorrhoeae*, β-lactam antibiotics at high concentration stimulated the synthesis of SDS-soluble peptidoglycan far in excess of any concomitant decrease in SDS-insoluble material whereas at low antibiotic concentrations the formulation of cross-linked material was increased (Brown and Perkins, 1979; Blundell and Perkins, 1981). Possibly the β-lactams, as analogs of acyl-D-alanyl-D-alanine, interact with an allosteric regulatory site on one or more of the biosynthetic enzymes to directly stimulate synthesis of the uncross-linked polymer. Enhanced synthesis of cross-linked peptidoglycan was reported earlier by Mirelman *et al.* (1976, 1977) in their study of peptidoglycan synthesis in *E. coli*. Using permeabilized cells of a thermosensitive division mutant, *E. coli* PAT 84, they found that filamentous organisms, grown at the restrictive temperature of 42°C, incorporated more peptidoglycan with a higher degree of cross-linkage than did organisms grown at 30°C. Treatment of organisms grown at the permissive temperature with low ($0.5\ \mu g\ ml^{-1}$) concentrations of ampicillin also increased the proportion of newly-synthesized peptidoglycan incorporated into the sacculus. These conditions, which cause filamentation *in vivo*, were shown to inhibit D,D-carboxypeptidase activity by 50% while transpeptidation remained unaffected. Other conditions which led to filament formation (i.e. naladixic acid or cephalexin treatment) also resulted in a decrease in the amount of D,D-carboxypeptidase activity detected when this was compared with transpeptidase activity. From these observations Mirelman and his colleagues (Mirelman, 1979) concluded that formation of the septum, and hence cell division, was dependant upon a balance between D,D-carboxypeptidase and transpeptidase activities. However, the construction of mutants of *E. coli* which apparently grow normally and yet lack most of their D,D-carboxypeptidase activity (Tamura *et al.*, 1976; Iwaya and Strominger, 1977; Matsuhashi *et al.*, 1977, 1978; Suzuki *et al.*, 1978) appears to rule out a physiological role for the carboxypeptidase and clearly conflicts with the above hypothesis. Possible explanations for this discrepancy were discussed by Mirelman (1979) in a recent review.

The effect on cross-linkage of similar changes in carboxypeptidase activity was studied more recently by De Pedro *et al.* (1980). They obtained results which also appear to rule out a regulatory role for the carboxypeptidase. Although in the absence of the enzyme (PBP-5) the number of pentapeptide side chains present in peptidoglycan showed a marked increase, the degree of cross-linkage was unaffected. Earlier, Sharpe *et al.* (1974) showed that treatment of 6-aminopenicillanic acid-resistant mutants of *B. subtilis* with high concentrations of the antibiotic reduced D,D-carboxypeptidase activity by more than 95% without affecting growth or cross-linkage of peptidoglycan.

Peptidoglycan biosynthesis by *P. aeruginosa* appeared to be similar in many respects to that observed in *E. coli* although in this case both transpeptidation and carboxypeptidase activity were inhibited by the same low (approximately $0.5\ \mu g\ ml^{-1}$ concentrations of many penicillins and cephalosporins (Mirelman and Nuchamowitz, 1979a,b; Moore *et al.*, 1979). Thus *in vivo* resistance of *P. aeruginosa* to these antibiotics appears to result from the inability of the β-lactams to penetrate the cell envelope and reach the sensitive enzymes rather than to any intrinsic resistance in the enzyme themselves. However, in contrast to the apparent situation in *E. coli* and *S. typhimurium* (Nikaido, 1979; Harder *et al.*, 1981) recent studies have suggested that the outer membrane of *P. aeruginosa* may not be the sole contributor to β-lactam antibiotic resistance in this organism (Hancock and Nikaido, 1978; Scudamore and Goldner, 1982). Because penetration of antibiotics into EDTA-treated Pseudomonads remained impaired, under conditions in which the outer membrane should be freely permeable, Scudamore and Goldner (1982) proposed the existence of an inner barrier which impeded access of the β-lactams to the penicillin-binding protein targets in the cytoplasmic membrane. Of the antibiotics tested, only rifampicin and aminoglycosides appeared to penetrate the 'inner barrier' efficiently. An alternative possibility whereby only a low proportion of the porin pores present in the outer membrane of *P. aeruginosa* are functional at any one time has been proposed (Benz and Hancock, 1981). The aminoglycosides, streptomycin and gentamycin were shown to cross the Pseudomonas outer membrane by a different mechanism to the hydrophilic (porin-mediated) pathway (Nikaido, 1979). A similar situation probably explains the observations of Scudamore and Goldner (1982) on the penetration of rifampicin and aminoglycosides.

The finding that none of the β-lactams examined completely inhibited cross-linking in *P. aeruginosa* suggests the involvement of multiple transpeptidases in the biosynthetic process. Mirelman and Nuchamowitz (1979b) proposed that a β-lactam-sensitive trans-peptidase catalyzed the attachment of newly-synthesized uncross-linked peptidoglycan to the pre-existing sacculus while a second transpeptidase, relatively resistant to β-lactams, was responsible for the cross-linkage of the soluble peptidoglycan. In fact this mechanism is more or less identical with that postulated to underly septum formation in *E. coli* (Mirelman, 1979).

However, these implications of complexity in the cross-linkage of newly-synthesized peptidoglycan to the wall may not represent the situation existing *in vivo*. Bacteria almost certainly have multiple transpeptidases some of which will act continuously to maintain the required degree of cross-linkage in the peptidoglycan while others may become activated for specific purposes such as septum formation. Evidence for multiple trans-peptidases in *E. coli* and *Staph. aureus* is discussed in more detail below.

3.3.2. *The Direction of Transpeptidation*

As stated above, the peptide side chains of nascent polymeric peptidoglycan can act as both acceptors and donors in transpeptidation reactions. Moreover not only can nascent peptidoglycan become cross-linked into the pre-existing wall but it can, in addition, form cross-links with itself. Such a reaction clearly occurs during protoplast reversion (Elliott *et al.*, 1975a,b). In liquid media protoplasts of *B. licheniformis* secrete soluble uncross-linked peptidoglycan which is often subject to attack by lytic enzymes. However, when incubated on the surface of hard agar, the protoplasts revert to normal bacteria. Clearly, at the start of this reversion process, cross-linkage must occur between side-chains of nascent peptidoglycan in the absence of pre-existing wall.

In contrast, during normal bacterial growth, nascent peptidoglycan is cross-linked into the pre-existing wall. Two possible mechanisms exist which determine the direction of this transpeptidation. In the first, the nascent peptidoglycan acts as the carboxyl donor through the terminal D-alanyl-D-alanine residues of the peptide side chains and the pre-existing wall acts as the amino acceptor. Alternatively the wall provides the donor peptide while the nascent peptidoglycan acts as the acceptor (Fig. 7).

The first mechanism occurs in *B. licheniformis* (Ward and Perkins, 1974), *B. megaterium* (Giles and Reynolds, 1979) and *P. aeruginosa* (Mirelman and Nuchamowitz, 1979a). Using wall–membrane preparations of *B. licheniformis* and UDP-*N*-acetylmuramoyl-penta-peptide in which the free amino group of diaminopimelic acid was blocked by acetylation, Ward and Perkins (1974) found that approximately half the newly-synthesized subunits

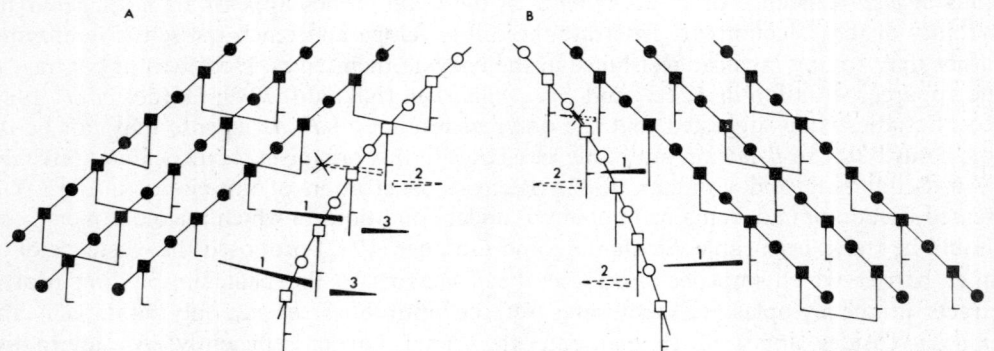

Fig. 7. Cross-linkage of newly-synthesized peptidoglycan to the pre-existing wall in *B. licheniformis* and *G. homari*. In *B. licheniformis* (A) the pre-existing wall ((–■–●–) acts as the acceptor and the newly synthesized peptidoglycan (–□–○–) as the donor in the transpeptidation reaction (——1——).

Prior D,D-carboxypeptidase activity (⸬⸬2⸬⸬) on the newly-synthesized peptidoglycan (–□–○–) will prevent subsequent cross-linkage. However, the ratio of D-alanine to D-glutamic acid in mature peptidoglycan suggests that carboxypeptidase action results in the removal of D-alanine residues not involved in cross-linkage (——3——). This direction of transpeptidation also occurs in other Bacilli and Gram-negative bacteria. In *G. homari* (B) the direction of transpeptidation is opposite. Thus, pentapeptide side-chains of the pre-existing wall (–■–●–) act as the donor, and tri- and tetrapeptide side-chains of the newly synthesized peptidoglycan (–□–○–) act as the acceptors in cross-linkage (——1——). Prior D,D and L,D-carboxypeptidase activity on the newly-synthesized polymer (⸬⸬2⸬⸬) is essential for transpeptidation to occur. However, some pentapeptide side-chains must be retained and incorporated into the wall for use as donor peptides in subsequent cross-linkage. The removal of one or both D-alanine residues from the pentapeptide side-chain (–□–○–) is shown diagrammatically (–□–○– = tetrapeptide and –□–○ = tripeptide).

polymerized were cross-linked dimers. Nascent peptidoglycan formed from this acetylated precursor cannot act as acceptor in a transpeptidase reaction. However, total incorporation of acetylated polymer was only 23% of that observed from unmodified precursor. This may reflect a decreased efficiency in the utilization of the acetylated pentapeptide by one of the biosynthetic enzymes or alternatively may mean cross-linkage between two newly-synthesized units is prevented. In B. *megaterium* the acetylated precursor was not utilized for peptidoglycan biosynthesis (Giles and Reynolds, 1979). Evidence for the direction of transpeptidation came from the observations that, while toluene-treated organisms utilized UDP-*N*-acetylmuramoyl-tetrapeptide at high efficiency for the formation of soluble uncross-linked peptidoglycan, none was cross-linked into the wall.

In contrast to the mechanism found in the Bacilli, *Gaffkya homari* was found to catalyze transpeptidation in the opposite direction (Hammes and Kandler, 1976, Hammes, 1976, 1978) (Fig. 7b). Thus the carboxyl-donor D-alanyl-D-alanine termini come from the pre-existing wall and the acceptor amino group from the nascent peptidoglycan. Wall–membrane preparations synthesized cross-linked peptidoglycan with equal efficiency from UDP-*N*-acetylmuramoyl-pentapeptide and UDP-*N*-acetylmuramoyl-tetrapeptide. While incorporation of the pentapeptide residues was inhibited by low concentrations of benzylpenicillin, the antibiotic had little effect on the cross linkage of tetrapeptide subunits. Thus the transpeptidase itself is resistant to inhibition by benzylpenicillin. In fact the peptide sidechains of nascent peptidoglycan acting as the amino acceptors in transpeptidation are tripeptides which arise by the combined action of a D,D- and L,D-carboxypeptidase (Hammes, 1978; Hammes and Seidel, 1978a,b). These enzymes act only on nascent peptidoglycan; the mature polymer and nucleotide-linked precursors are not substrates for either enzyme. Although both carboxypeptidases are inhibited by β-lactams it appears that the D,D-carboxypeptidase is the principal target. Thus in *G. homari*, the penicillin-sensitive D,D-carboxypeptidase appears to be essential for peptidoglycan synthesis in that it controls the ratio of penta- to tetra- and tripeptide residues in the nascent peptidoglycan. This ratio clearly influences both the extent of incorporation and the degree of cross-linkage in the mature peptidoglycan. A similar situation may exist in *S. faecalis* where D,D-carboxypeptidase activity appears 'important if not essential' for growth (Coyette *et al.*, 1978). Whether this means that both organisms have adopted a similar mechanism of peptidoglycan assembly will only become known with further study of *S. faecalis*. At present it seems likely that pre-existing peptidoglycan acting as the donor in transpeptidation is an unusual situation and that in most organisms nascent peptidoglycan will function in this role.

3.4. PENICILLIN-BINDING PROTEINS AS ENZYMES INVOLVED IN PEPTIDOGLYCAN BIOSYNTHESIS

Arising from the earlier studies of the biological effects of penicillin was the finding that sensitive bacteria irreversibly bound small amounts of the antibiotic (Cooper, 1956). Such an irreversible fixation supported the hypothesis of Tipper and Strominger (1965) that inhibition of transpeptidation resulted from penicilloylation of the enzyme and hence covalent-binding of the antibiotic to the membrane-bound protein. At this time the first *in vitro* demonstration of penicillin-sensitive transpeptidation and D,D-carboxypeptidase activity was made using membranes of *E. coli* (Araki *et al.*, 1966a,b; Izaki *et al.*, 1966). Tipper and Strominger (1965) had already suggested that covalent-binding of penicillin to membrane-bound transpeptidases and D,D-carboxypeptidase played an important role in the inhibition of peptidoglycan biosynthesis. These observations led to a considerable effort being put into studies of penicillin-binding proteins (PBPs, initially called penicillin binding components PBCs) both as potential transpeptidases and carboxypeptidases and in particular as targets for inhibition by β-lactam antibiotics. This review is not the place to discuss in detail the isolation and characterization of PBPs, these aspects were covered in several recent reviews (Blumberg and Strominger, 1974, Rogers *et al.*, 1980). However, it is particularly relevant in this chapter to consider the evidence that PBPs are enzymes involved in the terminal stages of peptidoglycan biosynthesis (Table 4).

TABLE 4. *Enzymic Activities of Some Purified Penicillin-Binding Proteins and their Suggested Roles in Peptidoglycan Biosynthesis*

Organism	PBP	Symbol	Apparent Molecular Wt × 10^{-3}	Enzyme Activity	Proposed Role in Peptidoglycan Biosynthesis	References
Gram-negative:						
E. coli	1a	pon A	91	Peptidoglycan polymerase transpeptidase }	Transpeptidase involved in peripheral wall extension	Suzuki *et al.*, 1978, 1980; Nakagawa *et al.*, 1979; Matsuhashi *et al.*, 1981
	1b	pon B/mrc	86.5–81.5			
	2	rod A	66	Transpeptidase	Maintenance of rod shape	Spratt, 1977a,c; Curtis and Strominger, 1981; Ishino *et al.*, 1982
	3	fts 1	60	Peptidoglycan polymerase and transpeptidase	Septum formation	Spratt, 1975, 1977a,c; Ishino and Matsuhashi, 1981
	4	dac B	49	Endopeptidase/D,D-carboxy-peptidase 1B	Secondary transpeptidase	Tamura *et al.*, 1976; Matsuhashi *et al.*, 1979
	5	dac A	42	D,D-carboxypeptidase 1A/UMT	D,D-carboxypeptidase	de Pedro and Schwartz, 1981 Amanuma and Strominger, 1980
	6	dac C	40	D,D-carboxypeptidase	?	Broome-Smith and Spratt, 1982; Amanuma and Strominger, 1980
S. typhimurium	4	—	52	D,D-carboxypeptidase/NMT/endopeptidase	?	Shepherd *et al.*, 1977
	5	—	38	D,D-carboxypeptidase/endopeptidase (little NMT activity)	?	Shepherd *et al.*, 1977
P. mirabilis	4	—		NMT/D,D-carboxypeptidase/NMT	} ?Transpeptidases in L forms	Schlif and Martin, 1980; Martin *et al.*, 1980
	5	—		D,D-carboxypeptidase/NMT		
P. vulgaris	4	—	46	D,D-carboxypeptidase/NMT	?	Rousset *et al.*, 1982
Gram-positive:						
B. megaterium	1	—	123	ND	Transpeptidase	Reynolds *et al.*, 1978
	3,4	—	83–70	ND	?	Chase, 1980
	4	—		Peptidoglycan polymerase	?	Taku *et al.*, 1982
	5	—	45	D,D-carboxypeptidase/UMT	?	Chase *et al.*, 1977
B. licheniformis	1	—	123	ND	Transpeptidase	Chase *et al.*, 1978
B. stearothermophilus	5	—	46.5	D,D-carboxypeptidase/UMT	?	Yocum *et al.*, 1974
B. subtilis	5	—	50	D,D-carboxypeptidase	?	Blumberg and Strominger, 1972; Umbriet and Strominger, 1973
B. coagulans	5	—	29	D,D-carboxypeptidase	?	McArthur and Reynolds, 1980
Staph. aureus	4	—	46	UMT/D,D-carboxypeptidase/β-lactamase	Secondary transpeptidase	Kozarich and Strominger, 1978; Wyke *et al.*, 1981
Strep. pneumoniae	3	—	43	D,D-carboxypeptidase	?	Hakenbeck and Kohiyama, 1982

ND, not determined. UMT and NMT, unnatural and natural model transpeptidases. The substrates used in the determination of these activities are described in the text.

Penicillin-binding proteins of many Gram-positive and Gram-negative bacteria have been extensively studied in recent years. Purification of these proteins was made possible by the observation that bound penicillin was released from PBPs of *B. subtilis* by treatment with neutral hydroxylamine yielding penicilloyl-hydroxmate and the active enzyme; in this case a D,D-carboxypeptidase (Lawrence and Strominger, 1970a,b). The reactivation of the enzyme was initially thought to involve the chemical hydrolysis of a thioester bond. However, Blumberg *et al.* (1974) found that denaturation of the penicilloylated enzyme with sodium dodecyl sulphate or by boiling prevented the hydroxylamine activated release of the antibiotic. It is now known that hydroxylamine acts as a nucleophilic agent to release the penicilloyl-residue in an enzyme catalyzed transpeptidation. Thus PBPs bound to penicillin or cephalosporin affinity columns could be released by hydroxylamine treatment, providing a rapid and effective purification procedure for these often minor membrane proteins. Selective purification can often be obtained, for example, by pretreatment of membrane preparations with β-lactams which bind selectively to some PBPs but only poorly to one or more others. Alternative methods include differential elution of PBPs from the affinity column and the use of mutants lacking one or more of the PBPs. A recent development in *E. coli* has been the cloning of individual PBPs on bacteriophage λ vectors and multicopy plasmids. The use of these has enabled strains to be constructed which overproduce, by as much as 100-fold, the amount of the PBPs found in the membrane (Spratt, 1980). Thus by using one or more of these techniques large numbers of PBPs have been purified and some shown to have *in vitro* enzyme activity.

The major advances in the study of the function of individual PBPs have been made using *E. coli*. Initially Spratt (1975, 1977a,b,c) used the dual approach of either examining the interaction of various penicillins and cephalosporins with PBPs or selecting mutants having growth characteristics similar to those of the antibiotic-treated organisms and examining such mutants for changes in their PBPs. By this time a correlation had already been made between the low molecular weight binding proteins and penicillin-sensitive D,D-carboxypeptidases. In fact the majority of isolated PBPs which possess enzyme activity *in vitro* catalyze this type of reaction although many also perform various 'unnatural model' transpeptidase reactions. This involves the replacement of the terminal D-alanyl residue of the peptide acyl-D-alanyl-D-alanine with a free amino acid such as glycine or D-alanine.

$$\text{acyl-D-ala-D-ala} + [^{14}\text{C}]\text{gly} \rightarrow \text{acyl-D-ala-}[^{14}\text{C}]\text{gly} + \text{D-alanine}$$

In *E. coli* PBPs 4, 5 and 6 were shown to be equivalent to D,D-carboxypeptidase 1A (PBP 5/6) and 1B (PBP 4) (Iwaya and Strominger, 1977; Matsuhashi *et al.*, 1977, 1979). These enzymes had previously been purified from *E. coli* membranes using conventional techniques and shown to possess additional unnatural model transpeptidase (1A) and endopeptidase (1B) activities (Tamura *et al.*, 1976). Mutants have been isolated which are grossly deficient in one or both carboxypeptidases (Suzuki *et al.*, 1978). At this time the only physiological response observed in the absence of PBP-4 (*dac B* mutants) was a reduced rate of lysis in the presence of ampicillin (Iwaya and Strominger, 1977). From this observation it was concluded that the *in vivo* function of PBP-4 was as an endopeptidase rather than as a carboxypeptidase. More recently De Pedro *et al.* (1980) have examined the degree of peptidoglycan cross-linkage in mutants lacking PBP 5/6 (*dac A*), PBP-4 (*dac B*) or both (*dac A dac B*). Other studies showed that newly-synthesized peptidoglycan of *E. coli* was less cross-linked and possessed a higher number of pentapeptide side chains than did the preexisting peptidoglycan (De Pedro and Schwarz, 1981). Because increased cross-linkage was not found in mutants lacking PBP-4, it was suggested that, *in vivo*, this PBP acts as a transpeptidase rather than as a carboxypeptidase or endopeptidase.

These studies also showed that cross-linkage increased in parallel with the attachment of lipoprotein to the peptidoglycan. More recently, it was suggested from pulse-labeling experiments and HPLC analysis of peptidoglycan from PBP-4⁻ and lipoprotein⁻ mutants of *E. coli*, that PBP-4 catalyzed the formation of the recently discovered diaminopimelyl-diaminopimelic acid cross-links (Glauner and Schwarz, 1983).

Evidence for the *in vivo* function of PBP 5/6 came from the finding that the number of pentapeptide residues in peptidoglycan was dramatically increased in mutants lacking these binding proteins. Thus, both *in vivo* and *in vitro*, PBP 5/6 appears to function as a carboxypeptidase converting newly-synthesized pentapeptide side chains into the tetra-peptides found in the mature polymer (De Pedro and Schwarz, 1981). Suprisingly double mutants (*dac A*, *dac B*) were found to have highly cross-linked peptidoglycan, an unexpected observation in view of the findings with the mutant lacking only PBP-4. The authors suggested that the large accumulation of pentapeptide subunits resulting from the lack of carboxypeptidase 1A favored an abnormal type of cross-linkage during the insertion of newly-synthesized peptidoglycan into the wall. This view is reminiscent of the postulated balance between carboxypeptidase and transpeptidase as a regulator of peptidoglycan biosynthesis discussed earlier in this section. However, in this case cell shape was normal.

More recently, Markiewicz *et al.* (1982) found that overproduction of PBP-5 in *E. coli* resulted in spherical growth of the organisms. The amount of PBP-5 in the mutant was approximately ten times that found in control cells while the D-alanine carboxypeptidase activity of isolated membranes showed a 3.7 fold increase. Moreover, the peptidoglycan of the mutant contained fewer pentapeptide side chains, a finding which supported the earlier conclusion (de Pedro *et al.*, 1980) that PBP-5 acts as a D,D-carboxypeptidase *in vivo*.

Markiewicz *et al.* (1982) suggested that spherical growth of *E. coli* could occur because excessive removal of D-alanine from the peptide side chains of peptidoglycan precursors prevented their utilization for cell elongation. However, the resulting tetrapeptides (and perhaps tripeptides) would be efficiently utilized by the peptidoglycan synthesizing enzymes involved in cell division (i.e. septum formation). Thus, cell division may require precursors with tetra- or tripeptide side chains to act as acceptors in transpeptidation reactions whereas, in cell elongation, pentapeptides would be required to act as donor peptides in cross-linkage. Spherical growth would result from an increased conversion of pentapeptide to tetrapeptide side chains, thereby stimulating cross-linking by the cell division system while suppressing cross-linking by the cell elongation system.

As mentioned briefly above, the relationship between selective binding of β-lactams to a particular PBP and characteristic morphological changes was first studied by Spratt (1975, 1977a). However, it had long been known that treatment of *E. coli* and related Gram-negative organisms with low concentrations of benzylpenicillin inhibited septation and resulted in continued growth of the bacteria as nonseptate filaments (Gardner, 1940; Lederberg, 1957). At slightly higher antibiotic concentrations, growth ceased and lysis ensued (Schwarz *et al.*, 1969). More recently, cephalosporins (particularly cephalexin and cefotaxime) were found that inhibited cell division only over much greater ranges of concentration. At the lowest concentration inhibiting cell division, cephalexin was found to bind specifically to PBP-3 (Spratt, 1977a). Confirmation of the role of PBP-3 in some aspect of septum formation came from the isolation of mutants thermosensitive in cell division. At the restrictive temperature, the inhibition of division resulting in filamentation was accompanied by the loss of the ability of PBP-3 to bind radioactive benzylpenicillin (Spratt, 1975, Suzuki *et al.*, 1978). The possibility that PBP-3 is a transpeptidase directly involved in septum formation is supported by the recent finding that purified PBP-3 catalyzes both transglycosylase and transpeptidase activities (Ishino and Matsuhashi, 1981). The enzyme(s) was isolated from a strain of *E. coli* carrying a plasmid encoding the structural gene for PBP-3 and was purified by affinity chromatography in the presence of *N*-formimidoylthienamycin which inhibited the binding of all other *E. coli* PBPs to the column. *In vitro* the purified protein catalyzed the formation of cross-linked peptidoglycan from undecaprenyl-P-P-disaccharide-pentapeptide (the disaccharide lipid intermediate). After lysozyme digestion of the newly-synthesized polymer and chromatographic separation of the products, cross-linkage was estimated to be 8–10%. This was significantly reduced by treatment with benzylpenicillin and cephalexin, antibiotics known to bind to

PBP-3 and cause filamentation *in vivo*, whereas treatment with others not giving the morphological response *in vivo* (e.g. *N*-formimidoylthienamycin, nocardicin A) were without effect on the *in vitro* enzyme activity.

The bifunctional aspect of certain penicillin-binding proteins from *E. coli* was established earlier in studies of PBP-1a and -1b. Initially PBP-1 (Spratt *et al.*, 1977a) showed a biphasic response to certain cephalosporins and with modified electrophoretic separation it was resolved into two components, PBP-1a and -1b (Spratt *et al.*, 1977a, Suzuki *et al.*, 1978). Subsequently Tamaki *et al.* (1977) and Suzuki *et al.* (1978) isolated mutants of *E. coli* lacking PBP-1b (*pon B*) and showed that membranes of such organisms were capable of synthesizing lipid intermediates but not peptidoglycan. Mutants lacking PBP-1a (*pon A*) were also isolated by Suzuki *et al.* (1978) but appeared unrelated to the initial thermosensitivity of the mutants. However, double mutants (*pon A, pon B*) could not be isolated and when one of the lesions was thermosensitive the organisms grew at the permissive temperature (30°C) but lysed when the temperature was raised to 42°C. Evidence that PBP-1a and 1b can intercompensate to maintain the necessary degree of peptidoglycan cross-linkage was obtained when pseudorevertants of PBP-1b⁻ organisms were found which possessed increased amounts of PBP-1a and PBP-2. More recently, Matsuhashi and his colleagues (Nakagawa *et al.*, 1979, Nakagawa and Matsuhashi, 1980, 1982; Ishino *et al.*, 1980; Matsuhashi *et al.*, 1981; Tomioka *et al*, 1982) have isolated and purified both PBP-1a and 1b's from membranes of *E. coli*. The purified proteins bound 0.35 (1a) and 0.06 (1b) mole of [^{14}C]benzylpenicillin per mole of protein (Matsuhashi *et al.*, 1981). Independently, Suzuki *et al.* (1980) also purified PBP-1b from a second strain of *E. coli*. In each case the isolated PBPs catalyzed the formation of peptidoglycan with a low degree of cross-linkage from the disaccharide lipid intermediate. The extent of cross-linkage produced by a particulate preparation from a mutant lacking both PBP-1b and the two D,D-carboxypeptidases described above (i.e. *pon B⁻, dac A⁻, dac B⁻*) was markedly increased when this preparation was incubated with purified PBP-1b (Suzuki *et al.*, 1980). More recently, improved reaction conditions have been described (Tomioka *et al.*, 1982) which resulted in the formation of hyper-cross-linked peptidoglycan by PBP-1a. In all these *in vitro* preparations, benzylpenicillin and certain other β-lactams inhibited cross-linkage and the release of D-alanine while the polymerization reaction (the transglycosylase) was inhibited by moenomycin, enduracidin and macarbomycin (Matsuhashi *et al.*, 1981; Suzuki *et al.*, 1980).

Penicillin-binding protein 2 of *E. coli* and other enteric bacteria specifically binds the 6-amidinopenicillanic acid derivative, mecillinam. Over a wide range of concentrations, treatment with this antibiotic results in conversion of the bacteria to osmotically-stable, ovoid cells. Only with relatively high concentrations and prolonged incubation was lysis observed (Lund and Tybring, 1972; Spratt, 1975, 1977a,b,c). Interestingly, more recent studies showed that clavulanic acid, thienamycin and a second aminopenicillanic also bound with highest affinity to PBP-2. However, with these antibiotics, the effective concentration range for the conversion to round cells was much smaller than with mecillinam and even the presence of relatively low concentrations resulted in lysis of the bacteria (Spratt 1977c, Spratt *et al.*, 1977b). In terms of structure–function relationships it is noteworthy that the β-lactam ring of all antibiotics showing preferential binding to PBP-2 is either unsubstituted or has an unusual form of substitution (Spratt *et al.*, 1977b).

The relationship of PBP-2 to cell shape determination was also established by the isolation of two classes of mutants. These were obtained in *E. coli* either as thermosensitive mutants which grew as rods at 30°C but were converted to osmotically-stable round cells at 42°C, or as mecillinam-resistant organisms (Spratt 1975, 1977b,c; Iwaya *et al.*, 1978). Studies of the binding of benzylpenicillin and mecillinam showed that PBP-2 was absent in the mecillinam-resistant organisms (or alternatively it was present but defective in function and β-lactam binding) and in the thermosensitive mutants grown at the restrictive temperature.

The nature of the enzyme activity catalyzed by PBP-2 remains unclear but a mecillinam-sensitive transpeptidation reaction was demonstrated in membranes of *E. coli* which contained increased amounts of PBP-2 (Ishino *et al.*, 1982). The membrane preparation, treated with cefmetazole to inhibit all other PBPs, catalyzed the formation of cross-linked peptidoglycan from nucleotide precursors. Cross-linkage was inhibited by concentrations of mecillinam similar to those concentrations inhibiting growth, whereas it was relatively resistant to other β-lactam antibiotics which do not bind readily to PBP-2.

Earlier suggestions that PBP-2 functioned as an LD-transpeptidase in the linkage of lipoprotein to peptidoglycan were disproved by Braun and Wolff (1975). Their findings suggested that PBP-2 is a transpeptidase involved in peripheral wall synthesis. A similar proposal was made recently by Markiewicz *et al.* (1982) on the basis of their finding that mecillinam treatment resulted in a 20% increase in cross-linkage of newly synthesized peptidoglycan. This change occurred within minutes following the addition of mecillinam and well before any shape change was observed. Similar results were obtained with the morphological mutants on transfer to the restrictive temperature. It was suggested that PBP-2 is a component of the enzyme system involved in the cross-linkage of new peptidoglycan for cell elongation. In the absence of PBP-2 activity peptidoglycan synthesis occurred entirely by the system responsible for cell division. Possibly the latter system, which involves PBP-3, inserts newly-synthesized peptidoglycan into the wall with a higher degree of cross-linkage. However this remains to be established.

PBP-2 was purified by affinity chromatography from *E. coli* membranes after pretreatment of the membrane with cephradine or cefoxitin (Curtis and Strominger, 1981), but *in vitro* activity was not detected.

Other purified PBPs in which the enzymic activity has been detected include the D,D-carboxypeptidase of *B. subtilis* (Blumberg and Strominger 1972, Umbreit and Strominger 1973, *B. stearothermophilus* (Yocum *et al.*, 1974) *B. megaterium* (Chase *et al.*, 1977; Chase, 1980) and *B. coagulans* (McArthur and Reynolds, 1980). Certain of these catalyze the unnatural model transpeptidation reaction discussed previously. However, the role of these enzymes *in vivo* remains unclear. The absence of terminal D-alanine residues in peptidoglycan of Bacilli implies that they function as D,D-carboxypeptidases.

Low molecular weight PBPs were also purified from *S. typhimurium* (Shepherd *et al.*, 1977) and *Proteus mirabilis* L-forms (Schlif and Martin, 1980; Martin *et al.*, 1980). PBP-4 catalyzed both natural model transpeptidation (i.e. the formation of cross-linked dimers from peptide substrates analogous to the peptide side chains of peptidoglycan) and endopeptidase activities in addition to being a D,D-carboxypeptidase, while PBP-5 was a much less efficient transpeptidase. Only PBP-4 and -5 were detected in L-forms of *P. mirabilis*. These organisms are produced on growth of the parent bacilli in the presence of one of a range of penicillins and cephalosporins. Suprisingly, they still contain cross-linked peptidoglycan. However, treatment of the L-forms with certain combinations of β-lactams (e.g. cefoxitin and benzylpenicillin) results in lysis.

Examination of the stabilities of the antibiotic-binding protein complexes showed that the cefoxitin–PBP-4 complex was labile whereas the complex with PBP-5 was quite stable. Opposite results were obtained with benzylpenicillin. Martin *et al.* (1980) postulated that, in the presence of either one of the antibiotics, the labile PBP complex retained sufficient enzymic activity to catalyze formation of cross-linked but defective peptidoglycan. When both antibiotics are present the stable-complexes formed are enzymically inactive and the L-forms cannot survive. Thus in L-forms both PBP-4 and -5 may act as transpeptidases, although the formation of mature and rod-shaped peptidoglycan requires the activity of other transpeptidases (PBPs).

A similar situation in which a low molecular weight PBP functions as a transpeptidase also exists in *Staph. aureus*. Earlier PBP-4, the binding protein of lowest molecular weight was purified and shown to catalyze D,D-carboxypeptidase, unnatural model transpeptidase and weak penicillinase activities (Kozarich and Strominger, 1978). The 'penicillinase' activity is clearly due to the lability of the PBP-4-benzylpenicillin complex which breaks down with a half-life of 5 min at 37°C. Since D,D-carboxypeptidase activity had not been detected in membranes of *Staph. aureus* the *in vivo* function of PBP-4 remained unknown. However, the peptidoglycan of mutants of *Staph. aureus* H lacking PBP-4 (and the enzymic activities associated with the isolated protein) was recently found to contain only 50% of the cross-links found in wild-type peptidoglycan (Wyke *et al.*, 1981) (Fig. 8). The mutants lacking PBP-4 showed increased sensitivity to β-lactams presumably as a consequence of the absence of the PBP. Revertants selected on the basis of increased resistance to β-lactams regained PBP-4, the enzymic activities *in vitro* and showed increased cross-linkage of their peptidoglycan. Moreover, the absence of PBP-4 could be mimicked by treatment of *Staph. aureus* with cefoxitin. At low concentrations this cephalosporin binds specifically and apparently irreversibly to PBP-4 (Curtis *et al.*, 1980). Thus in *Staph. aureus* PBP-4 apparently acts as a secondary transpeptidase whose function is required to maintain the high degree of cross-linkage found in staphylococcal peptidoglycan.

PBP-1 has been purified from *B. megaterium* (Reynolds *et al.*, 1978) and *B. licheniformis* (Chase *et al.*, 1978). However, in neither case was enzymic activity detected although comparison of the rate of breakdown of isolated benzylpenicillin–PBP complexes with the effects of the antibiotic on *in vitro* peptidoglycan biosynthesis implicated both binding proteins as transpeptidases. In *B. licheniformis* close agreement was found between the rate of recovery of peptidoglycan biosynthesis in whole cells pre-treated with benzylpenicillin (Tynecka and Ward, 1975) and the release of antibiotic from its complex with PBP-1. Similar results were obtained in *B. megaterium* when the formation of cross-linked dimers was followed in wall–membrane preparations.

The interaction of β-lactams with the soluble D,D-carboxypeptidases of Streptomyces has been the subject of extensive studies by Ghuysen and his colleagues. These enzymes, which also catalyze transpeptidation reactions with model peptide substrates, have been purified from *Streptomyces albus* G, strain R61, *S. rimosus* and *Actinomadura* R39. Detailed analysis has been made of substrate specificities, the kinetics of enzyme–substrate and enzyme–β-lactam interactions, the products arising from breakdown of the enzyme–penicillin complexes and the nature of the penicillin-binding site. More recently X-ray crystallographic studies of *S. albus* G and *Streptomyces* R61 enzymes have also been described (Dideberg *et al.*, 1980; Kelly *et al.*, 1982). The observations made with the soluble enzymes have now been extended to cover membrane-bound transpeptidases from several

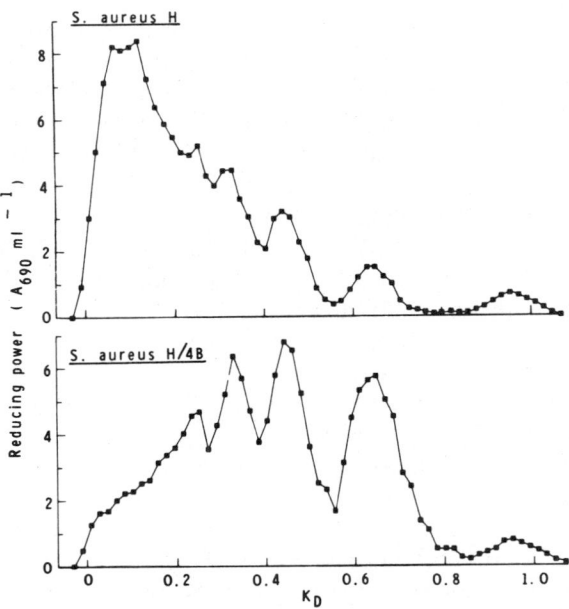

FIG. 8. Fractionation of the peptidoglycan of *Staph. aureus* H and a mutant lacking penicillin-binding protein 4. Peptidoglycan hydrolysed by treatment with *Charalopsis* B muramidase was fractionated by gel-filtration chromatography. Peptidoglycan of *Staph. aureus* H was highly cross-linked (oligomer, 67%; trimer, 16%; dimer, 11% and monomer 6%) whereas cross-linkage in the mutant lacking penicillin-binding protein 4 was much reduced (oligomer, 26%; trimer, 30%; dimer, 25.6% and monomer 28%) (Wyke *et al.*, 1981).

Streptomyces. These studies represent a major contribution in our understanding of the action of β-lactams at the molecular level. However, detailed consideration of the individual aspects of this work would be out of place in this chapter and the reader is directed to several excellent reviews by Ghuysen and his colleagues (Ghuysen, 1977a,b; Ghuysen, 1980; Ghuysen et al., 1979,1980).

Thus recent years have seen major advances in our understanding of the role of PBPs in peptidoglycan biosynthesis. Clearly, the mechanism of peptidoglycan assembly is very complicated and only preliminary investigations have been made of individual enzymic activities. Perhaps with increased knowledge of the enzymes and the substrates which themselves may be macromolecular precursors of peptidoglycan (i.e. partially cross-linked nascent peptidoglycan) a clearer picture will emerge.

3.5. O-Acetylation and De-N-Acetylation of Peptidoglycan

It has been known for many years that the N-acetylmuramoyl residues of the peptidoglycan of certain Gram-positive bacteria are also O-acetylated. In Staph. aureus approximately 50% of the muramic acid residues are present as the 4-N, 6-O-diacetyl derivative (Tipper et al., 1965; Tipper and Strominger, 1967) while the degree of substitution reaches nearly 70% in L. acidophilus (Coyette and Ghuysen, 1970). The presence of the O-acetyl substituent has the effect of making the peptidoglycan resistant to the endo-muramidase egg-white lysozyme (Brumfitt et al., 1958). More recently, 'O'-acetylation has been found in peptidoglycans of Gram-negative organisms including Proteus vulgaris, P. mirabilis, Neisseria perflava, N. gonorrhoeae, Moraxella glucidolytica and Pseudomonas alcaligenes (Fleck et al., 1971; Martin et al., 1973; Martin and Gmeiner, 1979; Blundell et al., 1980).

In P. mirabilis, peptidoglycan is synthesized from non-O-acetylated disaccharide pentapeptide subunits (Gmeiner and Kroll, 1981). Newly synthesized material, isolated from pulse-labeled cultures as polymer insoluble in hot detergent, contained significantly less O-acetyl substituents than did peptidoglycan from continuously-labeled organisms. However, during subsequent growth, O-acetylation of the peptidoglycan increased. From their detailed investigations Gmeiner and Kroll (1981) concluded that non-O-acetylated nascent peptidoglycan became cross-linked to O-acetylated polymer in the pre-existing sacculus. A second nascent chain of non-acetylated polymer was then cross-linked into the growing wall. Thus both types of peptidoglycan, whether O-acetylated or not, acted as acceptors in the transpeptidation reaction. Whether two separate transpeptidases catalyze these reactions remains to be established. Subsequently the newly-inserted peptidoglycan becomes partially O-acetylated. Among the products obtained by muramidase-treatment of peptidoglycan are dimers containing none, one or two O-acetyl substituents indicating that both O-acetylated and non-O-acetylated glycan chains (sections of chains) can be cross-linked. These products were also obtained from muramidase digests of N. gonor-rhoeae (Blundell and Perkins, 1981) suggesting that a similar process occurs in this organism. Treatment of both P. mirabilis and N. gonorrhoeae with β-lactam antibiotics caused a decrease in O-acetylation without greatly affecting the degree of peptidoglycan cross-linkage (Martin and Gmeiner, 1979; Blundell and Perkins, 1981). In P. mirabilis this result was obtained by comparing the peptidoglycan of untreated organisms with that of bacteria grown in the presence of benzylpenicillin. Although the degree of cross-linkage was essentially unchanged the morphology of the organisms (and hence the peptidoglycan sacculus) was clearly disturbed. Lear and Perkins (1983) followed the incorporation of [^{14}C]O-acetylated and non-O-acetylated subunits of N. gonorrhoeae peptidoglycan. The majority of cross-links were formed extremely rapidly (80% in 3 min) whereas only 65% of the final degree of O-acetylation had occurred in 10 min. Further cross-linkage and O-acetylation took place over the next 30–40 min (0.5 generations).

In general the observations made with the two organisms are in agreement. Newly-synthesized peptidoglycan appears to be non-O-acetylated and substitution takes place after transpeptidation of this component has occurred. The observations made following

β-lactam treatment suggest that the acetylation reaction is a highly-ordered process and that even quite subtle changes in the topology of the peptidoglycan may cause inhibition.

A second type of modification of peptidoglycan, the loss of N-acetyl groups, also occurs. This modification has been described in peptidoglycan of certain strains of *Bacillus cereus*, *B. megaterium* and *B. subtilis* (Araki *et al.*, 1972; Hayashi *et al.*, 1973; Westmacott and Perkins, 1979). In these organisms the extent of deacylation of N-acetylglucosamine residues ranged from approximately 20–80%. More recently, a high proportion of nonacetylated glucosamine residues were also found in the peptidoglycan of *Rhodopseudomonas viridis* (Schmelzer *et al.*, 1982) and *Clostridium perfringens* (Williamson and Ward, 1982). In each organism, de-N-acetylation of glucosamine resulted in the peptidoglycan being resistant to egg-white lysozyme, while N-acetylation with acetic anhydride restored lysozyme-sensitivity.

Although little is known concerning the biosynthesis of these peptidoglycans an enzyme which deacetylates N-acetylglucosamine residues in peptidoglycan of *B. cereus* has been described (Araki *et al.*, 1971). Thus, deacetylation probably occurs after the fully N-acetylated nascent peptidoglycan has become incorporated into the growing wall. In *C. perfringens* at least, the deacetylation does not appear to be affected by β-lactum antibiotics. Similar proportions of glucosamine residues were found in peptidoglycan of untreated and antibiotic treated organisms (Williamson and Ward, 1982).

3.6. REGULATION OF PEPTIDOGLYCAN SYNTHESIS

The importance of peptidoglycan as the wall polymer essential for maintaining the structural integrity of Gram-positive and Gram-negative bacteria has already been emphasized. However, in terms of the regulation of peptidoglycan synthesis this does not necessarily imply a static situation. The opposite appears to be true: the peptidoglycan is held in a dynamic equilibrium between synthesis and degradation through the action of autolysins. The synthesis of peptidoglycan has been described in detail and involves a complex series of enzymic activities leading from the cytoplasmic nuceotide-linked precursors to the insoluble cross-linked polymer. It seems likely that both the synthesis and the activity of each of these enzymes will also be regulated. While almost nothing is known concerning control over the formation of individual enzymes, some evidence (discussed in an earlier section) is available concerning the regulation of specific activities. In the latter stages of the biosynthetic process the regulation and balance of the various enzymes is maintained by unknown mechanisms. The recent evidence describing multiple penicillin-binding proteins and the finding that several of these catalyze transglycosylase and transpeptidase activities in *E. coli* shows the complexity of the situation. Moreover, the organisms appear to have established an equilibrium between the various enzymes allowing several alternate systems to function. The inhibition or loss of one enzyme is compensated by the activation of a second or third system to allow continued synthesis of peptidoglycan. Thus the integrity of the organism is maintained although in certain cases interference of this kind may lead to continued growth of the organism in a morphologically-disturbed form.

In addition evidence was recently presented that peptidoglycan biosynthesis in *E. coli* is under stringent control (Ishiguro and Ramey, 1976; Ishiguro, 1978; Ramey and Ishiguro 1978). Guanosine tetra- and pentaphosphates (ppGpp) and (pppGpp) which accumulate during amino acid starvation of stringently-controlled *E. coli* inhibited the synthesis of both nucleotide-linked precursors and peptidoglycan. Organisms labeled with [^{3}H]diaminopimelic acid were also shown to accumulate lipid intermediates suggesting the site of regulation involved the utilization of these precursors. More recently, the regulation of peptidoglycan biosynthesis was observed in other cultural conditions which lead to the accumulation of the guanosine derivatives. These include nutritional downshift (Ishiguro, 1979) and growth temperature upshift (Vanderwel and Ishiguro, 1982). Other studies (Ishiguro *et al.*, 1980) showed that amino-acid deprivation resulted in a marked decrease in both the D,D-carboxypeptidase activity and the ability to synthesize peptidoglycan in a stringent strain of *E. coli*. These changes were accompanied by an increase in the degree of cross-linkage of the peptidoglycan synthesized *in vitro* by ether-permeabilized cells of this strain. Amino acid starvation of *E. coli in vivo* also resulted in increased cross-linkage of peptidoglycan and resistance of the organisms to lysis (Goodell and Tomasz, 1980).

The role of autolytic enzymes in the regulation of peptidoglycan biosynthesis also remains unclear. In many organisms wall synthesis and degradation are balanced and 'turnover' of the wall ensues (for review see Rogers *et al.*, 1980). If wall synthesis is inhibited in such situations, without concomitant inhibition of either the formation or action of the autolysins, cell lysis occurs. Various amphipathic substances such as lipoteichoic acids, cardiolipin and the Forssman antigen from *S. pneumoniae* can strongly inhibit the action of certain autolysins of Gram-positive bacteria (Cleveland *et al.*, 1975, 1976; Holtje and Tomasz, 1975; Suginaka *et al.*, 1979). As yet similar inhibitors for Gram-negative autolysins have not been described. However, evidence has accumulated, again in *E. coli*, for oscillations during the cell cycle of synchronously-dividing cells, in the activity of both autolytic enzymes (including the penicillin-sensitive endopeptidase, PBP-4 described above) and peptidoglycan synthesizing activity. Included among these studies are investigations of the incorporation of D-[^{14}C]glutamic acid into peptidoglycan (Hoffman *et al.*, 1972), the ability of permeabilized *E. coli* PAT 84 to synthesize peptidoglycan *in vitro* (Mirelman *et al.*, 1976, 1977) and the activity of autolytic enzymes (Beck and Park, 1976; Hackenbeck and Messer, 1977). It is not yet clear whether the decreased activity of these various enzymes is due to inhibition of specific activities or to a lack of enzyme synthesis. Clearly, further studies of regulatory mechanisms in peptidoglycan biosynthesis are required before we can hope to understand this very complex aspect of wall formation.

REFERENCES

ALLEN, C. M., KEENAN, M. V. and SACK, J. (1976) *Lactobacillus plantarum* undecaprenyl pyrophosphate synthetase: purification and reaction requirements. *Archs Biochem. Biophys.* **175**: 236–248.
ALLEN, C. M. and MUTH, J. D. (1977) Lipid activation of undecaprenyl pyrophosphate synthetase from *Lactobacillus plantarum. Biochemistry* **16**: 2908–2915.
ALLEN, J. G., ATHERTON, F. R., HALL, M. J., HASSALL, C. H., HOLMES, S. W., LAMBERT, R. W., NISBET, L. J. and RINGROSE, P. S. (1978) Phosphonopeptides, a new class of synthetic antibacterial agents. *Nature, Lond.* **272**: 56–58.
ALLEN, J. G., ATHERTON, F. R., HALL, M. J., HASSALL, C. H., HOLMES, S. W., LAMBERT, R. W., NISBET, L. J. and RINGROSE, P. S. (1979) Phosphonopeptides as antibacterial agents: alaphosphin and related phosphonopeptides. *Antimicrob. Ag. Chemother.* **15**: 684–695.
AMANUMA, H., and STROMINGER, J. L., (1980) Purification and properties of penicillin-binding proteins 5 and 6 from *Escherichia coli* membranes. *J. biol. Chem.* **255**: 11171–11180.
ANDERSON, J. S., MATSUHASHI, M., HASKIN, M. A. and STROMINGER, J. L. (1965) Lipid-phosphoacetylmuramyl-pentapeptide and lipid-phosphodisaccharide-pentapeptide: presumed membrane transport intermediates in cell wall synthesis. *Proc. natn. Acad. Sci. U.S.A.* **53**: 881–889.
ANDERSON, J. S., MEADOW, P. M., HASKIN, M. A. and STROMINGER, J. L. (1966) Biosynthesis of the peptidoglycan of bacterial cell walls. 1. Utilization of uridine diphosphate acetylmuramyl pentapeptide and uridine diphosphate acetylglucosamine for peptidoglycan synthesis by particulate enzymes from *Staphylococcus aureus* and *Micrococcus lysodeikticus. Archs Biochem. Biophys.* **116**: 487–515.
ANWAR, R. A. and VLAOVIC, M. (1979) Purification of UDP-N-acetylenolpyruvyolglucosamine reductase from *Escherichia coli* by affinity chromatography, its subunit structure and absence of flavin as the prosthetic group. *Can. J. Biochem.* **57**: 188–196.
ARAKI, Y., FUKUOKA, S., OBA, S. and ITO, E. (1971) Enzymatic deacetylation of N-acetylglucosamine residues in peptidoglycan from *Bacillus cereus* cell walls. *Biochem. biophys. Res. Commun.* **45**: 751–758.
ARAKI, Y., NAKATANI, T., NAKAYAMA, K. and ITO, E. (1972) Occurrence of N-nonsubstituted glucosamine residues in peptidoglycan of lysozyme-resistant cell walls from *Bacillus cereus. J. biol. Chem.* **247**: 6312–6322.
ARAKI, Y., SHIMADA, A. and ITO, E. (1966a) Effect of penicillin on cell wall mucopeptide synthesis in an *Escherichia coli* particulate system. *Biochem. biophys. Res. Commun.* **23**: 518–525.
ARAKI, Y., SHIRAI, R., SHIMADA, A., ISHIMOTO, N. and ITO, E. (1966b) Enzymatic synthesis of cell wall mucopeptide in a particulate preparation of *Escherichia coli. Biochem. biophys. Res. Commun.* **23**: 466–472.
ATHERTON, F. R., HALL, M. J., HASSALL, C. H., LAMBERT, R. W., LLOYD, W. J. and RINGROSE, P. S. (1979) Phosphonopeptides as antibacterial agents: mechanism of action of alaphosphin. *Antimicrob. Ag. Chemother.* **15**: 696–705.
BECK, B. D. and PARK, J. T. (1976) Activity of three murein hydrolases during the cell division cycle of *Escherichia coli* K-12 as measured in toluene-treated cells. *J. Bacteriol.* **126**: 1250–1260.
BENZ, R. and HANCOCK, R. E. W. (1981) Properties of the large ion-permeable pores formed from protein F of *Pseudomonas aeruginosa* in lipid bilayer membranes. *Biochem. biophys. Acta* **646**: 298–308.

BLUMBERG, P. M. and STROMINGER, J. L. (1972) Five penicillin-binding components occur in *Bacillus subtilis* membranes. *J. biol. Chem.* **247**: 8107–8113.

BLUMBERG, P. M. and STROMINGER, J. L. (1974) Interaction of penicillin with the bacterial cell: penicillin-binding proteins and penicillin-sensitive enzymes. *Bacteriol. Rev.* **38**: 291–335.

BLUMBERG, P. M., YOCUM, R. R., WILLOUGHBY, E. and STROMINGER, J. L. (1974) Binding of [^{14}C] Penicillin G to the membrane-bound and the purified D-alanine carboxypeptidases from *Bacillus stearothermophilus* and *B. subtilis* and its release. *J. biol. Chem.* **249**: 6828–6835.

BLUNDELL, J. K. and PERKINS, H. R. (1981) Effects of β-lactam antibiotics on peptidoglycan synthesis in growing *Neisseria gonorrhoeae*, including changes in the degree of O-acetylation. *J. Bacteriol.* **147**: 633–641.

BLUNDELL, J. K., SMITH, G. J. and PERKINS, H. R. (1980) The peptidoglycan of *Neisseria gonorrhoeae*: O-acetyl groups and lysozyme sensitivity. *FEMS Microbiol. Lett.* **9**: 259–261.

BRAUN, V. and WOLFF, H. (1975) Attachment of lipoprotein to murein (peptidoglycan) of *Escherichia coli* in the presence and absence of penicillin FL 1060. *J. Bacteriol.* **123**: 888–897.

BROME-SMITH, J. K. and SPRATT, B. G. (1982) Deletion of the penicillin-binding protein 6 gene of *Eschericia coli*. *J. Bacteriol.* **152**: 904–906.

BROWN, C. A. and PERKINS, H. R. (1979) *In vitro* synthesis of peptidoglycan by β-lactam-sensitive and -resistant strains of *Neisseria gonorrhoeae*: effects of β-lactam and other antibiotics. *Antimicrob. Ag. Chemother.* **16**: 28–36.

BROWN, W. E., SEINEROVA, V., CHAN, W. M., LASKIN, A. I., LINNETT, P. and STROMINGER, J. L. (1974) Inhibition of cell wall synthesis by the antibiotics diaumycin and janiemycin. *Ann. N.Y. Acad. Sci.* **235**: 399–405.

BRUMFITT, W., WARDLAW, A. C. and PARK, J. T. (1958) Development of lysozyme-resistance in *Micrococcus lysodeikticus* and its association with an increased O-acetyl content of the cell wall. *Nature, Lond.* **181**: 1783–4.

BUMSTED, R. M., DAHL, J. L., SOLL, D. and STROMINGER, J. L. (1968) Biosynthesis of the peptidoglycan of bacterial cell walls. Further study of the glycyl transfer ribonucleic acids active in peptidoglycan biosynthesis in *Staphylococcus aureus*. *J. biol. Chem.* **243**: 779–782.

BUXTON, R. S. and WARD, J. B. (1980) Heat sensitive lysis mutants of *Bacillus subtilis* 168 blocked at three different stages of peptidoglycan synthesis. *J. gen. Microbiol.* **120**: 283–293.

CHASE, H. A. (1980) Purification of four penicillin-binding proteins from *Bacillus megaterium*. *J. gen. Microbiol.* **117**: 211–224.

CHASE, H. A., REYNOLDS, P. E. and WARD, J. B. (1978) Purification and characterization of the penicillin-binding proteins that is the lethal target of penicillin in *Bacillus megaterium* and *Bacillus licheniformis*. *Eur. J. Biochem.* **88**: 275–285.

CHASE, H. A., SHEPHERD, S. T. and REYNOLDS, P. E. (1977) Studies on the penicillin-binding components of *Bacillus megaterium*. *FEBS Lett.* **76**: 199–203.

CHATTERJEE, A. W., DOYLE, R. J. and STREIPS, U. N. (1977) A proposed functional role for bacterial N-acetylmuramyl-L-alanine amidases. *J. Theoret. Biol.* **68**: 385–390.

CHATTERJEE, A. N. and PARK, J. T. (1964) Biosynthesis of cell wall mucopeptide by a particulate fraction from *Staphylococcus aureus*. *Proc. natn. Acad. Sci. U.S.A.* **51**: 9–16.

CHRISTENSON, J. G., GROSS, S. K. and ROBBINS, P. W. (1969) Enzymatic synthesis of the antigen carrier lipid. *J. biol. Chem.* **244**: 5436–5439.

CLEVELAND, R. F., HOLTJE, J. V., WICKEN, A. J., TOMASZ, A., DANEO-MOORE, L. and SHOCKMAN, G. D. (1975) Inhibition of bacterial wall autolysins by lipoteichoic acids and related compounds. *Biochem. biophys. Res. Commun.* **67**: 1128–1135.

CLEVELAND, R. F., WICKEN, A. J., DANEO-MOORE, L. and SHOCKMAN, G. D. (1976) Inhibition of wall autolysis in *Streptococcus faecalis* by lipoteichoic acid and lipids. *J. Bacteriol.* **126**: 192–197.

COOPER, P. D. (1956) Site of action of radiopenicillin. *Bacteriol. Rev.* **70**: 28–48.

COYETTE, J. and GHUYSEN, J-M. (1970) Structure of the walls of *Lactobacillus acidophilus* strain AM Gasser. *Biochemistry*, **9**: 2935–2943.

COYETTE, J., GHUYSEN, J-M. and FONTANA, R. (1978) Solubilization and isolation of the membrane-bound DD-carboxypeptidase of *Streptococcus faecalis* ATCC 9790. *Eur. J. Biochem.* **88**: 297–305.

CURTIS, N. A. C., HAYES, M. V., WYKE, A. W. and WARD, J. B. (1980) A mutant of *Staphylococcus aureus* H lacking penicillin-binding protein 4 and transpeptidase activity *in vitro*. *FEMS Microbiol. Lett.* **9**: 263–266.

CURTIS, S. J. and STROMINGER, J. L. (1981) Purification of penicillin-binding protein 2 of *Escherichia coli*. *J. Bacteriol.* **145**: 398–403.

DE PEDRO, M. A. and SCHWARZ, U. (1981). Heterogeneity of newly-inserted and pre-existing murein in the sacculus of *Escherichia coli*. *Proc. natn. Acad. Sci. U.S.A.* **78**: 5856–5860.

DE PEDRO, M. A., SCHWARZ, U., NISHIMURA, Y. and HIROTA, Y. (1980) On the biological role of penicillin-binding proteins 4 and 5. *FEMS Microbiol. Lett.* **9**: 219–221.

DEZÉLÉE, P. and SHOCKMAN, G. D. (1975) Studies on the formation of peptide cross-links in the cell wall peptidoglycan of *Streptococcus faecalis*. *J. biol. Chem.* **250**: 6806–6816.

DIDEBERG, O., CHARLIER, P., DUPONT, L., VERMEIRE, M., FRERE, J. M. and GHUYSEN, J. M. (1980) The 4.5 Å resolution structure analysis of the exocellular D,D-carboxypeptidase of *Streptomyces albus* G. *FEBS Lett.* **117**: 212–214.

DIVEN, W. D. (1969) Studies on amino acid racemases II. Purification and properties of the glutamate racemase from *Lactobacillus fermenti*. *Biochem. biophys. Acta.* **191**: 702–706.

ELLIOTT, T. S. J., WARD, J. B. and ROGERS, H. J. (1975a). Formation of cell wall polymers by reverting protoplasts of *Bacillus licheniformis*. *J. Bacteriol.* **124**: 623–632.

ELLIOTT, T. S. J., WARD, J. B., WYRICK, P. B. and ROGERS, H. J. (1975b). Ultrastructural study of the reversion of protoplasts of *Bacillus licheniformis* to bacilli. *J. Bacteriol.* **124**: 905–917.

FLECK, J., MOCK, M., MINCK, R. and GHUYSEN, J-M. (1971) The cell envelope in *Proteus vulgaris* P18. Isolation and characterization of the peptidoglycan component. *Biochim. biophys. Acta* **233**: 489–503.

FLETCHER, G., IRWIN, C. A., HENSON, J. M., FILLINGIM, C., MALONE, M. M. and J. R. WALKER (1978)

Identification of the *Escherichia coli* cell division gene *sep* and organisation of the cell division-cell envelope genes in the sep-mur-FtsA-envA cluster as determined with specialized trandsducing lambda bacteriophages. *J. Bacteriol.* **133:** 91–100.

FORDHAM, W. D. and GILVARG, C. (1974) Kinetics of cross-linking of peptidoglycan in *Bacillus megaterium*. *J. biol. Chem.* **249:** 2478–2482.

FOX, S. M., WARD, J. B. and SARGENT, M. G. (1977) Glycan chain lengths of *Bacillus subtilis*. *Proc. Soc. gen. Microbiol.* **4:** 90.

FUCHS-CLEVELAND, E. and GILVARG, C. (1976) Oligomeric intermediate in peptidoglycan biosynthesis in *Bacillus megaterium*. *Proc. Natn. Acad. Sci. U.S.A.* **73:** 4200–4204.

GARDNER, A. D. (1940) Morphological effects of penicillin on bacteria. *Nature, Lond.* **146:** 837–838.

GEIS, A. and PLAPP, R. (1978) Phospho-*N*-acetylmuramoyl-pentapeptide-transferase of *Escherichia coli* K12. Properties of the membrane bound and the extracted and partially purified enzymes. *Biochim. biophys. Acta* **527:** 414–424.

GENNIS, R. B., SINENSKY, M. and STROMINGER, J. L. (1976) Activation of C_{55}-isoprenoid alcohol phosphokinase from *Staphylococcus aureus* II. Biophysical studies. *J. biol. Chem.* **251:** 1270–1276.

GENNIS, R. B. and STROMINGER, J. L. (1976a). Activation of C_{55}-isoprenoid alcohol phosphokinase from *Staphylococcus aureus*. 1. Activation by phospholipids and fatty acids. *J. biol. Chem.* **251:** 1264–1269.

GENNIS, R. B. and STROMINGER, J. L. (1976b) Activation of C_{55}- isoprenoid alcohol phosphokinase from *Staphylococcus aureus*. III. Activation by detergents. *J. biol. Chem.* **251:** 1277–1282.

GHUYSEN, J. M. (1968) The use of bacteriolytic enzymes in determination of wall structure and their role in cell metabolism. *Bact. Rev.* **32:** 425–464.

GHUYSEN, J-M. (1977a) The bacterial D,D-carboxypeptidase-transpeptidase enzyme system. A new insight into the mode of action of penicillin. *University of Tokyo Press.* pp. 162.

GHUYSEN, J-M. (1977b) The concept of the penicillin target from 1965 until today. *J. gen. Microbiol.* **101:** 13–33.

GHUYSEN, J-M. (1980) Antibiotics and peptidoglycan metabolism. *Top. Antibiot. Chem.* **5:** 9–117.

GHUYSEN, J-M., BRICAS, E., LACHE, M. and LEYH-BOUILLE M. (1968) Structure of the cell walls of *Micrococcus lysodeikticus*. III. Isolation of a new peptide dimer, N^{α}-[L-alanyl-γ-D-glutamyl glycine]-L-lysyl-D-alanyl-N^{α}-[L-alanyl-γ-D-glutamoyl glycine] -L-lysyl-D-alanine. *Biochemistry*, **7:** 1450–1460.

GHUYSN, J-M., FRERE, J. M., LEYH-BOUILLE M., COYETTE, J., DUSART, J. and NGUYEN-DISTECE M. (1979) Use of model enzymes in the determination of the mode of action of penicillins and Δ^{3}-cephalosporins. *A. Rev. Biochem.* **48,** 73–101.

GHUYSEN, J-M., FRERE, J. M., LEYH-BOUILLE, M., PERKINS, H. R. and NIETO, M. (1980) The active centres in penicillin-sensitive enzymes. *Phil. Trans. R. Soc. Lond.* B. **289:** 285–301.

GILES, A. F. and REYNOLDS, P. E. (1979) The direction of transpeptidation during cell wall peptidoglycan biosynthesis in *Bacillus megaterium*. *FEBS Lett.* **101:** 244–248.

GLAUNER, B. and SCHWARZ, U. (1983) The analysis of murein composition with high-pressure liquid chromatography. In: *The Target of Penicillin*, pp. 29–34, HAKENBECK, R., HOLTJE, J. V. and LABISCHINSK, H. (eds), Walter de Gruyter & Co. Berlin.

GMEINER, J. and KROLL, H. P. (1981) Murein biosynthesis and *O*-acetylation of *N*-acetylmuramic acid during the cell division cycle of *Proteus mirabilis*. *Eur. J. Biochem.* **117:** 171–177.

GOLDMAN, R. and STROMINGER, J. L. (1972) Purification and properties of C_{55}-isoprenylpyrophosphate phosphatase from *Micrococcus lysodiekticus*. *J. biol. Chem.* **247:** 5116–5122.

GOOD, C. M and TIPPER, D. J. (1972) Conditional mutants of *Staphylococcus aureus* defective in cell wall precursor synthesis. *J. Bacteriol.* **111:** 231–241.

GOODELL, E. W., MARKIEWICZ, Z. and SCHWARZ, U. (1983) Absence of oligomeric murein intermediates in *Escherichia coli*. *J. Bacteriol.* **156:** 130–135.

GOODELL, W. and TOMASZ, A. (1980) Alterations of *Escherichia coli* murein during amino acid starvation. *J. Bacteriol.* **144:** 1009–1016.

GREGORY, W. W. and GOODER, H. (1978) Inhibition of peptidoglycan biosynthesis at a postcytoplasmic reaction in a stable L-phase variant of *Streptococcus faecium*. *J. Bacteriol.* **135:** 900–910.

HAKENBECK, R. and KOHIYAMA M. (1982) Purification of penicillin-binding protein 3 from *Streptococcus pneumoniae*. *Eur. J. Biochem.* **127:** 231–236.

HACKENBECK, R. and MESSER, W. (1977) Activity of murein hydrolases in synchronized cultures of *Escherichia coli*. *J. Bacteriol.* **129:** 1239–1244.

HAMMES, W. P. (1976) Biosynthesis of peptidoglycan in *Gaffkya homari*. The mode of action of penicillin G and mecillinam. *Eur. J. Biochem.* **79:** 107–113.

HAMMES, W. P. (1978) The L,D-carboxypeptidase activity in *Gaffkya homari*. The target of the action of D-amino acids or glycine on the formation of wall-bound peptidoglycan. *Eur. J. Biochem.* **91:** 501–507.

HAMMES, W. P. and KANDLER, O. (1976) Biosynthesis of peptidoglycan in *Gaffkya homari*. The incorporation of peptidoglycan into the cell wall and the direction of transpeptidation. *Eur. J. Biochem.* **70:** 97–106.

HAMMES, W. P. and NEUHAUS, F. C. (1974a) On the specificity of phospho-*N*-acetylmuramyl-pentapeptide translocase. The peptide subunit of uridine diphosphate-*N*-acetylmuramyl-pentapeptide. *J. biol. Chem.* **249:** 3140–3150.

HAMMES, W. P. and NEUHAUS, F. C. (1974b) On the mechanism of action of vancomycin: inhibition of peptidoglycan synthesis in *Gaffkya homari*. *Antimicrob. Ag. Chemother.* **6:** 722–728.

HAMMES, W. P. and NEUHAUS, F. C. (1974c) Biosynthesis of peptidoglycan in *Gaffkya homari*: Role of the peptide subunit of uridine diphosphate-*N*-acetylmuramyl-pentapeptide. *J. Bacteriol.* **120:** 210–218.

HAMMES, W. P. and SEIDEL, H. (1978a) The activities *in vitro* of DD-carboxypeptidase and LD-carboxypeptidase of *Gaffkya homari* during biosynthesis of peptidoglycan. *Eur. J. Biochem.* **84:** 141–147.

HAMMES, W. P. and SEIDEL, H. (1978b) The LD-carboxypeptidase activity in *Gaffkya homari*. The target of the action of certain β-lactam antibiotics on the formation of wall-bound peptidoglycan. *Eur. J. Biochem.* **91:** 509–515.

HANCOCK, R. E. W. and NIKAIDO, H. (1978) Outer membranes of Gram-negative bacteria XIX. Isolation from

Pseudomonas aeruginosa PA01 and use in reconstitution and definition of the permeability barrier. *J. Bacteriol.* **136:** 381–390.

HARDER, K. J., NIKADO, H. and MATSUHASHI, M. (1981) Mutants of *Escherichia coli* that are resistant to certain β-lactam compounds lack the *omp F* porin. *Antimicrob. Ag. Chemother.* **20:** 549–552.

HAYASHI, H., ARAKI, Y. and ITO, E. (1973) Occurrence of glucosamine residues with free amino groups in cell wall peptidoglycan from bacilli as a factor responsible for resistance to lysozyme. *J. Bacteriol.* **113:** 592–598.

HAYASHI, S., KOCH, J. P. and LIN, E. C. C. (1964) Active transport of L-α-glycerophosphate in *Escherichia coli*. *J. biol. Chem.* **239:** 3098–3105.

HIGASHI, Y., SIEWERT, G. and STROMINGER, J. L. (1970) Biosynthesis of the peptidoglycan of bacterial cell walls. XIX. Isoprenoid alcohol phosphokinase. *J. biol. Chem.* **245:** 3683–3690.

HIGASHI, Y., STROMINGER, J. L. and SWEELEY, C. C. (1967) Structure of a lipid intermediate in cell wall peptidoglycan biosynthesis: a derivative of C_{55}-isoprenoid alcohol. *Proc. natn. Acad. Sci. U.S.A.* **57:** 1878–1884.

HILDERMAN, R. H. and RIGGS, H. G. (1973) Effect of glycyl-tRNA concentration on *in vitro* serine incorporation into the peptidoglycan of *S. epidermidis*. *Biochem. biophys. Res. Commun.* **50:** 1095–1103.

HOFFMANN, B., MESSER, W. and SCHWARZ, U. (1972) Regulation of polar cap formation in the life cycle of *E. coli*. *J. Supramolec. Struct.* **1:** 29–37.

HOLTJE, J. V. and TOMASZ, A. (1975) Lipoteichoic acid: a specific inhibitor of autolysin activity in pneumococcus. *Proc. natn. Acad. Sci. U.S.A.* **72:** 1690–1694.

ISHIGURO, E. E. (1978) Involvement of the *relA* gene product and feedback inhibition in the regulation of UDP-*N*-acetylmuramyl-peptide synthesis in *Escherichia coli*. *J. Bacteriol.* **135:** 766–774.

ISHIGURO, E. E. (1979) Regulation of peptidoglycan biosynthesis in *rel A*$^+$ and *rel A*$^-$ strains of *Escherichia coli* during diauxic growth on glucose and lactose. *Can. J. Microbiol.* **25:** 1206–1208.

ISHIGURO, E. E., MIRELMAN, D. and HARKNESS, R. F. (1980) Regulation of the terminal steps in peptidoglycan biosynthesis in ether-treated cells of *Escherichia coli*. *FEBS Lett.* **120:** 175–178.

ISHIGURO, E. E. and RAMEY, W. D. (1976) Stringent control of peptidoglycan biosynthesis in *Escherichia coli* K12. *J. Bacteriol.* **127:** 1119–1126.

ISHINO, F. and MATSUHASHI, M. (1981) Peptidoglycan synthetic enzyme activities of highly purified penicillin-binding protein 3 in *Escherichia coli*: a septum forming reaction sequence. *Biochem. biophys. Res. Commun.* **101:** 905–911.

ISHINO, F., MITSUI, K., TAMAKI, S. and MATSUHASHI, M. (1980) Dual enzyme-activities of cell wall peptidoglycan transglycosylase and penicillin-sensitive transpeptidase in purified preparations of *Escherichia coli* penicillin-binding protein 1A. *Biochem. biophys. Res. Commun.* **97:** 287–293.

ISHINO, F., TAMAKI S., SPRATT, B. G. and MATSUHASHI, M. (1982) A mecillinam-sensitive peptidoglycan cross-linking reaction in *Escherichia coli*. *Biochem. biophys. Res. Commun.* **109:** 689–696.

ITO, E. and STROMINGER, J. L. (1962) Enzymatic synthesis of the peptide in bacterial uridine nucleotides. II. Enzymatic synthesis and addition of D-alanyl-D-alanine. *J. biol. Chem.* **237:** 2696–2703.

ITO, E. and STROMINGER J. L. (1966) Enzymatic synthesis of the peptide in bacterial uridine nucleotides. III. Purification and properties of L-lysine adding enzyme. *J. biol. Chem.* **239:** 210–214.

ITO, E. and STROMINGER, J. L. (1973) Enzymatic synthesis of the peptide in bacterial uridine nucleotides. VII. Comparative biochemistry. *J. biol. Chem.* **248:** 3131–3136.

ITO, T., KODAMA, Y., KAWAMURA, K., SUZUKI, K., TAKATSUKI, A. and TAMURA, G. (1977) Structural elucidation of Tunicamycin. 1. Structure of tunicaminyl uracil a degradation product of tunicamycin. *Agric. Biol. Chem.* **41:** 2303–2305.

IWAYA, M., JONES, C. W., KORANA, J. and STROMINGER, J. L. (1978) Mapping of the mecillinam-resistant, round morphological mutants of *Escherichia coli*. *J. Bacteriol.* **133:** 196–202.

IWAYA, M. and STROMINGER, J. L. (1977) Simultaneous deletion of D-alanine carboxypeptidase 1B-C and penicillin-binding component IV in a mutant of *Escherichia coli* K12. *Proc. natn. Acad. Sci. U.S.A.* **74:** 2980–2984.

IZAKI, K., MATSUHASHI, M. and STROMINGER, J. L. (1966) Glycopeptide transpeptidase and D-alanine carboxy-peptidase: penicillin-sensitive enzymatic reactions. *Proc. natn. Acad. Sci. U.S.A.* **55:** 656–663.

IZAKI, K., MATSUHASHI, M. and STROMINGER, J. L. (1968) Biosynthesis of the peptidoglycan of bacterial cell walls XIII Peptidoglycan transpeptidase and D-alanine carboxypeptidase: Penicillin sensitive enzymatic reactions in strains of *Escherichia coli*. *J. biol. Chem.* **243:** 3180–3192.

JOHNSTON, L. S. and NEUHAUS, F. C. (1975) Initial membrane reaction in biosynthesis of peptidoglycan. Spin-labelled intermediates as receptors for vancomycin and ristocetin. *Biochemistry* **14:** 2754–2760.

KADNER R. J. and WINKLER, H. H. (1973) Isolation and characterization of mutations affecting the transport of hexose phosphate in *Escherichia coli*. *J. Bacteriol.* **113:** 895–900.

KAHAN, F. M., KAHAN, J. S., CASSIDY, P. J. and KROPP, H. (1974) The mechanisation of action of fosfomycin (phosphonomycin). *Ann. N.Y. Acad. Sci.* **235:** 364–386.

KALOMIRIS, E., BARDIN, C. and NEUHAUS, F. C. (1982) Biosynthesis of peptidoglycan in *Gaffkya homari*: reactivation of membranes by freeze-thawing in the presence and absence of walls. *J. Bacteriol.*, **150:** 535–544.

KAMIRYO, T. and MATSUHASHI, M. (1972) The biosynthesis of the cross-linking peptides in the cell wall peptidoglycan of *Staphylococcus aureus*. *J. biol. Chem.* **247:** 6306–6311.

KANEGASAKI, S. and WRIGHT, A. (1970) Mechanism of polymerization of the *Salmonella* O-antigen: utilization of lipid-linked intermediates. *Proc. natn. Acad. Sci. U.S.A.* **67:** 951–958.

KATZ, W., MATSUHASHI, M., DIETRICH, C. P. and STROMINGER, J. L. (1967) Biosynthesis of the peptidoglycan of bacterial cell walls IV. Incorporation of glycine in *Micrococcus lysodeikticus*. *J. biol. Chem.* **242:** 3207–3217.

KEENAN, M. V. and ALLEN, C. M. (1974) Characterization of undecaprenyl pyrophosphate synthetase from *Lactobacillus plantarum*. *Arch. biochem. Biophys.* **161:** 375–383.

KEGLEVIC, D., LADESIE, B., HADZIJA, O., TOMASIC, J., VALINGER, Z., POKOTNY, M. and NAUMSKI, R. (1974) Isolation and study of the composition of a peptidoglycan complex excreted by a biotin-requiring mutant of *Brevibacterium divaricatum* NRRL-2311 in the presence of penicillin. *Eur. J. Biochem.* **42:** 389–400.

KELLY, J. A., MOEWS, P. C., KNOX, J. R., FRERE, J. M. and GHUYSEN, J. M. (1982). Penicillin target enzyme and the antibiotic binding site. *Science* **218:** 479–481.

KOZARICH, J. W. and STROMINGER, J. L. (1978) A membrane enzyme from *Staphylococcus aureus* which catalyses transpeptidase, carboxypeptidase and penicillinase activities. *J. biol. Chem.* **253:** 1272–1278.

LAMBERT, M. P. and NEUHAUS, F. C. (1972) Mechanism of D-cycloserine action: alanine racemase from *E. coli* W. *J. Bacteriol.* **110:** 978–987.

LAWRENCE, P. J. and STROMINGER, J. L. (1970a) Biosynthesis of the peptidoglycan of bacterial cell walls XV. The binding of radioactive penicillin to the particulate enzyme preparation of *Bacillus subtilis* and its reversal with hydroxylamine or thiols. *J. biol. Chem.* **245:** 3653–3659.

LAWRENCE, P. J. and STROMINGER, J. L. (1970b) Biosynthesis of the peptidoglycan of bacterial cell walls XVI. The reversible fixation of radioactive penicillin G to the D-alanine carboxypeptidase of *Bacillus subtilis. J. biol. Chem.* **245:** 3660–3666.

LEAR, A. L. and PERKINS, H. R. (1983) Degrees of *O*-acetylation and cross-linking of the peptidoglycan of *Neisseria gonorrhoeae* during growth. *J. gen. Microbiol.,* **129:** 885–888.

LEDERBERG J. (1957) Mechanism of action of penicillin. *J. Bacteriol.* **73:** 144.

LEE, P. P., WEPPNER, W. A. and NEUHAUS, F. C. (1980) Initial membrane reaction in peptidoglycan synthesis. Perturbation of lipid-phospho-*N*-acetylmuramyl pentapeptide translocase interactions by n-butanol. *Biochem. biophys. Acta.* **597:** 603–613.

LINNETT, P. E., ROBERTS, R. J. and STROMINGER, J. L. (1974) Biosynthesis and cross-linking of the γ-glutamylglycine-containing peptidoglycan of vegetative cells of *Sporosarcina ureae. J. biol. Chem.* **249:** 2497–2506.

LUGTENBERG, E. J. J. and DE HAAN, P. G. (1971) A simple method for following the fate of alanine-containing components in murein synthesis in *Escherichia coli. Antonie van Leeuwenhoek J. Microbiol. Serol.* **37:** 537–552.

LUGTENBERG, E. J. J., DE HAAS-MENGER, L. and RUYTERS, W. H. M. (1972) Murein synthesis and identification of cell wall precursors of temperature-sensitive lysis mutants of *Escherichia coli. J. Bacteriol.* **109:** 326–335.

LUGTENBERG, E. J. J. and VAN SCHIJNDEL VAN DAM, A. (1972a). Temperature-sensitive mutants of *Escherichia coli* K-12 with low activities of the L-alanine adding enzyme and the D-alanyl-D-alanine adding enzyme. *J. Bacteriol.* **110:** 35–40.

LUGTENBERG E. J. J. and VAN SCHIJNDEL VAN DAM, A. (1972b) Temperature-sensitive mutants of *Escherichia coli* K-12 with low activity of the diaminopimelic acid adding enzyme. *J. Bacteriol.* **110:** 41–46.

LUGTENBERG, E. J. J. and VAN SCHIJNDEL VAN DAM, A. (1973) Temperature-sensitive mutant of *Escherichia coli* K-12 with impaired D-alanine: D-alanine ligase. *J. Bacteriol.* **113:** 96–104.

LUND, F. and TYBRING, L. (1972) 6β-Amidinopenicillanic acids—a new group of antibiotics. *Nature New Biol.* **236:** 135–137.

MAASS, D. and PELZER, H. (1981) Murein biosynthesis in ether permeabilized *Escherichia coli* starting from early peptidoglycan precursors. *Archs Microbiol.* **130:** 301–306.

MARKIEWICZ, Z., BROOME-SMITH, J. K., SCHWARZ, U. and SPRATT, B. G. (1982) Spherical *E. coli* due to elevated levels of D-alanine carboxypeptidase. *Nature, Lond.* **297:** 702–704.

MARTIN, H. H. (1964). Chemical composition of cell wall mucopolymer from penicillin spheroplasts and normal cells of *Proteus mirabilis. Abst. VI Internl. Cong. Biochem.* New York. VI: 70.

MARTIN, J. P., FLECK, J., MOCK, M. and GHUYSEN, J. M. (1973) The wall peptidoglycans of *Neisseria perflava, Moraxella glucidolytica, Pseudomonas alcaligenes* and *Proteus vulgaris* P18. *Eur. J. Biochem.* **38:** 301–306.

MARTIN, H. H. and GMEINER, J. (1979) Modification of peptidoglycan structure by penicillin action in cell walls of *Proteus mirabilis. Eur. J. Biochem.* **95:** 487–495.

MARTIN, H. H., TON-EHLERS, M. and SCHILF, W. (1980) Cooperation of benzylpenicillin and cefoxitin in bacterial growth inhibition. *Phil. Trans. R. Soc. Lond. B.* **289:** 365–367.

MARTINEZ-CARRION, M. and JENKINS, W. T. (1965) D-alanine-D-glutamate transaminase. 1. Purification and characterization. *J. biol. Chem.* **240:** 3538–3546.

MATSUHASHI, M., DIETRICH, C. P. and STROMINGER, J. L. (1967) Biosynthesis of the peptidoglycan of bacterial cell walls. III. The role of soluble ribonucleic acid and of lipid intermediates in glycine incorporation in *Staphylococcus aureus. J. biol. Chem.* **242:** 3191–3206.

MATSUHASHI, M., ISHINO, F., MAKAGAWA, J., MITSUI, K., NAKAJIMA-IIJIMA, S., TAMKI, S. and HASHIZUME, T. (1981) Enzymatic activities of penicillin-binding proteins of *Escherichia coli* and their sensitivities to β-lactam antibiotics. In: *β-Lactam Antibiotics—Mode of Action, New Developments and Future Prospects,* pp. 169–184 SALTON, M. J. R. and SHOCKMAN G. D. (eds), Academic Press.

MATSUHASHI, M., MARUYAMA, I. N., TAKAGAKI, Y., TAMAKI, S., NISHIMURA, Y. and HIROTA, Y. (1978) Isolation of a mutant of *Escherichia coli* lacking penicillin-sensitive D-alanine carboxypeptidase 1A. *Proc. natn. Acad. Sci. U.S.A.* **75:** 2631–2635.

MATSUHASHI, M., OHARA, I. and YOSHIYAMA, Y. (1970) Inhibition of bacterial cell wall synthesis *in vitro* by enduracidin, a new polypeptide antibiotic. *Progr. Antimicrob. Anticancer Chemother.* Proc. Int. Congr. Chemother. 6th 1969. Vol. 1. p. 226–229.

MATSUHASHI, M., TAKAGAKI, Y., MARUYAMA, I. N., TAMAKI, S., NISHIMURA, Y., SUZUKI, H., OGINO, U. and HIROTA, Y. (1977) Mutants of *Escherichia coli* lacking in highly penicillin-sensitive D-alanine carboxypeptidase activity. *Proc. natn. Acad. Sci. U.S.A.* **74:** 2976–2979.

MATSUHASHI, M., TAMAKI, S., CURTIS, S. J. and STROMINGER, J. L. (1979) Mutational evidence for identity of penicillin-binding protein 5 of *Escherichia coli* with the major D-alanine carboxypeptidase 1A activity. *J. Bacteriol.* **137:** 644–647.

MATSUZAWA, H., MATSUHASHI, M., OKA, A. and SUGINO, Y. (1969) Genetic and biochemical studies on cell wall peptidoglycan synthesis in *Escherichia coli* K-12. *Biochem. Biophys. Res. Commun.* **36:** 682–689.

McARTHUR, H. A. I. and REYNOLDS, P. E. (1980) Purification and properties of the D-alanyl-D-alanine carboxypeptidase of *Bacillus coagulans* NCIB 9635. *Biochem. biophys. Acta.* **612**, 107–118.

MESCHER, M. F. and STROMINGER, J. L. (1976) Bacitracin induces sphere formation in Halobacterium species which lack a wall peptidoglycan. *J. gen. Microbiol.* **89**: 375–378.

METT, H., BRACHA, R. and MIRELMAN, D. (1980) Soluble nascent peptidoglycan in growing *Escherichia coli* cells. *J. biol. Chem.* **255**: 9584–9890.

MIRELMAN, D. (1979) Biosynthesis and assembly of cell wall peptidoglycan. In: *Bacterial Outer Membranes*, pp. 115–166, INOUYE, M. (ed.), John Wiley and Sons, New York.

MIRELMAN, D. and BRACHA, R. (1974) Effect of penicillin on the *in vivo* formation of the D-alanyl-L-alanine peptide cross-linkage in cell walls of *Micrococcus luteus*. *Antimicrob. Ag. Chemother.* **5**: 663–666.

MIRELMAN, D., BRACHA, R. and SHARON, N. (1972) Role of the penicillin-sensitive transpeptidation reaction in attachment of newly-synthesized peptidoglycan to cell walls of *Micrococcus luteus*. *Proc. natn. Acad. Sci. U.S.A.* **69**: 3355–3359.

MIRELMAN, D., BRACHA, R. and SHARON, N. (1974) Penicillin-induced secretion of a soluble, uncross-linked peptidoglycan by *Micrococcus luteus* cells. *Biochemistry* **13**: 5045–5053.

MIRELMAN, D. and NUCHAMOWITZ, Y. (1979a) Biosynthesis of peptidoglycan in *Pseudomonas aeruginosa*. 1. The incorporation of peptidoglycan into the cell wall. *Eur. J. Biochem.* **94**: 541–548.

MIRELMAN, D. and NUCHAMOWITZ, Y. (1979b) Biosynthesis of peptidoglycan in *Pseudomonas aeruginosa*. 2. Mode of action of β-lactam antibiotics. *Eur. J. Biochem.* **94**: 549–556.

MIRELMAN, D. and SHARON, N. (1972) Biosynthesis of peptidoglycan by a cell wall preparation of *Staphylococcus aureus* and its inhibition by penicillin. *Biochem. biophys. Res. Commun.* **46**: 1909–1917.

MIRELMAN, D., YASHOUV-GAN, Y. and SCHWARZ, U. (1976) Peptidoglycan biosynthesis in a thermosensitive division mutant of *Escherichia coli*. *Biochemistry* **15**: 1781–1790.

MIRELMAN, D., YASHOUV-GAN, Y. and SCHWARZ, U. (1977) Regulation of murein biosynthesis and septum formation in filamentous cells of *Escherichia coli* PAT 84. *J. Bacteriol.* **129**: 1593–1600.

MIYAKAWA, T., MATSUZAWA, H., MATSUHASHI, M. and SUGINO, Y. (1972) Cell wall peptidoglycan mutants of *Escherichia coli* K-12: Existence of two clusters of genes *mra* and *mrb*, for cell wall peptidoglycan biosynthesis. *J. Bacteriol.* **112**: 950–958.

MOORE, B. A., JEVONS, S. and BRAMMER, K. W. (1979) Peptidoglycan transpeptidase inhibition in *Pseudomonas aeruginosa* and *Escherichia coli* by penicillins and cephalosporins. *Antimicrob. Ag. Chemother.* **15**: 513–517.

NAKAGAWA, J. and MATSUHASHI, M. (1980) Fragmentation of penicillin-binding protein—1Bs of *Escherichia coli* by proteolytic enzymes—a preliminary study in the location of the penicillin-binding site on the bifunctional peptidoglycan synthetase protein. *Agric. Biol. Chem.* **44**: 3041–3044.

NAKAGAWA, J. and MATSUHASHI, M. (1982) Molecular divergence of a major peptidoglycan synthetase with transpeptidase activities in *Escherichia coli* penicillin-binding proteins 1Bs. *Biochem. biophys. Res. Commun.* **105**: 1546–1553.

NAKAGAWA, J., TAMAKI, S. and MATSUHASHI, M. (1979) Purified penicillin-binding proteins 1Bs from *Escherichia coli* membrane showing activities of both peptidoglycan polymerase and peptidoglycan cross-linking enzyme. *Agric. Biol. Chem.* **43**: 1379–1380.

NEUHAUS, F. C. (1962a) The enzymatic synthesis of D-alanyl-D-alanine. I. Purification and properties of D-alanyl-D-alanine synthetase. *J. biol. Chem.* **237**: 778–786.

NEUHAUS, F. C. (1962b) The enzymatic synthesis of D-alanyl-D-alanine. II. Kinetic studies on D-alanyl-D-alanine synthetase. *J. biol. Chem.* **237**: 3128–3135.

NEUHAUS, F. C. (1972) Initial translocation reaction in the biosynthesis of peptidoglycan by bacterial membranes. *Acc. chem. Res.* **4**: 297–303.

NEUHAUS, F. C. and HAMMES, W. P. (1981) Inhibition of cell wall biosynthesis by analogues of alanine. *Pharmac. Ther.* **14**: 265–320.

NEUHAUS, F. C. and LYNCH, J. L. (1964) The enzymatic synthesis of D-alanyl-D-alanine III. On the inhibition of D-alanyl-D-alanine synthetase by the antibiotic D-cycloserine. *Biochemistry*, **3**: 471–480.

NIKAIDO, H. (1979) Nonspecific transport through the outer membrane. In: *Bacterial Outer Membranes*, pp. 361–407, INOUYE, M. (ed.), John Wiley and Sons, New York.

PARK, J. T. (1952a) Uridine-5'-pyrophosphate derivatives. I. Isolation from *Staphylococcus aureus*. *J. biol. Chem.* **194**: 877–884.

PARK, J. T. (1952b) Uridine-5'-pyrophosphate derivatives. II. A structure common to three derivatives. *J. biol. Chem.* **194**: 885–895.

PARK, J. T. (1952c) Uridine-5'-pyrophosphate derivatives. III. Amino acid-containing derivatives. *J. biol. Chem.* **194**: 897–904.

PELLON, G., BORDET, C. and MICHEL, G. (1976) Peptidoglycan synthesized by a membrane-preparation of *Micrococcus luteus*. *J. Bacteriol.* **125**: 509–517.

PERKINS, H. R. (1982) Vancomycin and related antibiotics. *Pharmac. Ther.* **16**: 181–197.

PETIT, J. F., STROMINGER, J. L. and SOLL, D. (1968) Biosynthesis of the peptidoglycan in bacterial cell walls. VII. Incorporation of serine and glycine into interpeptide bridges in *Staphylococcus epidermidis*. *J. biol. Chem.* **243**: 757–767.

PLAPP, R. and STROMINGER, J. L. (1970a) Biosynthesis of the peptidoglycan of bacterial cell walls. XVII. Biosynthesis of peptidoglycan and of inter-peptide bridges in *Lactobacillus viridescens*. *J. biol. Chem.* **245**: 3667–3674.

PLAPP, R. and STROMINGER, J. L. (1970b) Biosynthesis of the peptidoglycan of bacterial cell walls. XVIII. Purification and properties of L-alanyl transfer ribonucleic acid—Uridine diphosphate-*N*-acetylmuramyl-pentapeptide transferase from *Lactobacillus viridescens*. *J. biol. Chem.* **245**: 3675–3682.

PLESS, D. D. and NEUHAUS, F. C. (1973) Initial membrane reaction in peptidoglycan synthesis. Lipid dependence of phospho-*N*-acetylmuramyl-pentapeptide translocase (exchange reaction). *J. biol. Chem.* **248**: 1568–1576.

RAMEY, W. D. and ISHIGURO, E. E. (1978) Site of inhibition of peptidoglycan biosynthesis during the stringent response in *Escherichia coli*. *J. Bacteriol.* **135**: 71–77.

REISINGER P., SEIDL, H., TSCHESCHE, H. and HAMMES, W. P. (1980) The effect of nisin on murein synthesis. *Archs Microbiol.* **127**: 187–193.

REUSCH, V. V. and PANOS, C. (1976) Defective synthesis of lipid intermediates for peptidoglycan formation in a stabilized L-form of *Streptococcus pyogenes*. *J. Bacteriol.* **126**: 300–311.

REYNOLDS, P. E. (1971) Peptidoglycan synthesis in bacilli. II. Characteristics of protoplast membrane preparations. *Biochem. biophys. Acta.* **237**: 255–272.

REYNOLDS, P. E., SHEPHERD, S. T. and CHASE, H. A. (1978) Identification of the binding protein which may be the target of penicillin action in *Bacillus megaterium*. *Nature, Lond.* **271**: 568–570.

ROBBINS, P. W., BRAY, D., DANKERT, M. and WRIGHT, A. (1967) Direction of chain growth in polysaccharide synthesis. *Science* **158**: 1536–1542.

ROBERTS, R. J. (1972) Structures of two glycyl-tRNAs from *Staphylococcus epidermidis*. *Nature New Biol.* **237**: 44–45.

ROBERTS, W. S. L., PETIT, J. F. and STROMINGER, J. L. (1968b) Biosynthesis of the peptidoglycan of bacterial cell walls. VIII. Specificity in the utilization of L-alanyl transfer ribonucleic acid for interpeptide bridge synthesis in *Arthrobacter crystallopoietes*. *J. biol. Chem.* **243**: 768–772.

ROBERTS, W. S. L., STROMINGER, J. L. and SOLL, D. (1968a) Biosynthesis of the peptidoglycan of bacterial cell walls. VI. Incorporation of L-threonine into interpeptide bridges in *Micrococcus roseus*. *J. biol. Chem.* **243**: 749–756.

ROGERS, H. J. (1979) The function of bacterial autolysins. In: *Microbial Polysaccharides and Polysaccharases*, pp. 237–268, BERKELEY, R. C. W., GOODAY, G. W. and ELLWOOD, D. C. (eds), Academic Press.

ROGERS, H. J., PERKINS, H. R. and WARD, J. B. (1980) *Microbial Cell Walls and Membranes*, pp. 564, Chapman and Hall, London.

ROSENTHAL, R. S., JUNGKIND, D., DANEO-MOORE, L. and SHOCKMAN, G. D. (1975) Evidence for the synthesis of soluble peptidoglycan fragments by protoplasts of *Streptococcus faecalis*. *J. Bacteriol.* **124**: 398–409.

ROSENTHAL, R. S. and SHOCKMAN, G. D. (1975a) Characterization of the presumed cross-links in the soluble peptidoglycan fragments synthesised by protoplasts of *Streptococcus faecalis*. *J. Bacteriol.* **124**: 410–418.

ROSENTHAL, R. S. and SHOCKMAN, G. D. (1975b) Synthesis of peptidoglycan in the form of soluble glycan chains by growing protoplasts (autoplasts) of *Streptococcus faecalis*. *J. Bacteriol.* **124**: 419–423.

ROUSSET, A., NGUYEN-DISTECHE, M., MINCK, R. and GHUYSEN, J. M. (1982) Penicillin binding proteins and carboxypeptidase/transpeptidase activities in *Proteus vulgaris* P18 and its penicillin-induced stable L-form. *J. Bacteriol.* **152**: 1042–1048.

SANDERMANN, H. (1976a) A possible correlation between lipid hydration and lipid activation of the C_{55}-isoprenoid alcohol phosphokinase apoprotein. *Eur. J. Biochem.* **62**: 479–484.

SANDERMANN, H. (1976b) Interfacial regulation: influence of lipid polar group confirmation on lipid activation of C_{55}-isoprenoid alcohol phosphokinase apoprotein. *FEBS Lett.* **63**: 59–61.

SANDERMANN, H. and STROMINGER, J. L. (1972) Purification and properties of C_{55}-isoprenoid alcohol phosphokinase from *Staphylococcus aureus*. *J. biol. Chem.* **247**: 5123–5131.

SCHER, M., LENNARZ, W. J. and SWEELEY, C. C. (1968) The biosynthesis of mannosyl-l-phosphoryl-polyisoprenol in *Micrococcus lysodeikticus* and its role in mannan synthesis. *Proc. natn. Acad. Sci. U.S.A.* **59**: 1313–1320.

SCHLEIFER, K. H., HAMMES, W. P. and KANDLER, O. (1976) Effect of endogenous and exogenous factors on the primary structures of bacterial peptidoglycan. *Adv. Microbiol. Physiol.* **13**: 245–292.

SCHLEIFER, K. H., HUSS, L. and KANDLER, O. (1969) Effect of nutrition on amino acid sequence of serine containing murein of *Staphylococcus epidermidis* strain-24. *Arch. Mikrobiol.* **68**: 387.

SCHLEIFER, K. H. and KANDLER, O. (1972) Peptidoglycan types of bacterial cell walls and their taxonomic implications. *Bacteriol Rev.* **36**: 407–477.

SCHLIF, W. and MARTIN, H. H. (1980) Purification of two DD-carboxypeptidases/transpeptidases with different penicillin sensitivities from *Proteus mirabilus*. *Eur. J. Biochem.* **105**: 361–370.

SCHMELZER, E., WECKESSER, J., WARTH, R. and MAYER, H. (1982) Peptidoglycan of *Rhodopseudomonas viridis*: partial lack of N-acetyl substitution of glucosamine. *J. Bacteriol.* **149**: 151–155.

SCHRADER, W. P. and FAN, D. P. (1974) Synthesis of cross-linked peptidoglycan attached to previously formed cell wall by toluene-treated cells of *Bacillus megaterium*. *J. biol. Chem.* **249**: 4815–4818.

SCHWARZ, U., ASMUS, A. and FRANK, H. (1969). Autolytic enzymes and cell division of *Escherichia coli*. *J. molec. Biol.* **41**: 419–429.

SCUDAMORE, R. A. and GOLDNER, M. (1982) Limited contribution of the outermembrane penetration barrier towards intrinsic antibiotic resistance in *Pseudomonas aeruginosa*. *Can. J. Microbiol.* **28**: 169–175.

SHARPE, A., BLUMBERG, P. M. and STROMINGER, J. L. (1974) D-alanine carboxypeptidase and cell wall cross-linking in *Bacillus subtilis*. *J. Bacteriol.* **117**: 926–927.

SHEPHERD, S. T., CHASE, H. A. and REYNOLDS, P. E. (1977) The separation and properties of two penicillin-binding proteins from *Salmonella typhimurium*. *Eur. J. Biochem.* **78**: 521–532.

SIEWERT, G. and STROMINGER, J. L. (1967) Bacitracin: an inhibitor of the dephosphorylation of lipid pyrophosphate, an intermediate in biosynthesis of the peptidoglycan of bacterial cell walls. *Proc. natn. Acad. Sci. U.S.A.* **57**: 767–773.

SOMMA, S., MERATI, W. and PARENTI, F. (1977) Gardimycin, a new antibiotic inhibiting peptidoglycan synthesis. *Antimicrob. Ag. Chemother.* **11**: 396–401.

SOPER, T. S. and MANNING, J. M. (1981) Different modes of action of inhibitors of bacterial D-amino acid transaminase. *J. biol. Chem.* **256**: 4263–4268.

SOPER, T. S. and MANNING, J. M. (1982) Inactivation of pyridoxal phosphate enzymes by gabaculine. *J. biol. Chem.* **257**: 13930–13936.

SPRATT, B. G. (1975) Distinct penicillin binding proteins involved in the division, elongation and shape of *Escherichia coli* K12. *Proc. natn. Acad. Sci. U.S.A.* **72**: 2999–3003.

SPRATT, B. G. (1977a) Properties of the penicillin-binding proteins of *Escherichia coli* K12. *Eur. J. Biochem.* **72**: 341–352.

SPRATT, B. G. (1977b) Comparison of the binding properties of two 6-β-amidinopenicillanic acid derivatives that differ in the physiological effects in *Escherichia coli*. *Antimicrob. Ag. Chemother.* **11:** 161–166.

SPRATT, B. G. (1977c). Penicillin binding proteins of *Escherichia coli*: general properties and characterization of mutants. In: *Microbiology—1977*, pp. 182–190, SCHLESSINGER, D. (ed.), American Society for Microbiology, Washington, U.S.A.

SPRATT, B. G. (1980) Biochemical and genetical approaches to the mechanism of action of penicillin. *Phil. Trans. R. Soc. Lond. B.* **289:** 273–283.

SPRATT, B. G., JOBANPUTRA, V. and SCHWARZ, U. (1977a) Mutants of *Escherichia coli* which lack a component of penicillin-binding protein 1 are viable. *FEBS Lett.* **79:** 374–378.

SPRATT, B. G., JOBANPUTRA, V. and ZIMMERMANN, W. (1977b) Binding of thienamycin and clavulanic acid to the penicillin-binding proteins of *Escherichia coli* K12. *Antimicrob. Ag. Chemother.* **12:** 406–409.

STAUDENBAUER, W. and STROMINGER, J. L. (1972) Activation of D-aspartic acid for incorporation into peptidoglycan. *J. biol. Chem.* **247:** 5095–5102.

STICKGOLD, R. A. and NEUHAUS, F. C. (1967) On the initial stage in peptidoglycan synthesis. Effect of 5-fluorouracil substitution on phospho-N-acetylmuramyl-pentapeptide translocase (uridine-5'-phosphate). *J. biol. Chem.* **242:** 1331–1337.

SUGINAKA, H., SHIMATINI, M., OGAWA, M. and KOTANI, S. (1979) Prevention of penicillin-induced lysis of *Staphylococcus aureus* by cellular lipoteichoic acid. *J. Antibiot.* **32:** 73–77.

SUTHERLAND, I. W. (1977) Bacterial exopolysaccharides—their nature and production. In: *Surface Carbohydrates of the Prokaryotic Cell*, pp. 27–96, SUTHERLAND, I. W. (ed.), Academic Press, London and New York.

SUZUKI, H., NISHIMURA, Y. and HIROTA, Y. (1978) On the process of cellular division in *Escherichia coli*: a series of mutants of *E. coli* altered in the penicillin-binding proteins. *Proc. natn. Acad. Sci. U.S.A.* **75:** 664–668.

SUZUKI, H., VAN HEIJENOORT, Y., TAMURA, T., MIZOGUCHI, J., HIROTA, Y. and VAN HEIJENOORT, J. (1980) *In vitro* peptidoglycan polymerization catalysed by penicillin-binding protein 1b of *Escherichia coli* K-12. *FEBS Lett.* **110:** 245–249.

TAKATSUKI, A., KAWAMURA, K., OKINA, M., KODAMA, Y., ITO, T. and TAMURA, G. (1977) Structural elucidation of tumicamycin. *Agric. Biol. Chem.* **41:** 2307–2309.

TAKU, A. and FAN, D. P. (1976a) Purification and properties of a protein factor stimulating peptidoglycan synthesis in toluene and LiCl-treated *Bacillus megaterium* cells. *J. biol. Chem.* **251:** 1889–1895.

TAKU, A. and FAN, D. P. (1976b) Identification of an isolated protein essential for peptidoglycan synthesis as the N-acetylglucosaminyltransferase. *J. biol. Chem.* **251:** 6154–6156.

TAKU, A. and FAN, D. P. (1979) Dissociation and reconstitution of membranes synthesizing the peptidoglycan of *Bacillus megaterium*. A protein factor for the polymerization step. *J. biol. Chem.* **254:** 3991–3999.

TAKU, A., GARDNER, H. L. and FAN, D. P. (1975) Reconstitution of cell wall synthesis in toluene- and LiCl-treated *Bacillus megaterium* cells by addition of a soluble protein extract. *J. biol. Chem.* **250:** 3375–3380.

TAKU, A., GUNETILIKE, K. G. and ANWAR, R. A. (1970) Biosynthesis of uridine diphospho-N-acetylmuramic acid. III. Purification and properties of uridine-diphospho-N-acetylenolpyruvyl-glucosamine reductase. *J. biol. Chem.* **245:** 5012–5016.

TAKU, A., STUCKEY, M. and FAN, D. P. (1982) Purification of the peptidoglycan transglycosylase of *Bacilllus megaterium*. *J. biol. Chem.* **257:** 5018–5022.

TAMAKI, S., NAKAJIMA, S. and MATSUHASHI, M. (1977) Thermosensitive mutation in *Escherichia coli* simultaneously causing defects in penicillin-binding protein 1-Bs and in enzyme activity for peptidoglycan synthesis *in vitro*. *Proc. natn. Acad. Sci. U.S.A.* **74:** 5472–5476.

TAMURA, G., SASAKI, T., MATSUHASHI, M., TAKATSUKI, A. and YAMASAKI, M. (1976) Tunicamycin inhibits formation of lipid intermediate in cell-free peptidoglycan synthesis of bacteria. *Agric. Biol. Chem.* **40:** 447–449.

TAMURA, T., IMAE, Y. and STROMINGER, J. L. (1976) Purification to homogeneity and properties of two D-alanine carboxypeptidases I from *Escherichia coli*. *J. biol. Chem.* **251:** 414–423.

TANAKA, H., OIWA, R., MATSUKURA, S. and OMURA, S. (1978) Amphomycin inhibits phospho-N-acetylmuramoyl-pentapeptide translocase in peptidoglycan synthesis of Bacillus. *Biochem. biophys Res. Commun.* **86:** 902–908.

THORNDIKE, J. and PARK, J. T. (1969) A method for demonstrating the stepwise addition of glycine from transfer RNA into the murein precursor of *Staphylococcus aureus*. *Biochem. biophys. Res. Commun.* **35:** 642–647.

THORNE, K. J. I. and KODICEK, E. (1966) The structure of bactoprenol, a lipid formed by lactobacilli from mevalonic acid. *Biochem. J.* **99:** 123–127.

THORPE, S. J. and PERKINS, H. R. (1979) Deoxycholate enhancement of an intermediate of peptidoglycan synthesis in *Micrococcus luteus*. *FEBS Lett.* **105:** 151–154.

TIPPER, D. J. (1969) Studies on the cell wall peptidoglycans of *Staphylococcus epidermidis* Texas 26 and *Staphylococcus aureus* Copenhagen. II. Structure of neutral and basic peptides from hydrolysis with *Myxobacter* AL-1 peptide. *Biochemistry* **8:** 2192–2202.

TIPPER, D. J. and BERMAN, M. F. (1969) Structures of the cell wall peptidoglycan of *Staphylococcus epidermidis* Texas 26 and *Staphylococcus aureus* Copenhagen. Chain length and average sequence of cross-bridge peptides. *Biochemistry*, **8:** 2183–2192.

TIPPER, D. J., GHUYSEN, J. M. and STROMINGER, J. L. (1965) Structure of the cell wall of *Staphylococcus aureus* strain Copenhagen. III. Further studies of the disaccharides. *Biochemistry* **4:** 468–473.

TIPPER, D. J., KATZ, W., STROMINGER, J. L. and GHUYSEN, J. M. (1967) Substituents in the α-carboxyl group of D-glutamic acid in the peptidoglycan of several bacterial cell walls. *Biochemistry* **6:** 921–929.

TIPPER, D. J. and STROMINGER, J. L. (1965) Mechanism of action of penicillins: a proposal based on their structural similarity to acyl-D-alanyl-D-alanine. *Proc. natn. Acad. Sci. U.S.A.* **54:** 1133–1141.

TIPPER, D. J. and STROMINGER, J. L. (1967) Isolation of 4-O-β-N-O-acetylmuramyl-N-acetylglucosamine and 4-O-β-N, 6-O-diacetylmuramyl-N-acetylglucosamine and the structure of the cell wall polysaccharide of *Staphylococcus aureus*. *Biochem. biophys. Res. Commun.* **22:** 48–56.

TIPPER, D. J. and STROMINGER, J. L. (1968) Biosynthesis of the peptidoglycan of bacterial cell walls. XII.

Inhibition of cross-linking by penicillins and cephalosporins: studies in *Staphylococcus aureus in vivo*. *J. biol. Chem.* **243**: 3169–3179.

TIPPER, D. J. and WRIGHT, A. (1980) The structure and biosynthesis of bacterial cell walls. In: *The Bacteria*, Vol. 7, pp. 291–426, SOKATCH, J. R. and ORNSTON, L. N. (eds), Academic Press, New York and London.

TKACZ, J. S. (1981). Tunicamycin and related antibiotics. In: *Antibiotics VI Modes and Mechanisms of Microbial Growth Inhibitors*, pp. 255–278, HAHN, F. E. (ed.), Springer-Verlag.

TOMIOKA, S., ISHINO, F., TAMAKI, S. AND MATSUHASHI, M. (1982) Formation of hyper-cross-linked peptidoglycan with multiple cross-linkages by a pencillin-binding protein, 1A, of *Escherichia coli*. *Biochem. biophys. Res. Commun.* **106**: 1175–1182.

TOSCANO, W. H. and STORM, D. R. (1982) Bacitracin. *Pharmac. Ther.* **16**: 199–210.

TROY, F. A., VIJAY, I. K. and TESCHE, N. (1975) Role of undecaprenyl phosphate in synthesis of polymers containing sialic acid in *Escherichia coli*. *J. biol. Chem.* **250**: 156–163.

TYNECKA, Z. and WARD, J. B. (1975) Peptidoglycan synthesis in *Bacillus licheniformis*. The inhibition of cross-linking by benzylpenicillin and cephaloridine *in vivo* accompanied by the formation of soluble peptidoglycan. *Biochem. J.* **146**: 253–267.

UMBREIT, J. M. and STROMINGER, J. L. (1972) Isolation of polyisoprenyl alcohols from *Streptococcus faecalis*. *J. Bacteriol.* **112**: 1306–1309.

UMBREIT, J. N. and STROMINGER, J. L. (1973) D-alanine carboxypeptidase from *Bacillus subtilis* membranes. I. Purification and characterization. *J. biol. Chem.* **248**: 6759–6766.

VANDERWEL, D. and ISHIGURO, E. E. (1982) Regulation of peptidoglycan biosynthesis in *Escherichia coli* during growth temperature up-shift. *FEMS Microbiology Lett.* **13**: 43–46.

VALINGER, Z., KEGLERIC, D., WRISCHER, M. and NAUMSKI, R. (1982) *Brevibacterium divaricatum*: influence of nutritional conditions on the wall composition and release of uncross-linked peptidoglycan chains into medium. *Arch. Microbiol.* **132**: 280–284.

VAN HEIJENOORT, Y., DERRIEN, M. and VAN HEIJENOORT, J. (1978) Polymerization by transglycosylation in the biosynthesis of the peptidoglycan of *Escherichia coli* K-12 and its inhibition by antibiotics. *FEBS Lett.* **89**: 141–144.

VAN HEIJENOORT, Y. and VAN HEIJENOORT, J. (1980) Biosynthesis of the peptidoglycan of *Escherichia coli* K-12. Properties of the *in vitro* polymerization by transglycosylation. *FEBS Lett.* **110**: 241–244.

VENKATESWARAN, P. S. and WU, H. C. (1972) Isolation and characterization of a phosphonomycin-resistant mutant of *Escherichia coli* K-12. *J. Bacteriol.* **110**: 935–944.

VERWER, R. W. H., BEACHEY, E. H., KECK, W., STOHB, A. M. and POLERMANS J. E. (1980). Oriented fragmentation of *Escherichia coli* sacculi by sonication. *J. Bacteriol.* **141**: 327–332.

VERWER, R. W. H., NANNINGA, N., KECK, W. and SCHWARZ, U. (1978) Arrangement of glycan chains in the sacculus of *Escherichia coli*. *J. Bacteriol.* **136**: 723–729.

WAECHTER, C. J. and LENNARZ, W. J. (1976) The role of polyprenol-linked sugars in glycoprotein synthesis. *A. Rev. Biochem.* **196**: 95–112.

WANG, E. and WALSH, C. (1978) Suicide substrates for the alanine racemase of *Escherichia coli*. *Biochemistry*. **17**: 1313–1321.

WARD, J. B. (1973) The chain length of the glycans in bacterial cell walls. *Biochem. J.* **133**: 395–398.

WARD, J. B. (1974) The synthesis of peptidoglycan in an autolysin-deficient mutant of *Bacillus licheniformis* NCTC 6346 and the effect of β-lactam antibiotics, bacitracin and vancomycin. *Biochem. J.* **141**: 227–241.

WARD, J. B. (1975) Peptidoglycan synthesis in L-phase variants of *Bacillus licheniformis* and *Bacillus subtilis*. *J. Bacteriol.* **124**: 668–678.

WARD, J. B. (1977) Tunicamycin inhibition of bacterial wall polymer synthesis. *FEBS Lett.* **78**: 151–154.

WARD, J. B. (1981) Teichoic and teichuronic acids: biosynthesis assembly and location. *Microbiol. Rev.* **45**: 211–243.

WARD, J. B. and CURTIS, C. A. M. (1982) The biosynthesis and linkage of teichuronic acid to peptidoglycan in *Bacillus licheniformis*. *Eur. J. Biochem.* **122**: 125–132.

WARD, J. B. and PERKINS, H. R. (1973) The direction of glycan synthesis in a bacterial peptidoglycan. *Biochem. J.* **135**: 721–728.

WARD, J. B. and PERKINS, H. R. (1974) Peptidoglycan biosynthesis by preparations from *Bacillus licheniformis*: cross-linking of newly synthesized chains to preformed wall. *Biochem. J.* **139**: 781–784.

WAXMAN, D. J., YU, W. and STROMINGER, J. L. (1980) Linear uncross-linked peptidoglycan secreted by penicillin-treated *Bacillus subtilis*. *J. biol. Chem.* **255**: 11577–11587.

WEIDEL, W. and PELZER, H. (1964) Bag-shaped macromolecules—a new outlook on bacterial cell walls. *Adv. Enzymol.* **26**: 193–232.

WEPPNER, W. A. and NEUHAUS, F. C. (1978) Biosynthesis of peptidoglycan. Definition of the microenvironment of undecaprenyl diphosphate-*N*-acetylmuramyl-(5-dimethylaminonaphthalene-1-sulfonyl) pentapeptide by fluorescence spectroscopy. *J. biol. Chem.* **253**: 472–478.

WEPPNER, W. A. and NEUHAUS, F. C. (1979) Initial membrane reaction in peptidoglycan synthesis. Interaction of lipid with phospho-*N*-acetylmuramyl-pentapeptide translocase. *Biochem. biophys. Acta* **552**: 418–427.

WESTMACOTT, D. and PERKINS, H. R. (1979) Effects of lysozyme on *Bacillus cereus* 569: Rupture of chains of bacteria and enhancement of sensitivity to autolysins. *J. gen. Microbiol.* **115**: 1–11.

WESTON, A., WARD, J. B. and PERKINS, H. R. (1977) Biosynthesis of peptidoglycan in wall plus membrane preparations from *Micrococcus luteus*: direction of chain-extension, length of chains and effect of penicillin on cross-linking. *J. gen. Microbiol.* **99**: 171–181.

WICKUS, G. G. and STOMINGER, J. L. (1972) Penicillin-sensitive transpeptidation during peptidoglycan biosynthesis in cell-free preparations from *Bacillus megaterium*. I. Incorporation of free diaminopimelic acid into peptidoglycan. *J. biol. Chem.* **247**: 5297–5306.

WICKUS, G. G. and STROMINGER, J. L. (1973) Partial purification and properties of the pyruvate-uridine diphospho-*N*-acetylglucosamine transferase from *Staphylococcus epidermidis*. *J. Bacteriol.* **113**: 287–290.

WICKUS, G. G. and STROMINGER, J. L. (1974) Penicillin-sensitive transpeptidation during peptidoglycan biosynthesis in cell-free preparations from *Bacillus megaterium*. II. Effect of penicillins and cephalosporins on bacterial growth and *in vitro* transpeptidase. *J. biol. Chem.* **247**: 5307–5311.

WICKUS, G. G., RUBENSTEIN, P. A., WARTH, A. D. and STROMINGER, J. L. (1973) Partial purification and some properties of the uridine diphospho-*N*-acetylglucosamine-enolpuruvate reductase from *Staphylococcus epidermidis*. *J. Bacteriol.* **113**: 291–295.

WIJSMAN, H. J. W. (1972a) A genetic map of several mutations affecting the mucopeptide layer of *Escherichia coli*. *Genet. Res. Camb.* **20**: 65–74.

WIJSMAN, H. J. W. (1972b) The characterization of an alanine racemase mutant of *Escherichia coli*. *Genet. Res. Camb.* **20**: 269–277.

WILLIAMSON, R. and WARD, J. B. (1982) Benzylpenicillin-induced filament formation of *Clostridium perfringens*. *J. gen. Microbiol.* **128**: 3025–3035.

WILLOUGHBY, E., HIGASHI, Y., and STROMINGER, J. L. (1972) Isolation of C_{55}-isoprenylpyrophosphate from *Micrococcus lysodeikticus*. *J. biol. Chem.* **247**: 5113–5115.

WISE, E. M. and PARK, J. T. (1965) Penicillin: its basic site of action as an inhibitor of a peptide cross-linking reaction in cell wall mucopeptide synthesis. *Proc. natn. Acad. Sci. U.S.A.* **54**: 75–81.

WRIGHT, A., DANKERT, M., FENNESSEY, P. and ROBBINS, P. W. (1967) Characterization of a polyisoprenoid compound functional in O-antigen biosynthesis. *Proc. natn. Acad. Sci. U.S.A.* **57**: 1798–1803.

WU, H. C. and VENKATESWARAN, P. S. (1974) Fosfomycin-resistant mutant of *Escherichia coli*. *Ann. N.Y. Acad. Sci.* **235**: 587–592.

WYKE, A. W., WARD, J. B., HAYES, M. V. and CURTIS, N. A. C. (1981) A role *in vivo* for penicillin binding protein-4 of *Staphylococcus aureus*. *Eur. J. Biochem.* **119**: 389–393.

YAMASAKI, M., TAKATSUKI, A. and TAMURA, G. (1982) Tunicamycin in Microbiology. In: *Tunicamycin*, pp. 73–96, TAMURA, G. (ed.), Japan Societies Press, Tokyo.

YOCUM, R. R., BLUMBERG, P. M. and STROMINGER, J. L. (1974) Purification and characterization of the thermophilic D-alanine carboxypeptidase from membranes of *Bacillus stearothermophilus*. *J. biol. Chem.* **249**: 4863–4871.

ZEMELL, R. I. and ANWAR, R. A. (1975) Pyruvate-Uridine diphospho-*N*-acetylglucosamine transferase. Purification to homogeneity and feedback inhibition. *J. biol. Chem.* **250**: 3185–3192.

CHAPTER 2

INHIBITION OF CELL WALL BIOSYNTHESIS BY ANALOGUES OF ALANINE

Francis C. Neuhaus* and Walter P. Hammes†

*Department of Biochemistry and Molecular Biology, Northwestern University,
Evanston, IL 60201, U.S.A.
†Universität Hohenheim, 7000 Stuttgart 70, Federal Republic of Germany

1. INTRODUCTION

Many antibacterial agents owe their selective toxicity to the fact that their targets are structures which are only present in the sensitive bacterium. One of these structures is peptidoglycan. This cell wall polymer plays a vital role in protecting the bacterium from lysis in a hypotonic environment. A number of antibacterial agents, e.g. β-lactams, nisin, vancomycin, bacitracin, and moenomycin, interfere with the assembly of this peptidoglycan by inhibiting enzymic reactions involved in the final stages of assembly. This polymer contains a number of unique constituents that have also become the focus of research in chemotherapy. In 1958 Park suggested that these constituents, muramic acid, D-alanine and D-glutamic acid, offer the chemist an opportunity to design antimetabolites that interfere with the synthesis of this cell wall polymer. The discovery of the D-alanine analogues, D-cycloserine and O-carbamoyl-D-serine, provided examples of agents that interfere with the incorporation of D-alanine into the wall (Neuhaus, 1967). In recent years, the successes with fluoro-D-alanine by the Merck group, chloro-D-alanine by Manning and his coworkers, and alafosfalin by the Roche group have stimulated renewed interest in the search for analogues of alanine that inhibit the synthesis of functional peptidoglycan.

In our laboratories, we are concerned with defining new targets which can be used with alanine analogues to control the final stages of cell wall assembly. It is our goal to direct analogues, either as inhibitors or as replacements, against specific targets for the selective inhibition of peptidoglycan synthesis. Apart from the characterization of the features of these analogues which are responsible for their efficacy as inhibitors, these studies also contribute to a better understanding of wall assembly.

In this review we will describe three classes of alanine analogues and their target enzymes. They are: (1) those which inhibit alanine racemase, D-alanine:D-alanine ligase (ADP), and D-amino acid transaminase; (2) those which are incorporated via UDP-MurNAc-pentapeptide into nascent peptidoglycan where they exert their inhibitory effect in the final stages of cross-linking; (3) those which inhibit the LD-carboxypeptidase and DD-carboxypeptidase. In addition to these sites in peptidoglycan assembly, the use of analogues to inhibit D-alanyl-lipoteichoic acid (LTA) synthesis is discussed. At least three different stages of peptidoglycan synthesis can be distinguished by their location: (1) cytoplasmic synthesis of nucleotide-activated precursors; (2) synthesis of nascent peptidoglycan by the cytoplasmic membrane; (3) extramembranal processing of the nascent peptidoglycan for incorporation into wall. Thus, delivery of the analogue to the appropriate location where it is utilized or exerts its action is a significant feature in defining the antibacterial action of the analogue. For example, analogues in Classes 1 and 2

This review is dedicated to Professor Sir James Baddiley and Professor Otto Kandler, who introduced us to bacterial cell walls.

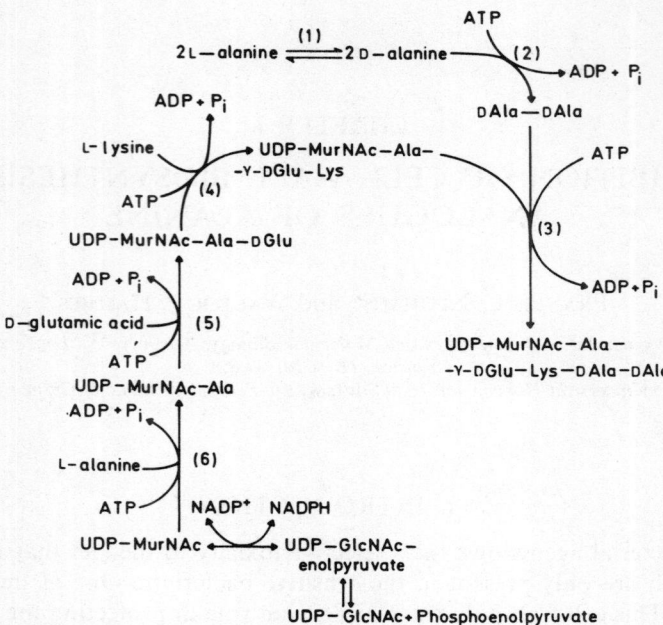

Fig. 1. The biosynthesis of UDP-MurNAc-Ala-DGlu-Lys-DAla-DAla. Enzymes 1 and 2 constitute the alanine branch of the pathway.

require active accumulation by transport systems. On the other hand, since the LD-carboxypeptidase and DD-carboxypeptidase function at extramembranal sites, active transport may not be a prerequisite for the action of analogues in Class 3.

In addition, we will summarize the utility of these alanine analogues as antimicrobial agents. This includes; consideration of selective toxicity, antibacterial spectra, release of the toxophore, synergistic combinations and acquisition of resistance. Finally, the *in vivo* use of these analogues requires acceptable pharmacokinetic properties in the host. Thus, it is our goal in this review to present some of the strategies leading to the development of analogues of this unique cell wall constituent, D-alanine.

2. ALANINE ANALOGUES AS INHIBITORS OF SPECIFIC TARGET ENZYMES

2.1. Inhibition of Alanine Racemase, D-Alanine:D-Alanine Ligase (ADP), and D-Amino Acid Transaminase (Class 1 Analogues).

The assembly of the peptidoglycan precursor, UDP-MurNAc-Ala-DGlu-Lys-DAla-DAla*, is catalyzed in the multienzyme pathway illustrated in Fig. 1. The two enzymes in this pathway, which constitute the alanine branch, are (1) alanine racemase (EC 5.1.1.1.) and (2) D-alanine:D-alanine ligase (ADP) (EC 6.3.2.4.). In 1960, Strominger and co-workers discovered that D-cycloserine, an analogue of D-alanine, is an effective inhibitor of reactions catalyzed by these enzymes. These observations provided the first example of an alanine analogue whose mechanism of action was established at the enzymic level (Strominger *et al.*, 1959, 1960).

In Table 1, analogues of alanine (Class 1) are summarized, together with their site(s) of action. These analogues of alanine can be divided into three categories based on their

---

*Unless stated, all abbreviations of residues denote the L-configuration. The omission of the hyphen, i.e. DAla-DAla, and the abbreviations conform with suggestions cited in *Biochemistry* 5, 2485 (1966). In UDP-MurNAc-pentapeptide the residues are numbered as follows: UDP-MurNAc-Ala^1-DGlu^2-Lys^3-DAla^4-DAla^5. Although not stated, the D-glutamic acid residue is linked through the γ-carboxyl group to the α-amino group of the diamino acid. Abbreviations used are: MurNAc, N-acetylmuramyl; GlcNAc, N-acetylglucosaminyl; UDP, uridine diphosphate; Nva, norvaline; Abu, α-amino-*n*-butyric acid; *m*-Dap, meso-α,ϵ-diaminopimelic acid. In peptides LAla(P) is used for L-1-aminoethylphosphonic acid. MIC is the minimal inhibitory concentration; K_m is the Michaelis constant and I_{50} is the concentration of inhibitor for 50% inhibition.

TABLE 1. *Class 1 Analogues of Alanine*

Analogue	Alanine Racemase	D-Alanine: D-Alanine ligase	D-Amino acid Transaminase	References
(1) D-Cycloserine	+[a]	+	+	Strominger *et al.* (1960) Neuhaus and Lynch (1964) Martinez-Carrion and Jenkins (1965) Neuhaus (1967, 1968) Yonaha *et al.* (1975)
(2) L-Cycloserine	+[b]	−	+[c]	Martinez-Carrion and Jenkins (1965) Neuhaus (1968) Lambert and Neuhaus (1972)
(3) O-Carbamoyl-D-serine	+	(S)[d]	?	Lynch and Neuhaus (1966) Shoji *et al.* (1968) Lambert and Neuhaus (1972) Wang and Walsh (1978)
(4) O-Carbamoyl-L-serine	+	?	?	Wang and Walsh (1978)
(5) β-Chloro-D-alanine	+	?	+	Manning *et al.* (1974) Yonaha *et al.* (1975) Kaczorowski *et al.* (1975) Henderson and Johnston (1976) Soper *et al.* (1977a) Wang and Walsh (1978) Soper and Manning (1978) Manning and Soper (1978)
(6) β-Chloro-L-alanine	+	?	?	Wang and Walsh (1978) Henderson and Johnston (1976)
(7) β-Fluoro-D-alanine	+	(S)[e]	?	Kahan and Kropp (1975) Kollonitsch and Barash (1976) Wang and Walsh (1978)
(8) β-Fluoro-L-alanine	+	?	?	Wang and Walsh (1978)
(9) β-Difluoro-D-alanine	+	?	?	Walsh *et al.* (1978)
(10) β-Trifluoro-DL-alanine	+	?	?	Silverman and Abeles (1976) Walsh *et al.* (1978)
(11) β-Bromo-D-alanine	?	?	+	Soper and Manning (1978) Manning and Soper (1978)
(12) L-1-Aminoethyl-phosphonic acid[f]	+	−	?	Johnston *et al.* (1968) Lambert and Neuhaus (1972) Adams *et al.* (1974) Lacoste *et al.* (1975) Allen *et al.* (1978) Atherton *et al.* (1979b)
(13) D-1-Aminoethyl-phosphonic acid	+	+	?	Lacoste *et al.* (1979) Atherton *et al.* (1979b)
(14) β-Aminoxy-D-alanine	+	(S)[d]	?	Neuhaus and Lynch (1964) Bisgard and Neuhaus (unpublished observations) Lambert and Neuhaus (1972)
(15) β-Aminoxy-L-alanine	+	?	?	Neuhaus (1968)
(16) O-Acetyl-D-serine	+	?	?	Shoji *et al.* (1968) Wang and Walsh (1978)

Continued overleaf

[a] The symbol + indicates that the analogue is an inhibitor of the enzyme. It does not indicate the effectiveness of the analogue.

[b] L-Cycloserine inhibits alanine racemase from *E. coli* and *B. subtilis* and not from *S. aureus* and *S. faecalis*.

[c] D-Cycloserine was a better inhibitor than L-cycloserine by a factor of 40.

[d] Analogue acts as a substrate for the synthesis of DAla-D-analogue.

[e] Analogue predicted to act as a substrate.

[f] L-1-Aminoethylphosphonic acid is a weak inhibitor of UDP-MurNAc:L-Alanine ligase (Atherton *et al.*, 1979b).

Table 1.—(continued)

Analogue	Alanine Racemase	D-Alanine: D-Alanine ligase	D-Amino acid Transaminase	References
(17) O-Acetyl-L-serine	+	?	?	Wang and Walsh (1978)
(18) D-Vinylglycine	?	?	+	Soper et al. (1977b)
(19) Acrylate	+	?	?	Adams et al. (1974)
(20) L-2-amino-3-butynoic acid	+	?	?	Kuroda et al. (1980a,b)
(21) 2-Bromo-propionate	+	?	?	Adams et al. (1974)

mechanism of inhibition (Table 2). Although each analogue is a competitive inhibitor of the target enzyme, the mechanism of inhibition can be distinguished. Category a and b inhibitors form Schiff bases with enzyme-bound pyridoxal phosphate followed by a time-dependent irreversible inactivation of the enzyme. The latter process is different in categories a and b. Category c inhibitors also compete with alanine for the enzyme binding site but do not show a time dependent irreversible inactivation.

Since many of the Class 1 analogues inhibit alanine racemase, a mechanistic description of this enzyme will be useful in interpreting their inhibitory activity. Of the purified alanine racemases, at least seven have been shown to require pyridoxal phosphate (Wood and Gunsalus, 1951; Rosso et al., 1969; Julius et al., 1970; Wang and Walsh, 1978; Diven et al., 1964; Johnston and Diven, 1969; Yonaha et al., 1975). The mechanism of enzymic racemization can be illustrated with the intermediates proposed by Metzler et al. (1954) for the non-enzymic racemization of amino acids by pyridoxal (Olivard et al., 1952). Reaction of amino acid and pyridoxal phosphate yields the aldimine (Schiff base) (I) which undergoes tautomerization labilizing the α-proton for release to the medium or a basic amino acid residue (B) (Fig. 2A). The symmetrical, planar ketimine (II) can add the proton from either side, generating either aldimine I or III. Hydrolysis of III yields the D-amino acid if the L-amino acid was used to generate I.

In two of the highly purified alanine racemases the stoichiometry of pyridoxal phosphate per catalytic site is one (Rosso et al., 1969; Wang and Walsh, 1978). However, separate substrate binding sites for D- and L-alanine have been implied from a variety of

Table 2. *Categories of Alanine Analogues in Class 1*

a. Alkylation of a nucleophile in the active site (pyridoxal phosphate dependent).[a]

1. β-Chloro-D-alanine
2. β-Chloro-L-alanine[b]
3. β-Fluoro-D-alanine
4. β-Fluoro-L-alanine
5. β-Bromo-D-alanine
6. O-acetyl-D-serine
7. O-carbamoyl-D-serine
8. D-Vinylglycine
9. β-Trifluoro-DL-alanine

b. Oxime formation with pyridoxal phosphate[a]

1. D-Cycloserine (alanine racemase)
2. β-Aminoxy-D-alanine

c. Reversible competitive inhibitors

1. L-1-Aminoethylphosphonic acid[c]
2. O-Carbamoyl-L-serine
3. O-Acetyl-L-serine
4. Acrylate
5. 2-Bromopropionate
6. D-Cycloserine (D-Alanine: D-alanine ligase (ADP))
7. D-1-Aminoethylphosphonic acid (D-Alanine:D-alanine ligase (ADP))

[a] Both category a and b inhibitors show competitive inhibition with D-alanine followed by time-dependent irreversible inactivation.

[b] With alanine racemase from *B. subtilis*, β-chloro-L-alanine is a noncompetitive inhibitor with L-alanine as the substrate (Henderson and Johnston, 1976).

[c] The alanine racemases from *E. coli* and *Pseudomonas aeruginosa* are inhibited reversibly whereas those from *S. aureus* and *S. faecalis* are inhibited irreversibly (Atherton et al., 1979b).

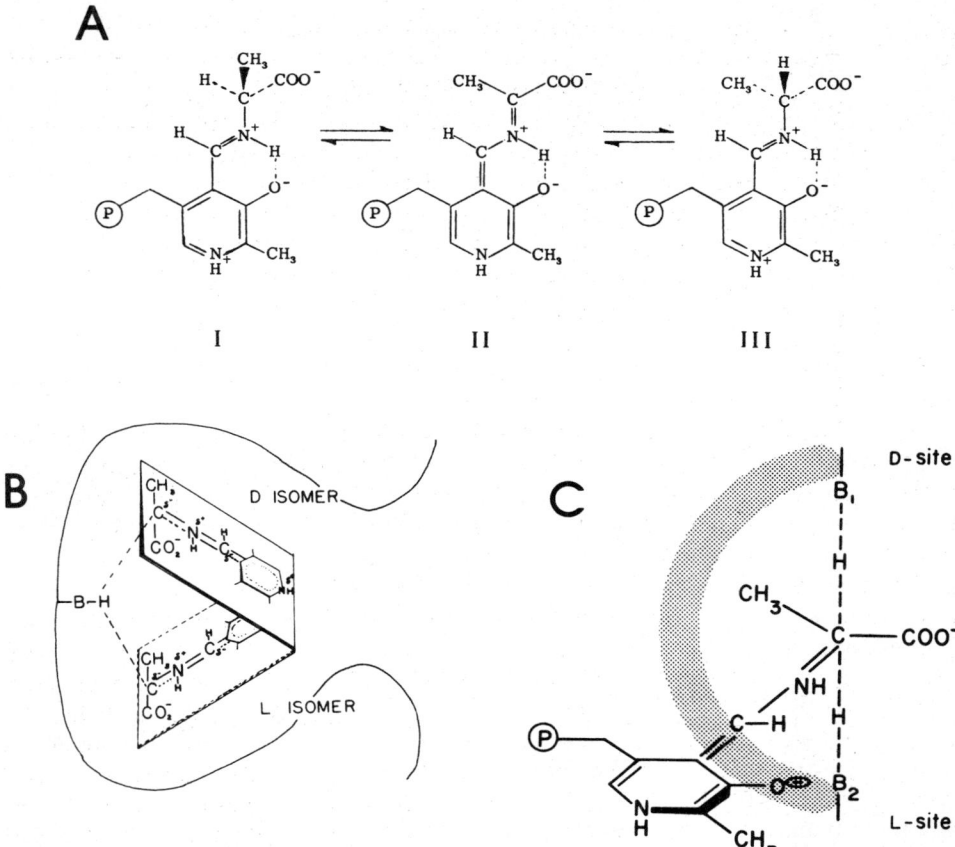

FIG. 2. (A) Mechanism of enzymic racemization adapted from model systems (Metzler *et al.*, 1954; Olivard *et al.*, 1952). (B) Schematic representation of the 'Swinging Door' mechanism of alanine racemase (Reprinted with permission from Henderson, L. L. and Johnston, R. B. *Biochem. Biophys. Res. Commun.* **68**: 793–798 (1976). Copyright 1976, Academic Press). (C) Proposed two-base (B) mechanism for racemization: proton addition from either B_1H or B_2H to the symmetrical ketimine intermediate (adapted from Adams, 1976).

experiments. For example, the asymmetry of the kinetic constants and differences in the pH activity curves for L- and D-alanine imply separate sites for the two enantiomers (Lambert and Neuhaus, 1972; Neuhaus *et al.*, 1972; Adams, 1976). This functional asymmetry has also been observed with a variety of enzyme inhibitors (Henderson and Johnston, 1976; Wang and Walsh, 1978). On the basis of these types of experiments Johnston (1980) proposed a 'swinging door' mechanism (Fig. 2B). In this mechanism, the planar pi system of the imine can swing to either the L- or the D-site. The position of the imine relative to the point of protonation will determine the resulting configuration. The specificity determinants of the two sites define the asymmetry of the kinetic constants, pH optima, and inhibitor constants which have been observed. In this model a single base (B) involved in protonation/deprotonation is proposed.

In a study of the α-H exchange reaction catalyzed by alanine racemase, it was recognized by Babu *et al.* (1975) and Dunathan *et al.* (1976) that the exchange process is also asymmetric. For example, in the L → D direction the rates of exchange and of racemization are equal whereas in the D → L direction the exchange rate significantly exceeds the racemization rate with two different alanine racemases. On the basis of these observations Adams (1976) proposed the two-base mechanism. The symmetrical intermediate is illustrated in Fig. 2C. Proton exchange with the solvent might be facilitated in one case and not in the other. This model differs from the 'swinging door' model proposed by Henderson and Johnston (1976) in that movement of the imine is not required in the

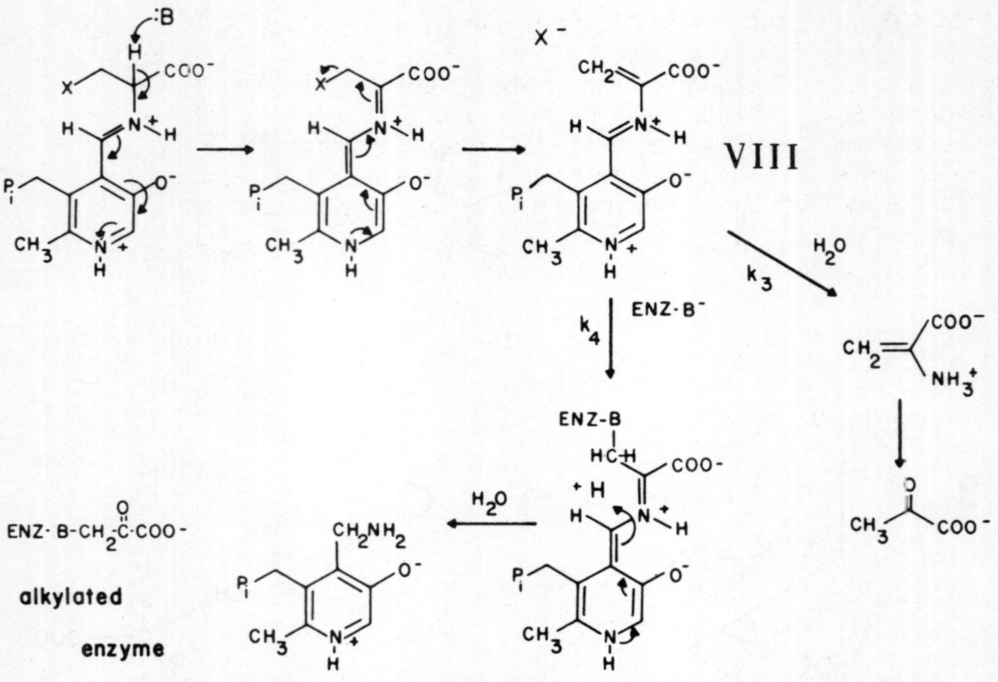

Fig. 3. Proposed scheme for the irreversible inactivation of alanine racemase by a suicide substrate, e.g. β-fluoro-D-alanine where X = F. Intermediate VIII is a common eneamino aldimine complex which alkylates Enz-B$^-$. (Reprinted with permission from Wang, E. and Walsh, C. *Biochemistry* **17**: 1313–1321 (1978). Copyright 1978, American Chemical Society.)

two-base mechanism. The mechanistic description of alanine racemase provides a model for interpreting the inhibitory activities of the analogues in the three categories.

Category *a* inhibitors have good leaving groups that generate by β-elimination an enzyme-bound electrophilic species that serves as an alkylating agent of a nucleophile in the active site. This type of inhibitor has been characterized as a 'suicide substrate' (Walsh, 1978) or 'suicide enzyme inactivator' (Abeles and Maycock, 1976). The mechanism of the irreversible inactivation can be illustrated with the scheme formulated by Wang and Walsh (1978) for alanine racemase (Fig. 3). The partition ratio k_3/k_4 is 830 for O-carbamoyl-D-serine (IV), O-acetyl-D-serine (V), β-chloro-D-alanine (VI) and β-fluoro-D-alanine (VII). This ratio indicates that 830 molecules of product (α,β-elimination), pyruvate, are formed on average per inactivation sequence (k_4). The same ratio is also observed for β-fluoro-L-alanine and β-chloro-L-alanine.

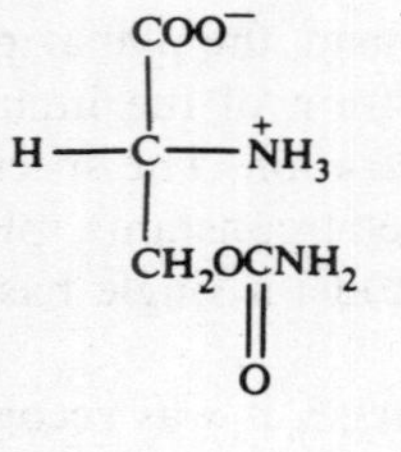

(IV) 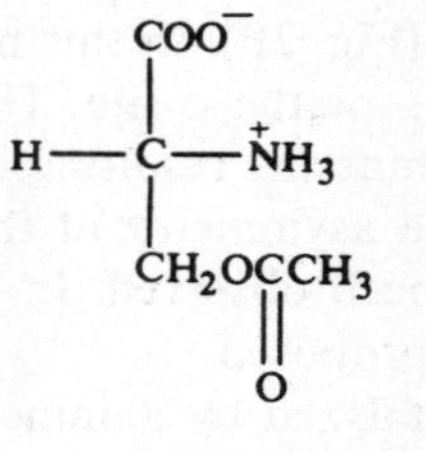   (V) 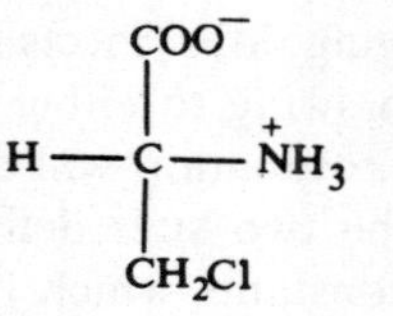   (VI) 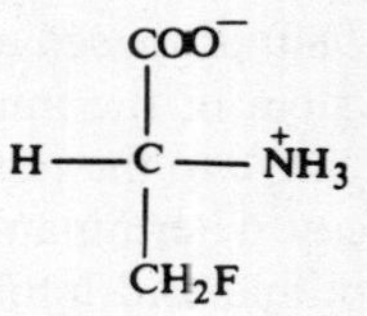   (VII)

O-Carbamoyl-L-serine and O-acetyl-L-serine also inhibit the racemase but apparently do not undergo catalysis (Wang and Walsh, 1978). Although O-phospho-D,L-serine and O-sulfo-D-serine have potential leaving groups, they do not inhibit or inactivate the enzyme. While many analogues inhibit racemase (Table 1), only alanine is a substrate for racemization (Adams, 1976).

The identical partition ratio for alanine analogues (IV, V, VI, VII) suggests that a common intermediate (VIII), the eneamino acid–pyridoxal complex, is the intermediate responsible for inactivation. In attempts to improve the electrophilicity of intermediate (VIII), β-trifluoro-D-alanine and β-difluoro-D-alanine have been compared with the β-fluoro-D-alanine (Walsh et al., 1978). For β-trifluoro-D-alanine the partition ratio decreases from 830 to <10. In contrast, with β-difluoro-D-alanine, this ratio increases to 10,000–100,000. Moreover, with the difluoro-amino acid the alkylated enzyme readily reactivates. Thus, the trifluoro-D-alanine is more effective in inactivating alanine racemase by alkylation than β-fluoro-D-alanine. The high ratio of $k_4 : k_3$ (Fig. 3) in which

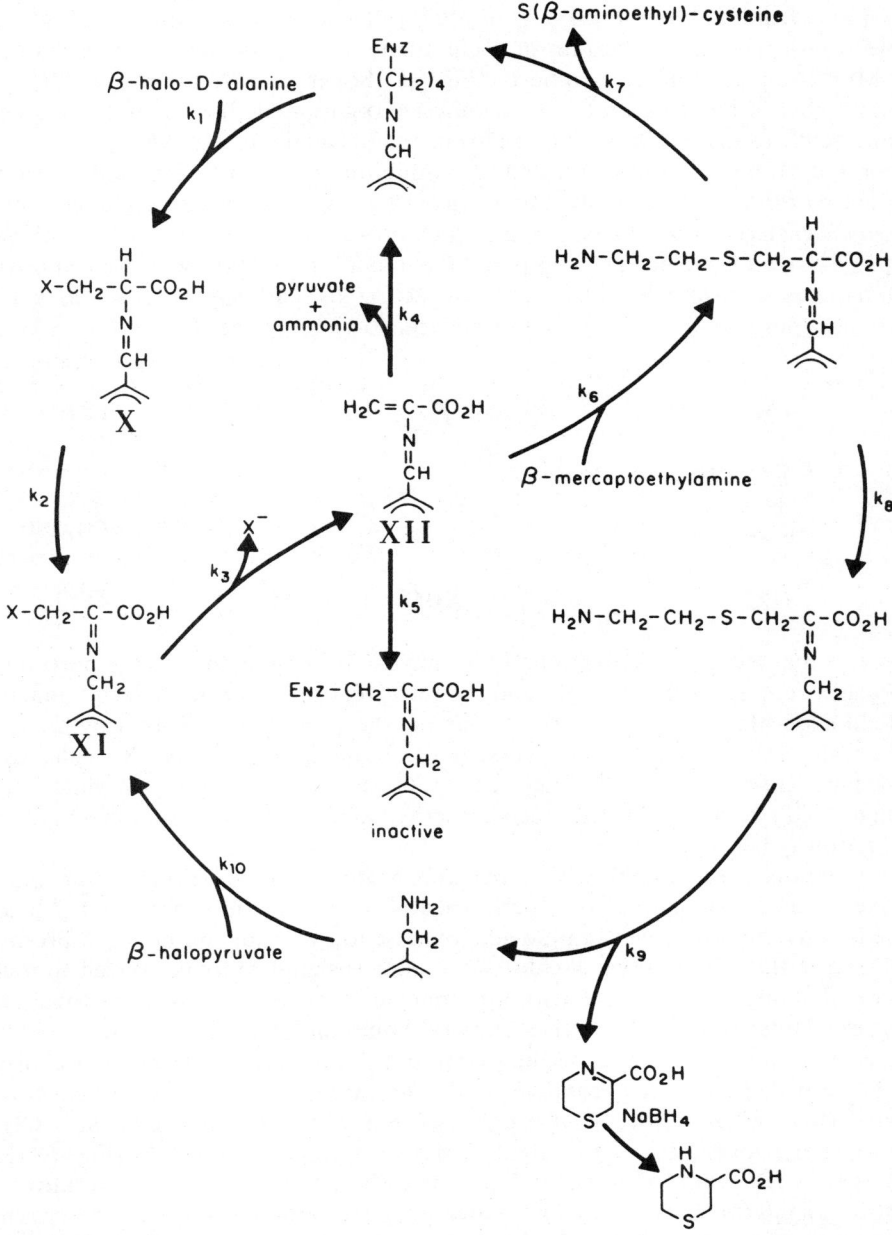

FIG. 4. Model of the β-elimination scheme and the trapping of intermediate XII during the reaction catalyzed by D-amino acid transaminase. (Reprinted with permission from Soper, T. S. and Manning, J. M. *Biochemistry* **17**: 3377–3384 (1978). Copyright 1978, American Chemical Society.) The topmost structure is the aldimine derivative formed between pyridoxal phosphate and a lysine residue in the active site.

the eneamine intermediate (VIII) is alkylatively captured in the inactivation sequence supports this conclusion. On the basis of these studies Wang and Walsh (1978) suggested that 'future antibiotic candidates targeted at alanine racemase might balance the features of being a D-amino acid isomer with a small good leaving group at the β-carbon, but one which when oxidized by an animal cell D-amino acid oxidase will yield a β-substituted α-keto acid of low reactivity (and toxicity)'.

The D-amino acid transaminase is also a target for analogues of D-alanine, e.g. D-cycloserine and β-chloro-D-alanine (Manning and Soper, 1978; Manning et al., 1974; Martinez-Carrion and Jenkins, 1965). In many species of bacteria this enzyme can provide D-glutamic acid with D-alanine as the donor substrate (Thorne and Molnar, 1955; Thorne et al., 1955; Hug and Werkman, 1957; Kuramitsu and Snoke, 1962; Martinez-Carrion and Jenkins, 1965; Yonaha et al., 1975). It was proposed that inhibition of this enzyme will deprive the bacterium of D-glutamate, one of the amino acids required for UDP-MurNAc-pentapeptide synthesis (Fig. 1) (Soper and Manning, 1978). Only a limited number of bacteria apparently synthesize D-glutamate from L-glutamate with the glutamic acid racemase (Glaser, 1960; Diven, 1969; Tanaka et al., 1961).

Soper and Manning (1978) described four inhibitors of the D-amino acid transaminase which act by three distinct catalytic pathways (Fig. 4): (1) a unimolecular β-elimination reaction characteristic of β-bromo-D- and β-chloro-D-alanine which act by pathway (k_1, k_2, k_3, k_4/k_5); (2) a bimolecular 'ping pong' β-elimination reaction with β-bromopyruvate which requires a D-amino acid cosubstrate acting by pathway (k_{10}, k_3, k_4/k_5); (3) a bimolecular 'ping-pong' transamination between D-vinylglycine (IX) and an α-keto acid

$$
\begin{array}{ccc}
\text{COO}^- & \text{H} & \text{COO}^- \\
| & | & | \\
\text{H}-\text{C}-\overset{+}{\text{N}}\text{H}_3 & \text{(XIII)} & \text{H}-\text{C}-\overset{+}{\text{N}}\text{H}_3 \\
| & & | \\
\text{HC}=\text{CH}_2 & & \text{CH}_2\text{ONH}_2 \\
\textbf{(IX)} & \textbf{(XIII)} & \textbf{(XIV)}
\end{array}
$$

cosubstrate that leads to inactivation of the enzyme. In these pathways the partition ratio is k_4/k_5 and represents the rate of catalytic turnovers per enzyme molecule inactivated. For β-chloro-D-alanine and β-bromo-D-alanine, the ratio is 350. With vinylglycine it is not clear whether the inactivation occurs via the aldimine intermediate X or the ketimine intermediate XI shown in Fig. 4. Intermediate XII (Fig. 4), the α-aminoacrylate-pyridoxal phosphate*, can be trapped with β-mercaptoethylamine to yield S-(β-aminoethyl)cysteine by the pathway (k_6, k_7).

As a potential alanine analogue, Soper and Manning (1978) favored β-bromo-D-alanine over β-chloro-D-alanine. This preference is based on the report that β-bromo-D-alanine is converted by renal D-amino acid oxidase to pyruvate and not to β-bromopyruvate (Dang et al., 1976) whereas β-chloro-D-alanine is significantly converted to β-chloropyruvate. β-Halopyruvates react with a number of enzymes and thus are toxic and not analogues of interest for antibacterial activity (Soper and Manning, 1978).

Category b inhibitors, D-cycloserine (XIII) and β-aminoxy-D-alanine (XIV), also form Schiff bases with pyridoxal phosphate of alanine racemase and D-amino acid transaminase. In the case of D-cycloserine, it is proposed that enzymic cleavage of the α-CH bond will lead to the formation of the highly reactive acylating agent XV (Fig. 5) (Rando, 1975). Species XV would then acylate an active site amino acid residue resulting in the formation of intermediate XVI (Fig. 5) and irreversible inactivation of the enzyme. An additional reaction may involve the formation of a substituted oxime (XVII) from intermediate XVI.

---

*Identical to VIII proposed for alanine racemase (Wang and Walsh, 1978).

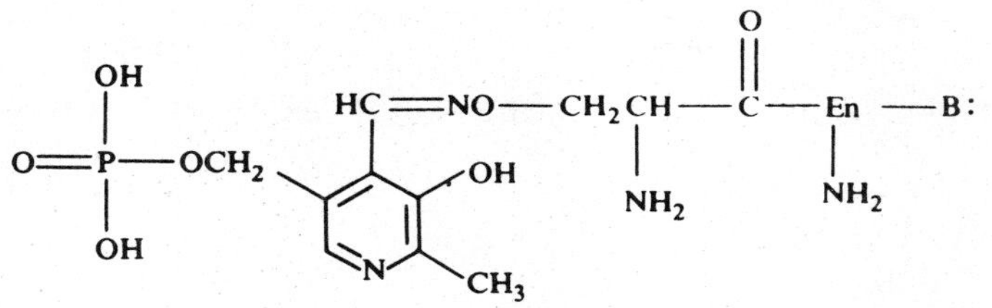

(XVII)

These proposals are based on the observations that D-cycloserine inactivates the racemase in a time dependent manner (Neuhaus, 1968; Wang and Walsh, 1978) and that this time-dependent phase is irreversible (Rando, 1975). Furthermore, this reaction scheme is based on the similar spectral changes observed with D-amino acid transaminase and the glutamic–aspartic transaminase upon addition of D-cycloserine (Martinez-Carrion and Jenkins, 1965; Karpeiskii *et al.*, 1963). In the case of β-aminoxy-D-alanine, only oxime formation would occur.

The distinguishing feature between category *a* and *b* inhibitors is the alkylation of an enzyme nucleophile for inhibitors in *a* and either substituted oxime formation and/or acylation of an enzyme amino acid residue for inhibitors in *b* (Table 2).

Category *c* inhibitors include L-1-aminoethylphosphonic acid (XVIII) derived from the antibacterial agent alafosfalin (XIX) (Allen *et al.*, 1978; Atherton *et al.*, 1979a,b; Allen *et al.*, 1979a,b). L-1-Aminoethylphosphonic acid is an analogue of L-alanine and is an excellent inhibitor of alanine racemase (Johnston *et al.*, 1968; Lambert and Neuhaus, 1972; Adams *et al.*, 1974; Atherton *et al.*, 1979b). The key to the use of this compound as an

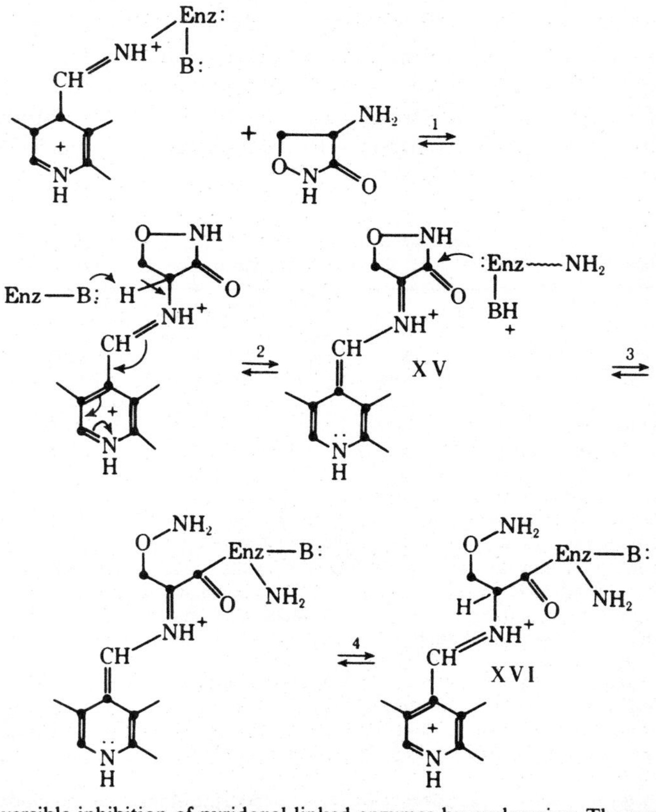

FIG. 5. Irreversible inhibition of pyridoxal-linked enzymes by cycloserine. The proposed scheme is based in part on experiments which show that D-cycloserine is an irreversible inhibitor of alanine racemase from *B. subtilis*. (Reprinted with permission from Rando, R. R. *Accounts Chem. Res.* **8**: 281–288 (1975). Copyright 1975, American Chemical Society.)

(XVIII)   **(XIX)**

antibacterial agent is the active transport and intracellular hydrolysis of either a dipeptide or an oligopeptide containing the analogue (Atherton *et al.*, 1979a) (see Sections 3.2., 3.3.). L-1-Aminoethylphosphonic acid that is not linked in a peptide shows no substantial uptake or antibacterial activity (Dulaney, 1970; Atherton *et al.*, 1979a). Two exceptions are *Proteus vulgaris* (Dulaney, 1970) and *Pseudomonas aeruginosa* (Lacoste *et al.*, 1975). The Roche group has shown that alanine racemase is one of the primary sites of action of this analogue resulting in an accumulation of UDP-MurNAc-Ala-DGlu-Lys (Atherton *et al.*, 1979b). The effect of L-1-aminoethylphosphonic acid on the activities of the racemases in Gram-positive and Gram-negative organisms differed greatly. Whereas the enzymes from *E. coli* and *Pseudomonas aeruginosa* were inhibited reversibly under the assay conditions employed, the enzymes from *S. faecalis* and *S. aureus* were inhibited irreversibly (Atherton *et al.*, 1979b). The mechanism of irreversible inactivation in these racemases has not been established. In addition, a second site of action is implied by the experiments of Atherton *et al.* (1979b). In Gram-negative organisms, UDP-MurNAc-L-Ala(P) is also accumulated in cells treated with alafosfalin. It has been shown that L-1-aminoethylphosphonic acid competes with L-alanine in the reaction catalyzed by the UDP-MurNAc:L-alanine ligase, as was observed with glycine (Hishinuma *et al.*, 1971) (Enzyme 6, Fig. 1). The resulting nucleotide containing L-1-aminoethylphosphonic acid is apparently not utilized by the UDP-MurNAc-Ala:D-glutamic acid ligase (Enzyme 5, Fig. 1). The more important effect of L-1-aminoethylphosphonic acid, however, appears to be the inhibition of alanine racemase. This conclusion was further supported by the marked

TABLE 3. *Effect of 5-Methyl Substitution of D-Cycloserine on D-Alanine: D-Alanine Ligase (ADP), Alanine Racemase, and the Growth of* S. faecalis R

	Ligase[a]		Racemase[b]	
Compound	K_I	K_{AI}	K_i	MIC[c]
	$(M \times 10^{-4})$		$(M \times 10^{-4})$	$(M \times 10^{-4})$
D-Cycloserine	0.22	1.4	2.4	1–2
cis-D-Cyclothreonine	1.2	1.9	20	5–6
trans-D-Cyclothreonine	5.4	5.6	>500	30–40

[a]For the D-alanine:D-alanine ligase (ADP) purified from *S. faecalis* R, the K_I is the inhibitor constant for the binding of *I* to the donor site while K_{AI} is the inhibitor constant for the binding of *I* to the acceptor site when the donor site binds a molecule of D-alanine. These constants were determined from kinetic data interpreted with a model that assumes an ordered sequence of substrate binding, i.e. (1) donor, (2) acceptor (Neuhaus and Lynch, 1964).

[b]For the racemase purified from *S. faecalis* R, the K_i is that concentration of compound which inhibits the enzyme 50%. It was established from a slope-replot derived from a series of Lineweaver–Burk plots at increasing concentrations of inhibitor (Bisgard, Bensman and Neuhaus, unpublished results).

[c]For growth studies, the effect of increasing concentrations of compounds were compared in cultures of *S. faecalis* R 8043 grown in medium containing 0.1% glucose (Neuhaus and Lynch, 1964). MIC is that concentration range that produces significant lysis of the culture and a 50% inhibition of total growth.

decrease in the intracellular pool of D-alanine when cells of *E. coli*, *S. aureus* and *Pseudomonas* were incubated with alafosfalin (Atherton *et al.*, 1979b).

Category *c* inhibitors (Table 2), which inhibit alanine racemase, also include O-carbamoyl-L-serine, O-acetyl-L-serine, acrylate and 2-bromopropionate (Adams *et al.*, 1974; Wang and Walsh, 1978). These inhibitors not only illustrate the latitude of binding specificity but indicate the limits which the enzyme imposes for initiating the covalent inactivation of the enzyme. A third example of a category *c* inhibitor relates to the action of D-cycloserine on D-alanine:D-alanine ligase (ADP) (Enzyme 2, Fig. 1). In contrast to the irreversible inactivation of the racemase, the inhibition of the ligase is reversible (Neuhaus and Lynch, 1964). D-Cycloserine competes with D-alanine at both the donor (N-terminal) and acceptor (C-terminal) sites of the ligase. A kinetic analysis of this enzyme reveals that the donor site has a higher 'affinity' for D-cycloserine than the acceptor site. Moreover, the donor site of the ligase has a higher affinity for D-cycloserine than does the alanine racemase. These constants are summarized in Table 3. Thus, the concentration for 50% inhibition of the ligase is one-tenth of that required to inhibit the racemase.

In addition, the effect of 5-methyl substitution of D-cycloserine on the racemase, on the D-alanine:D-alanine ligase, and on the MIC is shown in Table 3. *cis*-5-Methyl substitution affects binding of the D-cycloserine analogue at the donor site, whereas it appears to have almost no effect on binding at the acceptor site. In contrast, *trans*-5-methyl substitution hinders binding at both the donor and acceptor sites of the ligase. In the case of alanine racemase, a 10-fold higher concentration of *cis*-D-cyclothreonine (XX) is required

(XX)   **(XXI)**

to inhibit alanine racemase by 50%. Finally, the *trans*-5-methyl substituted cycloserine (*trans*-D-cyclothreonine) (XXI) does not inhibit alanine racemase to a significant extent (Table 3). Thus, there is a poor correlation between the inhibition of alanine racemase and the MIC. Moreover, there is a poor correlation between the inhibitor constants for the acceptor site of the ligase and the MIC. These studies further support the conclusion that the primary site of D-cycloserine action at low antibiotic concentrations in *S. faecalis* is the donor site of D-alanine:D-alanine ligase (Neuhaus, 1968). This proposal assumes that *S. faecalis* R is equally permeable to the two isomers of D-cyclothreonine and D-cycloserine. As discussed in Section 4.4., this proposal is of importance in describing the synergy of D-cycloserine with other D-alanine analogues.

As illustrated in Table 1, O-carbamoyl-D-serine and β-aminoxy-D-alanine are not only inhibitors of alanine racemase but they are substrates in the reaction catalyzed by D-alanine:D-alanine ligase (ADP). Thus, when these analogues are incubated with D-alanine, DAla-D-analogue is synthesized. These dipeptides are added to UDP-MurNAc-tripeptide resulting in the synthesis of UDP-MurNAc-pentapeptide with an analogue in position 5. Since these are probably incorporated into nascent peptidoglycan, they will also be considered briefly with the second class of inhibitors (see Section 2.2.). The importance of these analogues as substrates is illustrated with fluoro-D-alanine. Low concentrations of fluoro-D-alanine are bactericidal whereas high concentrations are auto-antagonistic (Kahan and Kropp, 1975). It is presumed that the D-alanine:D-alanine ligase utilizes fluoro-D-alanine for the synthesis of fluoro-DAla-fluoro-DAla which is used for UDP-MurNAc-pentapeptide synthesis. If this results in the synthesis of functional peptidoglycan, fluoro-D-alanine can antagonize its own inhibitory activity (see Section 4.4.).

2.2. Incorporation of d-Alanine Analogues into Nascent Peptidoglycan via UDP-MurNAc-pentapeptide (Class 2 Analogues)

A second class of D-alanine analogues includes those that are incorporated into nascent peptidoglycan (Fig. 6) via the precursor, UDP-MurNAc-pentapeptide. The best studied example of such an analogue is glycine. When bacteria are grown in media supplemented with elevated concentrations of glycine, growth inhibition with concomitant morphological changes, induction of spheroplast formation, decrease in crosslinkage of the peptidoglycan, and accumulation of UDP-MurNAc-pentapeptides can be observed (Schleifer et al., 1976). Since the morphological effects of glycine are similar to those of penicillin, it has been assumed that the cell wall is the main site of glycine action. The synthesis of peptidoglycan with decreased cross-linkage is accompanied by the synthesis and accumulation of a family of UDP-MurNAc-pentapeptides with partial replacement of both enantiomers of alanine by glycine (Hammes et al., 1973). Thus, incorporation of the alanine analogue, glycine, into nascent peptidoglycan, has specific and deleterious effects on the assembly of the cross-linked polymer.

A second example, which is also well-documented, is that of D-serine (Whitney and Grula, 1964, 1968; King and Grula, 1972; Yabu and Huempfner, 1974; Trippen et al., 1976; Schleifer et al., 1976). D-Serine is incorporated into peptidoglycan when bacteria are grown in the presence of this amino acid. As in the case of bacteria grown in the presence of glycine, the peptidoglycan of cells grown in the presence of D-serine is also less cross-linked. Thus, in both cases peptidoglycan is assembled that is less extensively cross-linked; as a result the cell may have a higher sensitivity to or a greater activity of autolysins.

In the case of glycine, alanine in positions 1, 4 and 5 of the peptide subunit of the nucleotide-activated precursor is partially replaced by glycine whereas, in the case of D-serine, D-alanine in positions 4 and 5 is partially replaced (Trippen et al., 1976; Hammes et al., 1973). The distribution of amino acid replacements in the families of nucleotides that accumulate indicate that precursors with glycine in position 5 do not accumulate to the same extent as those precursors with replacements at positions 1 and 4. The preferential utilization of the nucleotide with residue 5 replaced with glycine is the result of the discrimination exerted by phospho-MurNAc-pentapeptide translocase (1, Fig. 6), the first membrane enzyme involved in the synthesis of nascent peptidoglycan (Hammes and Neuhaus, 1974a). Specificity studies with UDP-MurNAc-peptides with replacements at positions 1 and 4 indicate that these are poorer substrates than those with replacements in position 5 for the synthesis of nascent peptidoglycan (Hammes and Neuhaus, 1974b). The specificity barriers exerted by these membrane enzymes are of primary importance in designing analogues that are utilized for nascent peptidoglycan synthesis but are not (or poorly) utilized for the assembly of cross-linked peptidoglycan (Fig. 6).

Since the cross-linked peptidoglycan formed from this modified nascent peptidoglycan has a decreased cross-linking (Hammes et al., 1973; Schleifer et al., 1976; Trippen et al., 1976), the replacement of D-alanine by an analogue in the peptide subunits can exert specific effects on the final assembly of this polymer. Schleifer and Kandler (1972) summarized the degree of amino acid variation among different bacterial species in the peptide subunit. Although there is significant variation in positions 1 and 3, position 4 and position 5 (where preservation in the wall allows analysis) are always occupied by D-alanine. The presence of D-alanine in positions 4 and 5 has been conserved in all bacterial species, suggesting that these residues play a key role in the final assembly process. Since the replacement of D-alanine in position 4 exerts the greatest inhibitory effect on cross-linked peptidoglycan synthesis, replacement in this position may provide an effective and specific means of inhibiting the cross-linking of the nascent peptidoglycan into the preexisting peptidoglycan of the wall.

The critical role of residue 4 in the cross-linking process is illustrated in Fig. 7. In *Gaffkya homari*, the donor peptide in this process is provided by the preexisting peptidoglycan of the cell wall (Hammes and Kandler, 1976). In the first round of cross-linking,

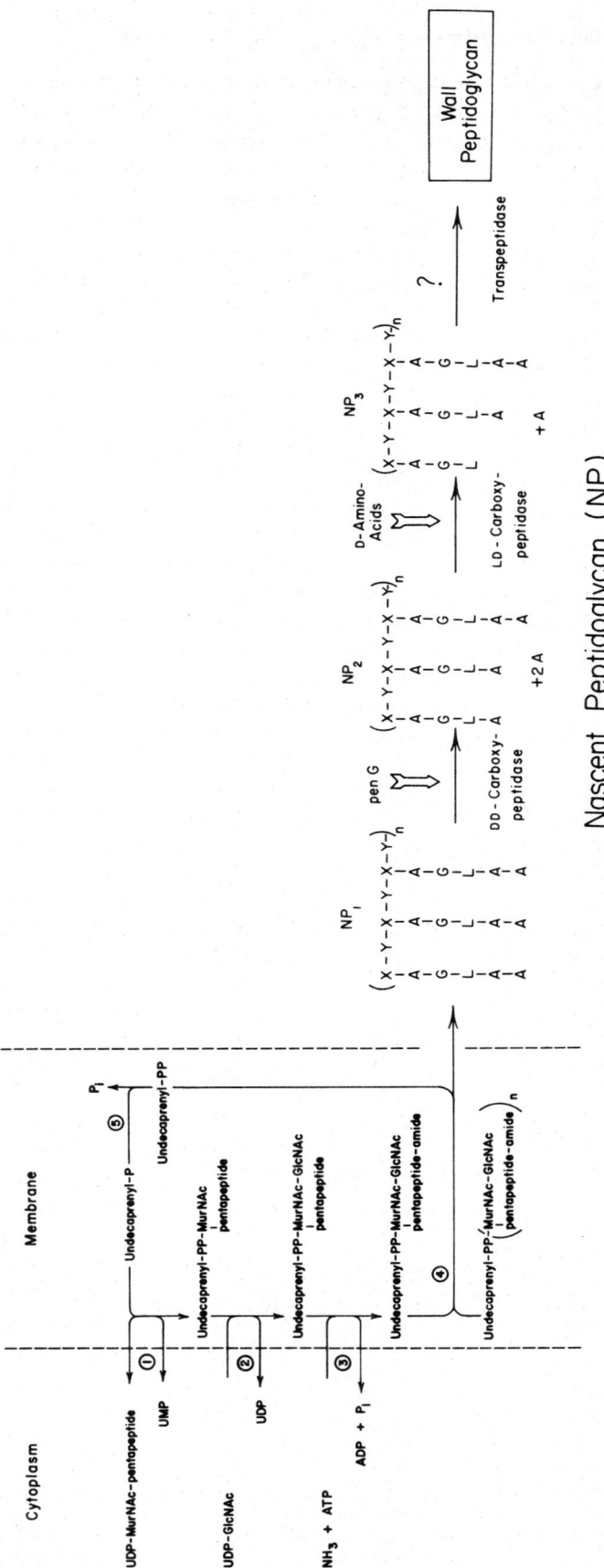

Fig. 6. Assembly of nascent peptidoglycan. In *G. homari* the nascent peptidoglycan is processed by DD-carboxypeptidase and LD-carboxypeptidase prior to incorporation into the preexisting peptidoglycan of the wall. In nascent peptidoglycan (NP), X is N-acetylmuramyl and Y is N-acetylglucosaminyl and A-G-L-A-A is Ala-DGlu-Lys-DAla-DAla.

analogue replacements will be found in the acceptor peptide subunits (nascent peptido-glycan) exclusively. As a result of one round of nascent peptidoglycan incorporation (round 1), analogue (X) is incorporated into preexisting peptidoglycan. Since this incorporation is inhibited by the analogue in position 4, one may assume that the acceptor binding site of the transpeptidase has a decreased affinity for peptide subunits which are modified in the neighborhood of the lysine residue involved in the cross-linking reaction. We also propose that the replacement of D-alanine by an analogue exerts a further inhibitory effect in the second round of peptidoglycan incorporation, i.e. when the modified donor peptide subunit-enzyme is formed. Thus, the inhibitory effects of this group of analogues may reflect one or more of the specificity determinants exerted by the transpeptidase.

An additional explanation for the inhibitory effect of residue 4 replacements can be proposed from studies of the carboxypeptidase activities of the peptidoglycan synthesizing system of this organism. It has been shown that DD-carboxypeptidase (Hammes and Kandler, 1976) and LD-carboxypeptidase (Hammes and Seidel, 1978a; Hammes, 1978) are both required for the synthesis of cross-linked peptidoglycan in *G. homari*. It is possible that analogue incorporation at position 4 and to a lesser extent at position 5 may also affect the activities catalyzed by these enzymes as well as that catalyzed by the transpeptidase. Studies on the penicillin-sensitive acyl-DAla-DAla carboxypeptidases from *Strepto-myces spp* show similar specificity for residues 4 and 5 of the model donor substrate for carboxypeptidase action or uncoupled transpeptidation, diacetyl-Lys^3-DAla^2-DAla^5 (reference peptide) (Leyh-Bouille *et al.*, 1972; Ghuysen, 1977). For example, when glycine or D-leucine replaces D-alanine in residue 4, V_{max}/K_m for the R39 carboxypeptidase is zero. When glycine or D-leucine replaces D-alanine in position 5, V_{max}/K_m is 9.8% and 78%, respectively, of that observed for the reference peptide. It was concluded that the

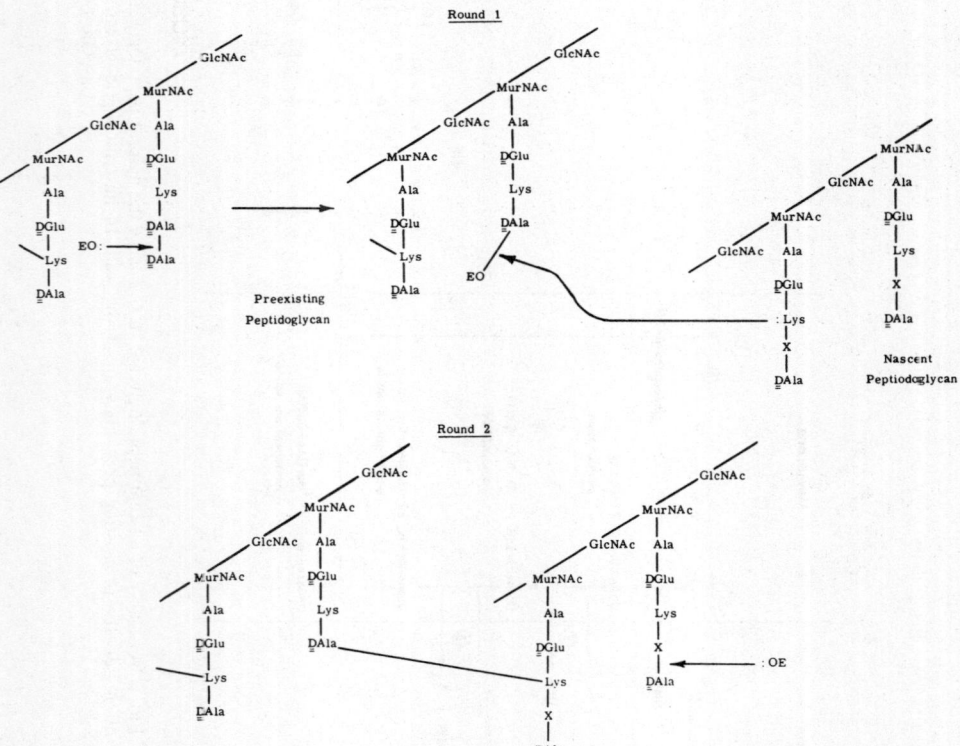

Fig. 7. Proposed mechanism for analogue inhibition in the reaction catalyzed by transpeptidase (EO:) in *G. homari*. This mechanism shows only the formation of bisdisaccharide dimers and not higher oligomers. In round 1 preexisting peptidoglycan refers to wall peptidoglycan. The amino acid in position 4 is represented as X, which may be D-alanine, another D-amino acid, or glycine.

carboxypeptidase exhibited considerable specificity for a C-terminal LR[3]-DAla[4]-D-amino acid[5] sequence. These results together with those found for the membrane DD-carboxypeptidase/transpeptidase from *Bacillus megaterium* (Marquet *et al.*, 1976) support the conclusions derived from the *G. homari* test system.

Exclusive incorporation of a D-alanine analogue into position 4 of the peptide subunit of nascent peptidoglycan is dependent on the specificity determinants of a variety of enzyme and transport systems. Thus, the analogue needs not only to be transported but also to be utilized in the alanine branch of peptidoglycan synthesis (Fig. 1). Incorporation requires its utilization by the D-alanine:D-alanine ligase (ADP) and UDP-MurNAc-tripeptide:DAla-DAla ligase (ADP) as well as by the membrane enzymes involved in the synthesis of nascent peptidoglycan (Fig. 6).

In *S. faecalis*, D-alanine:D-alanine ligase (ADP) has a high specificity for D-amino acids in the N-terminal site and a low specificity for D-amino acids in the C-terminal site (Neuhaus, 1962a,b). Thus, the enzyme is able to synthesize a wide variety of mixed dipeptides, e.g. DAla-DSer, DAla-DAbu, etc. The only D-alanine analogue besides glycine that is utilized at a significant rate for the N-terminal residue by the ligase is D-α-amino-*n*-butyric acid (DAbu). The high specificity for the N-terminal residue exerted by the ligase would appear to exclude this enzyme as a means for introducing the analogue specifically into position 4. Thus, the use of the D-alanine:D-alanine ligase (ADP) for the synthesis of D-alanine analogue-DAla is not likely to provide a successful approach for effecting the synthesis of a UDP-MurNAc-pentapeptide with a replacement in position 4. It appears, however, that the specificity profile of the ligase observed in studies with *S. faecalis* is not the same as in all bacteria. This can be concluded from the composition of the UDP-MurNAc-pentapeptides that are accumulated in *Bacillus subtilis* and *Corynebacterium callunae* when they are grown in the presence of D-serine at concentrations that partially inhibit growth (Trippen *et al.*, 1976). In these UDP-MurNAc-pentapeptides, 49 and 72% of the D-alanine residues in position 4 were replaced by D-serine in the respective organisms. In position 5, replacement was also observed in 82 and 67% of the D-alanine residues, respectively. Therefore, in some organisms it is possible to replace partially D-alanine residues in both positions 4 and 5.

To circumvent the specificity determinants exerted by D-alanine:D-alanine ligase (ADP), attention was directed to DD-dipeptides that have N-terminal D-alanine analogues. Specificity studies with UDP-MurNAc-Ala-DGlu-Lys:DAla-DAla ligase (ADP) from *S. faecalis* indicated that changes in the N-terminal residue of the dipeptide do not have a major effect on the activity catalyzed by the enzyme (Table 4; Neuhaus and Struve, 1965). In particular, CH_3CH_2- and $CH_3CH_2CH_2$- as R_n do not affect this activity. As a result of these studies, the use of DD-dipeptides of the type D-alanine analogue-DAla has been considered as a potential method for the specific incorporation of analogues into position 4 of the peptide subunit.

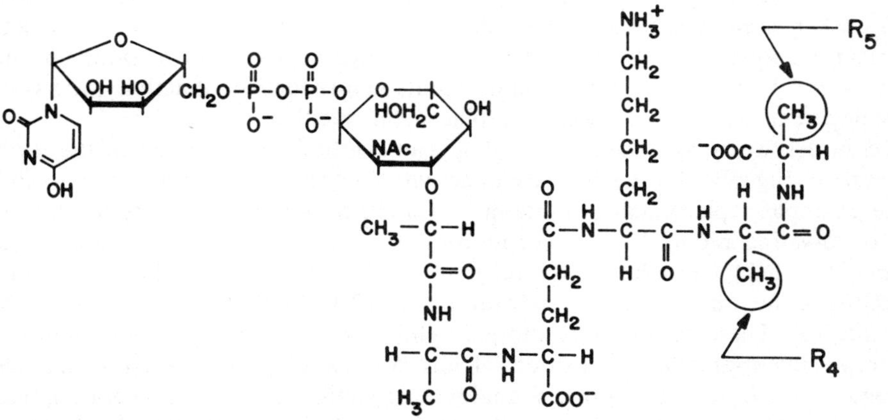

FIG. 8. Structure of UDP-MurNAc-Ala[1]-DGlu[2]-Lys[3]-DAla[4]-DAla[5]. Residues 4 and 5 are indicated.

TABLE 4. *Specificity Profile of UDP-MurNAc-Ala-DGlu-Lys:*
DAla-DAla Ligase (ADP) from S. faecalis[a]

$$R_n \!-\! \underset{H}{\overset{NH_3^+}{C}} \!-\! \overset{O}{\overset{\parallel}{C}} \!-\! \underset{H}{\overset{H}{N}} \!-\! \underset{H}{\overset{COO^-}{C}} \!-\! R_c$$

R_n	R_c	Km_i[b] $(M \times 10^{-4})$
CH₃CH₂—	—CH₃	0.9
CH₃CH₂CH₂—	—CH₃	1.2
CH₃—	—CH₃	1.6
HOCH₂—	—CH₃	2.6
(CH₃)₂CH—	—CH₃	3.9
CH₃CH₂—	—CH₂CH₃	7.0
CH₃—	—CH₂CH₃	7.6
CH₃—	—CH₂OH	9.1
CH₃—	—CH₂(CH₃)₂	26
CH₃—	—CH(OH)CH₃	33
CH₃—	—CH₂CH₂CH₃	>50

[a]Reprinted with permission from Neuhaus, F. C. and Struve, W. G. (1965) *Biochemistry* **4**: 120–131. Copyright 1965, American Chemical Society.
[b]Since $K_m = K_i$ in the ligase assay, and since some dipeptides were tested as substrates and some as inhibitors, the term Km_i is used for comparison. The assay for ligase measures the addition of labeled DAla-DAla to UDP-MurNAc-Ala-DGlu-Lys.

To assess the role of residues 4 and 5 in the assembly of cross-linked peptidoglycan, a series of UDP-MurNAc-pentapeptides (Fig. 8) was biosynthesized with these residues replaced singly by either D-α-amino-n-butyric acid, D-norvaline, or D-valine (Carpenter *et al.*, 1976). The testing of these analogues on cross-linked peptidoglycan synthesis has required the development of an *in vitro* system. For the system a membrane-wall preparation from *Gaffkya homari* that catalyzes the synthesis of cross-linked peptidoglycan was used. The advantages of this test system are:

(i) High specific activity.
(ii) Direct cross-linkage (A1α, Nᵉ-(DAla)-Lys (Schliefer and Kandler, 1972)).
(iii) 95% sensitivity of the *in vitro* system to benzylpenicillin at 10 μg/ml (Hammes, 1976; Carpenter *et al.*, 1976).
(iv) Absence of detectable autolytic activity.

The six nucleotides were compared with UDP-MurNAc-Ala-DGlu-Lys-DAla-DAla in both nascent peptidoglycan synthesis and in penicillin-sensitive peptidoglycan synthesis. In Fig. 9A nascent peptidoglycan synthesis that is catalyzed by membranes from this organism is shown with these nucleotides. Although replacement of D-alanine in either residue 4 or 5 by D-norvaline or D-valine results in a reduction of activity, the system has a low degree of selectivity between a replacement in either residue 4 or 5.

In contrast, when cross-linked peptidoglycan synthesis is examined in the membrane-wall system (Fig. 9B), a large decrease in activity is observed with replacements in residue 4. For example, replacement of D-alanine with either D-α-amino-n-butyric acid, D-norvaline, or D-valine reduced the incorporation to 153, 52 and 111 pmoles, respectively, compared with 2130 pmoles for the reference nucleotide at 30 min. For the replacements in residue 5, the amounts of incorporation were 1710, 1130 and 513 pmoles in the same time interval. These results were more carefully documented with D-α-amino-n-butyric acid replacing D-alanine in positions 4 and 5 separately. V_{max}/K_m for this residue 4 analogue relative to this residue 5 analogue is similar for nascent peptidoglycan synthesis, whereas for cross-linked peptidoglycan synthesis V_{max}/K_m for this residue 4 analogue is only 20% of that for the residue 5 analogue. Specifically, V_{max}/K_m and V_{max} for

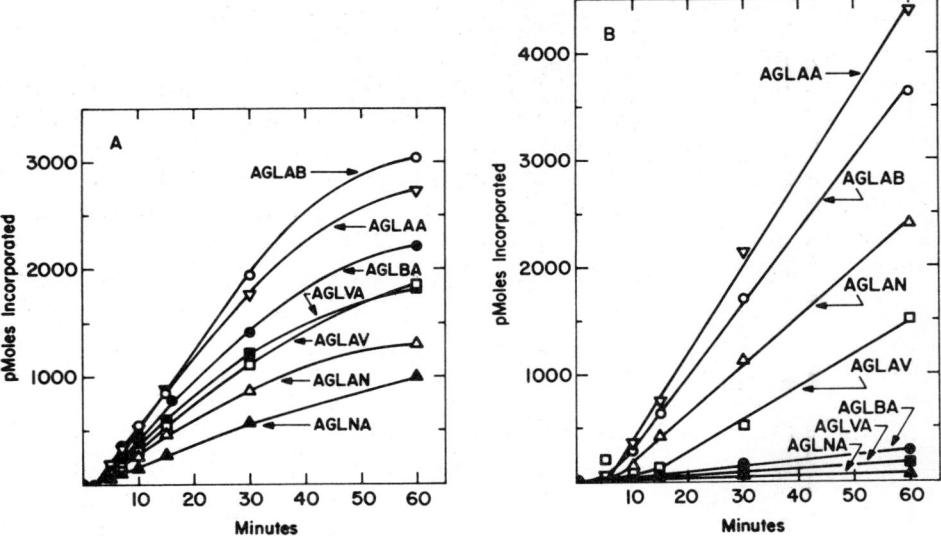

FIG. 9. Time courses of incorporation of [^{14}C]GlcNAc from UDP-[^{14}C]GlcNAc with analogues of UDP-MurNAc-Ala-DGlu-Lys-DAla-DAla (R$_4$ and R$_5$) into nascent peptidoglycan (A) and into wall (B). In A the assay for nascent peptidoglycan (chromatographically immobile) was used with membranes while in B the assay for wall-linked peptidoglycan (SDS-insoluble) was used with membrane-walls. The incorporations in A were penicillin insensitive whereas the incorporations in B were penicillin sensitive. Incorporation of [^{14}C]GlcNAc from UDP-[^{14}C]GlcNAc into SDS-insoluble material is considered to be a measure of transpeptidation. Thus, incorporations in A represent the synthesis of nascent, uncross-linked peptidoglycan while incorporations in B reflect the synthesis of cross-linked peptidoglycan. The abbreviations are: AGLAA, UDP-Mur-NAc-Ala-DGlu-Lys-DAla-DAla; AGLAB, UDP-MurNAc-Ala-DGlu-Lys-DAla-DAbu; AGLBA, UDP-MurNAc-Ala-DGlu-Lys-DAbu-DAla; AGLVA, UDP-MurNAc-Ala-DGlu-Lys-DVal-DAla; AGLAV, UDP-MurNAc-Ala-DGlu-Lys-DAla-DVal; AGLAN, UDP-MurNAc-Ala-DGlu-Lys-DAla-DNva; AGLNA, UDP-MurNAc-Ala-DGlu-Lys-DNva-DAla. (Reprinted with permission from Carpenter, C. V., Goyer, S. and Neuhaus, F. C. *Biochemistry* **15**: 3146–3152 (1976). Copyright 1976, American Chemical Society.)

UDP-MurNAc-Ala-DGlu-Lys-DAbu-DAla are 0.19 and 0.03 of that observed for the reference nucleotide, whereas V_{max}/K_m and V_{max} for UDP-MurNAc-Ala-DGlu-Lys-DAla-DAbu are 0.95 and 0.52 of that observed for the reference nucleotide. These data clearly illustrate the high degree of discrimination for the replacement of D-alanine by D-α-amino-*n*-butyric acid in position 4 in the membrane-wall system.

In a series of experiments with ether-treated cells of *E. coli*, Pelzer and Reuter (1980) have also examined analogues of DAla-DAla as potential inhibitors of cross-linked peptidoglycan synthesis. This system differs from that described by Carpenter *et al.* (1976) in that the analogue of UDP-MurNAc-peptide is biosynthesized *in situ*. Secondly, the ether-treated cells may represent a closer approximation to the events in the cell than the membrane-wall preparation utilized by Carpenter *et al.* (1976). Thirdly, the ether-treated cell preparations are incubated under conditions in which UDP-MurNAc-Ala-DGlu-*m*DAP-DAla-DAla is also synthesized. Thus, the results reflect the incorporation of an analogue into intermediates that contain significant amounts of normal pentapeptide residues. As shown in Table 5, large bulk substituents enhance the inhibitory activity of the analogues of DAla-DAla. Based on these data, analogues with substituted aromatic rings on the N-terminal residue may provide a broader basis for designing analogues with enhanced antimicrobial activity.

In an additional set of experiments, the effect of replacing alanine by glycine on the synthesis of cross-linked peptidoglycan was studied in *G. homari*. As shown in Table 6A, replacement of D-alanine in position 4 by glycine results in only 15% of the activity observed for D-alanine in this position. In contrast, replacement of D-alanine in position 5 by glycine gives 50% of the activity. Comparison of these data with those obtained for

TABLE 5. *Inhibition of SDS-Insoluble Peptidoglycan Synthesis by Analogues of DAla-DAla in* E. coli[a]

$$R_n - \overset{\overset{\displaystyle NH_3^+}{|}}{\underset{\underset{\displaystyle H}{|}}{C}} - \overset{\overset{\displaystyle O}{\|}}{C} - \overset{\overset{\displaystyle H}{|}}{N} - \overset{\overset{\displaystyle COO^-}{|}}{\underset{\underset{\displaystyle H}{|}}{C}} - R_c$$

R_n	Dipeptide Added R_c	I_{50}^b (M × 10^{-6})
biphenyl–CH$_2$–	–CH$_3$	3.5
indolyl–CH$_2$–	–CH$_3$	3.6
CH$_3$CH$_2$CH$_2$–	–CH$_3$	4.5
Br–phenyl–CH$_2$–	–CH$_3$	6.3
naphthyl–CH$_2$–	–CH$_3$	6.8
F–phenyl–CH$_2$–	–CH$_3$	7.1
cyclohexyl–CH$_2$–	–CH$_3$	7.2
HO–phenyl–CH$_2$–	–CH$_3$	9.1
CH$_3$CH$_2$CH$_2$CH$_2$–	–CH$_3$	10.6
Cl–phenyl–CH$_2$–	–CH$_3$	10.8
CH$_3$–phenyl–CH$_2$–	–CH$_3$	10.9
(CH$_3$)$_2$CH–CH$_2$–	–CH$_3$	11.7
(CH$_3$CH$_2$)(CH$_3$)CH–CH$_2$–	–CH$_3$	11.9

[a]Reprinted with permission from Pelzer, H. and Reuter, W. *Antimicrob. Agents Chemother.* **18:** 887–892 (1980). Copyright, 1980, American Society for Microbiology.
[b]I_{50} is defined as that concentration of analogue which inhibits the incorporation of [^{14}C]GlcNAc from UDP-[^{14}C]GlcNAc by 50% in the presence of 5.6 μM DAla-DAla and UDP-MurNAc-tripeptide in the assay for peptidoglycan synthesis using ether-treated (permeabilized) cells of E. coli.

nascent peptidoglycan synthesis and translocase activity gives a good correlation (Table 6A). This suggests that for glycine analogues, discrimination is exerted by phospho-MurNAc-pentapeptide translocase, the initial membrane enzyme involved in peptidoglycan synthesis (Hammes and Neuhaus, 1974a,b). An analysis of cross-linking (Table 6B), however, indicates an additional feature of analogue discrimination. Glycine residues in position 4 have a major effect on cross-linking, e.g. 16.7% of the cross-linking observed for UDP-MurNAc-Ala-DGlu-Lys-DAla-DAla. Thus, discrimination at the stage of transpeptidation, which is not revealed by the kinetic measurements, is indicated by cross-linked peptidoglycan synthesis. Alternatively, the degree of cross-linking may be adversely affected by the reduced rate of lipid precursor synthesis (Table 6A).

TABLE 6. *Effect of Replacing Alanine Residues in UDP-MurNAc-pentapeptide by Glycine on Peptidoglycan Synthesis in G.* homari

A. Comparison of activities for UDP-MurNAc-pentapeptides with alanine replaced by glycine.

Substrate	Phospho-MurNAc-pentapeptide translocase[a]	Peptidoglycan	
		nascent-[a]	wall-[b]
UDP-MurNAc-Ala-DGlu-Lys-DAla-DAla	1.0[c]	1.0[c]	1.0[c]
UDP-MurNAc-Gly-DGlu-Lys-DAla-DAla	0.24	0.30	0.40
UDP-MurNAc-Ala-DGlu-Lys-Gly-DAla	0.16	0.26	0.15
UDP-MurNAc-Ala-DGlu-Lys-DAla-Gly	0.65	0.50	0.50

B. Determination of the degree of cross-linking in the peptidoglycan formed from UDP-MurNAc-pentapeptides with D-Alanine replaced by glycine[d]

Substrate	Cross-linking[e] (%)
UDP-MurNAc-Ala-DGlu-Lys-DAla-DAla	100
UDP-MurNAc-Ala-DGlu-Lys-Gly-DAla	16.7
UDP-MurNAc-Ala-DGlu-Lys-DAla-Gly	70.8

[a]Nascent peptidoglycan represents uncross-linked peptidoglycan synthesized by membranes. Adapted from Hammes and Neuhaus, 1974b.

[b]Wall-linked peptidoglycan represents the synthesis of cross-linked peptidoglycan synthesized by membrane-walls. Hammes, unpublished observations.

[c]The values of V_{max}/K_m are normalized to that observed for UDP-MurNAc-DGlu-Lys-DAla-DAla.

[d]Hammes, unpublished results.

[e]Data are normalized to UDP-MurNAc-Ala-DGlu-Lys-DAla-DAla. The actual degree of cross-linking in *G. homari* is between 24 and 30%. The % cross-linking was established by the procedure of Hammes and Kandler (1976).

Theoretical studies describing the possible conformation of acyl-DAla-DAla (Fig. 10) give a good correlation between the % cross-linking calculated from the data of Carpenter *et al.* (1976) and the difference in energy (ΔV_{ex}) at $\phi_4 = 180°$ between the analogue and acyl-DAla-DAla (Virudachalam and Rao, 1978) (Table 7). The conformation chosen for acyl-DAla-DAla (Fig. 10B) is that most closely mimicking benzylpenicillin in solution (Virudachalam and Rao, 1977). The theoretical studies (Table 7) with analogues in positions 4 and 5 support the proposed conformation (Fig. 10B). Large values of ΔV_{ex} indicate that the analogue is unable to attain the favorable conformation shown for acyl-DAla-DAla that is hypothesized to be that required for activity in the DD-carboxypeptidase/transpeptidase system. Low values indicate that the analogue can assume a conformation similar to that of acyl-DAla-DAla in this system. For optimal binding, DD-carboxypeptidase/transpeptidase requires a conformation in which $\phi_4 \simeq 180°$, $\Psi_4 = 128°$, and $\phi_5 \simeq 150°$ of the fourth and fifth residues of the pentapeptide moiety (Fig. 10B). The biologically active conformation of acyl-DAla-DAla is shown. Energy calculations with glycine at either position 4 or 5 shows that ΔV_{ex} is negligible (R. Virudachalam, personal communication). However, the conformationally accessible area for glycine on the $(\phi\Psi)$ plane is about three times larger than that of alanine (Scheraga *et al.*, 1967). Because of this enhanced flexibility of the backbone, the concentration of the biologically active conformer of the analogue will be low even though it has a low ΔV_{ex} (R. Virudachalam, personal communication). Alternatively, replacement of D-alanine by glycine may result in poor 'induced fit' at the active site(s) of the DD-carboxypeptidase/transpeptidase. Thus, a theoretical analysis such as that described by Virudachalam and Rao (1978), when compared with the results from experimental systems, can provide some of the principles for the design of inhibitors of this system.

In recent years, many analogues of D-Ala-DAla have been synthesized as possible antibacterial agents. For example, Gale and Smith (1973) proposed that the α-methyl

A

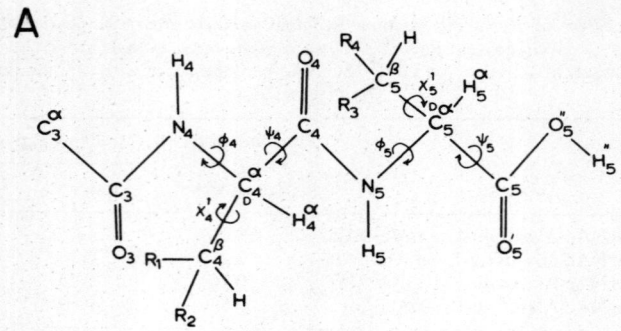

B

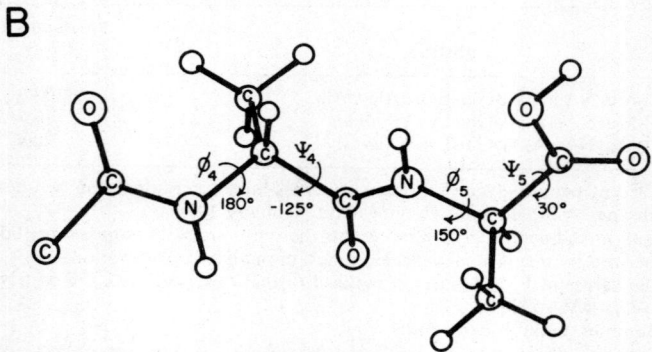

FIG. 10. Schematic representation of X-D-alanyl[4]-D-alanine[5] (A) and the biologically active conformation (B). In A, X-D-butyl[4]-D-alanine[5] $R_1 = CH_3$, $R_2 = R_3 = R_4 = H$); X-D-alanyl[4]-D-butyric acid[5] ($R_1 = R_2 = H$, $R_3 = CH_3$, $R_4 = H$); X-D-valyl[4]-D-alanine[5] ($R_1 = R_2 = CH_3$, $R_3 = R_4 = H$); X-D-alanyl[4]-D-valine[5] ($R_1 = R_2 = H$, $R_3 = R_4 = CH_3$). A: (Reprinted with permission from Virudachalam, R. and Rao, V. S. R. *Biopolymers* 17: 2251–2263 (1978). Copyright 1978, John Wiley and Sons.) B: (Reprinted with permission from R. Virudachalam, personal communication.)

TABLE 7. *Conformational Energy at $\phi_4 = 180°$ and Percentage Cross-Linking in Peptidoglycan Biosynthesis[a]*

Peptides	ΔV_{ex}(kcal/mol)[b]			Cross-linking[c] (%)
	χ_4^1 or χ_5^{1d} = 60°	= 180°	= −60°	
X[e]-DAla[4]-DAla[5]	0.0	—	—	100
X-Ala[4]-DAla[5]	>10.0	—	—	0
X-DAla[4]-Ala[5]	>10(4.12)[f]	—	—	14
X-DAbu[4]-DAla[5]	>10.0	−0.68	6.42	5
X-DAla[4]-DAbu[5]	0.12	0.12	1.12	76
X-DVal[4]-DAla[5]	>10.0	6.02	>10.0	4
X-DAla[4]-DVal[5]	3.50	2.02	3.26	14
X-DNva[4]-DAla[5]	—	—	—	1
X-DAla[4]-DNva[5]	—	—	—	61

[a]Reprinted with permission from Virudachalam, R. and Rao, V. S. R. *Biopolymers* 17: 2251–2263 (1978). Copyright 1978, John Wiley and Sons.

[b]ΔV_{ex} is the difference in energy between the analog and X-DAla[4]-DAla[5] ($\Delta V_{ex} = V_{ex}^{analogue} - V_{ex}^{substrate}$).

[c]Percentage cross-linking calculated from the data reported by Carpenter *et al.* (1976) and Marquet *et al.* (1976). Data are normalized to UDP-Mur-NAc-Ala-DGlu-Lys-DAla-DAla. See also footnote e, Table 6B.

[d]χ_4^1 and χ_5^1 are defined in Figure 10A and have no meaning for alanine. ϕ is 180° based on analogy to benzylpenicillin.

[e]X represents the remaining portion of the pentapeptide.

[f]The value within the parentheses denotes the energy value when $\phi_5 = 180°$.

derivatives of D-Ala-DAla might serve as antimetabolites. No activity was observed with either α-aminoisobutyryl-DAla or DAla-α-aminoisobutyric acid. Smissman *et al.* (1976) established that 2-(D-alanyl)-amino-3-butanone (XXII), DL-5-[α-(D-alanylamino)-ethyl]-1(2)H-tetrazole (XXIII) and DAla-D-alanine hydroxamic acid (XXIV) do not possess significant antibacterial activity. Stammer (Payne and Stammer, 1968; C. H. Stammer, personal communication) found that DAla-D-cycloserine (XXV) had no effect on bacterial

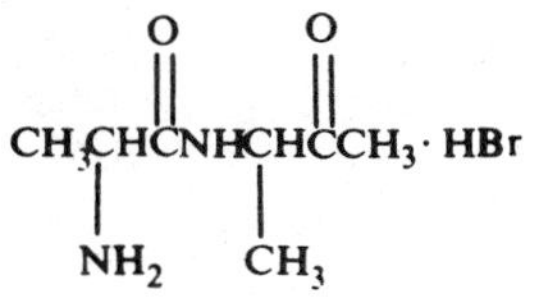

$$CH_3CHCNHCHCCH_3 \cdot HBr$$
$$NH_2 \quad CH_3$$

(XXII)

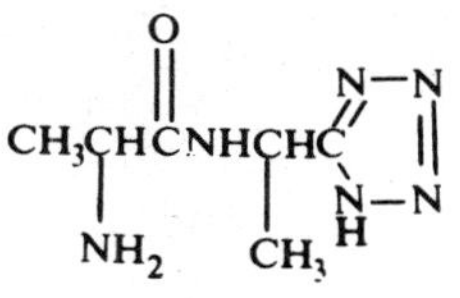

$$CH_3CHCNHCHC$$
$$NH_2 \quad CH_3$$

(XXIII)

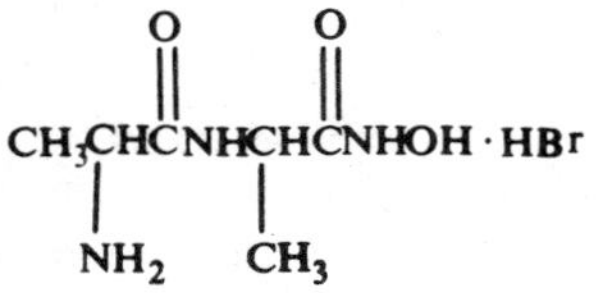

$$CH_3CHCNHCHCNHOH \cdot HBr$$
$$NH_2 \quad CH_3$$

(XXIV)

$$CH_3—CH—C—NH—CH$$
$$NH_2$$

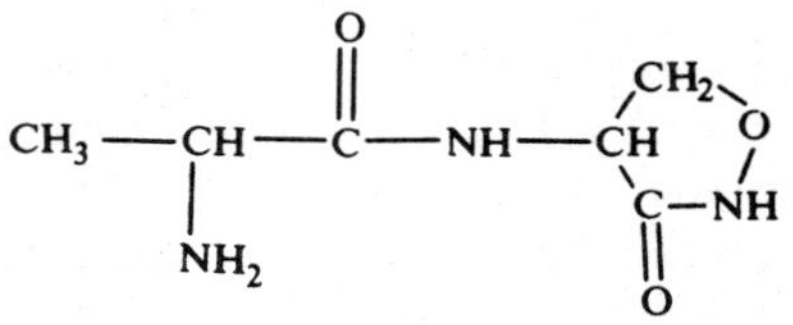

(XXV)

growth. A series of dipeptide analogues of DAla-DAla synthesized by Okada *et al.* (1976a,b, 1978) exhibited no antibacterial activity. In 1975, Huber *et al.* synthesized and evaluated DAla-DL-Ala(P) as an antibacterial agent. The only activity observed was against *Pseudomonas aeruginosa* and this activity was of the same order of magnitude as that shown by DL-1-aminoethylphosphonic acid. In an extensive study, the Roche group (Allen *et al.*, 1978) studied more than 300 di- to pentapeptide analogues related to DAla-DAla. No analogues of DAla-DAla were found to have antibacterial activity. However, during the course of this study, it was discovered that the L,L-dipeptide, Ala-LAla(P), possessed significant antibacterial activity (see Sections 3.2., 4.3).

The *in vitro* experiments described in this section with analogues of DAla-DAla containing steric substituents in the N-terminal residue provided a rational basis for designing an antibacterial agent, DNva-DAla, directed to the inhibition of the cross-linking process. This dipeptide had significant but relatively modest antibacterial activity against two strains of *E. coli*, *S. typhimurium* and *Klebsiella pneumoniae* (R. L. Girolami, personal communication). The primary limitation to this approach, however, is the discrimination exerted by the transport process, a feature that greatly limits the potential efficacy of this group of analogues (see Section 3.2).

2.3. INHIBITION OF LD-CARBOXYPEPTIDASE AND DD-CARBOXYPEPTIDASE (CLASS 3 ANALOGUES)

The third class of analogues comprises those amino acids that inhibit the cross-linking process by either reversal or inhibition of the reactions catalyzed by DD-carboxypeptidase, transpeptidase, or LD-carboxypeptidase. In addition to D-alanine, this class includes D-methionine, D-leucine and D-phenylalanine as well as D-serine, glycine, and D-threonine. The latter three amino acids were described in the previous section because they are also incorporated into peptidoglycan precursors, i.e. UDP-MurNAc-peptides. Several studies indicate that D-amino acids can exert their effect at extramembranal sites which may be similar or related to those affected by penicillin action (Lark and Lark, 1959, 1961; Michel and Hijmans, 1960). The fact that the effects of penicillin and D-methionine, as well as those of penicillin and D-alanine, are synergistic suggests that the sites of action of D-amino acids may actually be different from those of penicillin (Lark and Lark, 1961; Hammes and Seidel, 1978b). Although the concentrations of D-amino acids required to inhibit the synthesis of cross-linked peptidoglycan are in the millimolar range, inhibition at these target sites by D-amino acids may represent a unique approach for designing a class of antibacterial agents. Specificity studies may eventually lead to inhibitors that can exert their effects at lower concentrations or potentiate synergistically the effects of other antibacterial agents. An important feature of this class relates to the fact that active transport may not be required for their action at the extramembranal sites of peptidoglycan assembly, although permeation through the outer membrane in gram-negative bacteria is required.

A second feature of this class concerns the possible multiplicity and species variation of target enzymes for D-alanine analogues and their overlap with targets for β-lactam antibiotics. The targets of β-lactam antibiotic action are the penicillin binding proteins found in the cytoplasmic membrane. These proteins, a few of which have been identified as DD-carboxypeptidases, probably consist mostly of several transpeptidases with unique functions in bacterial growth and cell division. Multiple binding proteins have been found in every bacterial species examined. For example, in *E. coli* and *B. subtilis* higher molecular weight binding proteins are independent lethal targets for β-lactam antibiotics, whereas those of lower molecular weight can be genetically deleted (and presumably inhibited) without lethal effect. These latter binding proteins have been identified as DD-carboxypeptidases. However, in other organisms, e.g. *G. homari*, the assembly of cell wall peptidoglycan requires that nascent peptidoglycan be processed by at least two enzymes, DD-carboxypeptidase and LD-carboxypeptidase, prior to incorporation of the glycan into wall (Fig. 6). Inhibition of either of these enzymes results in a defective or poorly cross-linked peptidoglycan. It is thus apparent that D-alanine analogues, which may interact with penicillin-insensitive enzymes such as LD-carboxypeptidases, as well as with penicillin-sensitive DD-carboxypeptidases and transpeptidases, may act in combination with β-lactam antibiotics in a species-specific manner. This is equally true of the

TABLE 8. *Effect of Glycine, Alanine and their Derivatives on Cross-Linked Peptidoglycan Synthesis in B. megaterium*[a]

Compounds[b]	Cross-linking (%)
Glycine	14.1
Glycinamide	22.3
Glycine methyl ester	32.5
N-Acetylglycine	49.7
Glycylglycine	34.6
D-Alanine	17.5
L-Alanine	42.1
D-Alanine methyl ester	36.6
D-Alanine chloromethyl ketone	40.7
N-Acetyl(D,L)alanine	49.0
D-Alanyl-D-alanine	48.0
D-Valine	8.4
Racemic-Dpm	9.4
meso-Rich Dpm	11.4
None	51.3

[a]Reprinted with permission from Oka, T. *Antimicrob. Agents Chemother.* **10**: 579–591 (1976). Copyright 1976, American Society for Microbiology.
[b]The compounds were tested at 0.01 M in an assay for peptidoglycan synthesis using a particulate preparation from *B. megaterium* KM. Total peptidoglycan was isolated and digested with lysozyme. % cross-linking is the ratio of bisdisaccharide peptide (cross-linked) to the sum of bisdisaccharide peptide and disaccharide peptide.

action of these analogues alone or in combination with other inhibitors of peptidoglycan synthesis (see Section 4.4.).

The 'reversibility' of the transpeptidase was described by Izaki *et al.* (1966, 1968). Incubation of 40 mM D-amino acid in the peptidoglycan synthesizing system from *E. coli* inhibited the formation of cross-linked peptidoglycan and resulted in the formation of water soluble non-cross-linked peptidoglycan. Incubation of D-[^{14}C]alanine with UDP-MurNAc-Ala-DGlu-*m*[^{3}H]Dap-DAla-DAla and UDP-GlcNAc in the presence of membranes resulted in an incorporation into soluble peptidoglycan of 0.2 moles of D-[^{14}C]-alanine per mole of *m*-[^{3}H]Dap. It was suggested that this incorporation had taken place into position 5 of the peptide subunit. These experiments indicated that cross-linked peptidoglycan synthesis can be inhibited by 'reversing' or by inhibiting the action of the transpeptidase.

The inhibition of cross-linking by amino acids and alanine analogues has been studied in a particulate system from *Bacillus megaterium* (Oka, 1976) and in the membrane-wall system from *G. homari* (Hammes, 1978). As shown in Table 8, glycine, D-valine, *m*-Dap, and D-alanine (tested at 10^{-2} M) cause a significant reduction in the % cross-linking in *B. megaterium*. It is of interest that D-alanine chloromethyl ketone (XXVI) has no effect on

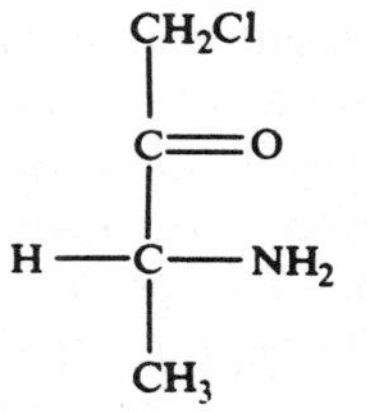

CH$_2$Cl
|
C=O
|
H —C— NH$_2$
|
CH$_3$

(XXVI)

this system (Nakamizo and Nakamura, 1978; Oka, 1976). Chloromethyl ketone analogues of substrates have been used as active-site directed inhibitors of a variety of serine proteases (Shaw, 1970). No attempt was made in the experiments described by Oka (1976) to establish whether the D-amino acids are incorporated into nascent or wall-linked peptidoglycan. In the synthesis of cross-linked peptidoglycan in *G. homari*, the I_{50} for D-alanine was found to be 5.6 mM. All D-amino acids with the exception of D-aspartic and D-glutamic are better inhibitors than D-alanine. These data are summarized in Table 9. Replacement of UDP-MurNAc-pentapeptide with UDP-MurNAc-tetrapeptide did not change the I_{50} values. Incorporation of radioactive D-alanine, D-leucine, or glycine was observed into SDS-soluble peptidoglycan, and, to a lower extent, into wall-bound peptidoglycan. An analysis of the modified peptidoglycan has clearly shown that the radioactive amino acids were incorporated into position 4 of the peptide subunits. Therefore, this incorporation is distinct from that observed by Izaki *et al.* (1966, 1968) in *E. coli*. Hammes (1978) has proposed that this incorporation is catalyzed by the LD-carboxypeptidase. An effect on LD-carboxypeptidase similar to that exerted by D-amino acids was also observed with two β-lactams, nocardicin A (XXVII) and cephalosporin C (XXVIII) (Hammes and Seidel, 1978b). Both are substituted with D-amino acids having free carboxyl and amino groups at the asymmetric C-atom. Cephalosporin C contains D-α-

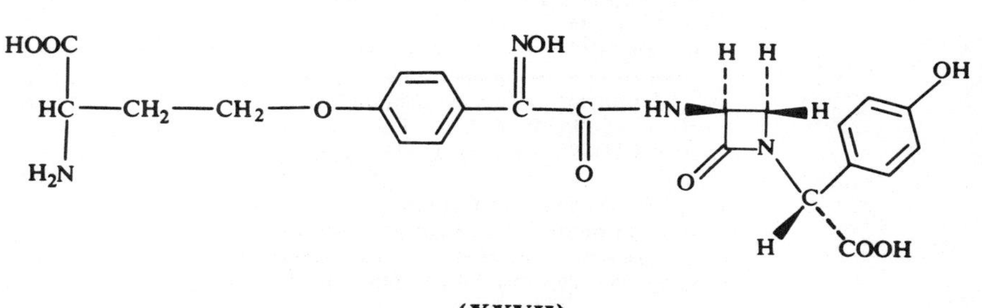

(XXVII)

(XXVIII)

aminoadipic acid and inhibits both DD-carboxypeptidase and LD-carboxypeptidase whereas nocardicin A contains D-homoserine and inhibits LD-carboxypeptidase exclusively. The inhibition of this carboxypeptidase results in fewer tripeptide subunits in the nascent peptidoglycan. It has been proposed by Hammes (1978) that nascent peptidoglycan deficient in these subunits is not an optimal substrate in the transpeptidation reaction. Thus, an essential role of the LD-carboxypeptidase in the processing of nascent peptidoglycan has been revealed in G. homari (Hammes, 1978).

Little is known about the role of the LD-carboxypeptidase. Clearly, its activity is required for the incorporation of nascent peptidoglycan into wall peptidoglycan in G. homari (Hammes and Seidel, 1978a). It has been concluded that the true substrate of this enzyme and of the DD-carboxypeptidase in G. homari is nascent peptidoglycan (Fig. 6). One function that is under consideration is its role in providing the proper population of pentapeptides, tetrapeptides, and tripeptides prior to incorporation of the nascent polymer into preexisting peptidoglycan. Tripeptide subunits have also been observed in the peptidoglycan of B. megaterium (Heijenoort et al., 1969), Bacillus sphaericus (Hungerer and Tipper, 1969), E. coli (Pelzer, 1963), Micrococcus roseus (Petit et al., 1966) and

TABLE 9. *Inhibition of Cross-Linked Peptidoglycan Synthesis in G. homari by D-Amino Acids*[a]

Amino acid[b]	Inhibition (%)
D-Alanine	52
D-α-NH₂-n-Butyric acid	53
D-Norleucine	70
D-Norvaline	70
D-Leucine	77
D-Valine	63
Glycine	41
D-Threonine	61
D-Serine	53
D-Cysteine	60
D-Methionine	73
D-Asparagine	55
D-Lysine	55
D-Ornithine	63
D-Phenylalanine	80
D-Histidine	63
Trifluoro-D-alanine	79
β-Chloro-D-alanine	60
D-Glutamate	3
D-Aspartate	9

[a]Reprinted with permission from Hammes, W. P. *Eur. J. Biochem.* **91**: 501–507 (1978). Copyright 1978, Springer-Verlag, New York.

[b]The D-amino acids were tested at a concentration of 8.3 mM in an assay for the synthesis of cross-linked wall peptidoglycan using membrane-walls from G. homari.

TABLE 10. *Inhibition by D-Methionine Analogues of Cross-Linked Peptidoglycan Synthesis in Membrane-Walls from G. homari*[a]

Analogue[b]	Inhibition (%)
D-Methionine	66
D-Ethionine	62
DL-Selenomethionine	76
DL-Methionine sulfone	52
DL-Methionine sulfoxide	61
DL-Methionine sulfoximine	32
DL-Allylglycine	61

[a]Neuhaus, unpublished observations.
[b]The analogues of D-methionine were tested at 5×10^{-4} M D-isomer in an assay for the synthesis of cross-linked wall peptidoglycan using membrane-walls from *G. homari*.

Corynebacterium diphtheriae (Kato *et al.*, 1968). These tripeptide subunits are thought to result from the action of DD-carboxypeptidase and LD-carboxypeptidase. A second role relates to the transpeptidation activity catalyzed by the LD-carboxypeptidase (Hammes, 1978; Coyette *et al.*, 1974). It has been suggested that this enzyme catalyzes the synthesis of the atypical cross bridges in *Mycobacterium smegmatis* (Wietzerbin *et al.*, 1974) and the attachment of lipoprotein to peptidoglycan in *E. coli* (Beck and Park, 1976). In *G. homari*, it has been concluded that this enzyme may be one of those responsible for the sulfhydryl sensitivity and heat lability of the membrane-wall preparation (Neuhaus *et al.*, 1980). In this bacterium the LD-carboxypeptidase may play a role in the relationship between membrane and wall. Part of the LD-carboxypeptidase from *B. megaterium*, which is similar to that described in *G. homari*, is an intrinsic part of the cell wall (DasGupta and Fan, 1979). Thus, the extramembranal location of this enzyme suggests that active transport may not be a prerequisite for activity of an inhibitor of this enzyme.

One of the more effective D-amino acids for spheroplast formation is D-methionine. Lark and Lark (1959, 1961) established that this D-amino acid is incorporated into cell wall material during this process. In an attempt to optimize the effect of those features in D-methionine which contribute to the inhibitory activity on peptidoglycan synthesis, a number of D-methionine analogues were examined as potential analogues of D-alanine for inhibition of the synthesis of cross-linked peptidoglycan (Table 10). Analogues which are significantly more effective than D-methionine have not been found. The I_{50} for D-methionine is 5×10^{-4} M. As in the case of *E. coli* (Izaki *et al.*, 1966), D-methionine also caused the formation of water-soluble peptidoglycan with membrane-walls synthesizing peptidoglycan from *G. homari* (Fig. 11).

In a series of specificity studies, Ghuysen and coworkers (Ghuysen, 1977) have established that the DD-carboxypeptidase from *Streptomyces* R61 catalyzes the efficient transpeptidation of Ac$_2$-Lys-DAla from Ac$_2$-Lys-DAla-DAla to acceptor compounds including D-cycloserine. The participation of D-cycloserine as an acceptor in this system may represent an additional facet of its mode of action. Acting as an acceptor in transpeptidation, it becomes an efficient inhibitor of the hydrolytic reaction catalyzed by the DD-carboxypeptidase from this strain of *Streptomyces*. It was proposed by Nieto *et al.* (1973) that donor substrate analogues functioning as inhibitors of the enzyme may have antibacterial activity. As illustrated in Table 11, a number of analogues are good inhibitors of the DD-carboxypeptidase, e.g. Ac$_2$-Lys-DAla-D-cycloserine and Ac-DAla-DAsp. The inhibitors of this DD-carboxypeptidase were without effect on the DD-carboxypeptidase from strain R39. This enzyme was inhibited by a different group of peptides which included ε-Gly-α-Ac-Lys and ε-DAla-α-Ac-Lys (Perkins *et al.*, 1981). However, none of the substrate analogues which inhibited the R61 enzyme showed growth inhibition of *Streptomyces* R61. Thus, although this approach did not produce an effective growth inhibitor

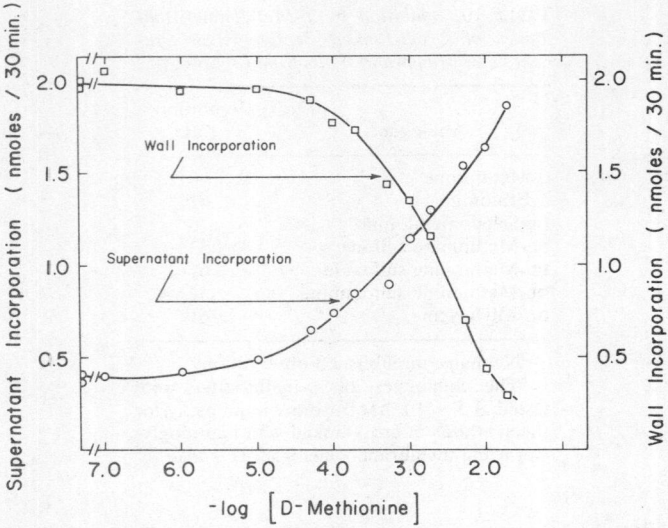

FIG. 11. Formation of water-soluble peptidoglycan in the presence of D-methionine. Increasing concentrations of D-methionine were incubated with membrane-walls from *G. homari* synthesizing wall peptidoglycan. Incorporation into the supernatant fraction (O——O) reflects the formation of water-soluble peptidoglycan. Wall incorporation (□——□) is the amount of SDS-insoluble peptidoglycan formed (F. C. Neuhaus and W. P. Hammes, unpublished observation).

of this organism, this approach might prove to be a productive one with other micro-organisms.

It is suggested that inhibition of either LD-carboxypeptidase or DD-carboxypeptidase by analogues of D-alanine represents a potential approach for designing agents that interfere with cell wall synthesis. Inhibition of these enzymes in organisms such as *G. homari* results in nascent peptidoglycan that is defective and hence cannot be cross-linked with the preexisting peptidoglycan of the cell wall. In the presence of glycine and a number of D-amino acids, nascent peptidoglycan is released as soluble peptidoglycan into the reaction medium, an observation similar to that of penicillin (Neuhaus and Hammes, unpublished observation).

TABLE 11. *Activity of the Exocellular* DD-*Carboxypeptidase from* Streptomyces *Strain R61 in the Presence of Peptide Inhibitors*

Peptide	Activity as substrate (%)	%[a] Inhibition	Molar ratio inhibitor/ substrate
Ac$_2$-Lys-DAla-DAla	100	—	
Ac-DAla-DAla	1	9	10
Suc$_2$-Lys-DAla-DAla	16	43	12
Ac-DAla-DGlu	0	25	10
Ac$_2$-Lys-DAla-DGlu	10	—	
Suc$_2$-Lys-DAla-DGlu	0	32–46	10
Ac-Gly-DAla-DGlu	0	25	10
Ac-DAla-DAsp	0	38	10
Ac-racemic-cyclodiaminoadipic acid	0	26	17
Ac$_2$-Lys-DAla-D-cycloserine	16	43	5
α-Ac-Lys-DGlu-DAla	0	33–35	11.6
Ac$_2$-Lys-DGlu-DAla	0	34–36	14

[a]The potential peptide inhibitor was incubated in the presence of Ac$_2$-Lys-DAla-DAla and the DD-carboxypeptidase. The following compounds were neither substrates nor inhibitors at a concentration of greater than 10 times that of the standard substrate (Ac$_2$-Lys-DAla-DAla): Suc-DAla-DGlu; α-Ac-Lys-DAla-DGlu; Ac-*meso*-cyclodiamino-adipic acid; Ac$_2$-Lys-racemic-cyclodiaminoadipic acid; D-cycloserine; Suc-D-cycloser-ine; Ac-DAla-D-cycloserine; Suc-DAla-D-cycloserine. Reprinted with permission from Nieto, M., Perkins, H. R., Leyh-Bouille, M., Frère, J.-M. and Ghuysen, J.-M. *Biochem. J.* **131**: 163–171 (1973).

2.4. INHIBITION OF D-ALANYL-LIPOTEICHOIC ACID SYNTHESIS

A potential target for D-alanine analogues, which is independent of those described in peptidoglycan assembly, is the incorporation of D-alanine into lipoteichoic and wall teichoic acids of many gram-positive organisms. The replacement of D-alanine by an analogue or the inhibition of the incorporation process by an analogue may provide the basis for designing compounds that inhibit or modify the function of the polymer.

Lipoteichoic acids (LTA) are linear polymers of poly(glycerol phosphate) covalently linked to glycolipid (Wicken and Knox, 1975; Archibald, 1974; Lambert et al., 1977). The poly(glycerol phosphate) portion is selectively acylated with D-alanine ester residues (XXIX), and in some cases it is also substituted with glycosyl groups. Recent findings

$$
\left[\begin{array}{c} H\;\;\;H\;\;\;H \\ -C-C-C-O-P-O- \\ H\;\;\;\;\;\;\;H \\ \;\;\;\;\;|\;\;\;\;\;\;\;\;\;|\;O^- \\ \;\;\;\;\;O \\ \;\;\;\;\;|\;\;\;\;\;\;\;\;\;O \\ \;\;\;\;\;C{=}O \\ \;\;\;\;\;| \\ H-C-\overset{+}{N}H_3 \\ \;\;\;\;\;| \\ \;\;\;\;\;CH_3 \end{array} \right]_n
$$

(XXIX)

indicate that LTA plays an important functional role in a variety of cellular processes. These include assembly of wall polymers (Fiedler and Glaser, 1974; Bracha and Glaser, 1976; Hancock and Baddiley, 1976; Fischer et al., 1980), regulation of autolytic activity (Cleveland et al., 1975, 1976; Höltje and Tomasz, 1975) and control of the Mg^{2+} ion concentration for membrane-associated enzymes (Archibald, 1974; Lambert et al., 1977; Naumova, 1978). In at least two of these functions, the D-alanine ester residues appear to have an important role in modulating the activity of the LTA. Baddiley and co-workers (Heptinstall et al., 1970; Hughes et al., 1973; Archibald, 1974; Lambert et al., 1977) have proposed that the negatively charged polymer serves to chelate Mg^{2+} and, therefore, to maintain a high concentration of this cation near the membrane. The capacity of the polymer to chelate Mg^{2+} is regulated in part by the D-alanine ester residues which neutralize the anionic nature of the phosphodiester links. Recently, it was established by Fischer and co-workers that LTA containing D-alanyl residues did not function as an LTA carrier (Fischer et al., 1980). Thus, the controlled incorporation of D-alanine into this polymer may be an important feature regulating its function. Because of the importance of D-alanine to the function of these polymers, it is proposed that analogues and inhibitors of D-alanine incorporation may inhibit or modify a functional property of the LTA.

An excellent example of this general approach was discovered by Tomasz and co-workers (Tomasz et al., 1975; Tomasz and Höltje, 1977). Teichoic acids of *Diplococcus pneumoniae* contain choline which can be replaced with ethanolamine by growing the bacterium in the presence of ethanolamine rather than choline. In contrast to choline grown cells, ethanolamine grown cells are not lysed by penicillin even though they maintain the high penicillin sensitivity. The cell wall containing ethanolamine is completely resistant to the hydrolytic action of the pneumococcal autolysin. Thus, the replacement of choline in the teichoic acid by ethanolamine has had a significant effect on the autolytic capacity of the cell and the penicillin induced lysis. In analogy to this modification of teichoic acid, replacement of the D-alanine or the inhibition of the incorporation of D-alanine may also provide a change in functional activity of the LTA.

In *Lactobacillus casei* the incorporation of D-alanine into LTA is accomplished in the following two-step reaction sequence (Baddiley and Neuhaus, 1960; Reusch and Neuhaus, 1971; Linzer and Neuhaus, 1973; Neuhaus *et al.*, 1974; Brautigan *et al.*, 1981). In reaction 1, D-alanine is activated in the presence of ATP and the D-alanine-activating enzyme to form an enzyme · AMP-D-alanine complex with the release of PP_i. In reaction 2, the activated D-alanine is covalently linked to membrane acceptor in the presence of the D-alanine:membrane acceptor ligase. Recently, definitive evidence that the *in vitro* system catalyzes the incorporation of D-alanine covalently linked to the poly(glycerol phosphate) of D-alanyl–LTA has been presented (Childs and Neuhaus, 1980).

$$\text{enzyme} + \text{D-alanine} + \text{ATP} \rightleftharpoons \text{enzyme} \cdot \text{AMP-D-alanine} + PP_i \qquad (1)$$

enzyme · AMP-D-alanine + membrane acceptor
$$\rightarrow \text{D-alanyl–membrane acceptor} + \text{enzyme} + \text{AMP} \qquad (2)$$

Specificity studies with the D-alanine activating enzyme (Reaction 1) isolated from *Lactobacillus plantarum* (Baddiley and Neuhaus, 1960) indicated an absolute specificity for amino acids of the D-configuration. In addition to D-alanine, the enzyme activates

TABLE 12. *Inhibitor and Substrate Specificity Profile of D-Alanyl-LTA Synthesis in* L. casei

A. Substrate specificity[a]

Substrate	Activity (pmol/hr)	K_m (μM)
D-[^{14}C]Alanine	23.8	18
L-[^{14}C]Alanine	0.6[b]	
DL-α-NH$_2$-n-[^{14}C]butyric acid	0.96	850
D-α-[^{14}C]Ala-D-α-[^{14}C]Ala	0.0	

B. Inhibitor specificity

Analogue[c,d]	(K_i/K_m)[e]
(1) D-α-NH$_2$-n-butyric acid	78
β-Fluoro-D-alanine[f]	290
β-Chloro-D-alanine[f]	1200
D-Serine	1900
D-Cycloserine	39,000
(2) D-Alanine hydroxamate	39
D-α-NH$_2$-n-butyric acid hydroxamate	390
D-Alaninol	3900
β-Alanine	12,000

[a]The alanine incorporation assay was used with membranes and supernatant fraction from *L. casei* and the labeled substrate (72 μM). The values of K_m were determined from Lineweaver–Burk plots. Reprinted with permission from Reusch, V. M. Jr. and Neuhaus, F. C. *J. Biol. Chem.* **246**: 6136–6143 (1971). Copyright 1971, American Society of Biological Chemists, Inc.

[b]The low activity with L-alanine is the result of alanine racemase. This activity is inhibited by D-cycloserine.

[c]Reprinted with permission from Reusch, 1971.

[d]The following compounds are inactive: O-carbamoyl-D-serine, DL-α-aminoethylphosphonic acid, β-aminoxy D-alanine, D-threonine, D-isoleucine, N-acetyl-D-alanine.

[e]K_i/K_m is the ratio of the inhibitor constant established from Lineweaver–Burk plots to the K_m of D-alanine in the incorporation system.

[f]Childs, Taron and Neuhaus, unpublished results.

D-α-NH$_2$-n-butyric acid (14.6%) and D-serine (7.5%) when compared with D-alanine at equimolar concentrations. No other D-amino acid tested was active in this reaction. In specificity studies of D-alanine incorporation into LTA, D-α-NH$_2$-n-butyric showed 4% of the activity observed with D-alanine when tested at equimolar concentrations (Table 12A). The K_m for D-alanine is 18 μM whereas the K_m for D-α-NH$_2$-n-butyric acid is 850 μM. These results indicate a high degree of specificity for D-alanine. Thus, the analogue, D-α-NH$_2$-n-butyric acid, can replace D-alanine only if high concentrations are present (Reusch and Neuhaus, 1971). The high specificity for D-alanine is further documented with inhibitor studies.

In Table 12B, an inhibitor specificity profile of the D-alanine incorporation system (reactions 1 and 2) is summarized. Most of these analogues have been established to be inhibitors of peptidoglycan synthesis (see Sections 2.1., 2.2.). For example, D-cycloserine, O-carbamoyl-D-serine, L- and D-1-aminoethylphosphonic acids, β-aminoxy-D-alanine, β-chloro-D-alanine and β-fluoro-D-alanine are effective inhibitors of alanine racemase. Two analogues, D-cycloserine and D-1-aminoethylphosphonic acid are effective inhibitors of D-alanine:D-alanine ligase. Each of these analogues is either inactive or poor as an inhibitor of incorporation of D-alanine into LTA. The relative values of K_i/K_m are summarized for several analogues. The only analogues that inhibit the incorporation of D-alanine into D-alanyl-LTA are D-α-NH$_2$-n-butyric acid, β-fluoro-D-alanine, D-alanine hydroxamate and D-α-NH$_2$-n-butyric hydroxamate. In each case, however, the inhibitory activity is poor. The conclusion from these studies is that the incorporation system has an extremely high degree of selectivity for D-alanine. Thus, the design of analogues of D-alanine, specific either for inhibition of incorporation or as replacements of the D-alanine residue, will be considerably more difficult than designing analogues of D-alanine as inhibitors for the assembly of peptidoglycan.

3. USE AND LIMITATIONS OF THE TRANSPORT SYSTEMS FOR ALANINE ANALOGUES

In order to reach their targets, those analogues of alanine that interfere with the alanine branch of peptidoglycan synthesis must be transported into the cell. The specificity determinants exerted by the respective transport systems are as important as those exerted by the target enzyme(s). Part of the success achieved with D-cycloserine, fluoro-D-alanine, and alafosfalin can be correlated with the efficient, active transport of these compounds. The transport systems that are critical to the action of these analogues are summarized in Table 13. Different bacterial sensitivities to an antimicrobial agent, even though the target enzyme has the same sensitivity, can be reconciled in many cases with differences in the specificity determinants exerted by the transport system (penetration barriers) (Franklin, 1973). Resistance to these analogues may reflect defects in the relevant transport system, as was observed with D-cycloserine (Wargel et al., 1971;

TABLE 13. *Transport Systems in E. coli for Alanine Analogues*

Systems	Analogue transported
(1) D-Alanine · glycine	D-Cycloserine, D-Serine, β-Fluoro-D-alanine[a] β-Chloro-D-alanine[a]
(2) Dipeptide system	Alafosfalin, DNva-DAla
(3) Oligopeptide system	Phosphono oligopeptides [(Amino acid)$_n$ − LAla(P)]

[a]Not established.

Reitz *et al.*, 1967). Clearly, the transport of the alanine analogue is of major importance in accounting for the bacterial specificity and effectiveness of these agents.

3.1. D-Alanine Transport System

The removal and reutilization of D-alanine from the extramembranal sites of wall assembly plays an important role in the cellular economy of the bacterium. D-Alanine occupies a unique position in the transport of amino acids. It is a product in the reactions catalyzed by peptidoglycan transpeptidase, DD-carboxypeptidase and LD-carboxypeptidase. Thus, it must be transported for reutilization by the cell (Chang, 1978). In *E. coli*, D-alanine is also a substrate for the D-alanine inducible dehydrogenase (Franklin and Venables, 1976; Wild *et al.*, 1974), one of the enzymes that is involved in driving active transport in this organism (Kaczorowski *et al.*, 1975a,b). Similarly, in *Bacillus subtilis* D-alanine is also required to support endogenous active transport under non-growing conditions (Clark and Young, 1978). It is concluded that the capacity for D-alanine transport is found in many genera of bacteria and that it is a prerequisite for the use of D-alanine analogues as antibacterial agents. The design of such analogues, which have their effect in the cytosol, must accommodate the specificity determinants that are exerted by this transport system. In the case of the D-alanine transport system, the latitude of specificity allows one to introduce only a limited number of D-alanine analogues into the cell.

In *E. coli*, the accumulation of D-alanine, L-alanine, and glycine is mediated by at least two transport systems. The systems for D-alanine and glycine are related, and are separate from that involved in the accumulation of L-alanine (Schwartz *et al.*, 1959; Kessel and Lubin, 1963; Piperno and Oxender, 1968; Wargel *et al.*, 1970; Robbins and Oxender, 1973; Cosloy, 1973; Halpern, 1974; Lee *et al.*, 1975). Mutants defective in the transport of D-alanine and glycine lose 20% of their ability to transport L-alanine. This suggests that this fraction of L-alanine is accumulated by the D-alanine · glycine system(s) whereas the remainder is accumulated by the L-alanine system (Wargel *et al.*, 1971). The role of these systems in the action of alanine analogues is summarized schematically in Fig. 12. In *Lactobacillus casei*, Leach and Snell (1960) established the existence of a transport system

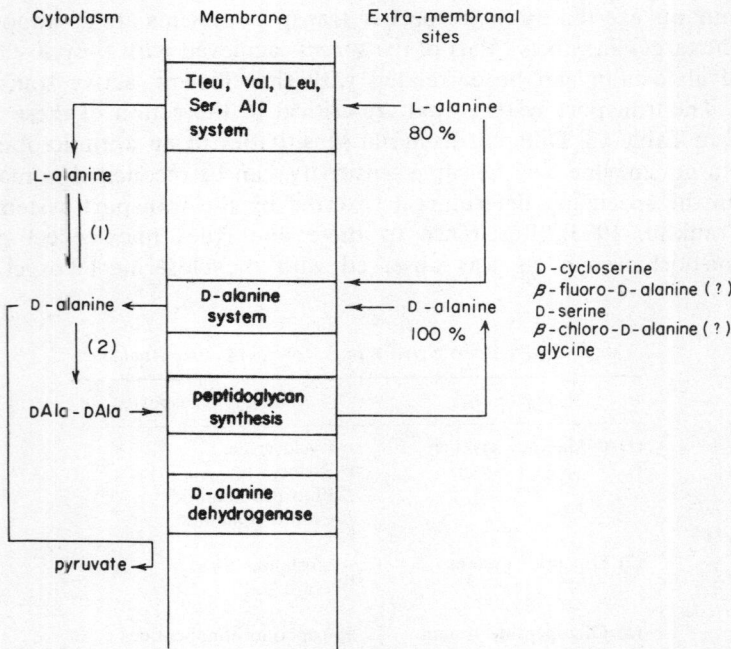

Fig. 12. The D-alanine-glycine transport system in *E. coli*. Enzyme (1) and (2) are alanine racemase and D-alanine:D-alanine ligase, respectively.

for L- and D-alanine and a separate system for D-alanine and glycine. A similar system for alanine and glycine also exists in *B. subtilis* (Clark and Young, 1974) which accumulates D-serine and D-cycloserine. In *M. tuberculosis* a single system transports D- and L-alanine, glycine, D-serine, D-cycloserine, and O-carbamoyl-D-serine (David, 1971). With *S. faecalis*, Mora and Snell (1963) concluded that a single transport system, which also accumulates D-cycloserine, is responsible for the accumulation of glycine, L-alanine and D-alanine. Membrane vesicles from *S. aureus* (Short *et al.*, 1972a,b), *B. subtilis* (Konings and Freese, 1972) and *E. coli* (Lombardi and Kaback, 1972) transport glycine, L- and D-alanine, and D-serine over a single system.

The importance of the specificity determinants exerted by the D-alanine transport system is further documented by the existence of analogues which are good enzyme inhibitors but show poor antibacterial activity. For example, O-carbamoyl-D-serine, which is a good inhibitor of alanine racemase (Lambert and Neuhaus, 1972), is a poor antibacterial agent because it is not accumulated by the D-alanine · glycine transport system (Wargel *et al.*, 1970). Apparently it is transported poorly by a different system. Another example of an alanine analogue that is poorly transported is O-acetyl-D-serine. Although it is an effective inhibitor of alanine racemase (Wang and Walsh, 1978), it shows no antibacterial activity (Shoji *et al.*, 1968). A similar situation exists for L- and D-1-aminoethylphosphonic acids. Only poor antibacterial activity (see exceptions 2.1) is observed for these isomers (Dulaney, 1970) even though these analogues are inhibitors of alanine racemase. D-1-Aminoethylphosphonic acid also inhibits D-alanine:D-alanine ligase (ADP) (see Section 2.1.). Holden *et al.* (1968) reported the active transport of DL-1-aminoethylphosphonic acid in *L. plantarum* and *S. faecalis*. Only by coupling the analogue with an amino acid or peptide is this analogue accumulated well. Thus, specificity determinants of the D-alanine transport system limit the potential number of D-alanine analogues which will be effective antibacterial agents.

3.2. DIPEPTIDE TRANSPORT SYSTEM

The dipeptide transport system(s) has become a focal point of interest in attempts to deliver analogues of alanine into the target cell. For example, one of the major factors in the efficacy of L-1-aminoethylphosphonic acid is its active accumulation as alafosfalin via the dipeptide transport system (Atherton *et al.*, 1979b). At least one naturally occurring antibiotic, bacilysin, requires its active accumulation via this system. Bacilysin (tetaine) (XXX) is a dipeptide of L-alanine and anticapsin (XXXI) that is actively accumulated. It is hydrolyzed to anticapsin, an inhibitor of glucosamine synthetase, and L-alanine (Kenig and Abraham, 1976; Kenig *et al.*, 1976; Chmara and Borowski, 1973; Perry and Abraham, 1979). The structure of this dipeptide bears some similarities to that of alafosfalin, i.e. the Ala-L-configuration of the dipeptide.

The similarities in antagonism specificities and resistance mechanisms suggest that bacilysin, alafosfalin, and the DAla-DAla analogue (DNva-DAla) are all actively accumulated via the dipeptide transport system.

The existence of a separate permease for dipeptides in *E. coli* is indicated by: (1) results of competition studies, (2) differences in structural requirements for the transport of

(XXX)   **(XXXI)**

dipeptides and oligopeptides and (3) the isolation of appropriate mutants coupled with genetic mapping (Payne and Gilvarg, 1971; Payne, 1975; Payne and Gilvarg, 1978). In competition studies it was found that dipeptides compete with tripeptide uptake whereas tripeptides do not compete with dipeptide uptake. Thus, the transport of dipeptides can be accomplished by both the dipeptide and oligopeptide transport systems. For active accumulation of a dipeptide, a free C-terminal carboxyl group is required. For the α-N-terminal, an N-alkyl substituent but not an N-acyl is tolerated. The dipeptide transport system prefers amino acid residues of the L-configuration (Kessel and Lubin, 1963; Payne, 1976; Payne and Gilvarg, 1971). However, prevention of either D-cycloserine or β-chloro-D-alanine induced lysis by DAla-DAla implies that this dipeptide is also taken up from the medium (Chambers *et al.*, 1963; Manning *et al.*, 1974). Moreover, the observation that DAla-DAla is an inhibitor of Gly-Gly transport (Kessel and Lubin, 1963) implies that DAla-DAla may be transported via the dipeptide system. The hetero-stereoisomers of alanyl-alanine, Ala-DAla and DAla-Ala, compete moderately well with Gly-Gly for uptake (Kessel and Lubin, 1963). Although the LL-stereoisomer is favored by the dipeptide system, changes in configuration in the two centers of asymmetry can be tolerated to some extent in the dipeptide transport system of *E. coli*. Thus, the specificity studies of dipeptide transport illustrate the degree of discrimination exerted against possible dipeptides containing an analogue of alanine. The use of DNva-DAla as a means of introducing D-norvaline into position 4 of the peptide subunit is subject to these specificity determinants (see section 2.2.).

Of three dipeptides with potential antimicrobial activity (DNva-DAla, DAbu-DAla, and DVal-DAla), only DNva-DAla inhibited the growth of *E. coli* K12 and W (Neuhaus *et al.*, 1977). The effect of increasing concentrations of DNva-DAla in the presence of 5×10^{-6} M D-cycloserine is illustrated (Fig. 13). Under these conditions, this concentration of D-cycloserine does not inhibit bacterial growth; however, it acts synergistically with the dipeptide, presumably by decreasing the synthesis of the normal dipeptide, DAla-DAla. In the absence of D-cycloserine, 2×10^{-3} M DNva–DAla is required to effect the same degree of growth inhibition as 2×10^{-4} M DNva-DAla in the presence of D-cycloserine (Fig. 13A,B).

It is of interest to ask which dipeptides will antagonize the effect exerted by DNva-DAla. Prevention of lysis with DD-dipeptides that are analogues of DAla-DAla is summarized in Table 14. Except for DVal-DAla and DAla-DVal each of the peptides has some

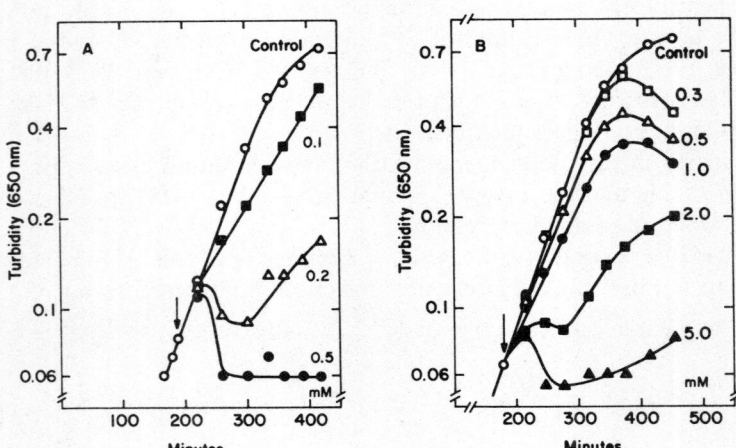

Fig. 13. Growth studies with *E. coli* W. Effect of increasing concentrations of DNva-DAla in the presence of 5×10^{-6} M D-cycloserine (A) and in the absence of D-cycloserine (B). (A) Concentrations of DNva-DAla were: 1×10^{-4} M (■), 2×10^{-4} M (△), and 5×10^{-4} M (●); (B) concentrations were: 3×10^{-4} M (□), 5×10^{-4} M (△), 1×10^{-3} M (●), 2×10^{-3} M (■) and 5×10^{-3} M (▲). (Reprinted with permission from Neuhaus, F. C., Goyer, S. and Neuhaus, D. W. *Antimicrob. Agents Chemother.* **11:** 638–644 (1977). Copyright 1977, American Society for Microbiology.)

TABLE 14. *Prevention of* DNva-DAla-*Induced Lysis in*
E. coli W[a]

Dipeptide addition	Growth response turbidity[b]
Expt 1.	
Control	0.64
DNva-DAla	0.05
DNva-DAla + DAbu-DAla	0.38
DNva-DAla + DAla-DAbu	0.53
DNva-DAla + DAla-DNva	0.48
DNva-DAla + DAla-DVal	0.10
DNva-DAla + DVal-DAla	0.08
DNva-DAla + DAla-DAla	0.64
Expt 2.	
Control	0.69
DNva-DAla	0.08
DNva-DAla + Gly-Gly	0.66
DNva-DAla + Ala-Ala	0.31
DNva-DAla + Nva-Ala	0.48

[a]Reprinted with permission from Neuhaus, F. C., Goyer, S. and Neuhaus, D. W. *Antimicrob. Agents Chemother.* **11**: 638–644 (1977). Copyright 1977, American Society for Microbiology.
[b]Turbidity represents the growth response in the presence of 5×10^{-6} M D-cycloserine 210 min after the addition of 5×10^{-4} M dipeptide.

ability to prevent DNva-DAla induced lysis when tested at equimolar concentrations. An interesting feature of this experiment is that DAla-DNva prevents the lytic action induced by DNva-DAla. The second part of this experiment indicates a more important aspect of this problem. The prevention of lysis is not restricted to dipeptides of the DD-configuration. Gly-Gly, Ala-Ala and Nva-Ala also have the ability to prevent the inhibitory activity exerted by DNva-DAla. Two interpretations of these data may be considered. The antagonizing dipeptide either inhibits the uptake of DNva-DAla or it effectively competes with DNva-DAla for addition to UDP-MurNAc-tripeptide in the reaction catalyzed by UDP-MurNAc-tripeptide:DAla-DAla ligase. However, since specificity studies with this enzyme eliminate LL-dipeptides as substrates for this enzyme, it would appear that these dipeptides inhibit the uptake of DNva-DAla.

The active accumulation of D[^{14}C]Ala-D[^{14}C]Ala is illustrated in Fig. 14A. The addition of either Ala-Ala or Gly-Gly markedly inhibits the uptake of D[^{14}C]Ala-D[^{14}C]Ala. Likewise, DNva-DAla inhibits the transport of this labeled dipeptide by 80%. In a similar experiment, the time course of [^{14}C]Gly-[^{14}C]Gly uptake was examined (Fig. 14B). Both DAla-DAla and DNva-DAla significantly reduce the accumulation of this dipeptide. On the basis of these results, it would appear that Gly-Gly and DAla-DAla are transported by a common system, a result that was implied from the inhibition data presented by Kessel and Lubin (1963). Additional specificity studies demonstrated that DVal-DAla was poorly transported relative to DNva-DAla, explaining why no antibacterial activity was observed with this analogue. These results as well as the results obtained in the study with the DD-dipeptide as an antibacterial agent suggest that the dipeptide transport system plays an essential role in the antibacterial action of DNva-DAla. However, the low antibacterial activity of DNva-DAla reflects the low rate of transport of the DD-dipeptide over the dipeptide transport system in *E. coli* W (Neuhaus *et al.*, 1977).

The dipeptide transport system plays a major role in the uptake of alafosfalin. In mutants lacking this dipeptide system, no transport of Ala-LAla(P) was detected; thus, no antibacterial activity was observed (Atherton *et al.*, 1979a). The involvement of the dipeptide system in the accumulation of alafosfalin was further supported by the finding that the antibacterial activity and transport was antagonized by Ala-Ala (Atherton *et al.*, 1979b). The tetrapeptide, (Ala)$_4$, and dipeptides containing D-amino acid residues did not

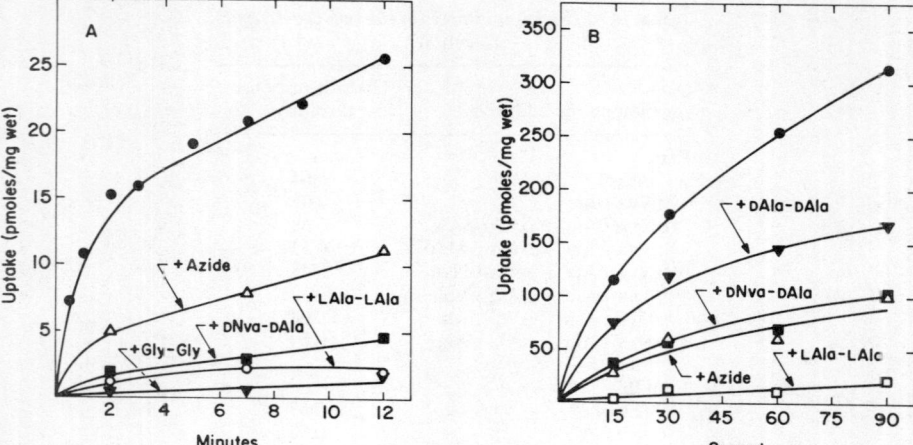

Fig. 14. Inhibition of DAla-DAla uptake (A) and Gly-Gly uptake (B) by dipeptide analogues and azide. (A) Concentration of D[^{14}C]Ala-D[^{14}C]Ala was 50 μM; (B) concentration of [^{14}C]Gly-[^{14}C]Gly was 50 μM. The concentration of sodium azide was 10 mM. In (A), either 10 mM DNva-DAla (■), 10 mM LAla-LAla (○), or 10 mM Gly-Gly (▼) was added; in (B), either 10 mM DAla-DAla (▼), 10 mM DNva-DAla (■), or 10 mM LAla-LAla (□) was added. (Reprinted with permission from Neuhaus, F. C., Goyer, S. and Neuhaus, D. W. *Antimicrob. Agents Chemother.* **11**: 638–644 (1977). Copyright 1977, American Society for Microbiology.)

compete at equimolar concentrations relative to alafosfalin (Atherton *et al.*, 1979*b*). Addition of D-alanine did not inhibit the active accumulation of Ala-LAla(P). From these data it may be concluded that the dipeptide system is responsible for accumulating alafosfalin.

3.3. Oligopeptide Transport System

During the past seven years, the oligopeptide transport system has also become a primary focus of interest in attempts at facilitating accumulation of analogues and substances that would otherwise be impermeant to the cell. For example, Fickel and Gilvarg (1973) and Ames *et al.* (1973) used this transport system to carry homoserine phosphate via the peptide, dilysyl-homoserine phosphate and histidinol phosphate via diglycyl-histidinol phosphate. These examples indicated a possible means for accumulating amino acid analogues as oligopeptidyl-analogues. Matthews and Payne (1975) coined the name "smugglins" for peptide complexes of this type. This approach was successfully used by Diddens *et al.* (1976, 1979) who accumulated (N$^{\epsilon}$-phosphono)methionine-S-sulfoximine via the tripeptide (N$^{\epsilon}$-phosphono)methionine-S-sulfoximinyl-Ala-Ala (XXXII). The methionine derivative is an inhibitor of glutamine synthetase. The Roche group has also successfully adapted this approach in designing carrier peptides for transporting L-1-aminoethylphosphonic acid into microbial cells.

Five characteristics of the transport process have been used to define the existence of a

(XXXII)

separate oligopeptide permease. These are: (1) distinct genetic loci for dipeptide per-mease(s) and oligopeptide permease genes; (2) oligopeptide permease mutants which still transport dipeptides; (3) dipeptides which use the oligopeptide permease but not vice versa; (4) the observation that the C-terminal carboxyl is only important in dipeptide transport and (5) the size restriction in oligopeptide transport (Payne and Gilvarg, 1971, 1978; Payne, 1975, 1976; Barak and Gilvarg, 1975). It was concluded that *E. coli* W, for example, has a single transport system that accommodates a wide variety of oligopeptides with only differences in affinity (Barak and Gilvarg, 1975). The size limit is generally manifested at the tetrapeptide, although it is strictly a function of the hydrodynamic volume (Barak and Gilvarg, 1975). Although hexaglycine is transported, the tetrapeptide, Lys-Lys-Lys-homoserine phosphate, is not. It is concluded that the limitation on size is imposed by pores of the outer membrane and not by the oligopeptide transport system in *E. coli* (Nikaido, 1980).

Another important feature of the oligopeptide transport system is its selectivity for the stereochemistry of the peptides. This feature must be considered in attempts at using the system to accumulate peptides with analogues of D-alanine. It was shown by Payne and Gilvarg (1971) that in a tripeptide, residues 1 and 2 must have the L-configuration whereas residue 3 may have either the L- or D-configuration. They indicated that 'steric wobble' may be accommodated in residue 3 of the tripeptide. This feature of the oligo-peptide transport system is important for designing peptides linked to analogues for accumulation by this system. In a study of *Pedicoccus cerevisiae*, Shankman *et al.* (1962) observed that Val-Val-DVal is transported by this organism whereas DVal-Val-Val and Val-DVal-Val appeared to be poorly transported by this organism.

In the case of the alanine analogue, L-1-aminoethylphosphonic acid, the covalent attachment of this compound to an oligopeptide, e.g. (Ala)$_{2-3}$, has increased its transport and antimicrobial activity in many organisms when compared to alafosfalin (Atherton *et al.*, 1979a). This increased antimicrobial activity reflects the enhanced accumulation of the analogue linked to the oligopeptide via the oligopeptide transport system (see Section 4.2.).

The results presented in this section clearly begin to define the scope and limitations which the transport systems impose on the types of analogues that can be accumulated. As will be described in Section 4, the selective cleavage of the analogue from the carrier peptide or amino acid will further restrict our ability to deliver an analogue via the dipeptide and oligopeptide transport systems. The following section will indicate how some of these restrictions can be circumvented and how some of the specificity features may be used to tailor an agent for a more defined antimicrobial spectrum. In summary, the challenge for the microbiologist is to rationally design agents around each of these restrictions.

4. ALANINE ANALOGUES AS ANTIBACTERIAL AGENTS

The search for new antibacterial agents is justified by our need for compounds with properties that are not found in the large number of those that are already available. These properties include: higher selective toxicity, broader or narrower antibacterial spectrum, lower degree of acquisition of resistance to the antibiotic, enhanced stability of the molecule, as well as more favorable pharmacokinetics. Our knowledge of the factors which determine these properties is limited; however, some important features have emerged which will help us to design more effective analogues of alanine as antibacterial agents.

4.1. SELECTIVE TOXICITY

Since the D-isomers of amino acids are not generally observed in eukaryotic metab-olism, one would expect that analogues of D-alanine should exert a higher degree of selective toxicity than the analogues of L-alanine. With D-cycloserine, however, neurotoxic side effects are shown that limit its usefulness as an antibacterial agent. Thus, the use of D-cycloserine has been minimal in view of the high dosage that is required for its therapeutic effectiveness. Dann and Carter (1964) attempted to correlate these neurotoxic effects with the marked increase of γ-aminobutyric acid in the brain upon administration of D-cycloserine. D-Cycloserine inhibits the γ-aminobutyric:α-ketoglutarate transaminase. However, it is highly probable that the mechanism of toxicity is more complex since the neurotoxicity is also associated with the urinary excretion of pyridoxine (Ito et al., 1958). This neurological toxicity can be partially reduced by the concomitant administration of large doses of pyridoxine with D-cycloserine.

In the case of fluoro-D-alanine, studies indicate that the tolerance of mice against the D-isomer (3.4 g/kg, per os) is at least 10-fold better than the L-isomer (Kollonitsch, 1978). The fluoro-D-alanine has been tested for safety in monkeys at up to 30 times the normal human dose without side effects (Kramer, 1975). The highly toxic fluoroacetyl-CoA, a possible degradation product of the fluoro-D-alanine, appears not to be formed. In fact, fluoride ions are excreted by rodents and Rhesus monkeys which are injected with fluoro-D-alanine, suggesting that the fluorine atom is removed in the degradation of the molecule (Kahan et al., 1975). Leung and Frey (1978) observed that the pyruvate dehydrogenase component of the pyruvate dehydrogenase complex from E. coli catalyzes the decomposition of fluoropyruvate to acetate and F^-. In a separate study of the pyruvate dehydrogenase complex, fluoropyruvate was shown to be a very strong competitive inhibitor of the reaction catalyzed by the complex (Bisswanger, 1980). These observations are consistent with the fact that fluoropyruvate is only one tenth as toxic as fluoroacetate in mice (Mager and Blank, 1954), and thus may explain why fluoro-D-alanine shows low toxicity.

Since L-alanine is a metabolite in all organisms, one would expect that analogues of the L-isomer might not be good candidates for the design of antimicrobial agents. However, the L-1-aminoethylphosphonic acid moiety of alafosfalin exhibits a surprisingly low order of toxicity (Allen et al., 1979b). For example, doses that would kill animals could not be determined because they exceeded the maximum amounts that could be administered per os (10,000 mg/kg in rats). Thus, one has to assume that L-1-aminoethylphosphonic acid specifically inhibits alanine racemase, an enzyme which is absent in eukaryotes, and that is not incorporated as an inhibitory L-alanine analogue into the metabolism of the host.

Each of these examples supports the conclusion that one cannot easily make predictions about selective toxicity of these analogues. In spite of the predicted specificity of the brain γ-aminobutyric-α-ketoglutaric transaminase, D-cycloserine is an effective inhibitor of this enzyme. The predicted selective toxicity of fluoro-D-alanine was in fact observed. On the other hand, the prediction that L-1-aminoethylphosphonic acid would be an antagonist of L-alanine metabolism in the host is incorrect. Apparently, there are few generalizations that one can draw concerning predictions of selective toxicity with these compounds.

4.2. ANTIBACTERIAL SPECTRA

D-Cycloserine, fluoro-D-alanine and alafosfalin each exhibit a characteristic antibacterial spectrum. For example, fluoro-D-alanine shows effective activity in inhibiting the growth of pathogenic bacteria of both gram-positive and gram-negative genera (Kahan, 1972; Kollonitsch et al., 1973). D-Cycloserine is also a "broad spectrum" antibiotic. In general, it is more effective against gram-positive bacteria than against gram-negative bacteria (Cuckler et al., 1955). Of particular importance was the discovery that D-cycloserine inhibits the growth of Mycobacterium tuberculosis. As a result it was observed by Epstein et al. (1955) and Lester et al. (1956) that D-cycloserine is effective in the treatment of tuberculosis in humans. However, because of the neurotoxicity of D-cycloserine at the required dose, D-cycloserine has been used only as an antibiotic of second or third

TABLE 15. *Antibacterial Activities of Alafosfalin and* LNva-LAla(P)[a]

Organism	MIC (μg/ml) Ala-LAla(P)	LNva-LAla(P)
E. coli NCIB 8879	1	0.03
K. aerogenes 331001	0.5	0.015
Enterobacter 250002	1	0.25
S. marcescens ATCC 14756	8	0.5
S. typhimurium 538003	4	0.25
H. influenzae NCTC 4560	32	4
P. mirabilis 502015	>128	16
P. aeruginosa NCIB 8295	>128	32
S. faecalis 585011	2	1
S. aureus NCIB 8625	32	8

[a]Reprinted with permission from Atherton, F. R., Hall, M. J., Hassall, C. H., Holmes, S. W., Lambert, R. W., Lloyd, W. J., and Ringrose, P. S. *Antimicrob. Agents Chemother.* **18:** 897–905 (1980). Copyright 1980, American Society for Microbiology.

choice. The combination of D-cycloserine with fluoro-D-alanine has been characterized as a "universal antibiotic" (Anon. 1975). Apparently, no bacterial strain has been found that is resistant to this combination, including *Pseudomonas aeruginosa* (Kropp *et al.*, 1975; Kramer, 1975; Kollonitsch, 1978).

Alafosfalin has a moderately broad spectrum of antibacterial activity, being more effective against gram-negative than gram-positive organisms. It is more active against *E. coli* than antibiotics commonly used in therapy and inhibits the growth of most strains resistant to agents such as ampicillin. Good levels of activity were found against *Klebsiella aerogenes, Enterobacter, Salmonella,* and *Serratia* species (Allen *et al.*, 1978; Traub, 1980). Generally strains of *Proteus* and *Pseudomonas* were less susceptible to alafosfalin than were other common gram-negative bacteria (Allen *et al.*, 1979a).

One of the unique features of L-1-aminoethylphosphonic acid as a toxophore of an antibacterial agent is the ability of the Roche group to modify its antibacterial spectrum. Thus, the covalent linking of L-1-aminoethylphosphonic acid to various carrier amino acids and peptides provides a new strategy in designing antibacterial agents with a specific antibacterial spectrum. As shown by Atherton *et al.* (1980) (Table 15), LNva-LAla(P) exhibits significantly higher antibacterial activity against a variety of organisms when compared with alafosfalin. For example, the activity against *Proteus* sp. was enhanced to an extent that this genus can be included into the sensitive organisms. It is

TABLE 16. *Antibacterial Activities of Phosphonodipeptides having the Formula* X-LAla(P) *in* E. coli NCIB 8879[a]

Residue X	MIC (μg/ml)	Residue X	MIC (μg/ml)
Orn	32	Cit	0.5
Gly	8	Met	0.25
αGlu	8	Arg	0.25
Gln	4	Leu	0.25
Ala	1	Abu	0.25
Ser	1	Nle	0.06
Trp	1	Nva	0.03
Tyr	1	Ahe[b]	0.03
His	0.5	Aoc[b]	0.015

[a]Reprinted with permission from Atherton, F. R., Hall, M. J., Hassall, C. H., Holmes, S. W., Lambert, R. W., Lloyd, W. J. and Ringrose, P. S., *Antimicrob. Agents Chemother.* **18:** 897–905 (1980). Copyright 1980, American Society for Microbiology.
[b]Abbreviations: Ahe, 2-aminoheptanoyl; Aoc, 2-amino-octanoyl.

TABLE 17. *Antibacterial Activity of Phosphono-Oligopeptides Y-(L-X)-LAla(P)*[a]

Organisms	Y^b = X =	Ala (−)	Ala $(Ala)_1$	Ala $(Ala)_2$	Sar $(Ala)_2$	Sar $(Nva)_2$	PGA $(Nva)_2$
E. coli NCIB 8879		0.5	0.5	0.12	0.03	0.25	0.03
K. aerogenes 331001		0.25	0.12	0.5	0.12	0.5	0.12
Enterobacter 250002		4	8		2	1	2
S. faecalis 585011		2	0.06	0.25	0.06	0.12	0.25
S. aureus NCIB 8625		32	8	32	>128	>128	4
S. marcescens ATCC 14756		8	4	4	1	8	4
S. typhimurium 538003		4	32	128	>128	8	2
H. influenzae NCTC 4560		32	<0.12	<0.12	0.03	0.03	0.06

The MIC (μg/ml) column group heads: Ala (−), Ala $(Ala)_1$, Ala $(Ala)_2$, Sar $(Ala)_2$, Sar $(Nva)_2$, PGA $(Nva)_2$.

[a]Reprinted with permission from Atherton, F. R., Hall, M. J., Hassall, C. H., Holmes, S. W., Lambert, R. W., Lloyd, W. J. and Ringrose, P. S., *Antimicrob. Agents Chemother.* **18**: 897–905 (1980). Copyright 1980, American Society for Microbiology.
[b]Abbreviations: L-sarcosyl, Sar; L-norvalyl, Nva; L-pyroglutamyl, PGA.

also of interest to compare the antibacterial activities of a series of phosphonodipeptides having the formula X-LAla(P). As shown in Table 16, in varying X from ornithine to 2-amino-octanoic acid, one can change the MIC from 32 μg to 0.015 μg/ml. These differences are most likely due to different rates of uptake and intracellular hydrolysis of the X-LAla(P).

In addition, marked effects on the antibacterial spectrum were also observed with different phosphono-oligopeptides (Atherton *et al.*, 1980). For example, although the activity against *Enterobacteriaceae* is often reduced, it is broadened to include high activity against *Haemophilus influenzae* and *Streptococcus faecalis* (Table 17) when compared with alafosfalin. Thus, the approaches used by the Roche group provide a rational basis for tailoring the antibacterial agent to a specific organism.

Nature has, in fact, anticipated the use of carrier peptides and amino acids as transport vehicles for toxophores (see Ringrose (1980) for a review). For example, bacilysin (see Section 3.2.) and plumbemycin A (XXXIII) (Park *et al.*, 1977) are two examples of inter-

(XXXIII)

est. The innovative adaptation of this principle to methionine analogues has been accomplished by Zähner and his colleagues (see Section 3.3.). Recently, Becker and his research group also used the peptide carrier concept to introduce analogues into yeast (Steinfeld *et al.*, 1979). Thus, the discovery by the Roche group of alafosfalin and the oligopeptide-LAla(P) represent additional examples of the practical utilization of the dipeptide and oligopeptide transport systems to accumulate analogues that would otherwise be impermeant to the cell.

4.3. Release of the Toxophore

The use of carriers for the accumulation of the toxophore in the bacterial cell requires the intracellular cleavage of the toxophore from the carrier. In the case of peptides, cleavage will be catalyzed by dipeptidases and aminopeptidases. This feature of specificity will severely limit our ability to transport and release D-toxophores by the carrier process. However, this procedure has been successfully applied to the accumulation of the L-toxophore, specifically L-1-aminoethylphosphonic acid.

The role of intracellular dipeptidases and aminopeptidases in the release of L-1-aminoethylphosphonic acid from alafosfalin is further confirmed by inhibition studies with bestatin, an inhibitor of aminopeptidase (Ringrose and Lloyd, 1979; Suda *et al.*, 1976). The intracellular cleavage of alafosfalin is inhibited by this compound. A survey of intracellular peptidases reveals little specificity for the particular L-amino acid residue (Miller, 1975). For example, dipeptides containing almost any of the standard L-amino acids or glycine can be hydrolyzed by whole cells, cell extracts and partially purified enzyme preparations from *E. coli* K and *E. coli* B. The most highly purified *E. coli* peptidase is aminopeptidase I which is similar to leucine aminopeptidase (Vogt, 1970). This enzyme will hydrolyze a variety of tripeptides and dipeptides at different efficiencies.

Microbial peptidases are generally specific for peptide bonds formed from L-amino acid residues (Payne and Gilvarg, 1978; Miller, 1975). The highly purified dipeptidase from *E. coli* B shows a wide specificity for L-amino acids. Dipeptides with D-amino acids, e.g. DLeu-Gly and Gly-DLeu, are competitive inhibitors (Patterson *et al.*, 1973). In a similar manner, the dipeptidocarboxypeptidase from *E. coli* does not cleave oligopeptides with D-alanine residues (Yaron *et al.*, 1972). There are few exceptions to this generalization. The importance of this specificity feature is illustrated from the observation of Shankman *et al.* (1960) that only one-half of the L-valine content of Val-Val-DVal is available for utilization. This observation implies that the resulting Val-DVal is not hydrolyzed by the two test organisms. *S. faecalis* and *L. plantarum.* Hanson *et al.* (1969) also concluded that dipeptides containing D-amino acids were not hydrolyzed. This selective discrimination by peptidase(s) is also illustrated with Ala-Ala-DAla-LAla(P). Although this oligopeptidyl-analogue is transported, the peptidase(s) does not release L-1-aminoethylphosphonic acid (Atherton *et al.*, 1979a). One exception to this generalization is the observation by Kihara *et al.* (1961) that *S. faecalis* shows good growth on DAla-Ala and DAla-Gly whereas no growth is observed for Ala-DAla. This result implies that these dipeptides are cleaved. Payne and Gilvarg (1978) indicated that there may be other interpretations for these results. The utilization of D-phenylglycyl-glycine by *E. coli* has been described by Pfeifer *et al.* (1980). This dipeptide containing a residue with the D-configuration is cleaved by a dipeptidase located either in the outer membrane, in the periplasmic space or at the outer surface of the cytoplasmic membrane. Additional exceptions to the above generalization include enzymes involved in peptidoglycan assembly, e.g. LD-carboxypeptidase and DD-carboxypeptidase (see section 2.3). Thus, it may be concluded that carrier peptides and amino acids linked to D-alanine analogues might be expected to lack antibacterial activity even though they are actively accumulated.

In spite of the conclusion developed in the previous paragraph, Neuhaus and co-workers have attempted to enhance the antimicrobial activity of DNva-DAla and O-carbamoyl-D-serine by linking these analogues to the carrier peptide Gly-Gly in an attempt to enhance accumulation of these analogues via the oligopeptide transport system. Each of these oligopeptides, Gly-Gly-DNva-DAla and Gly-Gly-O-carbamoyl-D-serine, showed no antibacterial activity. This lack of activity may be the result of either inability to accumulate the peptide or of inability to cleave the peptide to release the D-analogue. Thus, it has been tentatively concluded that the use of D-analogues linked to carrier peptides by peptide linkages is not a useful approach for transporting and releasing D-analogues into the cell.

A second consideration in the use of peptide carriers, which may limit the antibacterial efficacy of phosphonopeptides, concerns the liberation of the toxophore by peptidase action in the host. The release of the toxophore by intestinal peptidase(s) (first-pass metabolism) is lower in humans than in animals. In contrast, when alafosfalin is administered parenterally the increased plasma level per dose reflects the bypass of intestinal peptidases. A great variability in ED_{50} values in mouse septicemia can be observed by applying different L-X-LAla(P) phosphonodipeptides *per os* or *s.c.* In addition, substituting L-X- with either the sarcosyl or pyroglutamyl group enhanced the *in vivo* activity, presumably by limiting peptidase action in first-pass metabolism (Atherton *et al.*, 1980). As indicated previously, bacteria, e.g. *E. coli*, do not appear to have broad capacity to hydrolyze peptide bonds adjacent to D-amino acid residues. In contrast, kidney tissue has the enzymic capacity to hydrolyze certain peptides containing D-amino-acid residues, e.g. Gly-DLeu and DLeu-Gly (Felicetti and Hanson, 1970a,b). The highly purified renal dipeptidase from hog kidney is active on dipeptides in which the C-terminal amino acid has either the D- or L-configuration whereas it requires that the N-terminal amino acid has the L-configuration (Robinson *et al.*, 1953; Campbell *et al.*, 1966). Thus, metabolism in various tissues is a second feature that must be considered in the use of peptide carriers for transporting the toxophore to the target cell.

4.4. SYNERGISTIC COMBINATIONS

Combination therapy with two agents that act synergistically provides a useful approach for utilizing analogues that alone require relatively high concentrations for antibacterial activity. Table 18 summarizes some of the combinations that have been tested with emphasis on those combinations that have multiple targets in cell wall assembly.

Combinations of antibacterials are not only used to achieve potentiation of sensitivity to antibiotics, but also to reduce the probability of emergence of resistance. Moreover, combinations of antimicrobial agents can broaden the antibacterial spectrum in order to treat infections due to multiple causes. Finally, a major consideration for combination therapy is indicated when one of the agents is toxic in high levels. Thus, synergistic combinations of alanine analogues provide a promising approach for enhancing the clinical efficacy of these compounds (Stuart-Harris, 1979; Woodbine, 1977; Drews, 1979; Wise, 1979; Lacey, 1958) (see Section 4.6.).

The use of fluoro-D-alanine is limited by the high concentrations required to achieve antibacterial activity and by its autoantagonistic activity (Kollonitsch *et al.*, 1973). In the presence of D-cycloserine, the activity of fluoro-D-alanine is greatly potentiated. For example, complete inhibition of the growth of *E. coli* 2017 requires a minimum concentration of 25 μg/ml D-cycloserine and a minimum concentration of 3.12 μg/ml of β-fluoro-D-alanine (Kahan, 1972, 1977). In combination, complete inhibition is achieved with only 1.56 μg/ml of D-cycloserine and 1.56 μg/ml of β-fluoro-D-alanine. This represents a two-

TABLE 18. *Synergistic Combinations*[a]

1. β-Chloro-D-alanine	Penicillin	Soper and Manning (1976)
2. DNva-DAla	D-Cycloserine	Neuhaus *et al.* (1977)
3. DNva-DAla	β-Fluoro-D-alanine	Neuhaus (unpublished observation)
4. β-Fluoro-D-alanine	D-Cycloserine	Kahn (1977); Kropp *et al.* (1975)
5. Alafosfalin	D-Cycloserine	Allen *et al.* (1978)
6. Alafosfalin	Ampicillin Mecillinam Cephalexin	Allen *et al.* (1978; 1979a) Wise (1979) Greenwood and Vincent (1980)
7. D-Methionine	Penicillin	Lark and Lark (1959)
8. O-Carbamoyl-D-serine	D-Cycloserine	Tanaka and Umezawa (1964)
9. Mecillinam	Ampicillin	Baltimore *et al.* (1976) Grunberg *et al.* (1976)
10. L-Cycloserine	D-Cycloserine	Neuhaus (1967)
11. D-Cycloserine	Penicillin	Neuhaus (1967)
12. L-2-Amino-3-butynoic acid	D-Cycloserine	Kuroda *et al.* (1980a,b)

[a]This does not mean that this combination is synergistic for all bacteria.

fold reduction in the concentration of β-fluoro-D-alanine and a 15-fold reduction in the concentration of D-cycloserine. As a result of this decrease in D-cycloserine concentration, the neurotoxic side effects of this antibiotic may no longer limit its application. A second advantage to this combination derives from the inhibition of the autoantagonist (self reversal) activity of fluoro-D-alanine (Kahan, 1972, 1977). Although 3.2 μg/ml of fluoro-D-alanine completely inhibits growth of *E. coli* (2017), 50 μg/ml allows growth. Thus, even though alanine racemase (Enzyme 1, Fig. 1) is inhibited, the fluoro-D-alanine apparently participates in the reaction catalyzed by D-alanine:D-alanine ligase (Enzyme 2, Fig. 1). It is presumed that fluoro-DAla-fluoro-DAla is ligated to UDP-MurNAc-tripeptide for the synthesis of UDP-MurNAc-difluoro-pentapeptide (Kahan and Kropp, 1975). Thus, D-cycloserine was added to inhibit the autoantagonistic (self reversal) activity of the fluoro-D-alanine. This is possible since one of the primary sites of D-cycloserine action is D-alanine:D-alanine ligase (see Section 2.1). Thus, the combination of these analogues has achieved two results: (1) significant synergy resulting in significant reductions of both fluoro-D-alanine and D-cycloserine that are required; (2) inhibition of self-reversal by fluoro-D-alanine.

The second combination in this area that illustrates some unique features is the combination of alafosfalin and β-lactams. As summarized in Table 18, mecillinam, cephalexin and ampicillin have been combined individually with alafosfalin. In a study of 400 clinical isolates, gram-negative genera showed synergy (FIC index < 0.5) in about 25% of the strains (Hall *et al.*, 1979). The remainder showed weak synergy to additive effects. Little synergy was found with *S. faecalis* although with the other gram-positive genera synergy was greater than with *Enterobacteriaceae*. Synergy was observed in 15 to 83% of the different genera with the most effective synergism observed in *S. marcescens* SM7 (FIC index = 0.062) (Allen *et al.*, 1979a). An important consequence of the synergy of alafosfalin with β-lactams was the ability of the combination to lyse morphological variants which develop after treatment with β-lactams at sub-MIC levels (Greenwood, D. cited in Hall *et al.*, 1979). Another feature is that regrowth and hence resistance development can be largely prevented by combining phosphonopeptides with β-lactam antibiotics. This will be an important consideration in Section 4.5.

The enthusiasm generated by these two combinations, fluoro-D-alanine/D-cycloserine and alafosfalin/β-lactam, may be tempered as pharmacokinetic studies are published. Combinations which are synergistic in a test tube are not necessarily synergistic in a patient. Nevertheless, the potential clinical efficacy of such combinations warrants continued evaluation of this approach.

4.5. Acquisition of Resistance

The emergence of microbial strains that are resistant to antibacterial agents obviously limits the therapeutic value of these agents. This feature has been clearly demonstrated for penicillin. Thus, it becomes of some importance to establish the mechanisms by which these strains acquire resistance. With this information it then becomes necessary to either circumvent the process for selection of resistant strains or inhibit the enzymic process which confers resistance to the organism.

Of the various mechanisms by which bacteria may acquire resistance (see e.g. Davis and Maas, 1952; Moyed, 1964), only two appear to be relevant in our review of alanine analogues, namely decreased accumulation of the analogue and either increased concentration of the target enzyme or increased concentration of the competing substrate. The former may be more important, i.e. a defective transport system for the analogue. There is no indication that any of the resistance mechanisms for alanine analogues is determined by an R factor.

D-Cycloserine resistant mutants have been isolated from a variety of bacterial strains (Curtiss *et al.*, 1965; Howe *et al.*, 1964; Kessel and Lubin, 1965; Reitz *et al.*, 1967; Wargel *et al.*, 1971; Miller and Rheins, 1971; David, 1971). In the case of the D-cycloserine resistant mutants from *E. coli*, resistance generally results from a defective D-alanine–glycine

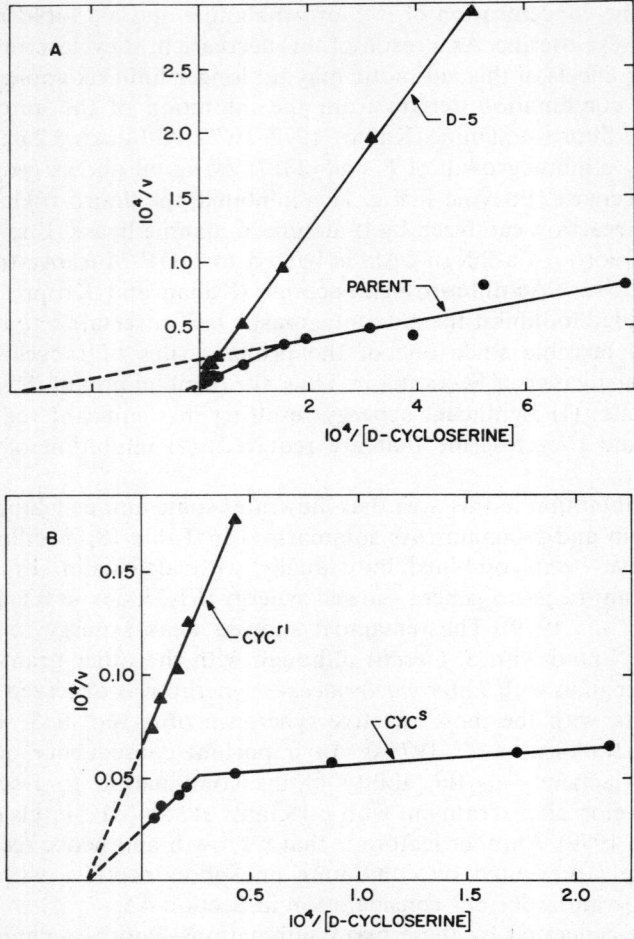

FIG. 15. Lineweaver–Burk plots of the uptake of D-[^{14}C]cycloserine in *E. coli* W and D-5(A) and in *E. coli* cyc^s and cyc^{rl}(B). D-5 is a multistep D-cycloserine resistant (80 fold) strain derived from *E. coli* W and cyc^{rl} is a single step D-cycloserine resistant (25 fold) strain derived from *E. coli* K-12 (cyc^s). (Reprinted with permission from Wargel, R. C., Shadur, C. A. and Neuhaus, F. C. *J. Bacteriology* **105**: 1028–1035 (1971). Copyright 1971, American Society for Microbiology.)

transport system (Wargel *et al.*, 1971). For example, a multistep mutant (D5, Fig. 15A) which is 80-fold resistant to D-cycloserine when compared with the parent, has lost >90% of its transport activity for D-alanine and glycine. A single step mutant (cyc^{rl}, Fig. 15B) from R. Curtiss with a 24-fold increase in D-cycloserine resistance has lost 70% of its transport capacity for these amino acids. The mutation conferring this resistance is located at min 83 on the *E. coli* K-12 genetic map (Russell, 1972). Thus, each of these mutants has lost a major part of its ability to transport D-cycloserine. A similar type of defective transport mutant was also isolated from *Streptococcus* strain Challis (Reitz *et al.*, 1967).

Other D-cycloserine resistant strains have been isolated which show a different mechanism of resistance. For example, from *Streptococcus* strain Challis one mutant was obtained with elevated levels of alanine racemase and D-alanine:D-alanine ligase. Transformation studies with the DNA from this mutant allowed one to select mutants in which either the racemase or the ligase is elevated (Reitz *et al.*, 1967). David (1971) also isolated mutants of *Mycobacterium tuberculosis* resistant to D-cycloserine. A D-cycloserine-resistant, permease competent (D-CS^r/perm$^+$) mutant and a D-cycloserine-resistant, permease-defective (D-CS^r/perm$^-$) mutant were isolated. A study of the first mutant suggested the presence of a mutation in the gene(s) controlling the enzyme D-alanine:D-alanine ligase. Recently Clark and Young (1977a) found that resistance to D-cycloserine in *Bacillus subtilis* 168 is inducible. Sensitivity to the antibiotic could be regained by growth in the absence of D-cycloserine. Resistance results from an apparent decrease in the accumulation of the antibiotic. It was proposed that D-cycloserine induces a new transport system in this strain which transports D-cycloserine at a lower rate relative to D-alanine and glycine (Clark and Young, 1977b).

In contrast to D-cycloserine, O-carbamoyl-D-serine resistant mutants had elevated levels of alanine racemase, the target enzyme. All mutants from *Streptococcus* strain Challis resistant to this analogue showed the same phenotype. When antibiotics with more than one site of action (e.g. D-cycloserine) are utilized, alterations in permeability may be more important than in those cases where the antibiotic has a single site of action (e.g. O-carbamoyl-D-serine). Decreased uptake of D-cycloserine would "protect" both enzymes, whereas a mutation which caused increased production of one of the sensitive enzymes would still find the biosynthetic pathway restricted by inhibition of the other sensitive enzyme (Reitz *et al.*, 1967).

In the case of alafosfalin, resistance also emerges (Hall *et al.*, 1979). After 11 passages of cultures in the presence of this phosphonopeptide, *E. coli* became resistant to 1000 µg/ml of this compound. Hall *et al.* (1979) proposed that these strains probably have a reduced uptake capacity for the compound. Most of this resistance (99.95%) was lost upon regrowth of a resistant population in alafosfalin-free media. Recently, Maruyama *et al.* (1979) also indicated that resistant cells of *E. coli* selected against alafosfalin did not show accumulation of this drug. In contrast, Lacoste *et al.* (1976) observed that alanine race-mase was derepressed in a mutant of *P. aeruginosa* that was resistant to 1-amino-ethylphosphonic acid.

An interesting example for comparison with alafosfalin is that of bacilysin, the dipep-tide of L-alanine and anticapsin (see Section 3.2.). Resistance to bacilysin is observed in mutants that are defective for a transport system, presumably the dipeptide system (Kenig *et al.*, 1976).

Combinations of these analogues, e.g. fluoro-D-alanine/D-cycloserine and alafosfalin/β-lactam, provide a useful approach for reducing the probability of selecting resistant strains. In the case of alafosfalin, the emergence of resistant organisms is suppressed by the combined application of this phosphonodipeptide and cephalexin. As illustrated in Figure 16, considerably more antibacterial activity is retained with the combination than with either agent alone (Hall *et al.*, 1979). This series of experiments clearly demonstrates that combinations of two agents not only may potentiate the effect of the components, but combinations have the additional advantage in not selecting for cells that are resis-tant to the individual components. This is only true in the absence of R-factor mediated resistance.

No data are available from the Merck group that would allow one to assess the emergence of resistant organisms against the combination of fluoro-D-alanine/D-cycloser-

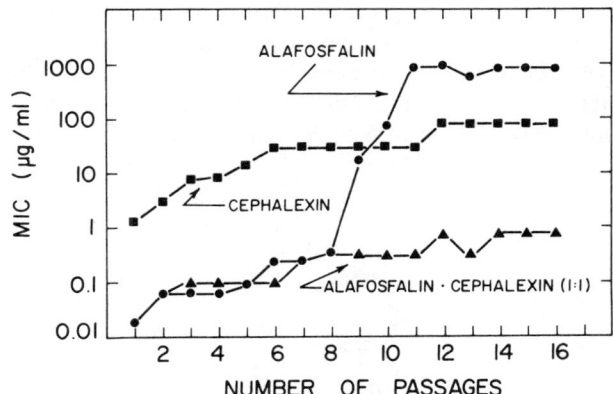

FIG. 16. Inhibition of resistance development with a combination of alafosfalin and cephalexin in
E. coli. (Reprinted with permission from C. H. Hassall, cited in Hall *et al.* (1979).)

ine. In contrast to the alafosfalin/β-lactam combination, the Merck combination may not show this added advantage. It is proposed that these analogues share the same transport system, i.e. the D-alanine–glycine transport system (see Section 3.1.). Thus, the use of these analogues in combination may tend to select for the same type of transport mutant.

The synergistic response (see Section 4.3.) as well as the suppression of resistance selection argues well for the use of combinations of these analogues. Whether these advantages outweigh some of the disadvantages encountered in pharmacokinetic experiments remains to be seen.

4.6. PHARMACOKINETICS

The efficacy of an alanine analogue or a combination of analogues depends not only on its ability to inhibit a target enzyme(s) and its accumulation by the target cell but also on its ability to reach the target cell in the host. This latter aspect involves the absorption, distribution, metabolism, and excretion of the analogue. The knowledge of these features, the pharmacokinetics, is essential for the proper use of these analogues. It is beyond the scope of this review to discuss all aspects of the pharmacokinetics of the alanine analogues. Rather, it is our purpose to discuss those aspects of D-cycloserine, fluoro-D-alanine, and alafosfalin as they relate to other sections of this review, and as they provide new strategies for therapy.

The pharmacokinetics of D-cycloserine are summarized by Otten et al. (1975a), Robson and Sullivan (1963), Kucers and Bennett (1975), and Curci (1970). In order to compare the available data for alafosfalin and fluoro-D-alanine, the following features of D-cycloserine should be indicated. Since absorption from both stomach and intestine takes place readily and nearly completely, parenteral application offers no advantage. Maximal concentrations are achieved in the serum within 1–4 hr (average 2). The half-life $(t_{\frac{1}{2}})$ is 8–12 hr (average 10) and 30–35% of the analogue is metabolized to antibiotically inactive compounds. The antibiotic diffuses well in all body fluids. The use of D-cycloserine in the chemotherapy of tuberculosis has been extensively described (Russell and Middlebrook, 1961).

One of the important considerations in choosing animal models to study the pharmacokinetics and efficacy of an alanine analogue concerns the presence of significant levels of D-alanine in the sera of rodent models. In contrast, sera from humans do not contain D-alanine (Hoeprich, 1965). The antagonistic effect of D-alanine on the alanine analogues described in this review will influence the efficacy of the analogue in rodent models. This feature provides an explanation why D-cycloserine is more effective against tuberculosis in humans and is less effective against experimental tuberculosis in mice and guinea pigs.

In order to enhance the stability of D-cycloserine and achieve better transport characteristics as well as lower neurotoxicity, the Merck group (Jensen et al., 1980; Kollonitsch et al., 1975) has developed a cycloserine prodrug (PCS) for use in their combination fluoro-D-alanine/D-cycloserine. The prodrug, (R)-4-[(1-methyl-3-oxo-1-butenyl)-amino]-3-isoxazolidinone (XXXIV), is the condensation product of acetylacetone and D-cycloserine. Hydrolysis of this conjugate to D-cycloserine is rapid in dilute solution below pH 6, but slow at pH 7.4 ($t_{\frac{1}{2}}$ = 70 min). This slower hydrolysis allows one to circumvent the prominent tubular reabsorption of D-cycloserine in man, a feature which is important

(XXXIV)

in eliminating the self-reversal of fluoro-D-alanine in the urinary tract. A similar approach was also used by Bonati *et al.* (1965). The condensation of D-cycloserine with terephthalaldehyde, terizidone (1,4-bis-D-3-oxo-4-izoxazolidinyl-iminomethyl)benzene (XXXV), shows enhanced stability and different pharmacokinetics in mice when compared with D-cycloserine (Adamek and Trnka, 1972; Otten *et al.*, 1975b).

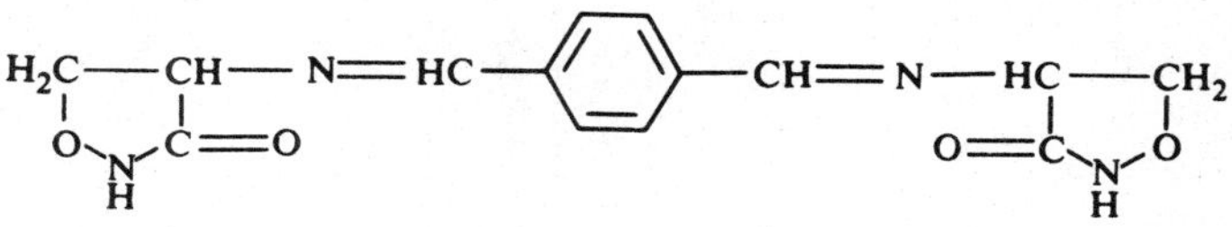

(XXXV)

In order to enhance the *in vivo* metabolic stability of β-fluoro-D-alanine to D-amino acid oxidase, Kollonitsch and Barash (1976) (Kollonitsch and Kahan, 1977) synthesized the α-*deutero* analogue of β-fluoro-D-alanine (DFA) (XXXVI). It was reasoned that the α-*deutero*-form would have increased stability due to the deuterium isotope effect on the

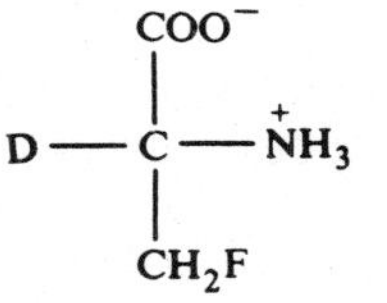

(XXXVI)

oxidase. The overall metabolism *in vivo* was reduced two to three-fold as judged from the proportion of fluoro-D-alanine and F^- excreted by the mouse, rat and Rhesus monkey and from serum F^- levels measured in monkey. The α-*protio*- and α-*deutero*-β-fluoro-D-alanine have equivalent *in vitro* antibacterial activities. Thus, the isotope effect on the oxidative reaction significantly improves the therapeutic index (Kahan *et al.*, 1975).

As indicated in Section 4.4, the combination of fluoro-D-alanine and D-cycloserine potentiates the individual activities of the analogues by factors of 2–10 and 4–20, respectively, both *in vitro* and *in vivo*. *In vivo* activity is optimal at body fluid fluoro-D-alanine:D-cycloserine ratios between 1:1 and 4:1. Most infections in mice were controlled by ED_{50}s < 6 mg/kg. *Per os* administration is 70% as efficient as *s.c.* injection. Activity against refractory infections, such as *Pseudomonas aeruginosa*, was exceeded only by that of gentamycin (Kropp *et al.*, 1975). It is likely that optimal ratios and systemic efficacy can be achieved with daily doses in adults of approximately 1500 mg DFA (XXXVI) and 300 mg PCS (XXXIV) (Kahan *et al.*, 1975).

The one disadvantage with this combination reflects the half-lives of the individual components. Fluoro-D-alanine is more rapidly excreted than D-cycloserine (Kahan, 1977). Thus, one has to conclude that the above ratios may be difficult to maintain in the host during combination therapy. The enhanced excretion of PCS (XXXIV) partially solves this problem. Thus, in certain therapies, it is proposed to administer the two components separately in order to maintain a favorable *in vivo* ratio (Kahan, 1977).

The pharmacokinetics of alafosfalin have been extensively studied in rats, baboons and humans (Allen *et al.*, 1979b; Lees *et al.*, 1979; Allen and Lees, 1980). In humans alafosfalin was rapidly absorbed after *i.m.* administration and peak concentrations were observed within 20–30 min. After *per os* administration the peak concentration was attained by 100 min. The phosphonodipeptide was rapidly cleared from the plasma with a half-life of 1 hr. In the case of *per os* administration, the alafosfalin was partially hydrolyzed to alanine and L-1-aminoethylphosphonic acid before it reached the general circulation (first-pass metabolism). Administration of 200 mg *i.m.* and 500 mg *per os* doses to humans produced plasma concentrations of alafosfalin which were in excess of the minimal

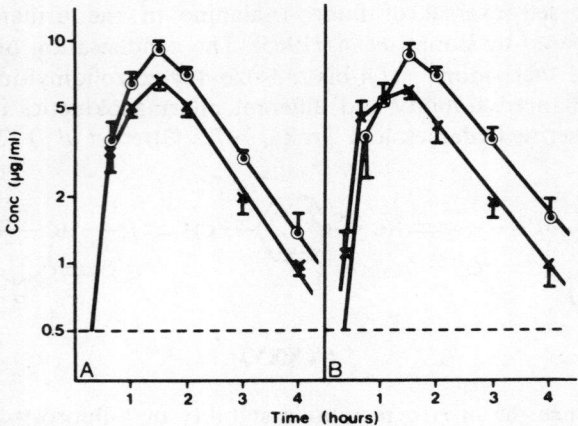

Fig. 17. Mean concentrations of cephalexin (250-mg Ceporex capsule; ⊙———⊙) and alafosfalin (500-mg tablet; ×———×) in plasma of human volunteers after administration together (A) and separately (B). (Reprinted with permission from Allen, J. G. and Lees, L. J. *Antimicrob. Agents Chemother.* **17**: 973–979 (1980). Copyright 1980, American Society for Microbiology.)

inhibitory concentration for many pathogenic organisms. The rate of absorption and elimination of this phosphonodipeptide is similar to that published for β-lactam antibiotics (Allen *et al.*, 1979b).

Administration of the combination, alafosfalin/cephalexin, in a 1:2 ratio to humans gave approximately equal concentrations in the plasma (Allen and Lees, 1980). The two antibacterial agents were absorbed, distributed and eliminated at virtually identical rates (Fig. 17). However, in the urine, the ratio of cephalexin to alafosfalin was not maintained because of significant hydrolysis of alafosfalin in the kidney. Thus, the alafosfalin/cephalexin combination, with matched pharmacokinetics in the human, appears to satisfy the requirement for synchronizing the actions of the two components (Gale *et al.*, 1972).

Although only a summary of the pharmacokinetics of D-cycloserine, β-fluoro-D-alanine, and alafosfalin is given, it is apparent that certain unique design features have resulted from the research of the Merck and Roche groups. These merit attention in our attempts to tailor these antibacterial agents in order to improve their pharmacokinetic characteristics. In the case of the Merck combination, the use of the prodrug of D-cycloserine to change absorption and release rates, and the use of the deuterium isotope effect to govern the rate of degradation of fluoro-D-alanine constitute innovative approaches to modulation of the *in vivo* ratio of the combination as well as the therapeutic index. In the case of the Roche combination, the ability to change the carrier peptide (amino acid) allows one to manipulate the antibacterial spectrum as well as the minimal inhibitory concentration. In addition, this ability also allows one to tailor the pharmacokinetics to match the characteristics of a second agent, e.g. in a synergistic combination.

5. CONCLUSION

One of the goals in this review is to present the rationale for the design of antibacterial agents directed at those target enzymes in cell wall assembly catalyzing reactions in which D-alanine is involved. Attaining this goal requires detailed analyses of these enzymes. Specificity and mechanism studies define some of the constraints and principles that must be satisfied when designing new analogues of D-alanine as inhibitors of this assembly process.

This review also focuses on the bacterial transport systems that are required to deliver the analogues to the target enzymes. The specificity constraints defined by these systems impose additional criteria which must also be satisfied in formulating new analogues. Finally, to be efficacious these analogues must not only satisfy the combination of specificity determinants defined by the target enzymes and the transport systems, but must also have acceptable pharmacokinetics. Certain design features are described which represent innovative approaches for modulating these kinetics.

Thus, the results from many laboratories have defined some of the principles for designing new analogues of alanine as antibacterial agents. They represent the initial stage in attaining the goal suggested by Park (1958) and illustrate the difficulties in designing efficacious analogues by a purely rational approach. Although the principles are numerous and complex, the results described in this review indicate that progress can be made and that we no longer need to be as pessimistic as in 1962 when H. J. Rogers assessed the field ... " in few fields have theoretical studies paid such poor dividends and the empirical approach been so triumphant as in the study of antibiotics." (Rogers, 1962). Rather, we should view the field from the perspective of the father of chemotherapy, Paul Ehrlich:

"Wenn diese eine Substanz, die sich bis jetzt am meisten bewährt hat, vielleicht für die Übertragung auf die menschliche Pathologie noch nicht geeignet sein sollte, so dürfen wir deswegen nicht die Flinte ins Korn werfen und unsere Hoffnungen aufgeben. Rom ist nicht an einem Tage erbaut! Dann müssen wir eben weiter auf dem Wege fortschreiten, der uns jetzt klar vorgezeichnet ist."

Über moderne Chemotherapie.
Vortrag gehalten in der X. Tagung der Deutschen
Dermatologischen Gessellschaft.
(Frankfurt am Main, 8. Juni 1908.)

Beiträge zur experimentellen Pathologie und Chemotherapie, Leipzig Akademische Verlagsgesellschaft m.b.H.
pp 165–202 (1909).

Acknowledgements—It is a pleasure to acknowledge the collaboration of our colleagues in this research. Their research, criticisms, and discussion have made many contributions to the success of this endeavor. Our research is supported by grant AI-04615 from the National Institute of Allergy and Infectious Diseases (F.N.) and the Deutsche Forschungsgemeinschaft (W.H.). Travel funds (F.N.) for preparing this manuscript were kindly provided from Boehringer Ingelheim and personal funds. We are indebted to H. Pelzer, C. H. Hassall, and J. M. Manning for manuscripts prior to publication. We are also indebted to R. Virudachalam, J. Martin, P. Ringrose, R. Johnston, R. L. Girolami and C. H. Stammer for comments and unpublished data.

REFERENCES

ABELES, R. H. and MAYCOCK, A. L. (1976) Suicide enzyme inactivators. *Accounts Chem. Res.* **9**: 313–319.

ADÁMEK, L. and TRNKA, L. (1972) Comparison of the antituberculotic efficiency of terizidone/Terivalidin, Bracco/and that of D-cycloserine both *in vitro* and *in vivo*. *Giorn. It. Mal. Torace* **26**: 241–247.

ADAMS, E. (1976) Catalytic aspects of enzymatic racemization. *Adv. Enzymol.* **44**: 69–138.

ADAMS, E., MUKHERJEE, K. L. and DUNATHAN, H. C. (1974) Alanine racemase of *Pseudomonas*: observations on substrate and inhibitor specificity. *Arch. Biochem. Biophys.* **165**: 126–132.

ALLEN, J. G., ATHERTON, F. R., HALL, M. J., HASSALL, C. H., HOLMES, S. W., LAMBERT, R. W., NISBET, L. J. and RINGROSE, P. S. (1978) Phosphonopeptides, a new class of synthetic antibacterial agents. *Nature* **272**: 56–58.

ALLEN, J. G., ATHERTON, F. R., HALL, M. J., HASSALL, C. H., HOLMES, S. W., LAMBERT, R. W., NISBET, L. J. and RINGROSE, P. S. (1979a) Phosphonopeptides as antibacterial agents: alaphosphin and related phosphonopeptides. *Antimicrob. Agents Chemother.* **15**: 684–695.

ALLEN, J. G., HAVAS, L., LEICHT, E., LENOX-SMITH, I. and NISBET, L. J. (1979b) Phosphonopeptides as antibacterial agents: metabolism and pharmacokinetics of alafosfalin in animals and humans. *Antimicrob. Agents Chemother.* **16**: 306–313.

ALLEN, J. G. and LEES, L. J. (1980) Pharmacokinetics of alafosfalin, alone and in combination with cephalexin, in humans. *Antimicrob. Agents Chemother.* **17**: 973–979.

AMES, B. N., AMES, G. F., YOUNG, J. D., TSUCHIYA, D. and LECOCQ, J. (1973) Illicit transport: the oligopeptide permease. *Proc. Natl. Acad. Sci. USA* **70**: 456–458.

ANON. (1975) Combination drug fights most bacteria. *Chem. Eng. News* **53**: no. 6, Oct. 6, 1975.

ARCHIBALD, A. R. (1974) The structure, biosynthesis and function of teichoic acid. *Adv. Microb. Physiol.* **11**: 53–95.

ATHERTON, F. R., HALL, M. J., HASSALL, C. H., LAMBERT, R. W. and RINGROSE, P. S. (1979a) Phosphonopeptides as antibacterial agents: rationale, chemistry, and structure-activity relationships. *Antimicrob. Agents Chemother.* **15**: 677–683.

ATHERTON, F. R., HALL, M. J., HASSALL, C. H., LAMBERT, R. W., LLOYD, W. J. and RINGROSE, P. S. (1979b) Phosphonopeptides as antibacterial agents: mechanism of action of alaphosphin. *Antimicrob. Agents Chemother.* **15**: 696–705.

ATHERTON, F. R., HALL, M. J., HASSALL, C. H., HOLMES, S. W., LAMBERT, R. W., LLOYD, W. J. and RINGROSE, P. S. (1980) Phosphonopeptide antibacterial agents related to alafosfalin: design, synthesis and structure-activity relationships. *Antimicrob. Agents Chemother.* **18**: 897–905.

Babu, U. M., Johnston, R. B. and McNeff, L. C. (1975) A general NMR method for the assay of racemase activity with optically active or optically inactive substrates. *Anal. Biochem.* **63**: 208–213.

Baddiley, J. and Neuhaus, F. C. (1960) The enzymic activation of D-alanine. *Biochem. J.* **75**: 579–587

Baltimore, R. S., Klein, J. O., Wilcox, C. and Finland, M. (1976) Synergy of mecillinam (FL 1060) with penicillins and cephalosporins against *Proteus* and *Klebsiella*, with observations on combinations with other antibiotics and against other bacterial species. *Antimicrob. Agents Chemother.* **9**: 701–705.

Barak, Z. and Gilvarg, C. (1975) Peptide transport. *Biomembranes* **7**: 167–218.

Beck, B. D. and Park, J. T. (1976) Activity of three murein hydrolases during the cell division cycle of *Escherichia coli* K-12 as measured in toluene-treated cells. *J. Bacteriol.* **126**: 1250–1260.

Bisswanger, H. (1980) Fluoropyruvate: a potent inhibitor of the bacterial and the mammalian pyruvate dehydrogenase complex. *Biochem. Biophys. Res. Commun.* **95**: 513–519.

Bonati, F., Bertoni, L., Rosati, G. and Zanichelli, V. (1965) Biological characteristics and antibacterial activity of Terizidone. *Il Farmaco, Prat.* **20**: 381–386.

Bracha, R. and Glaser, L. (1976) *In vitro* system for the synthesis of teichoic acid linked to peptidoglycan. *J. Bacteriol.* **125**: 872–879.

Brautigan, V. M., Childs, W. C. III, and Neuhaus, F. C. (1981) Biosynthesis of D-alanyl-lipoteichoic acid in *Lactobacillus casei*: D-alanyl-lipophilic compounds as intermediates. *J. Bacteriol.* **146**: 239–250.

Campbell, B. J., Lin, Y. C., Davis, R. V. and Ballew, E. (1966) The purification and properties of a particulate renal dipeptidase. *Biochim. Biophys. Acta* **118**: 371–386.

Carpenter, C. V., Goyer, S. and Neuhaus, F. C. (1976) Steric effects on penicillin-sensitive peptidoglycan synthesis in a membrane-wall system from *Gaffkya homari. Biochemistry* **15**: 3146–3152.

Chambers, P., Bing, J., Lynch, J., Neuhaus, F. C., Brockman, R. W. (1963) Effects of cycloserine and related compounds on cell wall synthesis in sensitive and resistant *Escherichia coli. Bacteriol. Proc.* **119**: 98.

Chang, M.-S. (1978) The relationship of the D-alanine transport system to the cross-linking of peptidoglycan in *Escherichia coli* W. Ph.D. Thesis, Northwestern University.

Childs, W. C. III and Neuhaus, F. C. (1980) Biosynthesis of D-alanyl-lipoteichoic acid: characterization of ester-linked D-alanine in the *in vitro*-synthesized product. *J. Bacteriol.* **143**: 293–301.

Chmara, H. and Borowski, E. (1973) Antibiotic tetaine, a new inhibitor of murein precursors synthesis in *Escherichia coli* K-12. *Biochem. Biophys. Res. Commun.* **52**: 1381–1387.

Clark, V. L. and Young, F. E. (1974) Active transport of D-alanine and related amino acids by whole cells of *Bacillus subtilis. J. Bacteriol.* **120**: 1085–1092.

Clark, V. L. and Young, F. E. (1977a) Inducible resistance to D-cycloserine in *Bacillus subtilis* 168. *Antimicrob. Agents Chemother.* **11**: 871–876.

Clark, V. L. and Young, F. E. (1977b) D-Cycloserine-induced alterations in the transport of D-alanine and glycine in *Bacillus subtilis* 168. *Antimicrob. Agents Chemother.* **11**: 877–880.

Clark, V. L. and Young, F. E. (1978) D-Alanine incorporation into macromolecules and effects of D-alanine deprivation on active transport in *Bacillus subtilis. J. Bacteriol.* **133**: 1339–1350.

Cleveland, R. F., Holtje, J.-V., Wicken, A. J., Tomasz, A., Daneo-Moore, L. and Shockman, G. D. (1975) Inhibition of bacterial wall lysins by lipoteichoic acids and related compounds. *Biochem. Biophys. Res. Commun.* **67**: 1128–1135.

Cleveland, R. F., Wicken, A. J., Daneo-Moore, L. and Shockman, G. D. (1976) Inhibition of wall autolysis in *Streptococcus faecalis* by lipoteichoic acid and lipids. *J. Bacteriol.* **126**: 192–197.

Cohen, A. (1969) Pyridoxine in the prevention and treatment of convulsions and neurotoxicity due to cycloserine. *Ann. N.Y. Acad. Sci.* **166**: 346–349.

Cosloy, S. D. (1973) D-Serine transport system in *Escherichia coli* K-12. *J. Bacteriol.* **114**: 679–684.

Coyette, J., Perkins, H. R., Polacheck, I., Shockman, G. D. and Ghuysen, J.-M. (1974) Membrane-bound DD-carboxypeptidase and LD-transpeptidase of *Streptococcus faecalis* ATCC 9790. *Eur. J. Biochem.* **44**: 459–468.

Cuckler, A. C., Frost, B. M., McClelland, L. and Solotorovsky, M. (1955) The antimicrobial evaluation of oxamycin (D-4-amino-3-isoxazolidone), a new broad-spectrum antibiotic. *Antibiotics and Chemotherapy* **5**: 191–197.

Curci, C. (1970) Pharmacological considerations on cycloserine. *Scand. J. Resp. Dis. Suppl.* **1970**: 51–60.

Curtiss, R., III, Charamella, L. J., Berg, C. M. and Harris, P. E. (1965) Kinetic and genetic analyses of D-cycloserine inhibition and resistance in *Escherichia coli. J. Bacteriol.* **90**: 1238–1250.

Dang, T.-Y., Cheung, Y. F. and Walsh, C. (1976) Reactions of β-fluoroalanine and β-bromoalanine with D-amino acid oxidase. *Biochem. Biophys. Res. Commun.* **72**: 960–968.

Dann, O. T. and Carter, C. E. (1964) Cycloserine inhibition of γ-amino-butyric-α-ketoglutaric transaminase. *Biochem. Pharmacol.* **13**: 677–684.

DasGupta, H. and Fan, D. P. (1979) Purification and characterization of a carboxypeptidase-transpeptidase of *Bacillus megaterium* acting on the tetrapeptide moiety of the peptidoglycan. *J. Biol. Chem.* **254**: 5672–5683.

David, H. L. (1971) Resistance to D-cycloserine in the tubercle bacilli: mutation rate and transport of alanine in parental cells and drug-resistant mutants. *Appl. Microbiol.* **21**: 888–892.

Davis, B. D. and Maas, M. K. (1952) Analysis of the biochemical mechanism of drug resistance in certain bacterial mutants. *Proc. Natl. Acad. Sci. USA* **38**: 775–785.

Diddens, H., Dorgerloh, M. and Zähner, H. (1979) Metabolic products of microorganisms 176. on the transport of small peptide antibiotics in bacteria. *J. Antibiotics* **32**: 87–90.

Diddens, H., Zähner, H., Kraas, E., Göhring, W. and Jung, G. (1976) On the transport of tripeptide antibiotics in bacteria. *Eur. J. Biochem.* **66**: 11–23.

Diven, W. F. (1969) Studies on amino acid racemases: II. Purification and properties of the glutamate racemase from *Lactobacillus fermenti. Biochim. Biophys. Acta* **191**: 702–706.

Diven, W. F., Scholz, J. J. and Johnston, R. B. (1964) Purification and properties of the alanine racemase from *Bacillus subtilis. Biochim. Biophys. Acta* **85**: 322–332.

Drews, J. (1979) *Grundlagen der Chemotherapie*, Springer-Verlag, Wien.

DULANEY, E. L. (1970) 1-Aminoethylphosphonic acid, an inhibitor of bacterial cell wall synthesis. *J. Antibiotics* **23**: 567–568.

DUNATHAN, H. C., HINDENLANG, D. M. and ADAMS, E. (unpublished observations) cited in: Catalytic Aspects of Enzymatic Racemization. E. ADAMS. *Advances in Enzymology* **44**: 69–138.

EPSTEIN, I. G., NAIR, K. G. S. and BOYD, L. J. (1955) Cycloserine in the treatment of human pulmonary tuberculosis. Transactions of the 14th conference on the chemotherapy of tuberculosis. Veterans Administration—Armed Forces, Washington, DC: 326.

FELICETTI, D. and HANSON, H. (1970a) Charakterisierung einer D-leucylglycin spaltenden Aktivität aus menschlichen Nieren. *Hoppe–Seyler's Z. Physiol. Chem.* **351**: 1253–1259.

FELICETTI, D. and HANSON, H. (1970b) Charakterisierung einer Glycyl-D-leucin spaltenden Präparation aus menschlichen Nieren. *Hoppe–Seyler's Z. Physiol. Chem.* **351**: 1260–1267.

FICKEL, T. E. and GILVARG, C. (1973) Transport of impermeant substances in *E. coli* by way of oligopeptide permease. *Nature New Biol.* **241**: 161–163.

FIEDLER, F. and GLASER, L. (1974) The synthesis of polyribitol phosphate II. On the mechanism of polyribitol phosphate polymerase. *J. Biol. Chem.* **249**: 2690–2695.

FISCHER, W., KOCH, H. U., RÖSEL, P. and FIEDLER, F. (1980) Alanine ester-containing native lipoteichoic acids do not act as lipoteichoic acid carrier. Isolation, structural and functional characterization. *J. Biol. Chem.* **255**: 4557–4562.

FRANKLIN, F. C. H. and VENABLES, W. A. (1976) Biochemical, genetic, and regulatory studies of alanine catabolism in *Escherichia coli* K12. *Molec. gen. Genet.* **149**: 229–237.

FRANKLIN, T. J. (1973) Antibiotic transport in bacteria. *Crit. Rev. Microbiol.* **2**: 253–272.

GALE, E. F., CUNDLIFFE, E., REYNOLDS, P. E., RICHMOND, M. H. and WARING, M. J. (1972) In: *The Molecular Basis of Antibiotic Action*, Chapter 8: Perspectives. p. 419, John Wiley, London.

GALE, G. R. and SMITH, A. B. (1973) Insensitivity of bacteria to proposed antimetabolites of D-alanyl-D-alanine. *J. Bacteriol.* **114**: 460–461.

GHUYSEN, J. M. (1977) The DD-carboxypeptidase–transpeptidase system: interaction with carbonyl donor and amino acceptor substrates. In: *The Bacterial DD-Carboxypeptidase–transpeptidase Enzyme System: A New Insight into the Mode of Action of Penicillin*, pp. 43–112. E. R. Squibb Lectures on Chemistry of Microbial Products. University of Tokyo Press.

GLASER, L. (1960) Glutamic acid racemase from *Lactobacillus arabinosus*. *J. Biol. Chem.* **235**: 2095–2098.

GREENWOOD, D. and VINCENT, R. (1980) Interactions between alafosfalin and other inhibitors of bacterial cell wall synthesis. Current Chemotherapy Infectious Diseases, *Proc. 11th ICC and 19th ICAAC*, pp. 360–361. American Soc. for Microbiology.

GRUNBERG, E., CLEELAND, R., BESKID, G. and DeLORENZO, W. F. (1976) *In vivo* synergy between 6β-amidinopenicillanic acid derivatives and other antibiotics. *Antimicrob. Agents Chemother.* **9**: 589–594.

HALL, M. J., ARISAWA, M., HOLMES, S. W., MARUYAMA, H. B. and NISBET, L. J. (1979) The *in vitro* and *in vivo* properties of some novel phosphonopeptides alone and in combination with β-lactam antibiotics. Abstracts 19th Interscience Conference on Antimicrobial Agents and Chemotherapy, (Oct., 1979), Boston, MA. No. 238.

HALPERN, Y. S. (1974) Genetics of amino acid transport in bacteria. *Ann. Rev. Genet.* **8**: 103–133.

HAMMES, W. P. (1976) Biosynthesis of peptidoglycan in *Gaffkya homari*: The mode of action of penicillin G and mecillinam. *Eur. J. Biochem.* **70**: 107–113.

HAMMES, W. P. (1978) The LD-carboxypeptidase activity in *Gaffkya homari*. The target of the action of D-amino acids or glycine on the formation of wall-bound peptidoglycan. *Eur. J. Biochem.* **91**: 501–507.

HAMMES, W. P. and KANDLER, O. (1976) Biosynthesis of peptidoglycan in *Gaffkya homari*: The incorporation of peptidoglycan into the cell wall and the direction of transpeptidation. *Eur. J. Biochem.* **70**: 97–106.

HAMMES, W. P. and NEUHAUS, F. C. (1974a) On the specificity of phospho-N-acetylmuramyl-pentapeptide translocase. The peptide subunit of uridine diphosphate-N-acetylmuramyl-pentapeptide. *J. Biol. Chem.* **249**: 3140–3150.

HAMMES, W. P. and NEUHAUS, F. C. (1974b) Biosynthesis of peptidoglycan in *Gaffkya homari*: Role of the peptide subunit of uridine diphosphate-N-acetylmuramyl-pentapeptide. *J. Bacteriol.* **120**: 210–218.

HAMMES, W. P., SCHLEIFER, K. H. and KANDLER, O. (1973) Mode of action of glycine on the biosynthesis of peptidoglycan. *J. Bacteriol.* **116**: 1029–1053.

HAMMES, W. P. and SEIDEL, H. (1978a) The activities *in vitro* of DD-carboxypeptidase and LD-carboxypeptidase of *Gaffkya homari* during biosynthesis of peptidoglycan. *Eur. J. Biochem.* **84**: 141–147.

HAMMES, W. P. and SEIDEL, H. (1978b) The LD-carboxypeptidase activity in *Gaffkya homari*. The target of the action of certain β-lactam antibiotics on the formation of wall-bound peptidoglycan. *Eur. J. Biochem.* **91**: 509–515.

HANCOCK, I. and BADDILEY, J. (1976) *In vitro* synthesis of the unit that links teichoic acid to peptidoglycan. *J. Bacteriol.* **125**: 880–886.

HANSON, H., FRITSCHE, M. and IWIG, K. (1969) Stereospezifität und Aktivität einiger Exopeptidasen und Azylase von gram-positiven Bakterien unter besonderer Berücksichtigung des Zellalters. *Acta biol. med. germ.* **22**: 507–517.

HEIJENOORT, J. V., ELBAZ, L., DEZÉLÉE, P., PETIT, J.-F., BRICAS, E. and GHUYSEN, J.-M. (1969) Structure of the meso-diaminopimelic acid containing peptidoglycans in *Escherichia coli* B and *Bacillus megaterium* KM. *Biochemistry* **8**: 207–212.

HENDERSON, L. L. and JOHNSTON, R. B. (1976) Inhibition studies of the enantiomers of β-chloroalanine on purified alanine racemase from *B. subtilis*. *Biochem. Biophys. Res. Commun.* **68**: 793–798.

HEPTINSTALL, S., ARCHIBALD, A. R. and BADDILEY, J. (1970) Teichoic acids and membrane function in bacteria. *Nature (Lond)* **225**: 519–521.

HISHINUMA, F., IZAKI, K. and TAKAHASHI, H. (1971) Inhibition of L-alanine adding enzyme by glycine. *Agric. Biol. Chem.* **35**: 2050–2058.

Hoeprich, P. D. (1965) Alanine: cycloserine antagonism: VI. Demonstration of D-alanine in the serum of guinea pigs and mice. *J. Biol. Chem.* **240**: 1654–1660.

Höltje, J.-V. and Tomasz, A. (1975) Lipoteichoic acid: a specific inhibitor of autolysin activity in pneumococcus. *Proc. Natl. Acad. Sci. USA* **72**: 1690–1694.

Holden, J. T., van Balgooy, J. N. A. and Kittredge, J. S. (1968) Transport of aminophosphonic acids in *Lactobacillus plantarum* and *Streptococcus faecalis*. *J. Bacteriol.* **96**: 950–957.

Howe, W. B., Melson, G. L., Meredith, C. H., Morrison, J. R., Platt, M. H. and Strominger, J. L. (1964) Stepwise development of resistance to D-cycloserine in *Staphylococcus aureus*. *J. Pharmacol. Exptl. Therap.* **143**: 282–284.

Huber, J. W. III, Gilmore, W. F. and Robertson, L. W. (1975) Synthesis and antimicrobial evaluation of N-D-alanyl-1-aminoethylphosphonic acid. *J. Med. Chem.* **18**: 106–108.

Hug, D. H. and Werkman, C. H. (1957) Transamination in *Rhodospirillum rubrum*. *Arch. Biochem. Biophys.* **72**: 369–375.

Hughes, A. H., Hancock, I. C. and Baddiley, J. (1973) The function of teichoic acids in cation control in bacterial membranes. *Biochem. J.* **132**: 83–93.

Hungerer, K. D. and Tipper, D. J. (1969) Cell wall polymers of *Bacillus sphaericus* 9602. I. Structure of the vegetative cell wall peptidoglycan. *Biochemistry* **8**: 3577–3587.

Ito, F., Ryuichi, A., Hayaski, A., Yuasa, M., Tone, K. and Nishio, K. (1958) cited in Cohen, A. C. (1969) Pyridoxine in the prevention and treatment of convulsions and neurotoxicity due to cycloserine. *Ann. N.Y. Acad. Sci.* **166**: 346–349.

Izaki, K., Matsuhashi, M. and Strominger, J. L. (1966) Glycopeptide transpeptidase and D-alanine carboxypeptidase: penicillin-sensitive enzymatic reactions. *Proc. Natl. Acad. Sci. USA* **55**: 656–663.

Izaki, K., Matsuhashi, M. and Strominger, J. L. (1968) Biosynthesis of the peptidoglycan of bacterial cell walls. XIII. Peptidoglycan transpeptidase and D-alanine carboxypeptidase: penicillin-sensitive enzymatic reaction in strains of *Escherichia coli*. *J. Biol. Chem.* **243**: 3180–3192.

Jensen, N. P., Friedman, J. J., Kropp, H. and Kahan, F. M. (1980) Use of acetylacetone to prepare a prodrug of cycloserine. *J. Med. Chem.* **23**: 6–8.

Johnston, M. M. and Diven, W. F. (1969) Studies on amino acid racemases: 1. Partial purification and properties of the alanine racemase from *Lactobacillus fermenti*. *J. Biol. Chem.* **244**: 5414–5420.

Johnston, R. B., Scholz, J. J., Diven, W. F. and Shepherd, S. (1968) Some further studies on the purification and mechanism of the action of alanine racemase from *B. subtilis*. In: *Pyridoxal Catalysis: Enzymes and Model Systems*, Snell E. E., Braunstein, A. E., Severn, E. E. and Torchinsky, Y. M. (eds.), I.U.B. Symposium Series **35**, pp. 537–547, John Wiley, New York.

Johnston, R. B. (1980) The mechanism of vitamin B_6 in the action of amino acid racemases. In: *Vitamin B_6 Metabolism and Role in Growth*. Tryfiates, G. P. (Ed.), pp. 257–286. Food and Nutrition Press, Westport, CT.

Julius, M., Free, C. A. and Barry, G. T. (1970) Alanine racemase (*Pseudomonas*) In: *Methods in Enzymology: Metabolism of Amino Acids and Amines*. Tabor and Tabor (eds.), **17A**, pp. 171–176. Academic Press, New York.

Kaczorowski, G., Shaw, L., Laura, R. and Walsh, C. (1975a) Active transport in *Escherichia coli* B membrane vesicles. Differential inactivating effects from the enzymatic oxidation of β-chloro-L-alanine and β-chloro-D-alanine. *J. Biol. Chem.* **250**: 8921–8930.

Kaczorowski, G., Shaw, L., Fuentes, M. and Walsh, C. (1975b) Coupling of alanine racemase and D-alanine dehydrogenase to active transport of amino acids in *Escherichia coli* B membrane vesicles. *J. Biol. Chem.* **250**: 2855–2865.

Kahan, F. M. (1972) Antibacterial composition and process. Republic of South Africa patent 730761 (Dec. 15, 1972).

Kahan, F. M. (1977) Antibacterial composition comprising 3-fluoro-D-alanine or deutero analogue in combination with auto-antagonist inhibitor. United States patent 4, 031, 231 (June 21, 1977).

Kahan, F. M. and Kropp, H. (1975) MK641/MK642 A fixed-ratio combination (1): rationale; The sequential blockade of bacterial cell-wall biosynthesis. Abstracts, 15th Interscience Conference on Antimicrobial Agents and Chemotherapy, Washington, D.C., Sept. 1975, No. 100.

Kahan, F. M., Kropp, H., Onishi, H. R. and Jacobus, D. P. (1975) MK641/MK642 A fixed-ratio combination antimicrobial (4): Advantages over the FA/CS prototype. Abstracts, 15th Interscience Conference on Antimicrobial Agents and Chemotherapy, Washington, D.C., Sept. 1975, No. 103.

Karpeiskii, M. Ya., Breusov, Yu. N., Khomutov, R. M., Severin, E. S. and Polyanovskii, O. L. (1963) The mechanism of reaction of cycloserine and related compounds with aspartate-glutamate transaminase. *Biokhimiya* **28**: 345–352.

Kato, K., Strominger, J. L. and Kotani, S. (1968) Structure of the cell wall of *Corynebacterium diphtheriae*. I. Mechanism of hydrolysis by the L-3 enzyme and the structure of the peptide. *Biochemistry* **7**: 2762–2773.

Kenig, M. and Abraham, E. P. (1976) Antimicrobial activities and antagonists of bacilysin and anticapsin. *J. Gen. Microbiol.* **94**: 37–45.

Kenig, M., Vandamme, E. and Abraham, E. P. (1976) The mode of action of bacilysin and anticapsin and biochemical properties of bacilysin-resistant mutants. *J. Gen. Microbiol.* **94**: 46–54.

Kessel, D. and Lubin, M. (1963) On the distinction between peptidase activity and peptide transport. *Biochim. Biophys. Acta* **71**: 656–663.

Kessel, D. and Lubin, M. (1965) Stability of α-hydrogen of amino acids during active transport. *Biochemistry* **4**: 561–565.

King, R. D. and Grula, E. A. (1972) Condition of cell-wall mucopeptide in dividing and non-dividing cells of *Micrococcus lysodeikticus* dis-IIp⁺. *Canadian J. Microbiol.* **18**: 519–529.

Kihara, H., Ikawa, M. and Snell, E. E. (1961) Peptides and bacterial growth: X. Relation of uptake and hydrolysis to utilization of D-alanine peptides for growth of *Streptococcus faecalis*. *J. Biol. Chem.* **236**: 172–176.

KOLLONITSCH, J. (1976) 3-Fluoro-D-alanine and pharmacologically acceptable esters and pharmacologically acceptable salts thereof. United States patent 3, 956, 367 (May 11, 1976).

KOLLONITSCH, J. (1978) Novel methods for selective fluorination of organic compounds: design and synthesis of fluorinated antimetabolites. *Isr. J. Chem.* **17**: 53–59.

KOLLONITSCH, J., BARASH, L., KAHAN, F. M. and KROPP, H. (1973) New antibacterial agent *via* photofluorination of a bacterial cell wall constituent. *Nature* **243**: 346–347.

KOLLONITSCH, J., BARASH, L., JENSEN, N. P., KAHAN, F. M., MARBURG, S., PERKINS, L., MILLER, S. M. and SHEN, T. Y. (1975) MK641/MK642 A fixed-ratio combination antimicrobial (3): Improved derivatives of 3-fluoro-D-alanine and cycloserine. Abstracts, 15th Interscience Conference on Antimicrobial Agents and Chemotherapy (Sept. 1975), Washington, D.C., No. 102.

KOLLONITSCH, J. and BARASH, L. (1976) Organofluorine synthesis via photofluorination: 3-Fluoro-D-alanine and 2-deuterio analogue, antibacterials related to the bacterial cell wall. *J. Am. Chem. Soc.* **98**: 5591–5593.

KOLLONITSCH, J. and KAHAN, F. M. (1977) Fluorinated amino acids. United States patent 4, 028, 405 (June 7, 1977).

KONINGS, W. N. and FREESE, E. (1972) Amino acid transport in membrane vesicles of *Bacillus subtilis. J. Biol. Chem.* **247**: 2408–2418.

KRAMER, B. (1975) Merck and Co. develops combination drug that seems to work against all bacteria. Wall Street Journal (September 27, 1975).

KROPP, H., KAHAN, F. M. and WOODRUFF, H. B. (1975) MK641/MK642 A fixed-ratio combination antimicrobial (2): Laboratory evaluation of antibacterial activity. Abstracts, 15th Interscience Conference on Antimicrobial Agents and Chemotherapy, Washington, DC. Sept. 1975, No. 101.

KUCERS, A. and BENNETT, N. M. (1975) Cycloserine. In: *The Use of Antibiotics: A Comprehensive Review with Clinical Emphasis.* pp. 271–275, Heinemann, London.

KURAMITSU, H. K. and SNOKE, J. E. (1962) The biosynthesis of D-amino acids in *Bacillus licheniformis. Biochim. Biophys. Acta* **62**: 114–121.

KURODA, Y., OKUHARA, M., GOTO, T., IGUCHI, E., KOHSAKA, M., AOKI, H. and IMANAKA, H. (1980a) FR-900130, A novel amino acid antibiotic. I. Discovery, taxonomy, isolation, and properties. *J. Antibiotics* **33**: 125–131.

KURODA, Y., OKUHARA, M., GOTO, T., KOHSAKA, M., AOKI, H. and IMANAKA, H. (1980b) FR-900130, A novel amino acid antibiotic. II. Isolation and structure elucidation of the acetyl derivative of FR-900130. *J. Antibiotics* **33**: 132–136.

LACOSTE, A. M., CASSAIGNE, A. and NEUZIL, E. (1975) Acides aminés phosphoniques et croissance de *Pseudomonas aeruginosa. Comptes Rendus de l'Académie des Sciences,* Paris, Series **D280**: 1173–1176.

LACOSTE, A. M., POULSEN, M., CASSAIGNE, A. and NEUZIL, E. (1976) Recherches sur l'action antibiotique de l'acide DL-1-amino éthyl phosphonique. Journées Biochimiques Franco-Belges 24–26 Juin 1976. Résumés p. 46.

LACOSTE, A.-M., POULSEN, M., CASSAIGNE, A. and NEUZIL, E. (1979) Inhibition of D-alanyl-D-alanine ligase in different bacterial species by amino phosphonic acids. *Current Microbiology* **2**: 113–117.

LACEY, B. W. (1958) Mechanisms of chemotherapeutic synergy. *Symp. Soc. Gen. Microbiol.* **8**: 247–287.

LAMBERT, M. P. and NEUHAUS, F. C. (1972) Mechanism of D-cycloserine action: alanine racemase from *Escherichia coli* W. *J. Bacteriol.* **110**: 978–987.

LAMBERT, P. A., HANCOCK, I. C. and BADDILEY, J. (1977) Occurrence and function of membrane teichoic acids. acids. *Biochim. Biophys. Acta* **472**: 1–12.

LARK, C., BRADLEY, D. and LARK, K. G. (1963) Further studies on the incorporation of D-methionine into the bacterial cell wall. Its incorporation into the R-layer and the structural consequences. *Biochim. Biophys. Acta* **78**: 278–288.

LARK, C. and LARK, K. G. (1959) The effects of D-amino acids on *Alcaligenes fecalis. Can. J. Microbiol.* **5**: 369–379.

LARK, C. and LARK, K. G. (1961) Studies on the mechanism by which D-amino acids block cell wall synthesis. *Biochim. Biophys. Acta* **40**: 308–322.

LEACH, F. R. and SNELL, E. E. (1960) The absorption of glycine and alanine and their peptides by *Lactobacillus casei. J. Biol. Chem.* **235**: 3523–3531.

LEE, M., ROBBINS, J. C. and OXENDER, D. L. (1975) Transport properties of merodiploids covering the *dag A* locus in *Escherichia coli* K-12. *J. Bacteriol.* **122**: 1001–1005.

LEES, L. J., ALLEN, J. G., CARS, O., HENNING, C. and LEICHT, E. (1979) The bioavailability and tissue distribution of alafosfalin and combinations in man and animals. Abstracts, 19th Interscience Conference on Antimicrobial Agents and Chemotherapy (Oct. 1979) Boston, MA. No. 240.

LESTER, W., SALOMIN, A., REIMANN, A. F., SHULRUFF, E. and GERG, G. S. (1956) Cycloserine therapy in tuberculosis in humans. *Am. Rev. Tuberc.* **74**: 121–127.

LEUNG, L. S. and FREY, P. A. (1978) Fluoropyruvate: an unusual substrate for *Escherichia coli* pyruvate dehydrogenase. *Biochem. Biophys. Res. Commun.* **81**: 274–279.

LEYH-BOUILLE, M., NAKEL, M., FRÈRE, J.-M., JOHNSON, K., GHUYSEN, J.-M., NIETO, M. and PERKINS, H. R. (1972) Penicillin-sensitive DD-carboxypeptidases from *Streptomyces* strains R39 and K11. *Biochemistry* **11**: 1290–1298.

LINZER, R. (1973) The biosynthesis of teichoic acid: a role for the D-alanine activating enzyme. Ph.D. Thesis, Northwestern University.

LINZER, R. and NEUHAUS, F. C. (1973) Biosynthesis of membrane teichoic acid: a role for the D-alanine activating enzyme. *J. Biol. Chem.* **248**: 3196–3201.

LOMBARDI, F. J. and KABACK, H. R. (1972) Mechanisms of active transport in isolated bacterial membrane vesicles. VII. The transport of amino acids by membranes prepared from *Escherichia coli. J. Biol. Chem.* **247**: 7844–7857.

LYNCH, J. L. and NEUHAUS, F. C. (1966) On the mechanism of action of the antibiotic O-carbamoyl-D-serine in *Streptococcus faecalis. J. Bacteriol.* **91**: 449–460.

Mager, J. and Blank, I. (1954) Synthesis of fluoropyruvic acid and some of its biological properties. *Nature* **173**: 126–127.

Manning, J. M., Merrifield, N. E., Jones, W. M. and Gotschlich, E. C. (1974) Inhibition of bacterial growth by β-chloro-D-alanine. *Proc. Natl. Acad. Sci. USA* **71**: 417–421.

Manning, J. M. and Soper, T. S. (1978) Inactivation of D-amino acid transaminase and the antibacterial action of β-haloderivatives of D-alanine. In: *Enzyme-Activated Irreversible Inhibitors*. Seiler, N., Jung, M. J. and Koch-Weser, J. (eds). pp. 163–176, Proceedings of the International Symposium on Substrate Induced Irreversible Inhibition of Enzymes, Stockholm 1978, Elsevier/North-Holland Biomedical Press, Amsterdam.

Marquet, A., Nieto, M. and Diaz-Maurino, T. (1976) Membrane-bound DD-carboxypeptidase and transpeptidase activities from *Bacillus megaterium* KM at pH 7. General properties, substrate specificity and inhibition by β-lactam antibiotics. *Eur. J. Biochem.* **68**: 581–589.

Martinez-Carrion, M. and Jenkins, W. T. (1965) D-Alanine-D-glutamate transaminase. II. Inhibitors and the mechanism of transamination of D-amino acids. *J. Biol. Chem.* **240**: 3547–3552.

Maruyama, H. B., Arisawa, M. and Sawada, T. (1979) Alafosfalin, a new inhibitor of cell wall biosynthesis: *in vitro* activity against urinary isolates in Japan and potentiation with β-lactams. *Antimicrob. Agents Chemother.* **16**: 444–451.

Matthews, D. M. and Payne, J. W. (1975) Occurrence and biological activities of peptides. In: *Peptide Transport in Protein Nutrition*, pp. 392–463, Matthews, D. M. and Payne, J. W. (eds), North Holland/American Elsevier.

Metzler, D. E., Ikawa, M. and Snell, E. E. (1954) A general mechanism for vitamin B_6-catalyzed reactions. *J. Am. Chem. Soc.* **76**: 648–652.

Michel, M. F. and Hijmans, W. (1960) The additive effect of glycine and other amino acids on the induction of the L-phase of group A β-haemolytic streptococci by penicillin and D-cycloserine. *J. Gen. Microbiol.* **23**: 35–46.

Miller, C. G. (1975) Peptidases and proteases of *Escherichia coli* and *Salmonella typhimurium*. *Ann. Rev. Microbiol.* **29**: 485–504.

Mora, J. and Snell, E. E. (1963) The uptake of amino acids by cells and protoplasts of *S. faecalis*. *Biochemistry* **2**: 136–141.

Moyed, H. S. (1964) Biochemical mechanisms of drug resistance. *Ann. Rev. Microbiol.* **18**: 347–366.

Nakamizo, N. and Nakamura, M. (1978) Synthetic inhibitors of enzymes involved in peptidoglycan biosynthesis. I. Preparation of D-alanine chloromethylketones. *Chem. Pharm. Bull.* **26**: 2233–2235.

Naumova, I. B. (1978) Teichoic acids in the regulation of biochemical processes in microorganisms. *Biokhimiya* **43**: 195–207.

Neuhaus, F. C. (1962a) The enzymatic synthesis of D-alanyl-D-alanine. I. Purification and properties of D-alanyl-D-alanine synthetase. *J. Biol. Chem.* **237**: 778–786.

Neuhaus, F. C. (1962b) The enzymatic synthesis of D-alanyl-D-alanine. II. Kinetic studies on D-alanyl-D-alanine synthetase. *J. Biol. Chem.* **237**: 3128–3135.

Neuhaus, F. C. (1967) D-Cycloserine and O-carbamoyl-D-serine. In: *Antibiotics: Mechanism of Action*, vol. 1, pp. 40–83, Gottlieb, D. and Shaw, P. D. (eds), Springer, Heidelberg.

Neuhaus, F. C. (1968) Selective inhibition of enzymes utilizing alanine in the biosynthesis of peptidoglycan. Antimicrobial Agents and Chemotherapy (1967) 304–313.

Neuhaus, F. C., Carpenter, C. V., Lambert, M. P. and Wargel R. J. (1972) D-Cycloserine as a tool in studying the enzymes in the alanine branch of peptidoglycan synthesis. In: *Molecular Mechanisms of Antibiotic Action on Protein Biosynthesis and Membranes*. Muñoz, E., Garcia-Ferrandiz, F. and Vasquez, D. (eds), pp. 339–362, Elsevier, Amsterdam.

Neuhaus, F. C., Goyer, S. and Neuhaus, D. W. (1977) Growth inhibition of *Escherichia coli* W by D-norvalyl-D-alanine: an analogue of D-alanine in position 4 of the peptide subunit of peptidoglycan. *Antimicrob. Agents Chemother.* **11**: 638–644.

Neuhaus, F. C., Linzer, R. and Reusch, V. M. Jr. (1974) Biosynthesis of membrane teichoic acid: Role of the D-alanine-activating enzyme and D-alanine:membrane acceptor ligase. *Ann. N.Y. Acad. Sci.* **235**: 502–518.

Neuhaus, F. C. and Lynch, J. L. (1964) The enzymatic synthesis of D-alanyl-D-alanine. III. On the inhibition of D-alanyl-D-alanine synthetase by the antibiotic D-cycloserine. *Biochemistry* **3**: 471–480.

Neuhaus, F. C. and Struve, W. G. (1965) Enzymatic synthesis of analogues of the cell-wall precursor. I. Kinetics and specificity of uridine diphospho-N-acetylmuramyl-L-alanyl-D-glutamyl-L-lysine:D-alanyl-D-alanine ligase (adenosine diphosphate) from *Streptococcus faecalis* R. *Biochemistry* **4**: 120–131.

Neuhaus, F. C., Tobin, C. E. and Ahlgren, J. A. (1980) Membrane-wall interrelationship in *Gaffkya homari*: sulfhydryl sensitivity and heat lability of nascent peptidoglycan incorporation into walls. *J. Bacteriol.* **143**: 112–119.

Nieto, M., Perkins, H. R., Leyh-Bouille, M., Frère, J.-M. and Ghuysen, J.-M. (1973) Peptide inhibitors of *Streptomyces* DD-carboxypeptidases. *Biochem. J.* **131**: 163–171.

Nikaido, H. (1980) Nonspecific transport through the outer membrane. In: *Bacterial Outer Membranes; Biogenesis and Functions*. pp. 361–407, Inouye, M. (ed), John Wiley, New York.

Oka, T. (1976) Mode of action of penicillins *in vivo* and *in vitro* in *Bacillus megaterium*. *Antimicrob. Agents Chemother.* **10**: 579–591.

Okada, Y., Iguchi, S., Okinaka, M., Yagyu, M., Sano, K. and Otani, M. (1978) Amino acids and peptides. III. Synthesis of stereoisomeric alanine containing peptide derivatives and their effects on germination of *Bacillus thiaminolyticus* spores. *Chem. Pharm. Bull.* **26**: 3588–3591.

Okada, Y., Okinaka, M., Yagyu, M., Watabe, K., Sano, K. and Kakiuchi, Y. (1976b) Amino acids and peptides. II. Synthesis of stereoisomeric alanine containing peptide derivatives and their effects on germination of *Bacillus thiaminolyticus* spores. *Chem. Pharm. Bull.* **24**: 3081–3084.

Okada, Y., Tani, S., Yawatari, Y. and Yagyu, M. (1976a) Synthesis of stereoisomeric alanine containing peptide derivatives. *Chem. Pharm. Bull.* **24**: 1925–1927.

OLIVARD, J., METZLER, D. E. and SNELL, E. E. (1952) Catalytic racemization of amino acids by pyridoxal and metal salts. *J. Biol. Chem.* **199**: 669–674.

OTTEN, H., PLEMPEL, M. and SIEGENTHALER, W. (1975a) Cycloserin. In: *Antibiotika-Fibel: Antibiotika und Chemotherapeutika Therapie mikrobieller Infektionen.* pp. 583–587, Georg Thieme Verlag, Stuttgart.

OTTEN, H., PLEMPEL, M. and SIEGENTHALER, W. (1975b) Terizidon. In: *Antibiotika-Fibel: Antibiotika und Chemotherapeutika Therapie mikrobieller Infektionen.* pp. 587–589. Georg Thieme Verlag, Stuttgart.

PARK, B. K., HIROTA, A. and SAKAI, H. (1977) Structure of plumbemycin A and B, antagonists of L-threonine from *Streptomyces plumbeus. Agric. Biol. Chem.* **41**: 573–579.

PARK, J. T. (1958) Selective inhibition of bacterial cell-wall synthesis: its possible applications in chemotherapy. *Symp. Soc. Gen. Microbiol.* **8**: 49–61.

PATTERSON, E. K., GATMAITAN, J. S. and HAYMAN, S. (1973) Substrate specificity and pH dependence of dipeptidases purified from *Escherichia coli* B and from mouse ascites tumor cells. *Biochemistry* **12**: 3701–3709.

PAYNE, J. W. (1975) Transport of peptides in microorganisms. In: *Peptide Transport in Protein Nutrition.* pp. 283–364. MATTHEWS, D. M. and PAYNE, J. W. (eds), Elsevier/North-Holland, Amsterdam.

PAYNE, J. W. (1976) Peptides and micro-organisms. *Adv. Microbiol. Physiol.* **13**: 55–113.

PAYNE, J. W. and GILVARG, C. (1971) Peptide transport. *Adv. Enzymol.* **35**: 187–244.

PAYNE, J. W. and GILVARG, C. (1978) Transport of peptides in bacteria. In: *Bacterial Transport.* pp. 325–369. ROSEN, B. P. (ed), Marcel Dekker, New York.

PAYNE, R. A. and STAMMER, C. H. (1968) Cycloserine peptides. *J. Org. Chem.* **33**: 2421–2425.

PELZER, H. (1963) Mucopeptidhydrolasen in *Escherichia coli* B. Nachweis und Wirkungsspezifität. *Z. Naturforschung* **18B**: 950–956.

PELZER, H. and REUTER, W. (1980) Inhibition of peptidoglycan synthesis in ether-permeabilized cells of *Escherichia coli* by structural analogues of D-alanyl-D-alanine. *Antimicrob. Agents Chemother.* **18**: 887–892.

PERKINS, H. R., FRÈRE, J.-M. and GHUYSEN, J.-M. (1981) Synthetic peptide inhibitors of transpeptidation by the exocellular DD-carboxypeptidase-transpeptidase from *Actinomadura* R39. *FEBS Lett.* **123**: 75–78.

PERRY, D. and ABRAHAM, E. P. (1979) Transport and metabolism of bacilysin and other peptides by suspensions of *Staphylococcus aureus. J. Gen. Microbiol.* **115**: 213–221.

PETIT, J.-F., MUNOZ, E. and GHUYSEN, J.-M. (1966) Peptide cross-links in bacterial cell wall peptidoglycans studied with specific endopeptidases from *Streptomyces albus* G. *Biochemistry* **5**: 2764–2776.

PFEIFER, D., KELLEY, J. and PLAPP, R. (1980) Utilization of D-phenylglycylglycine in *Escherichia coli. Arch. Microbiol.* **127**: 203–207.

PIPERNO, J. R. and OXENDER, D. L. (1968) Amino acid transport systems in *Escherichia coli* K12. *J. Biol. Chem.* **243**: 5914–5920.

RANDO, R. (1975) Mechanisms of action of naturally occurring irreversible enzyme inhibitors. *Accounts Chem. Res.* **8**: 281–288.

REITZ, R. H., SLADE, H. D. and NEUHAUS, F. C. (1967) The biochemical mechanisms of resistance by Streptococci to the antibiotics D-cycloserine and O-carbamyl-D-serine. *Biochemistry* **6**: 2561–2570.

REUSCH, V. M. JR (1971) The biosynthesis of teichoic acid: the formation of alanyl ester linkages by D-alanine: membrane acceptor ligase. Ph.D. Thesis, Northwestern University.

REUSCH, V. M., JR. and NEUHAUS, F. C. (1971) D-Alanine:membrane acceptor ligase from *Lactobacillus casei. J. Biol. Chem.* **246**: 6136–6143.

RINGROSE, P. S. (1980) Peptides as antimicrobial agents. In: *Microorganisms and Nitrogen Sources: Transport and Utilization of Amino Acids, Peptides, Proteins and Related Substrates.* pp. 641–692. PAYNE, J. W. (ed). John Wiley, New York.

RINGROSE, P. S. and LLOYD, W. J. (1979) Permease-exploitation by the antibacterial peptide mimetic alafosfalin. Abstracts, 11th International Congress of Biochemistry (1979), Toronto, No. 06-8-R69.

ROBBINS, J. C. and OXENDER, D. L. (1973) Transport systems for alanine, serine, and glycine in *Escherichia coli* K12. *J. Bacteriol.* **116**: 12–18.

ROBINSON, D. S., BIRNBAUM, S. M. and GREENSTEIN, J. P. (1953) Purification and properties of an aminopeptidase from kidney cellular particulates. *J. Biol. Chem.* **202**: 1–26.

ROBSON, J. M. and SULLIVAN, F. M. (1963) Antituberculosis drugs. *Pharmacol. Rev.* **15**: 169–212.

ROGERS, H. J. (1962) Mode of action of the penicillins. In: *Resistance of Bacteria to the Penicillins.* DEREUCK, A. V. S. and CAMERON, M. P. (eds) Ciba Foundation Study Group No. 13. pp. 25–55, J. & A. Churchill, London.

ROSSO, G., TAKASHIMA, K. and ADAMS, E. (1969) Coenzyme content of purified alanine racemase from *Pseudomonas. Biochem. Biophys. Res. Commun.* **34**: 134–140.

RUSSELL, R. R. B. (1972) Mapping of a D-cycloserine resistance locus in *Escherichia coli* K-12. *J. Bacteriol.* **111**: 622–624.

RUSSELL, W. F. JR and MIDDLEBROOK, G. (1961) *Chemotherapy of Tuberculosis*, Charles C. Thomas, Springfield, IL.

SCHLEIFER, K. H., HAMMES, W. P. and KANDLER, O. (1976) Effect of endogenous and exogenous factors on the primary structures of bacterial peptidoglycan. *Adv. Microbiol. Physiol.* **13**: 245–292.

SCHLEIFER, K. H. and KANDLER, O. (1972) Peptidoglycan types of bacterial cell walls and their taxonomic implications. *Bacteriol. Rev.* **36**: 407–477.

SCHWARTZ, J. H., MAAS, W. K. and SIMON, E. J. (1959) An impaired concentrating mechanism for amino acids in mutants of *Escherichia coli* resistant to L-canavanine and D-serine. *Biochim. Biophys. Acta* **32**: 582–583.

SHANKMAN, S., GOLD, V., HIGA, S. and SQUIRES, R. (1962) On the mode of action of a peptide inhibitor of growth in *P. cerevisiae. Biochem. Biophys. Res. Commun.* **9**: 25–31.

SHANKMAN, S., HIGA, S., FLORSHEIM, H. A., SCHVO, Y. and GOLD, V. (1960) Peptide studies. II. Growth-promoting activity of peptides of L-leucine and L- and D-valine for lactic acid bacteria. *Arch. Biochem. Biophys.* **86**: 204–209.

SHAW, E. (1970) Chemical modification by active-site-directed reagents. In: *The Enzymes*, vol. 1, pp. 91–146, BOYER, P. D. (ed). Academic Press, New York.

SCHERAGA, H. A., SCOTT, R. A., VANDERKOOI, G., LEACH, S. J., GIBSON, K. D., OOI, T. and NEMETHY, G. (1967) Calculations of polypeptide structures from amino acid sequence. In: *Conformation of Biopolymers* vol. 1, pp. 43–60, RAMACHANDRAN, G. N. (ed.) Academic Press, London.

SHOJI, J.-I., EBATA, M. and OTSUKA, H. (1968) Studies on the action of O-carbamyl-D-serine in *Bacillus subtilis*. *J. Antibiotics* 21: 170–178.

SHORT, S. A., WHITE, D. C. and KABACK, H. R. (1972a) Active transport in isolated bacterial membrane vesicles. V. The transport of amino acids by membrane vesicles prepared from *Staphylococcus aureus*. *J. Biol. Chem.* 247: 298–304.

SHORT, S. A., WHITE, D. C. and KABACK, H. R. (1972b) Mechanisms of active transport in isolated bacterial membrane vesicles. IX. The kinetics and specificity of amino acid transport in *Staphylococcus aureus* membrane vesicles. *J. Biol. Chem.* 247: 7452–7458.

SILVERMAN, R. B. and ABELES, R. H. (1976) Inactivation of pyridoxal phosphate dependent enzymes by mono- and polyhaloalanines. *Biochemistry* 15: 4718–4723.

SMISSMAN, E. E., TERADA, A. and EL-ANTABLY, S. (1976) Synthesis of inhibitors of bacterial cell wall biogenesis. Analogues of D-alanyl-D-alanine. *J. Med. Chem.* 19: 165–167.

SOPER, T. S., JONES, W. M., LERNER, B., TROP, M. and MANNING, J. M. (1977a) Inactivation of bacterial D-amino acid transaminase by β-chloro-D-alanine. *J. Biol. Chem.* 252: 3170–3175.

SOPER, T. S. and MANNING, J. M. (1976) Synergy in the antimicrobial action of penicillin and β-chloro-D-alanine *in vitro*. *Antimicrob. Agents Chemother.* 9: 347–349.

SOPER, T. S. and MANNING, J. M. (1978) β-Elimination of β-halo substrates by D-amino acid transaminase associated with inactivation of the enzyme. Trapping of a key intermediate in the reaction. *Biochemistry* 17: 3377–3384.

SOPER, T. S., MANNING, J. M., MARCOTTE, P. A. and WALSH, C. T. (1977b) Inactivation of bacterial D-amino acid transaminases by the olefinic amino acid D-vinylglycine. *J. Biol. Chem.* 252: 1571–1575.

STEINFELD, A. S., NAIDER, F. and BECKER, J. M. (1979) Anticandidal activity of 5-fluorocytosine-peptide conjugates. *J. Med. Chem.* 22: 1104–1109.

STROMINGER, J. L., ITO, E. and THRENN, R. H. (1960) Competitive inhibition of enzymatic reactions by oxamycin. *J. Am. Chem. Soc.* 82: 998–999.

STROMINGER, J. L., THRENN, R. H. and SCOTT, S. S. (1959) Oxamycin, a competitive antagonist of the incorporation of D-alanine into a uridine nucleotide in *Staphylococcus aureus*. *J. Am. Chem. Soc.* 81: 3803.

STUART-HARRIS, C. (1979) Antibiotic interactions. In: *Antibiotic Interactions*, pp. 1–9, WILLIAMS, J. D. (ed). Academic Press, London.

SUDA, H., AOYAGI, T., TAKEUCHI, T. and UMEZAWA, H. (1976) Inhibition of aminopeptidase B and leucine aminopeptidase by bestatin and its stereoisomer. *Arch. Biochem. Biophys.* 177: 196–200.

TANAKA, M., KATO, Y. and KINOSHITA, S. (1961) Glutamic acid racemase from *Lactobacillus fermenti*: purification and properties. *Biochem. Biophys. Res. Commun.* 4: 114–117.

TANAKA, N. and UMEZAWA, H. (1964) Synergism of D-4-amino-3-isoxazolidone and O-carbamyl-D-serine. *J. Antibiotics*, Ser. A17: 8–10.

THORNE, C. B., GÓMEZ, C. G. and HOUSEWRIGHT, R. D. (1955) Transamination of D-amino acids by *Bacillus subtilis*. *J. Bacteriol.* 69: 357–362.

THORNE, C. B. and MOLNAR, D. M. (1955) D-Amino acid transamination in *Bacillus anthracis*. *J. Bacteriol.* 70: 420–426.

TOMASZ, A. and HOLTJE, J. V. (1977) Murein hydrolases and the lytic and killing action of penicillin. In: *Microbiology—1977*, pp. 209–215. SCHLESSINGER, D. (ed), American Society for Microbiology, Washington, D.C.

TOMASZ, A., WESTPHAL, M., BRILES, E. B. and FLETCHER, P. (1975) On the physiological functions of teichoic acids. *J. Supramolec. Struct.* 3: 1–16.

TRAUB, W. H. (1980) *In vitro* evaluation of alaphosphin (Ro 03-7008) against *Serratia marcescens*. *Chemotherapy* 26: 103–110.

TRIPPEN, B., HAMMES, W. P., SCHLEIFER, K.-H. and KANDLER, O. (1976) Die Wirkung von D-aminosäuren auf die Struktur und Biosynthese des Peptidoglycans. *Arch. Microbiol.* 109: 247–261.

VIRUDACHALAM, R. and RAO, V. S. R. (1977) Theoretical studies on β-lactam antibiotics. I. Conformational similarity of penicillins and cephalosporins to X-D-alanyl-D-alanine and correlations of their structure with activity. *Int. J. Peptide Protein Res.* 10: 51–59.

VIRUDACHALAM, R. and RAO, V. S. R. (1978) Theoretical studies of peptidoglycans. I. Effect of L-alanyl, D-butyl, or D-valyl residues at the positions 4 or 5 of the pentapeptide moiety of peptidoglycan on the cross-linking reaction. *Biopolymers* 17: 2251–2263.

VOGT, V. M. (1970) Purification and properties of an aminopeptidase from *Escherichia coli*. *J. Biol. Chem.* 245: 4760–4769.

WALSH, C. T. (1978) Chemical approaches to the study of enzymes catalyzing redox transformations. *Ann. Rev. Biochem.* 47: 881–931.

WALSH, C., JOHNSTON, M., MARCOTTE, P. and WANG, E. (1978) Studies on suicide substrates for pyridoxal-P and flavin-linked enzymes. In: *Enzyme-Activated Irreversible Inhibitors*. pp. 177–185. SEILER, N., JUNG, M. J. and KOCH-WESER, J. (eds), Proceedings of the International Symposium on Substrate Induced Irreversible Inhibition of Enzymes, Stockholm, 1978, Elsevier/North-Holland, Amsterdam.

WANG, E. and WALSH, C. (1978) Suicide substrates for the alanine racemase of *Escherichia coli* B. *Biochemistry* 17: 1313–1321.

WARGEL, R. J., SHADUR, C. A. and NEUHAUS, F. C. (1970) Mechanism of D-cycloserine action: Transport systems for D-alanine, D-cycloserine, L-alanine, and glycine. *J. Bacteriol.* 103: 778–788.

WARGEL, R. J., SHADUR, C. A. and NEUHAUS, F. C. (1971) Mechanism of D-cycloserine action: Transport mutants for D-alanine, D-cycloserine, and glycine. *J. Bacteriol.* 105: 1028–1035.

WHITNEY, J. G. and GRULA, E. A. (1964) Incorporation of D-serine into the cell wall mucopeptide of *Micrococcus lysodeikticus*. *Biochem. Biophys. Res. Commun.* **14**: 375–381.

WHITNEY, J. G. and GRULA, E. A. (1968) A major attachment site for D-serine in the cell wall mucopeptide of *Micrococcus lysodeikticus*. *Biochim. Biophys. Acta* **158**: 124–129.

WICKEN, A. J. and KNOX, K. W. (1975) Lipoteichoic acids: a new class of bacterial antigen. *Science* **187**: 1161–1167.

WIETZERBIN, J., DAS, B. C., PETIT, J.-F., LEDERER, E., LEYH-BOUILLE, M. and GHUYSEN, J.-M. (1974) Occurrence of D-alanyl-(D)-*meso*-diaminopimelic acid and *meso*-diaminopimelyl-*meso*-diaminopimelic acid interpeptide linkages in the peptidoglycan of *Mycobacteria*. *Biochemistry* **13**: 3471–3476.

WILD, J., WALCZAK, W., KRAJEWSKA-GRYNKIEWICZ, K. and KLOPOTOWSKI, T. (1974) D-Amino acid dehydrogenase: The enzyme of the first step of D-histidine and D-methionine racemization in *Salmonella typhimurium*. *Molec. Gen. Genet.* **128**: 131–146.

WISE, R. (1979) Antimicrobial potentiating agents. *J. Antimicrob. Chemother.* **5**: 121–128.

WOOD, W. A. and GUNSALUS, I. C. (1951) D-Alanine formation: a racemase in *Streptococcus faecalis*. *J. Biol. Chem.* **190**: 403–416.

WOODBINE, M. (1977) A synergic perspective. In: *Antibiotics and Antibiosis in Agriculture with Special Reference to Synergism*, pp. 27–56, WOODBINE, M. (ed). Butterworths, London.

YABU, K. and HUEMPFNER, H. R. (1974) Inhibition of growth of *Mycobacterium smegmatis* and of cell wall synthesis by D-serine. *Antimicrob. Agents Chemother.* **6**: 1–10.

YARON, A., MLYNAR, D. and BERGER, A. (1972) A dipeptidocarboxypeptidase from *E. coli*. *Biochem. Biophys. Res. Commun.* **47**: 897–902.

YONAHA, K., MISONO, K., YAMAMOTO, T. and SODA, K. (1975) D-Amino acid aminotransferase of *Bacillus sphaericus*. Enzymologic and spectrometric properties. *J. Biol. Chem.* **250**: 6983–6989.

YONAHA, K., YORIFUJI, T., YAMAMOTO, T. and SODA, K. (1975) Alanine racemase of *Bacillus subtilis* var. *aterrimus*. *J. Ferment. Technol.* **53**: 579–587.

CHAPTER 3

BACITRACIN

WILLIAM A. TOSCANO, Jr.† and DANIEL R. STORM§

†Charles A. Dana Laboratory of Toxicology, Harvard University School of Public Health, Boston, MA 02115 and
§Department of Pharmacology, University of Washington School of Medicine, Seattle, WA 98195

1. INTRODUCTION

The bacitracin peptides were first discovered and identified in 1945 as a product of a *Bacillus licheniformis* strain isolated from a tibial wound sustained by a patient named Margaret Tracy (Johnson *et al.*, 1945). Over the past forty-odd years a major effort has been directed toward elucidating the mechanisms of antibiotic action of the bacitracins. Even though the antimicrobial activity of the bacitracins has been known for some time, the mechanism of antibiotic activity has not been unambiguously defined. Indeed, although the effect of bacitracins on cell wall peptidoglycan biosynthesis is probably the major cause of its antibiotic activity, bacitracins affect a number of biochemical processes. Aside from the antibiotic activity of the bacitracins, these peptides have proven useful as a tool for investigating lipid–protein interactions at the molecular level.

The primary goal of this article is to review current literature on the mechanism of action of the bacitracins, with special emphasis on physico–chemical studies. The timeliness of this review is dictated by recent advances in the structure–function relationships of bacitracin.

2. ISOLATION AND SEPARATION

Bacitracin was initially isolated by butanol extraction of a cell free extract of *B. licheniformis* grown on tryptone or beef infusion media (Johnson *et al.*, 1945). Bacitracin was found to be water soluble, resistant to acidic pH, boiling, and pepsin or trypsin digestion. It was soon recognized that bacitracin isolated in this manner was not a single molecular species but a heterogeneous mixture of related peptides. Resolution of this mixture was first effected by counter-current distribution which demonstrated that commercial bacitracin is composed of at least nine separable components (Craig *et al.*, 1952, 1969; Newton and Abraham, 1953). Ion exchange chromatography was useful in only a partial resolution of components (Konigsberg and Craig, 1959; Storm and Strominger, 1973). Chromatography on carboxymethyl cellulose (CMC) columns yielded only six components without resolving bacitracin A and B. High performance liquid chromatography (HPLC) appears to be the most promising technique for resolving the various components of bacitracin. Using a one-meter column packed with Bondapak C_{18}/Dorasil, commercial preparations of bacitracin have been resolved into twenty-two components in fewer than 40 min (Tsuji *et al.*, 1974, 1975). A comparison of elution profiles from HPLC and CMC chromatography is given in Fig. 1. Chromatography on CMC results in the separation of three major bands, I: desamidobacitracin; II: bacitracin F; III: bacitracin A + bacitracin B (Fig. 1, upper panel). As shown in the lower panel HPLC yields good resolution of bacitracins A, B and B_2, as well as other forms of the antibiotic. Even though the resolution afforded by HPLC is powerful as an analytical technique, its applicability as a tool in preparation of purified components needs further development. In this regard, fast protein liquid chromatography (FPLC) appears to be a technique that affords the separating power of HPLC on a preparative scale, and will no doubt be soon utilized to prepare large quantities of highly purified bacitracin (Suelter, 1985).

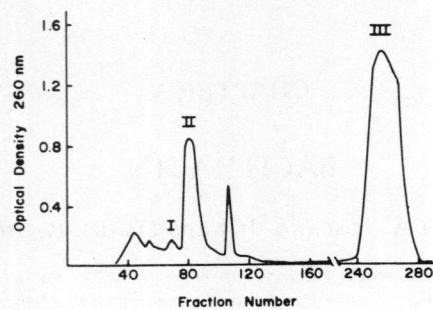

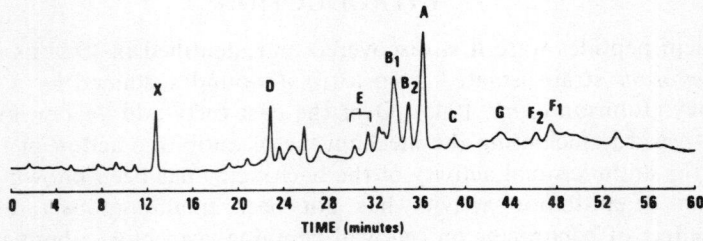

FIG. 1. Separation of components from commercial bacitracin by ion-exchange and high perform-ance liquid chromatography. *Top*: Commercial bacitracin (130 mg) was dissolved in 1 ml of 0.06 M pyridine-acetate buffer, pH 4.9, and applied to a CM-cellulose column (2 × 100 cm). The column was washed with 800 ml of the same buffer, and the eluant collected in 5 ml fractions. At fraction 160 the buffer was changed to 0.006 M pyridine/0.06 M acetic acid. pH 3.4. Fraction I: desamido-bacitracin; Fraction II: bacitracin F; Fraction III: bacitracin A + bacitracin B. (Reprinted with permission from Storm and Strominger, 1973.) *Bottom*: An HPLC chromatogram of a commercial bacitracin preparation showing the separation of bacitracin components using a μ Bondapak C_{18} column (300 × 4 mm). Elution was achieved using a convex gradient from 5% methanol to 50% methanol/20% acetonitrile in 10 mM phosphate buffer, pH 4.5. Bacitracin com-ponents are: A, B, B_2, C, D, E, F_1, F_2, G and X. (Reprinted with permission from Tsuji *et al.*, 1975.)

The reasons for the heterogeneity observed with commercial bacitracin isolated from *B. licheniformis* are not fully understood, and will become more clear when the structures of all the bacitracin peptides have been determined. Several of the bacitracins differ by only a few amino acids. This may be due to errors in synthesis by the multi-enzyme complex of bacitracin synthetase (Bernlohr and Novelli, 1960; Froyshov and Laland, 1974; Ishihara and Shimura, 1974).

3. STRUCTURE

Bacitracin A makes up between 60–80% of commercial bacitracin, and it is this component which is responsible for antibiotic activity. Bacitracin A is a small peptide composed of a seven membered cyclic peptide and a tail comprised of five amino acids (Fig. 2) (Galardy *et al.*, 1971). As with other peptide antibiotics, bacitracin A contains a number of amino acids not normally found in proteins, including D amino acids, and ornithine. Several unique structural features are apparent, including a thiazoline ring formed between the terminal isoleucine and cysteine residues as well as an amide bond between the ε-amino group of lysine and asparagine. The N-terminal leucine residue has the L-configuration. Ionizable groups on the peptide include the amino group at this N-terminus, glutamic and aspartic carboxyl groups, the δ-amino group of ornithine, and the imidazole nitrogen of histidine. The peptide is relatively non-polar, which may be a contributing factor in the high affinity of bacitracin A for membrane lipids (Lyerla and Freedman, 1972).

Upon treatment of bacitracin A under neutral or slightly basic conditions a transform-ation to bacitracin F occurs (Abraham, 1957; Regna, 1959; Weinberg, 1967). Bacitracin F

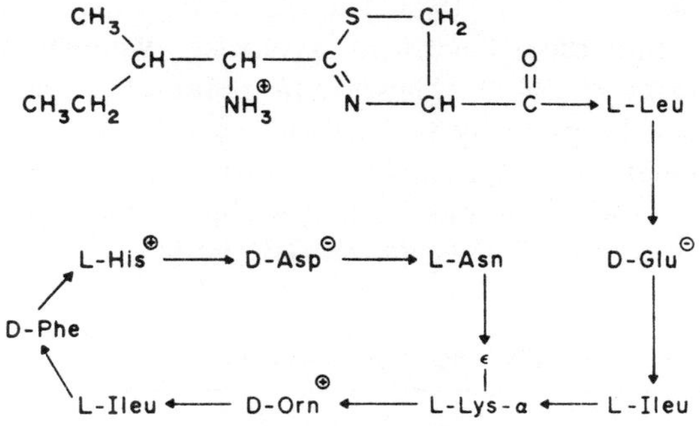

FIG. 2. Structure of bacitracin A. (Reprinted with permission from Scogin *et al.*, 1980.)

is similar to bacitracin A except that the thiazoline ring has been oxidatively deaminated. Bacitracin F exhibits 20–30-fold lower potency toward *Micrococcus lysodeikticus* than bacitracin A (Storm and Strominger, 1973). Bacitracin B is a result of the replacement of isoleucine by valine in bacitracin A (Abraham, 1957).

4. BIOSYNTHESIS

The biosynthesis of bacitracin is catalyzed by a multienzyme complex known as bacitracin synthetase, rather than by utilization of normal protein synthesis machinery. The complex has been partially purified in several laboratories (Pfaender *et al.*, 1973; Simlot *et al.*, 1973; Froyshov and Laland, 1974; Ishihara and Shimura, 1974; Rieder *et al.*, 1975). The complex contains specific activating enzymes for each of the amino acids of bacitracin. Once charged with the respective amino acid, the enzymes catalyze the exchange of ATP with inorganic pyrophosphate suggesting the involvement of aminoacyl adenosine intermediates. There is evidence that the amino acids and intermediate peptides are covalently attached to the bacitracin synthetase complex via this ester bond (Froyshov, 1975). Several of the covalently attached peptide intermediates have been identified by Froyshov as bacitracin intermediates: these include Ile–Cys, Ile–Cys–Leu and Ile–Cys–Leu–Glu. Froyshov's data indicate that bacitracin synthesis proceeds toward the C-terminus as in protein synthesis and in the synthesis of the nucleotide pentapeptide precursor of bacterial cell wall peptidoglycan. Vitkovic and Sadoff (Vitkovic and Sadoff, 1977a) have identified an exocellular protease, designated CMC_{III} which is released concomitantly with bacitracin. Synthesis of bacitracin *in vitro* indicated that CMC_{III} may play some role in the formation of the bacitracin peptides (Vitkovic and Sadoff, 1977b), however the role of this serine protease in cleaving bacitracin from bacitracin synthetase needs further clarification.

Bacitracin synthesis is initiated in the early exponential phase of vegetative growth, reaching a constant rate in the stationary phase of growth. Metabolic regulation of bacitracin synthetase is in itself an interesting problem. In general, bacitracin synthesis parallels growth of vegetative cells in synthetic media lacking glucose (Snoke and Cornell, 1965; Haavik, 1974; Hanlon and Hodges, 1981; Hanlon *et al.*, 1982). Addition of glucose inhibits bacitracin synthesis, however this inhibition is not a result of catabolite repression, but of a decrease in the pH of the growth medium, presumably as a result of accumulation of pyruvate and acetate (Haavik, 1974). This apparent inhibition can be overcome by the addition of $CaCO_3$, or increasing the buffering capacity of the growth medium. It has been postulated that the molecular basis for carbon metabolite regulation of bacitracin synthesis may be related to growth rate control (Martin and Demain, 1980). This possibility was suggested because the glucose experiments (Haavik, 1974) were conducted under conditions that could result in an enhanced rate of growth (Hanlon *et al.*, 1982). Experiments have been conducted to examine whether amino acid pool compositions exert a regulatory action on the production of bacitracin in both wild type and mutant strains of

B. licheniformis (Haavik and Vessia, 1978; Haavik, 1981; Supek et al., 1985). L-Histidine and L-phenylalanine stimulated bacitracin synthesis, whereas D-phenylalanine was strongly inhibitory (Haavik, 1981). These data point to interesting possibilities for examining regulation of the pathway to bacitracin synthesis. Analysis of the effects of metabolites on the regulation of bacitracin synthesis awaits the ultimate purification of bacitracin synthetase. Although it has been postulated that bacitracin is a structural component of the spore coat of B. licheniformis (Bernlohr and Novelli, 1964), analysis of

TABLE 1. Synergism between Bacitracin and Polymyxin–Agarose

Bacitracin (μg/ml)	Growth*	
	Without polymyxin–agarose	With polymyxin–agarose† (0.2 mg/ml)
0	210	210§
5	200	200
10	210	210
25	208	18
50	210	19
100	210	19
200	210	19

*All cultures inoculated with E. coli SC 9251 (5×10^6 cells/ml). Growth of the cultures was monitored by light scattering after 14 hr. Growth is reported by Klett units.
†Dry polymyxin–agarose was allowed to swell for 2 hr in media prior to incubation.
§Growth was preceded by a 2.0 hr lag period.

hydrolysates of purified spore coats showed only trace quantities of ornithine, indicating bacitracin to be only a minor component of the spore coat (Marshke and Bernlohr, 1970). Furthermore, a mutant of B. licheniformis has been isolated which is capable of sporulation although deficient in bacitracin synthesis, indicating that bacitracin is not an essential component of the spore coat (Haavik and Thomassen, 1966; Haavik and Froyshov, 1975).

5. ANTIMICROBIAL SPECTRUM

Bacitracin is a potent antibiotic against gram-positive cocci, staphylococci, streptococci, corynebacteria, Treponema pallidum, T. vincenti, Actinomyces israeli, anaerobic cocci, clostridia, neisseria, including most gonococci and meningococci, but it is relatively ineffective against most gram-negative bacteria (Weinberg, 1967; Jawetz, 1970; Storch and Krogstad, 1981; Gotz and Rand, 1982; Hackenbeck et al., 1983; Garcia-Patrone, 1985; Maddox et al., 1985).

In general, bacitracin is an ineffective agent against anaerobic infections (Nord and Olsson-Liljequist, 1985). However, recent studies have demonstrated that the group of anaerobes that synthesize methane, the Archaebacteria, are sensitive to the actions of bacitracin (Hammes et al., 1979). Of this group, Methanobacterium arbophilicum, M. M.O.H., M. O.H.G. and M. formicium showed inhibition by bacitracin while Methanospirilum and Methanosarcina were insensitive to the antibiotic.

The mechanism of the antibiotic action of bacitracin against the Archaebacteria is not yet clearly understood. The antibiotic sensitive strains of Methanobacterium sp. and Methanobrevibacter sp. contain the peptidoglycan-like substance, pseudomurein, in the cell wall and it has been proposed that bacitracin sensitivity is due to inhibition of dephosphorylation of a polyisoprenyl pyrophosphate precursor of pseudomurein (Hammes et al., 1979). The insensitive genera, Methanospirillum, and Methanosarcina, lack pseudomurein in their cell walls which are composed of protein subunits with an external sheath (Kandler and Konig, 1978) and a heteropolysaccharide (Kandler and Hipp, 1977), respectively. Strains of the genera Methanococcus and Halococcus, which also lack pseudomurein, are sensitive to bacitracin (Mescher *et al.*, 1974; Mescher and Strominger, 1978; Hammes *et al.*, 1979). Early studies suggested that bacitracin inhibited synthesis of a glycoprotein forming the rigid cell wall (Mescher and Strominger, 1975), however neither *Methanococcus sp.*, nor *Halococcus sp.* contain such a glycoprotein envelope. Bassinger and Oliver (1979) have proposed that bacitracin sensitivity of these organisms is due to the inhibition of dephosphorylation of an isoprenyl pyrophosphate precursor of ether lipids common to these genera. Clearly, more studies are necessary to elucidate the molecular mechanism of sensitivity toward bacitracin of this unique family of bacteria.

The insensitivity of gram negative organisms may be due to the outer membrane structure, which serves as a barrier against permeation by some antibiotics, since gram-negative bacteria, like gram-positive organisms, have bacitracin sensitive target sites on the inner membrane surface (Brown and Richards, 1965; Leive, 1974). This hypothesis was tested by utilizing polymyxin B bound to agarose together with bacitracin in growth inhibition of *Escherichia coli*. When *E. coli* SC 9251 was treated with bacitracin in the presence of polymyxin–agarose, the bactericidal effect of bacitracin was greatly enhanced (Rosenthal and Storm, 1977). It was postulated that the enhanced action of bacitracin on *E. coli* is due to disruption of its outer membrane by polymyxin B (Storm *et al.*, 1977), even when polymyxin has been covalently linked to agarose beads (La Porte *et al.*, 1977). The coupled polymyxin had no effect on growth by itself, presumably because it was unable to reach the cytoplasmic membrane. The synergistic effect of bacitracin and covalently attached polymyxin B is shown in Table 1. These experiments illustrated that bacitracin at concentrations greater than 200 μg/ml had no effect on growth of the organism. However, when polymyxin–agarose was added in the presence of 20 μg/ml bacitracin, growth was completely inhibited. These data strongly suggest that the insensitivity of gram-negative strains is due to the inability of the peptide to penetrate the outer membrane to interact with sensitive targets.

6. MECHANISM OF ACTION

Bacitracin affects a number of biochemical processes in bacteria, including metal ion transport (Haavik, 1976), peptidoglycan synthesis (Abraham and Newton, 1958; Park, 1958, 1960; Mandelstam and Rogers, 1959; Siewert and Strominger, 1967), membrane permeability (Crawford and Abraham, 1957; Smith and Weinberg, 1962; Snoke and Cornell, 1965; Harrington and Baddiley, 1983), and biosynthesis of inducible enzymes (Creaser, 1955; Gale and Folkes, 1955; Smith and Weinberg, 1962). Peptidoglycan biosynthesis and membrane permeability appear to be the cellular processes most sensitive to antibiotic action, which probably lead to the inhibition of cell growth (Storch and Krogstad, 1981; Bertram *et al.*, 1981). Even though bacitracin may have several sites of action, the current working hypothesis is that its influence on membrane permeability and peptidoglycan biosynthesis share a common molecular basis (Storm and Strominger, 1974; Bertram *et al.*, 1981).

6.1. INTERACTION WITH DIVALENT CATIONS

Divalent metal cations are required for the antibiotic activity of bacitracin. It has been shown that the antimicrobial activity of bacitracin toward *Staphylococcus aureus* is inhibited by EDTA (Adler and Snoke, 1962), but EDTA inhibition can be overcome by the addition of Ca^{2+}, Mn^{2+}, or Zn^{2+}. Weinberg has reported that Zn^{2+} is the most effective cation in stimulation of the antimicrobial action of bacitracin (Weinberg, 1958). It has been proposed that bacitracin may act in transporting potentially toxic divalent cations from the surface of *B. licheniformis* to the cytoplasm (Haavik, 1975). Since Mn^{2+}, Zn^{2+} and Cd^{2+} are highly toxic it is argued that transport of these ions by bacitracin enhances their toxicity. A mutant strain incapable of producing bacitracin was not affected by Mn^{2+} at concentrations which inhibited the growth of bacitracin-producing strains. However, when bacitracin was added to the medium, Mn^{2+} toxicity was restored to the

TABLE 2. *Comparison of pK Values from NMR and Direct Titration of Bacitracin A**

| Group | pK Value | |
	NMR	Direct titration
Asp COO^-	4.0	4.1
Glu COO^-	4.3	4.5
His imidazole	6.7	6.7
Ile NH_3^+	7.9	7.7
Orn $\delta\text{-}NH_3^+$	—	10.0

*The direct titration was performed as previously described (Scogin *et al.*, 1980) in H_2O. The pK values were not significantly altered when the titration was performed in D_2O. Data taken from Mosberg *et al.*, 1980.

non-producing strain (Haavik and Froyshov, 1975). The proposal that bacitracin participates in metal ion transport by *B. licheniformis* is potentially interesting, but no direct evidence has been put forth to demonstrate the peptide actually catalyzes the uptake of metal ions in bacteria. The role that bacitracin plays in metal ion transport remains to be clearly defined.

Direct interaction between bacitracin A and divalent metal ions has been observed by several techniques including potentiometry and optical and magnetic resonance spectroscopy (Wasylishen and Graham, 1974). Titration studies gave an apparent order of binding of $Cu^{2+} > Ni^{2+} > (Co^{2+}, Zn^{2+}) > Mn^{2+}$ (Garbutt *et al.*, 1961). Titration binding of Zn^{2+} and Ni^{2+} to bacitracin A was monitored by ultraviolet absorbance changes as well as by measuring proton release concomitant with metal binding. It was found that both Ni^{2+} and Zn^{2+} form 1:1 complexes with bacitracin A in solution (Scogin *et al.*, 1980; 1983). On the basis of these data it has been proposed that the metal coordinates directly to the carboxyl of glutamate, histidine imidazole, and the thiazoline ring. No involvement of the N-terminal amino group or the aspartate carboxyl was observed. The data further indicated that the pK of the N-terminal amino shifts from 7.7 to 5.7 upon complex formation. High resolution NMR has been used to assess Zn^{2+} binding to bacitracin in an effort to describe complex formation in molecular terms (Mosberg *et al.*, 1980). Assignments of resonances affected by metal ion binding were made by monitoring the pH dependence of proton resonance shifts, and by homonuclear decoupling at 270 MHz.

The pK values obtained from direct titration and from NMR are in close agreement (Table 2). Analysis of the NMR data once again indicate Zn^{2+} binding to the thiazoline ring, the histidine imidazole, and the glutamic acid carboxyl. The model deduced from NMR and titration data is given in Fig. 3. This model is consistent with earlier ORD spectral measurements performed by Cornell and Guiney (1970), in which it was proposed that the thiazoline ring provides one coordination site for Zn^{2+}.

6.2. EFFECTS ON MEMBRANE PERMEABILITY

Two mechanisms have been proposed as the major action of bacitracin in eliciting bactericidal effects: (1) perturbation of selective membrane permeability, and (2) inhibition of peptidoglycan biosynthesis. There is a large body of evidence that bacitracin affects the permeability of protoplast membranes prepared from gram-positive bacteria. Bacitracin has been shown to cause rapid lysis of protoplasts prepared from *B. licheniformis* and *M. lysodeikticus* when either zinc or cadmium was present in the incubation mixtures (Snoke and Cornell, 1965). The ratio of antibiotic to protoplasts required for this lytic action was comparable to the ratio of antibiotic per cell necessary to inhibit bacterial growth. It must be noted, however, that protoplasts are often unstable and susceptible to surface active agents. In order to circumvent this problem, Reynolds has developed a so-called reconditioning system for protoplasts prepared from *B. megaterium*

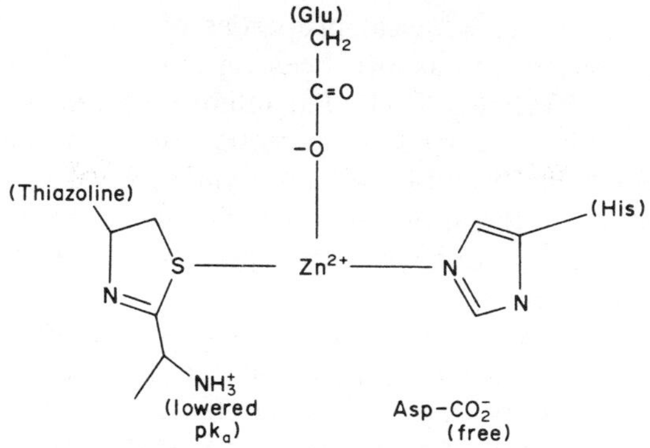

FIG. 3. Schematic model proposed for Zn^{2+}-bacitracin A. The same model would apply to the complexes formed with Ni^{2+} or Co^{2+} and bacitracin. (Reprinted with permission from Scogin et al., 1980.)

strain KM (Reynolds, 1971). Protoplasts 'reconditioned' by incubation in growth medium for 30 min at 37°C were capable of peptidoglycan synthesis, however, peptidoglycan biosynthesis was not a requisite for protoplast growth. For example, D-cycloserine and penicillin did not inhibit protoplast growth (Hancock and Fitz-James, 1964). Bacitracin, however, did inhibit protoplast growth when present in concentrations similar to the minimal inhibitory concentration for whole cells. Similar results were found for *Streptococcus faecalis* protoplasts (Shockman and Lampen, 1962), and L-forms of some *S. aureus* strains (Williams, 1963; Molander et al., 1964). It has been reported that methicillin, oxacillin, and cephalothin will induce L-forms of *S. aureus* whereas bacitracin will not (Molander et al., 1964). Group A *Streptococci*, however, will produce L-forms indistinguishable from those produced by penicillin when treated with bacitracin (Rotta et al., 1965), indicating that the toxic effect of bacitracin on *Streptococci* is due to its effect on cell wall integrity. Direct evidence for bacitracin-induced structural changes in plasma membranes has been demonstrated by electron microscopy (Sleytr et al., 1976).

Pronounced structural changes in the form of rods of 25–30 nm in length were observed on freeze fractured plasma membranes which had been treated with bacitracin. Even though the above evidence indicates that bacitracin affects the structure and permeability of protoplasts of most bacteria, the relationship between these phenomena and the effects of bacitracin on intact bacteria is not yet clear.

It was observed by MacDonald and co-workers that bacitracin at concentrations between 10^{-3} and 10^{-4} M stimulated the release of low molecular weight markers trapped in phospholipid liposomes (MacDonald et al., 1974). Cadmium ions specifically enhanced this release. Since the concentration of bacitracin employed in the experiments was several orders of magnitude greater than that required for inhibition of bacterial growth, the physiological significance of these observations is open to question. Even though bacitracin at 5×10^{-4} M did lower the conductance of planar lipid bilayers, Mueller and Rudin (1969) observed no clear influence of bacitracin on conductance measurements. Further model membrane studies are required to draw definite conclusions regarding the physiological significance of bacitracin-induced permeability changes.

6.3. INHIBITION OF PEPTIDOGLYCAN SYNTHESIS

Inhibition of peptidoglycan biosynthesis by bacitracin has been demonstrated in a number of studies. Bacitracin has been shown to inhibit the accumulation of uridine nucleotides (Abraham and Newton, 1958) and to inhibit the incorporation of radiolabeled amino acids into peptidoglycans without affecting amino acid incorporation into cellular proteins (Park, 1958, 1960; Mandelstam and Rogers, 1959). In addition, bacitracin induced protoplast formation in *S. aureus* (Abraham, 1957) and L-form formation from strains of Group A *Streptococci* (Rotta et al., 1965). There were virtually no differences in morphological or bacteriological properties of the L-forms induced by either penicillin or bacitracin. Bacitracin has also been reported to inhibit peptidoglycan biosynthesis in *B. megaterium* (Reynolds, 1971). The inhibition of peptidoglycan biosynthesis in the afore-mentioned studies occurred at antibiotic concentrations similar to the minimum inhibitory concentrations. Peptidoglycan biosynthesis was not completely inhibited *in vivo* at any concentration of the antibiotic used. The incomplete inhibition of peptidoglycan biosynthesis was rationalized when the specific bacitracin-sensitive step in cell wall biosynthesis was identified.

The bacitracin-sensitive step of peptidoglycan biosynthesis was first identified when Siewart and Strominger (1967) demonstrated that ^{14}C labeled peptidoglycan could be synthesized *in vitro* when (^{14}C pentapeptide)-disaccharide $[^{32}P]$–PP–C_{55}-isoprenol was used as a substrate in the presence of membranes from *M. lysodeikticus*. $^{32}P_i$ was released at the same time. Peptidoglycan was still synthesized in the presence of bacitracin, however, $^{32}P_i$ was not released, and a ^{32}P-labeled lipid, assumed to be C_{55}-isoprenyl-pyrophosphate, accumulated at higher levels.

These results suggested that bacitracin inhibited the enzymatic conversion of C_{55}-isoprenyl pyrophosphate to C_{55}-isoprenyl phosphate. This conversion is catalyzed by a membrane associated pyrophosphatase which is essential for *in-vivo* peptidoglycan biosynthesis, since only the monophosphate form of the lipid can react with UDP-acetylmuramylpentapeptide. The inability of bacitracin to completely inhibit *in-vitro* peptidoglycan synthesis is explained because the incorporation of the pool of precursors, linked to the pyrophosphate form of the lipid carrier, would not be inhibited. Eventual inhibition of peptidoglycan biosynthesis would occur because bacitracin inhibits the recycling of C_{55}-isoprenylpyrophosphate. This proposal was verified by demonstration that dephosphorylation of C_{55}-isoprenyl pyrophosphate by membranes from *M. lysodeikticus* was inhibited by bacitracin (Siewert and Strominger, 1967). Inhibition of this *in-vitro* reaction required bacitracin concentrations similar to the minimum inhibitory concentration for growth of *M. lysodeikticus*. Phosphomonoesterase from *E. coli* or alkaline phosphatase from calf intestinal mucosa also catalyzed dephosphorylation of C_{55}-isoprenyl pyrophosphate. These activities were inhibited by bacitracin suggesting specificity for the substrate rather than the enzyme. It was proposed that the antibiotic forms a complex with the lipid, and this was verified directly (Stone and Strominger, 1971; Storm and Strominger, 1973).

Formation of a complex between C_{55}-isoprenyl pyrophosphate and the components of commercial bacitracin was first demonstrated qualitatively by the Hummel–Dryer column binding method (Stone and Strominger, 1972). Subsequent studies, using highly purified bacitracin components and various isoprenyl pyrophosphates, characterized the effects on binding of divalent cations, pH, and variations in lipid and peptide structure (Storm and Strominger, 1973). It was demonstrated that bacitracin A and C_{55}-isoprenyl pyrophosphate form a 1:1 complex with an apparent K_a of 6.5×10^{-5} M^{-1} at pH 8.5 in the presence of 1 mM Mg^{2+} at a constant ionic strength of 0.08.

The pH dependency of binding was bell shaped. Binding was maximal at pH 7.0–7.5, indicating that a specific ionization state of the peptide and/or lipid is required for maximum stability of the complex. Two inflections in the pH profile were observed, the first at pH 6, and the second between pH 8.5 and 9.0. The only groups on bacitracin A which titrate at pH 6.0 are the histidine imidazole nitrogen (see Table 2) and the third ionization of the lipid pyrophosphate moiety. It is not possible to distinguish between the two groups on the basis of titration data alone. The second inflection, occurring between pH 8.5 and 9.0, reflects ionization of the α-amino group of the N-terminal isoleucine and the δ-amino group of ornithine (Table 2). While conclusions drawn from pH studies are largely inferential, the data suggest that polar or electrostatic interactions contribute to the stability of the bacitracin-A–C_{55} isoprenyl pyrophosphate complex, which involves divalent metal ion (see below).

In order to assess whether a correlation exists between *in-vitro* binding constants and antibiotic activity, binding between C_{55}-isoprenyl pyrophosphate and several derivatives

TABLE 3. *Binding Constant for Various Bacitracin Species with the C_{55}-isoprenyl Pyrophosphate*

Bacitracin	MIC†	K (M^{-1})§	K(M^{-1})(EDTA)§
Desamido bacitracin	7×10^{-4}	1.4×10^3	2×10^3
Bacitracin F	5×10^{-5}	9.8×10^3	6.3×10^3
Mono-DNP-bacitracin	3×10^{-7}	2.8×10^4	—
Bacitracin A, B	2×10^{-7}	1.0×10^6	—
Bacitracin A	1×10^{-7}	1.1×10^6	5.2×10^3

†MIC = minimal growth inhibitory concentration.

§Association constants (K) were determined in 0.1 M Tris-Cl-buffer (pH 7.5) in the presence of 1 mM MgCl$_2$, 0.05 mM mercaptoethanol, ionic strength at 0.08 M, in the absence of (K) or presence (K) (EDTA) of 5 mM EDTA.
(Adapted with permission from Mosberg *et al.*, 1980.)

of bacitracin A was examined. The binding constants determined at pH 7.5 in the presence of 1 mM Mg^{2+}/0.05 mM 2-mercaptoethanol at constant ionic strength are summarized in Table 3. Complete inhibition of *M. lysodeikticus* growth occurred at a bacitracin A concentration of 1×10^{-7} M, and an association constant of 1×10^{-6} M was observed in the presence of Mg^{2+}. Inclusion of 1 mM Zn^{2+} ion resulted in a three-fold increase in the binding constant, while EDTA lowered the binding constant 200-fold, indicating the importance of divalent metal ion in the binding of bacitracin A to the lipid-pyrophosphate. Monodinitrophenylation of the δ-amino group of ornithine in bacitracin reduced antibiotic activity of bacitracin A by 66% and lowered the binding constant by 40-fold. Bacitracin F shows relatively poor antibiotic activity and its K_a for binding was 100-times lower than bacitracin A. Since EDTA had little effect on binding between bacitracin F and C$_{55}$-isoprenyl pyrophosphate, a metal ion is probably not a requirement for this interaction. Finally, the desamido derivative was the poorest antibiotic tested and showed the weakest interaction with lipid. Bacitracin A, bacitracin F and the desamido derivative all had comparable affinities for the lipid in the presence of EDTA, suggesting some basal level of binding by bacitracin peptides in the absence of metal ions. It has been postulated that a ternary complex is formed between lipid pyrophosphate, metal ion and bacitracin peptide, and that if capacity to form this ternary complex is eliminated, residual binding is driven by secondary hydrophobic forces. Binding studies using a number of C$_{55}$-isoprenyl pyrophosphate structural analogues lends credence to the above models. As shown in Table 4, both the pyrophosphate function and alkyl side chain are required for optimum binding. For example, farnesyl monophosphate binds approximately 200 times less strongly than farnesyl pyrophosphate or C$_{55}$-isoprenyl pyrophosphate. In the same manner, inorganic pyrophosphate complexes approximately 20 times more strongly than inorganic phosphate. The data in Table 4 also indicate that a minimum hydrocarbon chain of 2 or 3 isoprene units is required for efficient binding, strengthening the proposed role of hydrophobic interactions of bacitra-

TABLE 4. *Binding Constants for Interaction of Lipid Analogs with Bacitracin A*

Substrate	K (M^{-1})
Inorganic phosphate	483
Inorganic pyrophosphate	10.400
Isopentenyl pyrophosphate	8.090
Farnesyl phosphate	5.590
Farnesyl pyrophosphate	829.000
C$_{55}$-isoprenyl pyrophosphate	1.050.000

Association constants (K) were determined at pH 7.5 (0.1 M Tris), 1 mM MgCl$_2$, 0.05 mM mercaptoethanol, ionic strength at 0.08 M.

TABLE 5. *Metal Ion Specificity for Binding of Bacitracin A to* PP_i

Metal ion added	$K(\text{M}^{-1})$
None	< 100
Cu^{2+}	1,780
Hg^{2+}	3,040
Co^{2+}	3,720
Ni^{2+}	4,000
Mg^{2+}	4,740
Cd^{2+}	6,800
Zn^{2+}	17,800

Association constants (K) for bacitracin A and inorganic pyrophosphate were determined in 0.1 M Tris-HCl (pH 7.5), 0.05 mM 2-mercaptoethanol. Bacitracin A was pretreated with EDTA to remove divalent cations. EDTA was separated from bacitracin A by chromatography on Bio-Gel P-2. Divalent cations were added in the chloride form to a concentration of 1 mM.

cin with lipid. Hydrophobic interactions have been further implicated by NMR studies (Storm, 1974).

Since bacitracin is capable of binding various divalent cations, the interaction between metal-free bacitracin A and inorganic pyrophosphate was examined in the presence of various ions. The data summarized in Table 5 shows that the association constants varied over a 10-fold range with the K_a in the presence of Zn^{2+} being approximately four-fold greater than that found in the presence of Mg^{2+}.

The data summarized above supports the hypothesis that the antibiotic action of bacitracin A is due to interaction with C_{55}-isoprenyl pyrophosphate and inhibition of peptidoglycan biosynthesis. There is an excellent correlation between the concentration dependence of growth inhibition of *M. lysodeikticus* and both inhibition of peptidoglycan biosynthesis *in vitro* and inhibition of dephosphorylation of C_{55}-isoprenyl pyrophosphate *in vitro*. The divalent cation requirement for maximum binding to lipid, $Zn^{2+} > Cd^{2+} > Mg^{2+}$, is similar to that shown for antibiotic activity (Weinberg, 1958), and the pH maximum for binding and antibiotic activity are the same.

Further support for the above proposal was obtained from binding studies of [³H]-bacitracin to cells and protoplast preparations of *M. lysodeikticus* (Storm and Strominger, 1974). The K_m for bacitracin binding to cells was 3.7×10^{-6} M, which is in close agreement with *in vitro* binding studies for interaction of bacitracin A and C_{55}-isoprenyl pyrophosphate. These data strongly suggest that permeability changes caused by bacitracin arise from interactions of bacitracin A and C_{55}-isoprenyl pyrophosphate, and may be secondary to the lethal effects of this interaction on peptidoglycan biosynthesis.

7. CONCLUSIONS

Although the mechanism of the antibiotic activity of bacitracin has not been unambiguously defined, it is clear that many of the biological properties of the peptide can be attributed to its high affinity for polyisoprenyl pyrophosphates. If indeed the antibiotic activity of bacitracin is due to interactions with C_{55}-isoprenyl pyrophosphate, this system offers a rare opportunity for studying interactions between an antibiotic and its 'receptor' in considerable detail. Bacitracin and the isoprenyl pyrophosphates are readily available in purified form and it should be possible to define, by various physical techniques, the chemical interactions contributing to the stability of the complex. It is also notable that this complex represents one of the most specific lipid–peptide interactions of biological significance that has thus far been described.

If binding of bacitracin to this complex is responsible for the action of bacitracin in sensitive organisms, then acquisition of resistance by an organism through mutational modification of the drug target seems highly improbable because of the lack of specific cell protein targets. It is possible that an inactivation of the drug, or more likely, reduced target access due to changes in cell wall permeability would be more likely mechanisms of acquired resistance.

REFERENCES

ABRAHAM, E. P. (1957) Biochemistry of some peptide and sterol antibiotics. pp. 69–73, John Wiley, New York.

ABRAHAM, E. P. and NEWTON, G. G. F. (1958) Structure and function of some sulfur-containing peptides. *CIBA Found. Symp. Amino Peptides Antimetab.* pp. 205–225.

ADLER, R. H. and SNOKE, J. E. (1962) Requirement of divalent metal ions for bacitracin activity. *J. Bact.* **83**: 1315–1317.

BASSINGER, G. W. and OLIVER, J. D. (1979) Inhibition of *Halobacterium cutirubrum* lipid biosynthesis by bacitracin. *J. gen. Microbiol.* **111**: 423–427.

BERNLOHR, R. W. and NOVELLI, G. D. (1960) Some characteristics of bacitracin production by *Bacillus licheniformis. Archs Biochem. Biophys.* **87**: 232–238.

BERNLOHR, R. W. and NOVELLI, G. D. (1964) Bacitracin biosynthesis and spore formation: The physiological role of an antibiotic. *Archs Biochem. Biophys.* **103**: 94–104.

BERTRAM, K. C., HANCOCK, I. C. and BADDILEY, J. (1981) Synthesis of teichoic acid by *Bacillus subtilis* protoplasts. *J. Bact.* **148**: 406–412.

BROWN, M. R. W. and RICHARDS, R. M. E. (1965) Effect on the resistance of *Pseudomonas aeruginosa* to antimicrobial agents. *Nature (London)* **207**: 1391–1393.

CORNELL, N. W. and GUINEY, D. G. (1970) Binding sites for zinc (II) in bacitracin. *Biochem. biophys. Res. Commun.* **40**: 530–536.

CRAIG, L. C., WEISIGER, J. R., HAUSMAN, W. and HARFENIST, E. J. (1952) The separation and characterization of bacitracin polypeptides. *J. biol. Chem.* **199**: 259–266.

CRAIG, L. C., PHILLIPS, W. F. and BURACHIK, M. (1969) Bacitracin A. Isolation by counter-current distribution and characterization. *Biochemistry.* **8**: 2348–2356.

CRAWFORD, K. and ABRAHAM, E. E. (1957) The synergistic action of cephalosporin C and benzyl-penicillin against a penicillinase-producing strain of *Staphylococcus aureus. J. gen. Microbiol.* **16**: 604–613.

CREASER, E. H. (1955) The induced biosynthesis of galactosidase in *Staphylococcus aureus. J. gen. Microbiol.* **12**: 288–297.

FROYSHOV, O. (1975) Enzyme-bound intermediates in the biosynthesis of bacitracin. *Eur. J. Biochem.* **59**: 201–206.

FROYSHOV, O. and LALAND, S. G. (1974) On the biosynthesis of bacitracin by a soluble enzyme complex from *B. licheniformis. Eur. J. Biochem.* **42**: 235–242.

GALARDY, R. E., PRINZ M. P. and CRAIG, L. C. (1971) Tritium-Hydrogen exchange of bacitracin A. Evidence for an intramolecular hydrogen bond. *Biochemistry* **10**: 2429–2436.

GALE, E. F. and FOLKES, J. P. (1955) The assimilation of amino acids by bacteria. *Biochem. J.* **59**: 675–684.

GARBUTT, J. T., MOREHOUS, A. L. and HANSON, A. M. (1961) Metal binding properties of bacitracin. *Agric. Food Chem.* **9**: 285–289.

GARCIA-PATRONE, M. (1985) Bacitracin increases size of parasporal crystals and spores in *Bacillus thruingiensis. Mol. Cell. Biochem.* **68**: 131–137.

GOTZ, V. P. and RAND, K. H. (1982) Medical management of antimicrobial associated diarrhea and colitis. *Pharmacotherapy* **2**: 100–109.

HAAVIK, H. I. (1974) Formation of bacitracin by *Bacillus licheniformis*, effect of glucose. *J. gen. Microbiol.* **81**: 383–390.

HAAVIK, H. I. (1975) Effect of bacitracin and manganese (II) ions upon the producer strain *Bacillus licheniformis. Acta path. micribiol. scand.* **83B**: 513–518.

HAAVIK, H. I. (1976) On the role of bacitracin peptides in trace metal transport by *Bacillus licheniformis. J. gen. Micribiol.* **96**: 393–396.

HAAVIK, H. I. (1981) Effects of amino acids upon bacitracin production by *Bacillus licheniformis. FEMS Microbiol. Lett.* **10**: 111–114.

HAAVIK, H. I. and FROYSHOV, O. (1975) Function of peptide antibiotics in producer organisms. *Nature (London)* **254**: 79–82.

HAAVIK, H. I. and THOMASSEN, S. (1966) A bacitracin-negative mutant of *Bacillus licheniformis* which is able to sporulate. *J. gen. Microbiol.* **76**: 451–454.

HAAVIK, H. I. and VESSIA, B. (1978) Bacitracin production by the high-yielding mutant *Bacillus licheniformis* strain AL: Stimulating effect of L-leucine. *Acta Path. Microbiol. Scand. Sect. B.* **86**: 67–70.

HAKENBECK, R., MARTIN, C. and MORELLI, G. (1983) *Streptococcus pneumoniae* proteins released into medium upon inhibition of cell wall biosynthesis. *J. Bact.* **155**: 1372–1381.

HAMMES, W. P., WINTER, J. and KANDLER, O. (1979) The sensitivity of pseudomurein-containing genus *Methanobacterium* to inhibitors of murein synthesis. *Archs Microbiol.* **123**: 275–279.

HANCOCK, R. and FITZ-JAMES, P. C. (1964) Some differences in the action of penicillin, bacitracin and vanomycin of *B. megaterium. J. Bact.* **87**: 1044–1050.

HANLON, G. W. and HODGES, N. A. (1981) Bacitracin and protease production in relation to sporulation during exponential growth of *Bacillus licheniformis* on poorly utilized carbon and nitrogen sources. *J. Bact.* **147**: 427–431.

HANLON, G. W., HODGES, N. A. and RUSSELL, A. D. (1982) The influence of glucose, ammonium and magnesium availability of the production of protease and bacitracin by *Bacillus licheniformis*. *J. gen. Microbiol.* **128**: 845–851.

HARRINGTON, C. R. and BADDILEY, J. (1983) Peptidoglycan synthesis by partly autolyzed cells of *Bacillus subtilis* W23. *J. Bact.* **155**: 776–792.

ISHIHARA, H. and SHIMURA, K. (1974) Biosynthesis of bacitracins. *Biochim. biophys. Acta* **338**: 588–600.

JAWETZ, E. (1970) Polymyxins, colistin, bacitracin, ristocetin and vanomycin. In: *Antimicrbiol Therapeutics*, p. 91, KAGAN B. (ed). Benjamin N. Saunders, Philadelphia.

JOHNSON, B. A., ANKER, H. and MELENEY, F. L. (1945) Bacitracin: a new antibiotic produced by a member of the *B. subtilis* group. *Science* **102**: 376–377.

KANDLER, O. and HIPP, H. (1977) Lack of peptidoglycan in the cell walls of *Methanosarcina barkeri*. *Archs Microbiol.* **113**: 57–60.

KANDLER, O. and KONIG, H. (1978) Chemical composition of the peptidoglycan free cell walls of methanogenic bacteria. *Archs Microbiol.* **118**: 141–152.

KONIGSBERG, W. and CRAIG, L. C. (1959) Cellulose ion exchange and rotary dispersion studies with bacitracin polyeptides. *J. Am. chem. Soc.* **81**: 3452–3458.

LAPORTE, D. C., ROSENTHAL, K. S. and STORM, D. R. (1977) Inhibition of *E. coli* growth and respiration by polymyxin covalently attached to agarose. *Biochemistry* **16**: 1642–1648.

LEIVE, L. (1974) The barrier function of the gram negative envelope. *Ann. N.Y. Acad. Sci.* **235**: 109–129.

LYERLA, J. R. and FREEDMAN, M. H. (1972) Spectral assignment and conformational analysis of cyclic peptides by carbon-13 NMR. *J. biol. Chem.* **247**: 8183–8192.

MACDONALD, R. I., MACDONALD, R. C. and CORNELL, N. W. (1974) Perturbation of liposomal and planar lipid bilayer membranes by bacitracin. *Biochemistry* **13**: 4018–4024.

MADDOX, J. S., WARE, J. C. and DILLON, H. C., Jr. (1985) The natural history of streptococcal skin infection: Prevention with topical antibiotics. *J. Am. Acad. Dermatol.* **13**: 207–212.

MANDELSTAM, J. and ROGERS, H. J. (1959) The incorporation of amino acids into the cell-wall mucopeptide of staphylococci and the effect of antibiotics on the process. *Biochem. J.* **72**: 654–662.

MARSCHKE, C. K. and BERNLOHR, R. W. (1970) Reevaluation of bacitracin as a spore coat component. *J. Bact.* **102**: 283–284.

MARTIN, J. F. and DEMAIN, A. L. (1980) Control of antibiotic biosynthesis. *Microbiol. Revs.* **44**: 230–251.

MESCHER, M. F. and STROMINGER, J. L. (1975) Bacitracin induces sphere formation in halobacterium species which lack a wall peptidoglycan. *J. gen. Microb.* **89**: 375–378.

MESCHER, M. F. and STROMINGER, J. L. (1978) The cell surface protein of *Halobacterium salinarium*. In: *Energetics and Structure of Halophile Organisms*, pp. 503–511, CAPLAN, S. R. and GINZBURG. M. (eds). Elsevier, Amsterdam.

MESCHER, M. F., STROMINGER, J. L. and WATSON, S. W. (1974) Protein and carbohydrate composition of the cell envelope of *Halobacterium salinarium*. *J. Bact.* **120**: 945–954.

MOLANDER, C. W., KAGAN, B. M., WEINBERGER, H. J., HEIMLICH, E. M. and BUSSER, R. J. (1964) Induction by antibiotics and comparative sensitivity of L-phase variants of *S. aureus*. *J. Bact.* **88**: 591–594.

MOSBERG, H. I., SCOGIN, D. A., STORM, D. R. and GENNIS, R. B. (1980) Proton nuclear magnetic resonance studies on bacitracin A and its interaction with zinc ion. *Biochemistry* **19**: 3353–3357.

MUELLER, P. and RUDIN, D. O. (1969) In: *Current Topics in Bioenergetics*, pp. 157, SANADI, D. R. (ed). Academic Press, New York.

NEWTON, G. G. F. and ABRAHAM, E. P. (1953) Some properties of the bacitracin polypeptides. *Biochem. J.* **53**: 597–604.

NORD, C. E. and OLSSON-LILJEQUIST, B. (1985) Comparative *in vitro* activity of SCH 34343 and other antimicrobial agents against anaerobic bacteria. *J. Antimicrobial Chemotherapy Suppl C* **15**: 183–188.

PARK, J. T. (1958) Inhibition of cell-wall synthesis in *Staphylococcus aureus* by chemicals which cause accumulation of wall precursors. *Biochem. J.* **70**: 2P.

PARK, J. T. (1960) Inhibition of synthesis of bacterial mucopeptide or protein by certain antibiotics and its possible significance for microbiology and medicine. *Antimicrob. Agents Annu.* 338–343.

PFAENDER, P., SPECHT, D., HEINRICH, G., SCHWARZ, E., KUHN, E. and SIMLOT, M. M. (1973) Enzymes of *Bacillus licheniformis* in the biosynthesis of bacitracin A. *Febs Lett.* **32**: 100–104.

REGNA, P. P. (1959) The chemistry of antibiotics. In: *Antibiotics, their Chemistry and Nonmedical Uses*, pp. 58, D. van Nostrand, New York.

REYNOLDS, P. E. (1971) Peptidoglycan synthesis in Bacilli II. Characteristics of protoplast membrane preparations. *Biochim. biophys. Acta* **237**: 255–272.

RIEDER, H., HEINRICH, G., BREUKER, E., SIMLOT, M. M. and PFAENDER, P. (1975) Bacitracin synthetase. *Methods Enzymol.* **43**: 548–559.

ROSENTHAL, K. S. and STORM, D. R. (1977) Disruption of the *Escherichia coli* outer membrane permeability barrier by immobilized polymyxin. *Br. J. Antibiot.* **30**: 1087–1092.

ROTTA, J., KARAKAWA, W. W. and KRAUSE, R. M. (1965) Isolation of L forms from group A streptococci exposed to bacitracin. *J. Bact.* **89**: 1581–1585.

SCOGIN, D. A., MOSBERG, H. I., STORM, D. R. and GENNIS, R. B. (1980) Binding of nickel and zinc ions to bacitracin A. *Biochemistry* **19**: 3348–3352.

SCOGIN, D. A., BALDWIN, T. O. and GENNIS, R. B. (1983) Studies on the complex formed between bacitracin A and divalent cations. *Biochim. biophys. Acta* **742**: 184–188.

SHOCKMAN, G. D. and LAMPEN, J. O. (1962) Inhibition by antibiotics of the growth of bacterial and yeast protoplasts. *J. Bact.* **84**: 508–512.

SIEWERT, G. and STROMINGER, J. L. (1967) Bacitracin: an inhibitor of the dephosphorylation of lipid pyrophosphate, an intermediate in biosynthesis of the peptidoglycan of bacterial cell walls. *Proc. natn. Acad. Sci. U.S.A.* **57**: 767–773.

SIMLOT, M. M., PFAENDER, P. and SPECHT, D. (1973) Synthesis of antibiotics by enzymes from altered growth conditions by *Bacillus licheniformis*. *FEBS Lett.* **35**: 231–235.

SLEYTR, U. B., OLIVER, T. C. and THORNE, K. J. I. (1976) Bacitracin-induced changes in bacterial plasma membrane structure. *Biochim. biophys. Acta* **419**: 570–573.

SMITH, J. L. and WEINBERG, E. D. (1962) Mechanisms of antibacterial action of bacitracin. *J. gen. Microbiol.* **28**: 559–569.

SNOKE, J. E. and CORNELL, N. (1965) Protoplast lysis and inhibition of growth of *Bacillus licheniformis* by bacitracin. *J. Bact.* **89**: 415–420.

STONE, K. J. and STROMINGER, J. L. (1971) Mechanism of action of bacitracin: Complexation with metal ion and C_{55}-isoprenyl pyrophosphate. *Proc. natn. Acad. Sci. U.S.A.* **68**: 3223–3227.

STONE, K. J. and STROMINGER, J. L. (1972) Inhibition of sterol biosynthesis by bacitracin. *Proc. Natn. Acad. Sci. U.S.A.* **69**: 1287–1289.

STORCH, G. A. and KROGSTAD, D. J. (1981) Antibiotic-induced lysis of enterococci. *J. Clin. Invest.* **68**: 639–645.

STORM, D. R. (1974) Mechanism of bacitracin action, a specific lipid-peptide interaction. *Ann. N.Y. Acad. Sci.* **235**: 387–398.

STORM, D. R. and STROMINGER, J. L. (1973) Complex formation between bacitracin peptides and isoprenyl pyrophosphates. *J. biol. Chem.* **248**: 3940–3945.

STORM, D. R. and STROMINGER, J. L. (1974) Binding of bacitracin to cells and protoplasts of *Micrococcus lysodeikticus*. *J. biol. Chem.* **249**: 1823–1827.

STORM, D. R., SWANSON, P. E. and ROSENTHAL, K. S. (1977) Polymyxin and related peptide antibiotics. *A. Rev. Biochem.* **46**: 723–763.

SUELTER, C. H. (1985) *A Practical Guide to Enzymology*, New York, Wiley-Interscience, pp. 110–116.

SUPEK, V., GAMULIN, S. and DELIĆ, V. (1985) Enhancement of bacitracin biosynthesis by branched-chain amino acids in a regulatory mutant of *Bacillus licheniformis*. *Folia Microbiol.* (Prague) **30**: 342–348.

TSUJI, K., ROBERTSON, J. H. and BACH, J. Z. (1974) Quantitative high pressure liquid chromatographic analysis of bacitracin, a peptide antibiotic. *J. Chromatogr.* **99**: 597–608.

TSUJI, K., ROBERTSON, J. H. and BACH, J. Z. (1975) Quantitative high pressure liquid chromatographic method for polypeptide antibiotics and its application to study the effects of treatments to reduce microbial levels in bacitracin powder. *J. Chromatogr.* **112**: 663–672.

VITKOVIC, L. and SADOFF, H. L. (1977a) *In vitro* production of bacitracin by proteolysis of vegetative *Bacillus licheniformis* cell protein. *J. Bact.* **131**: 897–905.

VITKOVIC, L. and SADOFF, H. L. (1977b) Purification of the extracellular protease of *Bacillus licheniformis* and its inhibition by bacitracin. *J. Bact.* **131**: 891–896.

WASYLISHEN, R. E. and GRAHAM, M. R. (1975) A nuclear magnetic resonance study of the metal binding sites in bacitracin. *Can. J. Biochem.* **53**: 1250–1254.

WEINBERG, E. D. (1958) Enhancement of bacitracin by the metallic ions of group II B. *Antibiotic. Annu.* 924–929.

WEINBERG, E. D. (1967) Bacitracin, gramicidin and tyrocidine. *Antibiotics* **II**: 240–253.

WILLIAMS, R. E. O. (1963) L forms of *Staphylococcus aureus*. *J. gen. Microbiol.* **33**: 325–334.

CHAPTER 4

VANCOMYCIN AND RELATED ANTIBIOTICS

H. R. PERKINS

Department of Microbiology, University of Liverpool, Liverpool L69 3BX, England

Abstract

Vancomycin, ristocetin and related glycopeptide antibiotics combine non-covalently with certain peptide sequences in bacterial wall peptidoglycan, notably acyl-D-alanyl-D-alanine. By this means biosynthesis of peptidoglycan is inhibited; current thoughts on the mode of action are detailed. Studies by X-ray crystallography and NMR have elucidated the structure of the binding sites and can largely account for their chemical specificity. The mechanism by which ristocetin (but not vancomycin) induces platelet aggregation in normal human plasma but not in some von Willebrand patients is discussed. The revival of clinical interest in this group of antibiotics for the treatment of intransigent infections is also described.

1. INTRODUCTION

Vancomycin and ristocetin are related glycopeptide antibiotics that were discovered in the mid-fifties, being respectively isolated from *Streptomyces orientalis* (McCormick *et al.*, 1956) and from *Nocardia lurida* (Grundy *et al.*, 1957). Ristomycin was independently isolated from *Proactinomyces fructiferi* var. *ristomycini* (Brazhnikova *et al.*, 1963) but has since been identified with ristocetin (Sztaricskai *et al.*, 1980). The earliest investigations showed that these substances were more active against gram-positive than against gram-negative bacteria, with minimum inhibitory concentrations (MIC values) of as little as 0.1 μg/ml of ristocetin or 0.25 μg/ml of vancomycin for the most sensitive bacteria such as the streptococci (see Lightbown, 1964). Both antibiotics were bacteriostatic and there was some evidence that higher concentrations could be bactericidal in particular instances. Vancomycin came to be used clinically, particularly in the period before β-lactamase-resistant penicillins such as methicillin became available. Therapeutic doses could be given, sufficient to be bactericidal against streptococci, staphylococci, corynebacteria and clostridia, but only bacteriostatic for enterococci. Gram-negative bacteria, with the exception of some strains of *Neisseria*, were resistant and so too were mycobacteria and fungi (Kucers and Bennett, 1975). In the early years, considerable problems with toxicity were encountered, but at least some of these have subsequently been attributed to impurities in the preparations, now largely eliminated (Riley, 1970). Because of the development of ever more resistances to β-lactam and other antibiotics there has been a resurgence of clinical interest in vancomycin as a drug that can offer potential cures in specific conditions where β-lactams are contra-indicated (Esposito and Gleckman, 1977; Cook and Farrar, 1978). One of the attractions of vancomycin, evident at an early stage and borne out since, is that resistances to it do not readily develop. Its mode of action, by which it sequestrates intermediates of peptidoglycan synthesis rather than interfering directly with one of the biosynthetic enzymes (see below), could well account for the failure to develop resistance.

2. COMPOSITION AND STRUCTURE

Early information about the chemical composition of these antibiotics was very limited. Thus, for instance, it was known that vancomycin contained organic chlorine,

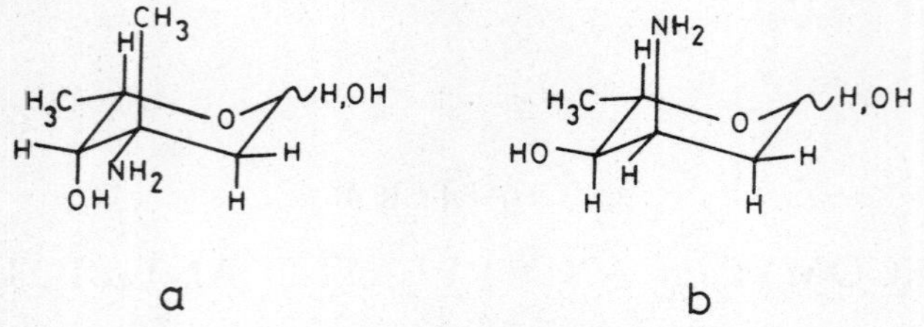

FIG. 1. Structures of (a) Vancosamine and, (b) Ristosamine.

carboxyl, amino and phenolic groups and that on hydrolysis it yielded aspartic acid, glucose and N-methyl-leucine (Johnson, 1962).

Later, Marshall (1965) published investigations from which a structure containing phenols and chlorophenols could be deduced. He also described a crystalline degradation product CDP-I, which was produced by keeping vancomycin at pH 4.2 and 60–70°C for 40 hr and consisted of heavy amber crystals devoid of antibiotic activity (Marshall, 1965). It was this crystalline product that subsequently permitted a successful X-ray crystallographic resolution of the structure of CDP-I, and by implication of vancomycin (Sheldrick et al., 1978).

Antibiotics of the vancomycin group all seem to contain unusual amino sugars, although recent deductions of the overall structures have indicated that these residues occupy different sites. The first of these sugars to be tentatively identified was ristosamine from ristomycin (ristocetin), though it was not fully characterized until 1974 (Bognar et al., 1974) (Fig. 1). Meanwhile, the amino sugar peculiar to vancomycin had been described and characterized as vancosamine (Weringa et al., 1972; Johnson et al., 1972) (Fig. 1).

Apart from these amino sugars, the antibiotics also typically contain residues of neutral sugars, which often vary even within isolates from a particular organism (Bardone et al., 1978). Thus ristocetins A and B differ solely by the size of the carbohydrate chain attached (Fig. 2). It was apparent at an early stage that the sugar residues were not essential for antibiotic activity, and indeed in some cases they could be removed with benefit. Thus acid hydrolysis removed the sugars from the ristocetins and at the same time gave enhanced antibacterial activity (Philips et al., 1960).

Progress towards full structural formulae for these antibiotics was inevitably slow, since conventional degradative procedures yielded rather uninformative fragments. The problem of the aglycone of vancomycin, begun by Johnson (1962) and Marshall (1965), was driven towards a credible solution by the ingenious combination of chemical degradation and substitutions such as methylation with the application of proton and ^{13}C-NMR. Smith et al., (1974) were able to identify five benzene rings in the molecule, two of them linked as chlorophenols by phenolic ether linkages to another non-chlorinated phenol, itself in turn glycosylated at its remaining phenolic oxygen by 2-vancosaminyl-glucose. Other evidence suggested that the remaining benzene rings were present as a biphenyl system, again with additional OH-groups. Further progress was reported by Smith et al., (1975), whose work suggested that the phenolic units were in fact components of hitherto unknown α-amino acids joined by amide linkages and coupled in the same way to D-aspartic acid and N-methyl-D-leucine. At this stage it became clear that the biphenyl unit was in fact a component of the diamino-dicarboxylic acid actinoidinic acid, originally isolated from actinoidin (Lomakina et al., 1972). This structure has now been found as a common feature in all these antibiotics.

The final assembly into the first complete three-dimensional structure for any member of the group was achieved by X-ray crystallography of the vancomycin degradation product CDP-I, which differs in composition from its parent antibiotic by the loss of a single amide group (Sheldrick et al., 1978). The structure proposed for CDP-I is shown in Fig. 3a and at the time it was thought to correspond to the correct structure for vancomycin, which would be the amidated version. Recently, however, Williamson and Williams (1981b) have used the technique of nuclear Overhauser effect difference spectroscopy to re-examine vancomycin and have come to the conclusion that the native antibiotic differs from CDP-I in the orientation of one of the chlorinated aromatic rings. They propose that during the long incubation at pH 4.2 used to release the amide nitrogen and thus to convert vancomycin to CDP-I, the bond between C_2 and C_3 of the β-hydroxy-chlorotyrosine residue connecting the aspartic acid and N-methylleucine residues becomes broken and reforms with the chlorophenyl part of the molecule rotated through approximately 180°. The revised structure for vancomycin would therefore be as in Fig. 3b. This structure takes into account the earlier results, acquired particularly by ^{1}H-NMR (Williams and Kalman, 1977; Convert $et\ al.$, 1980) and ^{13}C-NMR (Bongini $et\ al.$, 1981).

More recently Harris $et\ al.$ (1983) re-examined the rearrangement proposals of Williamson and Williams (1981b) and obtained results that led to a new proposal for vancomycin structure (Fig. 3c). They reasoned that vancomycin might contain asparagine rather than isoasparagine at region c of Fig. 2, and that in the conditions required to produce CDPI the asparagine would lose its amide NH_2 and rearrange to aspartic acid. They produced evidence that the aspartic residue of vancomycin was indeed present as asparagine and that CDPI formation involved a degradative reaction whereby the peptide amide nitrogen of asparagine attacked the β-carboxamide to give a succinimide intermediate. This in turn led by hydrolysis to CDPI, of which the minor component had the Cl substituent as shown in Fig. 3b and the major one as in Fig. 3a. The conclusions of Harris $et\ al.$ (1983) would also require a modification of Fig. 5b, which would make it more closely resemble Fig. 5a.

Structural work on the other members of the vancomycin family is also proceeding apace. It is not proposed to trace here the early developments but rather to present the structures currently accepted. Thus the structure of ristocetin A is now considered to be as in Fig. 2 (Kalman and Williams, 1980a; Williamson and Williams, 1980; Sztaricskai $et\ al.$, 1980). The comparison with vancomycin is very clear: in ristocetin, didechlorovancomycinic acid replaces vancomycinic acid, the phenolic group on its central benzene ring is glycosylated by a different oligosaccharide, ristosamine and D-mannose are attached at other parts of the structure where vancomycin was unsubstituted, and the parts of the peptide chain formed in vancomycin by D-asparagine and N-methyl-D-leucine are replaced by the diphenolic ether diaminodicarboxylic acid called ristomycinic acid. The only other difference is the methyl esterification of the C-terminus of the peptide chain. In both antibiotics the central nucleus consists of didechlorovancomycinic acid peptide linked to actinoidinic acid in exactly the same way.

The related antibiotic avoparcin, (Kunstmann $et\ al.$, 1969), which has been used in animal feedstuffs, has been allocated a related partial structure (McGahren $et\ al.$, 1979, 1980). The structures proposed for avoparcin α and avoparcin β are shown in Fig. 2. Once more the vancomycinic acid-actinoidinic acid nucleus is proposed (in this case with a single chlorine substituent on the vancomycinic acid moiety) and the place held by ristomycinic acid in ristocetin is taken by two unlinked p-hydroxyphenylglycine residues, one of which is chlorinated in the β form of the antibiotic and the other substituted glycosidically by L-rhamnose. In addition the complete molecule contains two residues of ristosamine and one each of D-mannose and D-glucose, the last-named being substituted at its 2-position by one residue of ristosamine, a feature similar to that found in vancomycin. Further studies (Ellestad $et\ al.$, 1983; Fesik $et\ al.$, 1984a) by NMR and other methods have provided more detail for the structure, which very closely resembles others in this group of antibiotics. Conformational changes at the amino terminal end of the peptide chain (i.e. around the d region of Fig. 2) produced great differences in antibacterial activity against $Staphylococcus\ aureus$ (Smith). Thus the MIC of β-avoparcin was some 60-fold lower than that of epi-β-avoparcin, the only difference being epimerization around the chiral centre in region d (Fig. 2). The close structural similarity of this group of antibiotics, no doubt related to the precise stereochemical requirements of their mode of action (see below), is thus apparent.

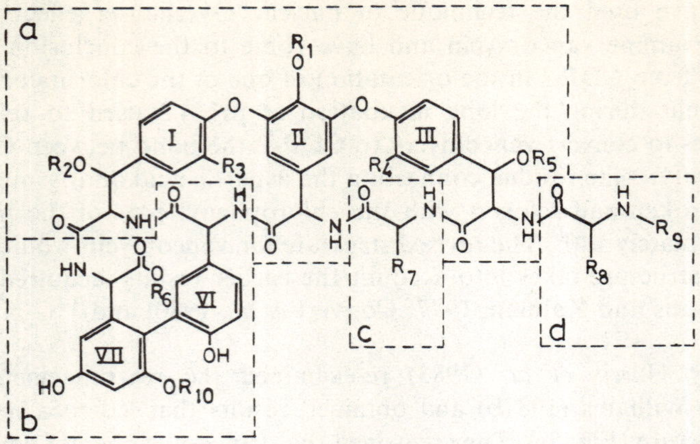

FIG. 2. Generalized structure of the vancomycin group of antibiotics. *a* is the vancomycinic acid region, *b* the actinoidinic acid region. Regions *c* and *d* differ according to the particular antibiotic (see below).

Vancomycin

R_1 = 2-α-L-vancosaminyl-β-D-glucosyl-

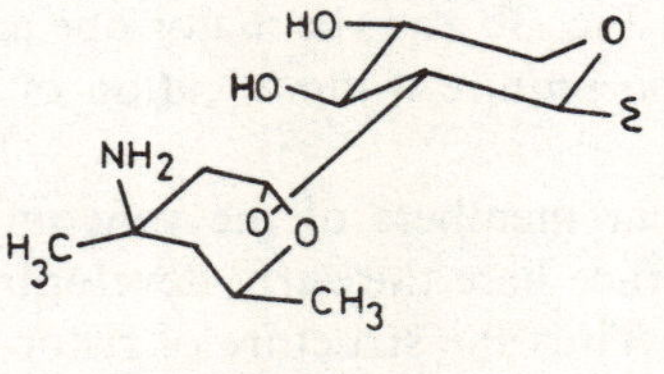

$R_2 = R_5 = R_{10}$ = H
$R_3 = R_4$ = Cl
R_8 = isobutyl -CH$_2$CH(CH$_3$)$_2$
R_9 = CH$_3$ hence region *d* = N-methyl-D-leucyl

Region *c*, D-isoasparaginyl =

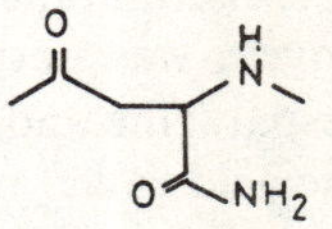

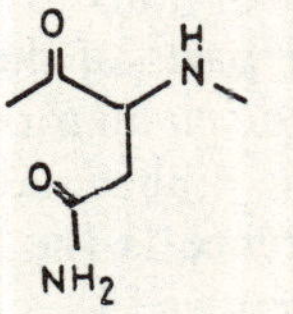

Williamson and Williams (1981)

D-asparaginyl =

Harris *et al.* (1983)

Ristocetin (Ristomycin)
Ristocetin A
R_1 = 2-α-[2-α-D-arabinofuranosyl-α-D-mannopyranosyl]-6α-L-rhamnopyranosyl-β-D-glucosyl-

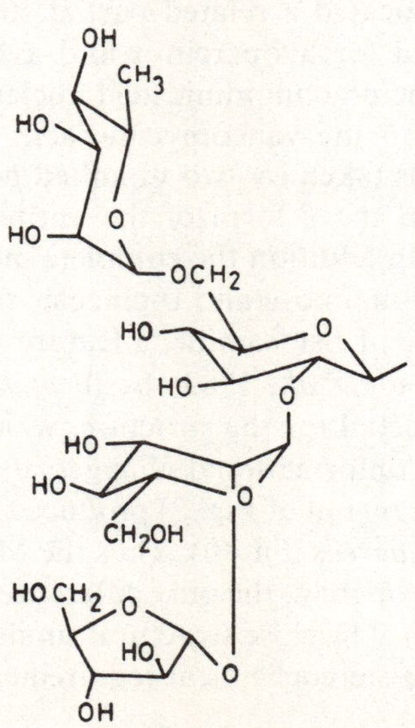

Ristocetin B
R_1 = 6-α-L-rhamnopyranosyl-β-D-glucosyl-
R_2 = α-L-ristosaminyl-
R_3 = R_4 = R_5 = R_9 = H
R_6 = CH_3
R_7 and R_8 are supplied by ristomycinic acid, which thus links regions c and d.

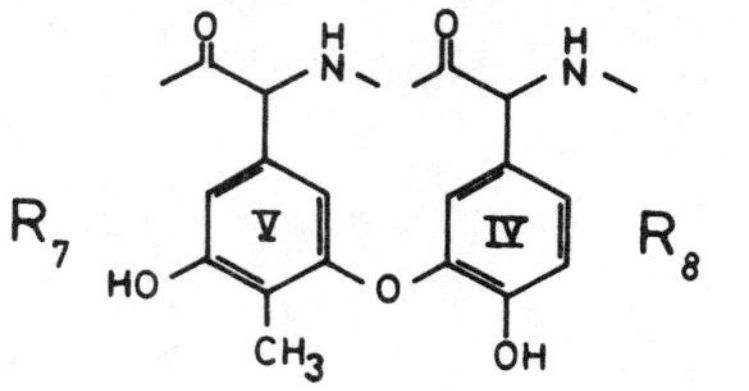

R_7 R_8

R_{10} = β-D-mannosyl

Avoparcin
R_1 = 2-α-L-ristosaminyl-β-D-glucosyl
R_5 = α-D-mannosyl
R_2 = α-L-ristosaminyl
R_3 = Cl }
R_4 = H }
R_6 = R_{10} = H
R_7 =

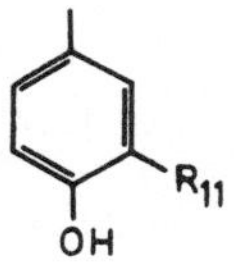

R_{11} where R_{11} = H in avoparcin α, and Cl in avoparcin β. Hence c = p-hydroxyphenyl-glycyl with or without chloro substitution.

R_8 =

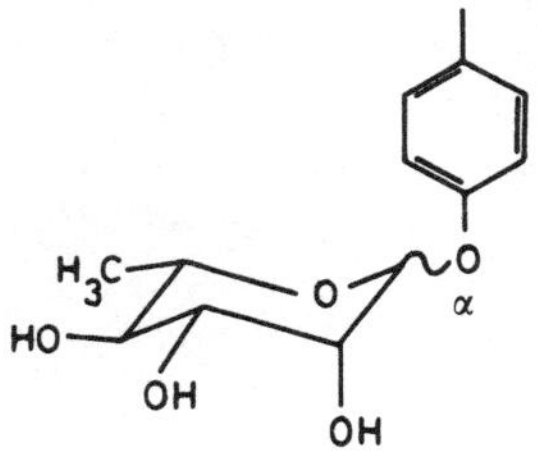

Hence d = the O-α-L-rhamnoside of p-hydroxyphenylglycyl
R_9 = CH_3 In avoparcin β, the configuration around the carbon atom attached to R_N and NH-R_9 is R, and in avoparcin epi-β the configuration is S (Ellestad *et al.*, 1983).

A relative newcomer to this group of antibiotics is teicoplanin (formerly teichomycin) (Bardone *et al.*, 1978), which is unlike all other members of the group in having an acyl aliphatic chain (Williams and Grüneberg, 1984). It is active against most of the organisms susceptible to vancomycin, sometimes at lower concentrations (Grüneberg *et al.*, 1983), but its action on enterococci has attracted particular attention. Against these species it is much more active than vancomycin and is even more active than ampicillin (Pallanza *et al.*, 1983). Teicoplanin appears to be much more protective than vancomycin in mice infected with *S. aureus* (Pallanza *et al.*, 1983).

3. MODE OF ACTION

The first hint that these antibiotics acted by interfering in some way with bacterial wall synthesis came from the work of Reynolds (1961) and Jordan (1961), both of whom showed that vancomycin inhibition of gram-positive bacteria was accompanied

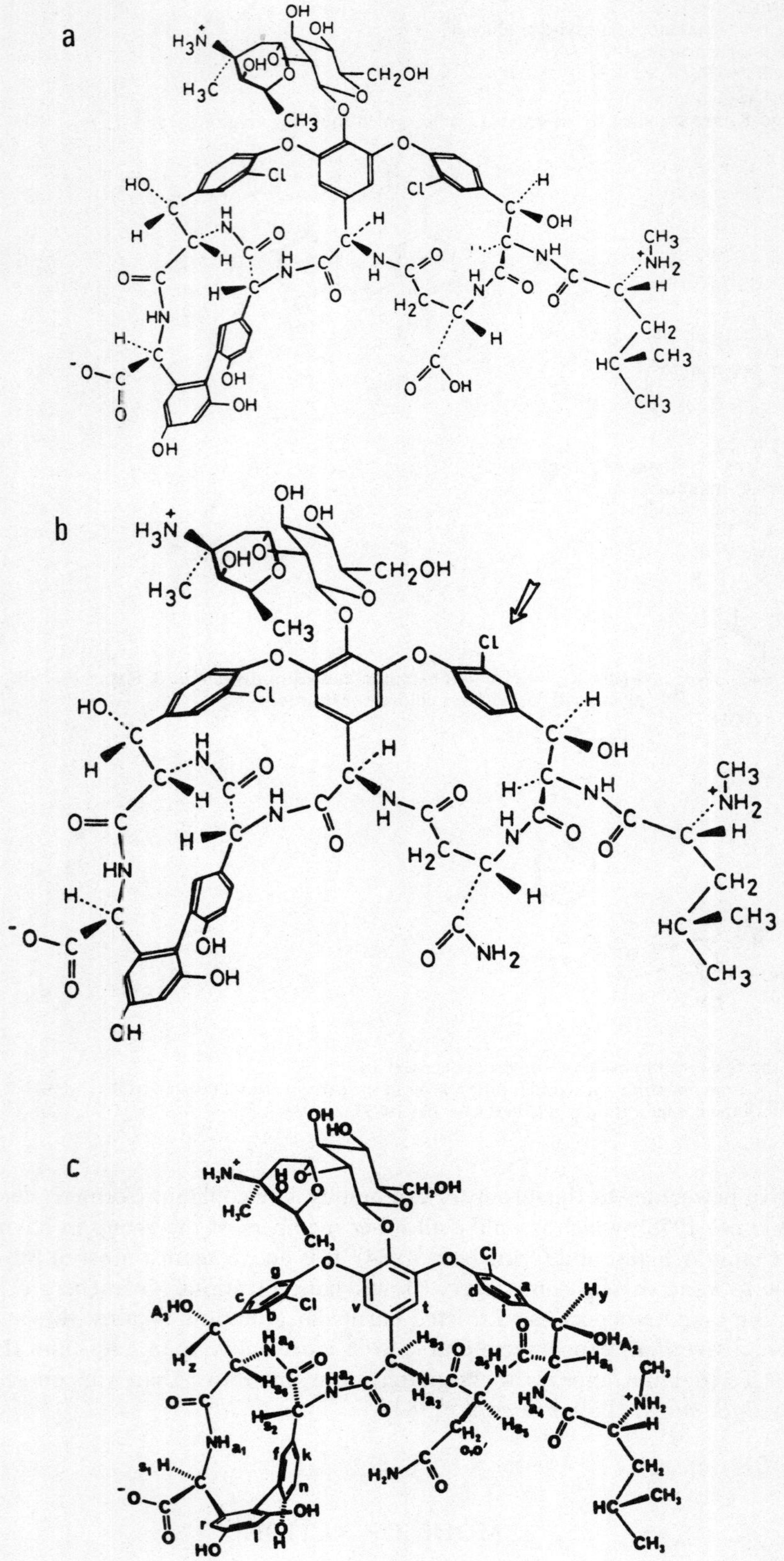

FIG. 3. (a) Structure of vancomycin CDP-I (Sheldrick *et al.*, 1978). (b) Structure proposed for vancomycin by Williamson and Williams (1981b). Difference arrowed. (c) Structure proposed by Harris *et al.* (1983).

by the accumulation of the same type of nucleotide-linked wall intermediate first found by Park (1952) in penicillin-treated *Staphylococcus aureus* H, namely UDP-*N*-acetylmuramyl–L-alanyl–D-isoglutamyl–L-lysyl–D-alanyl–D-alanine (UDP-Mur-Ac-pentapeptide). Similar results for ristocetin soon followed (Wallas and Strominger, 1963).

Further evidence of involvement in wall biosynthesis came from early *in vitro* studies with membrane preparations, in which it was shown that vancomycin and ristocetin caused 50% inhibition of peptidoglycan synthesis at the same concentrations needed to cause 50% growth inhibition in the same organisms (Anderson *et al.*, 1965, 1967). The formation of lipid intermediates, as shown in the outline of the sequence of peptidoglycan synthesis given in Fig. 4, was not inhibited by these antibiotics and indeed was even enhanced, so that their action had to occur at a later stage in synthesis. Since in the membrane preparations used by Anderson *et al.*, (1965, 1967), and by others at the time, no cross-linking of the peptidoglycan synthesized *in vitro* occurred, it follows that the inhibition by vancomycin must have taken place at the level of glycan chain polymerization, although, of course, this does not necessarily indicate that polymerization is the only target process in intact, growing bacteria.

An independent set of results implicating bacterial walls in the action of these antibiotics came from observations, first that vancomycin was rapidly bound by bacteria and could not easily be released (Jordan, 1965; Reynolds, 1966) and second that isolated walls of *S. aureus* (Jordan, 1965) and *Bacillus subtilis* (Best and Durham, 1965) would also bind the drug. The intracellular distribution of the absorbed antibiotic was followed by the use of (^{125}I)-iodinated vancomycin (Perkins and Nieto, 1970; Bordet and Perkins, 1970). In *B. subtilis* and *M. luteus*, each subjected to the lowest concentration of labelled antibiotic

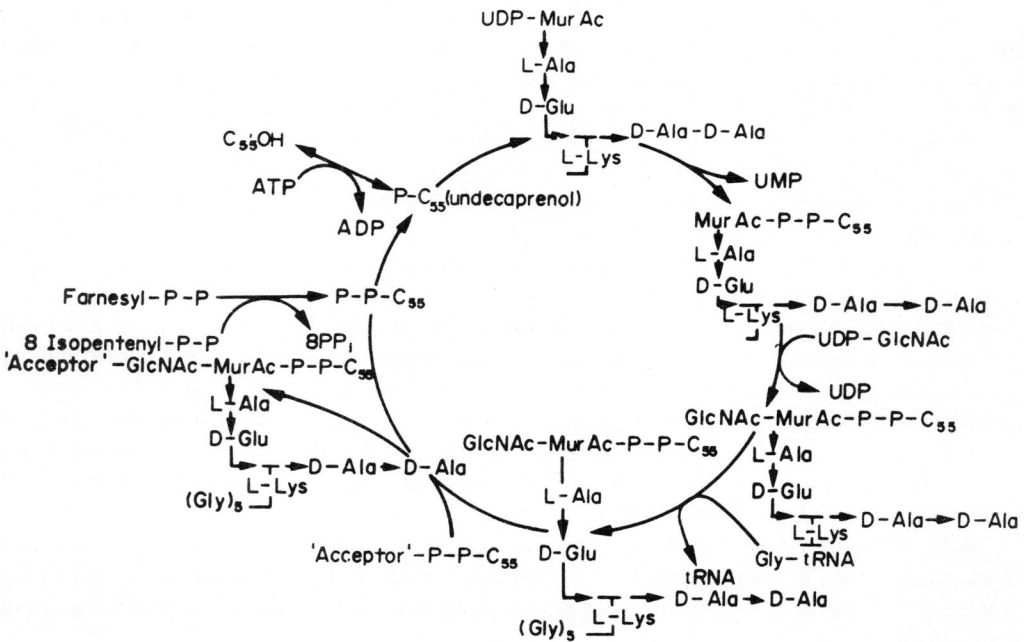

FIG. 4. The biosynthesis of linear uncross-linked peptidoglycan in *S. aureus*. Phospho-*N*-acetyl-muramyl-pentapeptide is translocated to the membrane-bound lipid carrier, undecaprenyl phosphate (C_{55}-P) followed by the transfer of *N*-acetylglucosamine to complete the disaccharide repeating unit. Addition of the five glycine residues of the cross-bridge and the amidation of the α-COOH group of D-glutamate (not shown) then occur before the disaccharide-peptide becomes polymerized. Polymerization is shown to occur while the nascent peptidoglycan remains attached to undecaprenyl-phosphate. Subsequent events include the formation of cross-links by transpeptidation and in most organisms the removal of uncross-linked D-alanine residues by carboxypeptidase activity. (Taken, with permission, from Rogers *et al.*, 1980).

required to inhibit growth, most of the radioactivity was found in the cell walls, although some appeared in the membrane fraction. The latter proportion increased during longer incubations with iodovancomycin, but pre-formed protoplasts absorbed very little of the antibiotic. Binding of both vancomycin and ristocetin to UDP-MurAc-pentapeptides was first shown by Chatterjee and Perkins (1966) and later it became clear that simple addition of the antibiotics to solutions of UDP-MurAc-pentapeptides led instantaneously to tight binding for which the integrity of the acyl-D-alanyl–D-alanine terminus was essential (Perkins, 1969). Furthermore, it was shown that both of the alanine residues needed to have the D-configuration and the terminal carboxyl group had to be free. Thus vancomycin and ristocetin each bound to peptides with the same C-terminal structure found in both the cytoplasmic and the membrane-bound intermediates of peptidoglycan synthesis. There was therefore a *prima facie* case that this binding underlay their mode of action as antibiotics.

The precise specificity of this unusual binding between an antibiotic and a metabolic intermediate, was examined by Nieto and Perkins (1971a,b,c), with the results shown in Table 1. By the method used, namely the examination of u.v. difference spectra, no binding could be demonstrated if the C-terminal or C-sub-terminal residue of the peptide was L-alanine, but peptides with D-alanine or glycine in these positions would all bind. Calculation of the energy changes occurring on binding was used to measure the effect of changes in structure at specific points in the peptide: thus for instance, comparison of the free energy of binding of Ac_2-L-Lys–D-Ala–D-Ala with that for Ac_2-L-Lys–D-Ala–Gly was taken to indicate the effect of introducing a methyl group in the D-configuration at the C-terminal residue. In fact the simplest possible peptide used, representing a backbone without any side-chains (acetyltetraglycine), showed appreciable affinity for both antibiotics, which could be enhanced by introducing "D" side-chains in either the first or second residue from the C-terminus or "L" side-chains in the third position. There were, however, noticeable differences between vancomycin and ristocetin in their response to the introduction of particular side-chains. Thus methyl side-chains in the D-configuration at the C-terminus (D-Ala) produced greatly increased binding for both antibiotics, a long chain such as 2-methylpropyl (D-Leu) markedly decreased binding to vancomycin but did not affect ristocetin and 4-aminobutyl (D-Lys) again had a more deleterious effect with the former than the latter antibiotic. In the sub-C-terminal position D-substituents were beneficial for binding of both antibiotics, but bulky side-chains such as 2-methylpropyl (D-Leu) were obstructive for ristocetin but still somewhat conducive to the binding of vancomycin. The third position from the C-terminus gave better binding with a long-chain L-substituent, particularly to vancomycin, but detailed changes were not so important and even a D-substituent (as in Ac-D-Ala–D-Ala–D-Ala) did not prevent binding.

Another important observation from this study of peptide binding was that certain peptides such as Ac-L-Ala–D-Glu–Gly, representing analogs of part of the peptidoglycan structure not at the terminus of the original biosynthetic precursor UDP-MurAc-pentapeptide, would also bind to the antibiotics—well to vancomycin and poorly to ristocetin. This was taken to explain the known fact that the peptidoglycan of *Micrococcus luteus*, which contains many –L-Ala–D-Glu–Gly termini, will bind vancomycin extremely well and ristocetin somewhat less readily.

Work with the u.v. difference spectra, circular dichroism (C.D.) and optical rotatory dispersion (O.R.D.) (Nieto and Perkins, 1971a,c) gave not only a measure of binding affinities but also an indication of the parts of the antibiotic molecule that were immediately involved.

Evidence was presented for ionic interaction, formation and possibly breakage of hydrogen bonds, steric repulsion and hydrophobic bond formation. There was no doubt that the phenolic groups of vancomycin and ristocetin were close to the binding site, since it was their absorptions that were greatly affected. However, C.D. and O.R.D. suggested that no great alteration of structure occurred during the binding event.

At the time that the binding data summarized in Table 1 were accumulated the structural chemistry of the antibiotics was not sufficiently advanced to provide a rational

TABLE 1. *Association constants and free energy changes for the combination of vancomycin and ristocetin B with peptides (Nieto and Perkins, 1971c). Reproduced with permission from the version of Rogers et al. (1980)*

	Vancomycin		Ristocetin B	
	K_a(l/mol)	ΔG(cal/mol)	K_a(l/mol)	ΔG(cal/mol)
Changes in Residue 1				
Ac$_2$-L-Lys–D-Ala–D-Ala	1.5×10^6	-8400	5.9×10^5	-7850
Ac$_2$-L-Lys–D-Ala–Gly	1.3×10^5	-6950	2.2×10^4	-5900
Ac$_2$-L-Lys–D-Ala–D-Leu	9.2×10^3	-5390	6.1×10^5	-7860
Ac$_2$-L-Lys–D-Ala–D-Lys	1.4×10^4	-5620	1.0×10^5	-6800
Ac$_2$-L-Lys–D-Ala–L-Ala	no combination		no combination	
Ac-D-Ala–D-Ala	2.0×10^4	-5840	7.2×10^4	-6600
Ac-D-Ala–Gly	5.4×10^3	-5070	1.9×10^3	-4470
Changes in Residue 2				
Ac$_2$-L-Lys–Gly–D-Ala	9.4×10^4	-6760	1.6×10^5	-7070
Ac$_2$-L-Lys–D-Leu–D-Ala	2.9×10^5	-7420	5.8×10^4	-6470
Ac$_2$-L-Lys–L-Ala–D-Ala	no combination		no combination	
Ac$_2$-L-Lys–Aib–Gly†	no combination		no combination	
Ac-Gly–D-Ala	1.1×10^4	-5500	4.9×10^4	-6390
Changes in Residue 3				
Ac-Gly–D-Ala–D-Ala	9.4×10^4	-6760	1.6×10^5	-7070
Ac-L-Ala–D-Ala–D-Ala	3.1×10^5	-7450	2.2×10^5	-7270
N-Ac-L-Tyr–D-Ala–D-Ala	1.9×10^5	-7180	2.9×10^5	-7430
Ac-D-Ala–D-Ala–D-Ala	5.0×10^4	-6380	1.3×10^5	-6960
Ac$_2$-L-Dbu–D-Ala–D-Ala	7.7×10^5	-8000		
Ac$_2$-L-Orn–D-Ala–D-Ala	1.3×10^4	-8320		
Ac$_2$-L-Lys–D-Ala–D-Ala‡	1.1×10^6	-8220		
Myristoyl-D-Ala–D-Ala‡	5.0×10^4	-6500		
Influence of Free Amino Groups				
L-Lys–D-Ala–D-Ala	1.2×10^4	-5510	8.2×10^3	-5320
α-Ac-L-Lys–D-Ala–D-Ala	4.7×10^5	-7700	1.9×10^5	-7200
Other Peptides				
Ac-L-Ala–Gly–Gly	4.9×10^3	-5200	2.5×10^3	-4620
Ac-Gly–Gly–Gly–Gly	1.5×10^3	-4300	8.0×10^2	-3950
Ac-L-Ala–D-Glu–Gly	4.8×10^5	-7720	6.8×10^2	-3850
C. poinsettiae dimer§	9.4×10^4	-6760	9.8×10^5	-8150
Ac$_2$-L-Lys–D-Leu–D-Leu	5.0×10^3	-5000		
Ac$_2$-L-Lys–L-Ala–L-Ala	no combination			
Influence of Peptide Chain Length				
D-Glu–γ-L-Lys–D-Ala–D-Ala	7.6×10^5	-8000		
D-Glu(α-Bzl)–γ-L-Lys–D-Ala–D-Ala	3.2×10^5	-7670		
L-Ala–D-Glu–γ-L-Lys–D-Ala–D-Ala	6.3×10^5	-7870		
L-Tyr–D-Glu–γ-L-Lys–D-Ala–D-Ala	8.3×10^5	-8050		
UDP–MurAc–L-Ala–D-Glu–γ-L-A$_2$pm–D-Ala–D-Ala	7.2×10^5	-7960		

†Abbreviations: A$_2$pm, α,α'-diaminopimelic acid; Hsr, homoserine; Mur, muramic acid; Dbu, 2,4-diaminobutyric acid; Aib, α-aminoisobutyric acid; Bzl, benzyl.
‡Experiment performed in 50% ethanol.
§Structure of dimer:

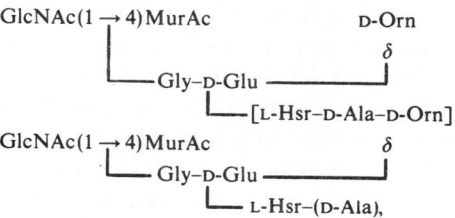

which represents a mixture of molecules with and without the (D-Ala) residue. The region that should form complexes with the antibiotics is enclosed within square brackets.

explanation. Since then, however, an enormous amount of structural information has been acquired, including the identification of many hitherto unknown components, as set out in an earlier section (Figs 2 and 3).

Simultaneously, more sophisticated physical techniques than simple difference spectroscopy or circular dichroism and optical rotatory dispersion (Nieto and Perkins, 1971a,c) were applied to the examination of the antibiotic–peptide complexes. Thus Brown et al. (1975a,b) used proton NMR spectroscopy at 100 MHz to study the binding of Ac-D-Ala–D-Ala to vancomycin by following the chemical shifts of the three methyl resonances of the peptide. The CH_3 resonance of the C-terminal D-alanine residue sustained a relatively large shift to higher field during complex formation, thus giving an indication that this group must lie over the face of one of the aromatic rings in the antibiotic. Much more detailed evidence, by NMR and nuclear Overhauser effects, has since defined the binding complexes with great specificity.

The interaction between the advances in understanding of ristocetin and vancomycin has been considerable. Naturally, the establishment of a structure for CDP-I from vancomycin by X-ray crystallography provided the first firm basis for detailed proposals of how acyl-D-Ala–D-Ala peptides could bind (Sheldrick et al., 1978). This information helped in the elucidation of the ristocetin structure and it was in fact the peptide-complex with ristocetin that was first unravelled (Kalman and Williams, 1980a,b). The structure of ristocetin currently agreed between the various workers active in the field is shown in Fig. 2. Much of the detail was established by the examination of nuclear Overhauser effects (NOEs) when the antibiotic and its complex with Ac-D-Ala–D-Ala were studied in Me_2SO-d_6 solution (Williams et al., 1979). Under these conditions the exchange rate between complex and its free components was sufficiently slow at 30°C to permit each species (ristocetin, peptide, complex) to give a characteristic spectrum in the presence of the other components, when antibiotic and peptide were mixed in overall ratios of say 1:2 or 2:1. Information on the conformation of the bound peptide was derived from negative intermolecular NOEs and the $J_{\alpha,NH}$ coupling constants. The nature of the binding site was then deduced from the temperature coefficients and chemical shifts of the amide NH resonances, in conjunction with model-building studies (Kalman and Williams, 1980b). The nature of the binding site was confirmed by the observation of four intermolecular NOEs between the protons of the peptide on the one hand and ristocetin on the other. A simplified diagram of the binding region given by Kalman and Williams (1980b) is shown in Fig. 5. The NMR data also indicated a high rigidity of binding and suggested that the bound peptide was in an extended conformation similar to that found in X-ray crystallographic studies of trialanine. The structural picture deduced provided an explanation for the specific restrictions of binding observed earlier by Nieto and Perkins (1971c) (Table 1). The ristocetin structure could accommodate larger side-chains of the D-configuration on the C-terminal residue, since this side-chain projects above ring II. In vancomycin the bulky chlorine substituents interfere (Kalman and Williams, 1980b; Sheldrick et al., 1978). The proposals for the binding interactions have been confirmed by ^{13}C-NMR methods, which also showed that the sugars of ristocetins A or B are not involved in the binding. The ring carbons underwent chemical shift changes that were relatively large and to high field, observations that suggested that one of the rings may lie above a plane defined by the three atoms of the carboxylate anion of the peptide (Williamson and Williams, 1981a).

The methods involving peptide binding in Me_2SO-d_6 at 30°C, described above for ristocetin, have now been further adapted and applied to vancomycin (Williams and Butcher, 1981). Study of NOEs has resulted in a revision of the earlier proposal (Sheldrick et al., 1978) for the structure of the antibiotic–peptide complex, which failed to explain the increased binding of peptide with its C-terminal carboxyl group in an anionic state and the N-methylleucine of vancomycin in its cationic state (Convert et al., 1980). By using Me_2SO containing 30% carbon tetrachloride Williams and Butcher (1981) were able to cool the solutions to 0°C and so decrease the unimolecular rate constant for dissociation of the complex. Their results showed that the carboxylate anion of Ac-D-

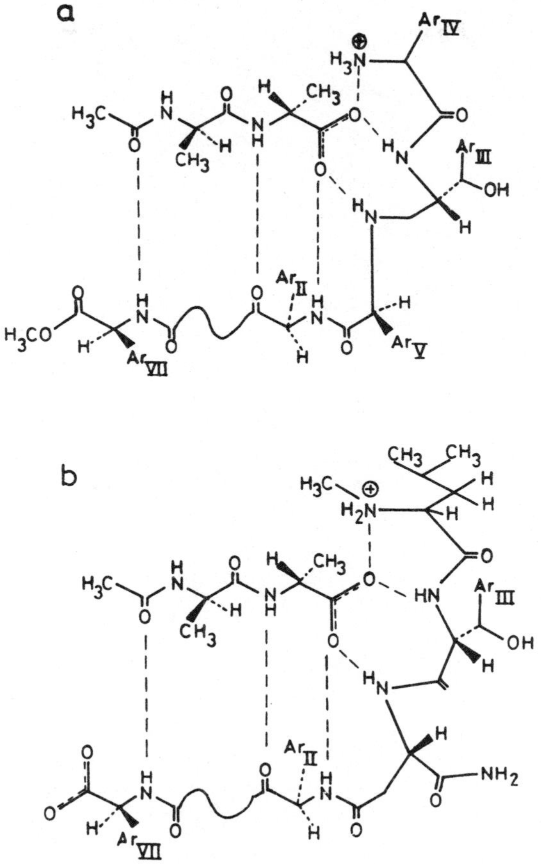

FIG. 5. Proposed binding interactions between acetyl-D-alanyl D-alanine (upper left) and (a) risto-cetin A (Kalman and Williams, 1980b); (b) vancomycin (Williams and Butcher, 1981). The portions of the antibiotic peptide backbones not involved in hydrogen-binding to the wall analog are indicated by wavy lines.

Ala–D-Ala must be hydrogen bonded to the amide NH group linked to the β-carboxyl group of the D-aspartyl residue of vancomycin. This led to the conclusion that vancomycin in the complex must undergo a profound conformational change, at least relative to its structure in crystalline CDP-I. These changes, which involve isoasparagine, N-methylleucine and the β-hydroxy-chlorotyrosine unit between them, give rise to a carboxylate anion 'receptor pocket', in which vancomycin can form two further hydrogen bonds and a salt bridge to aid the binding of acyl-D-alanyl-D-alanine termini. This pocket closely resembles that found in ristocetin (Fig. 5). The exact detail around the D-aspartyl residue would need to be modified in the light of the finding that it is an asparaginyl rather than an isoasparaginyl group (Harris *et al.* 1983).

Subsequent NMR studies on the binding of β-avoparcin and epi-β-avoparcin (Fesik *et al.*, 1984b) to Ac-D-Ala-D-Ala and to Ac₂-LLys-D-Ala-D-Ala have essentially supported the general pattern of binding, although as will be seen by comparing Fig. 6 with Fig. 5, there are some differences of detail. Interestingly, epi-β-avoparcin, which has far lower antibacterial activity than β-avoparcin, bound Ac-D-Ala-D-Ala hardly at all and bound the tripeptide less well by an order of magnitude than did β-avoparcin.

4. MECHANISM OF INTERFERENCE WITH PEPTIDOGLYCAN SYNTHESIS

Although the antibiotics clearly interfere with peptidoglycan synthesis because of their ability to form complexes with biosynthetic intermediates possessing –D-Ala–D-Ala

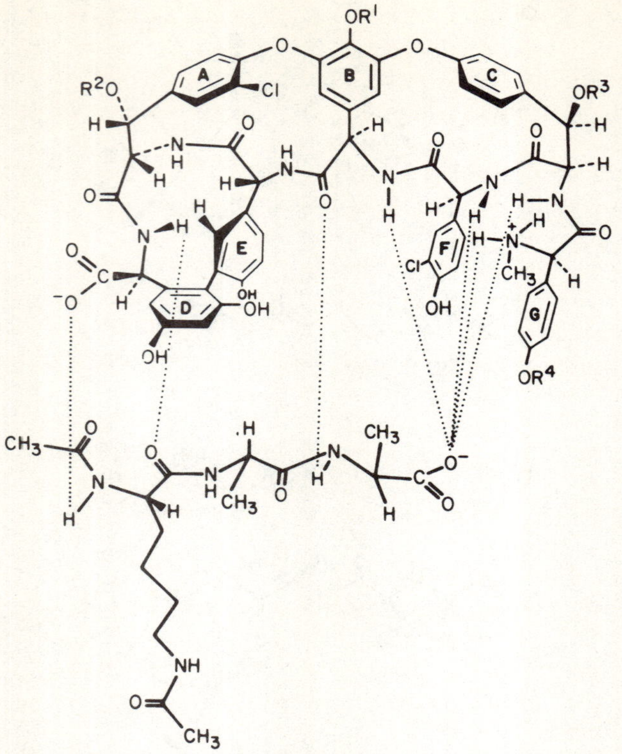

FIG. 6. Proposed model of the structure of the β-avoparcin:Ac$_2$-L-Lys-D-Ala-D-Ala complex obtained from NOE and ^{1}H chemical shift data (Fesik *et al.*, 1984).

termini, the precise method of intervention has not proved easy to establish. Early evidence that the same binding site was indeed involved was obtained by Nieto *et al.* (1972) who showed that vancomycin complexed with a suitable exogenous binding peptide was relatively ineffective in inhibiting bacterial growth or *in-vitro* peptidoglycan synthesis. The same investigation also studied the retention of ^{125}I-iodovancomycin during growth inhibition and recovery of sensitive Gram-positive bacteria. The concentration of antibiotic present in the cells when growth inhibition initially occurred was no greater than when growth resumed, a result leading to the conclusion that in the intervening period iodovancomycin had in some way been transferred from inhibitory sites to sites that were not involved in peptidoglycan synthesis. Alternatively new, unaffected, sites must have been created during the period of bacteriostasis.

A possible point of action during the formation of mature peptidoglycan would be prevention of the modification of –D-Ala–D-Ala termini by DD-carboxypeptidases. The soluble DD-carboxypeptidases secreted by *Streptomyces albus* G (Leyh-Bouille *et al.*, 1970) and by *E. coli* (Izaki and Strominger, 1968; Bogdanovsky *et al.*, 1969) were inhibited by vancomycin and ristocetin. Since the antibiotics compete with the enzyme for the same binding site on the peptide this result is hardly surprising. A somewhat more complicated interaction has been investigated in the rather unusual biosynthetic system involved in the production of peptidoglycan by *Gaffkya homari*. In this organism it is possible to obtain *in vitro* biosynthetic systems that will polymerize peptidoglycan not only from UDP-MurAc-pentapeptide but also from the same precursor deprived of either one or both of its terminal D-alanine residues (Hammes and Neuhaus, 1974). Synthesis of peptidoglycan from either truncated precursor was totally unaffected by vancomycin. The enhancement by vancomycin of the accumulation of the lipid intermediate MurAc(-pentapeptide)-P-P-undecaprenol was not observed when the precursors no longer contained a terminus such as –D-Ala–D-Ala that could be recognized by the antibiotic. So long as the complete pentapeptide side-chain was present, vancomycin also inhibited the

UMP exchange reaction UMP-P-MurAc(pentapeptide) + P-undecaprenol $\rightleftharpoons$ UMP + MurAc(pentapeptide)–P–P–undecaprenol (Hammes and Neuhaus, 1974). These authors also showed that peptidoglycan synthesis from precursor analogues, in which either of the D-alanine residues was replaced by glycine, was equally sensitive to vancomycin, whereas the physical studies of Nieto and Perkins (1971b) would have predicted a decreased effect. A precursor with a glycine residue next to the muramic acid instead of L-alanine permitted peptidoglycan synthesis that was exceptionally sensitive to vancomycin, suggesting that at least in nucleotide precursors even the fifth residue from the C-terminus may influence binding by the antibiotic. So far, interaction at this residue has not been accounted for in the physical studies and model building.

The influence of vancomycin at various stages of peptidoglycan biosynthesis was also considered by Ward (1974), who used a membrane preparation from an autolysin-deficient mutant of *Bacillus licheniformis*. The concentration at which vancomycin inhibited peptidoglycan synthesis or enhanced lipid intermediate production by 50% was only 0.08 mol. prop. relative to the amount of added UDP-MurAc-pentapeptide precursor, a result which suggested that the key intermediate responsible for the antibiotic effects must be other than the nucleotide itself. For the DD-carboxypeptidase, also present in the enzyme preparation and monitored by the release of D-alanine, a 50% inhibition was exerted by 0.32 mol. prop. of vancomycin.

Polymerization of N-acetylglucosaminyl–N-acetylmuramyl-pentapeptide sub-units to make linear peptidoglycan from the disaccharide(pentapeptide)–P–P–undecaprenol precursor was studied directly by Van Heijenoort *et al.* (1978), the enzyme being a membrane preparation from *E. coli*. Vancomycin and ristocetin both inhibited the transglycosylation reaction by approximately 50% at concentrations of about 0.05 and 0.1 mol. prop. respectively. Again the implication would appear to be that the lipid intermediate itself is not the molecular species that governs the inhibitory action of these antibiotics.

The association of lipid intermediate with vancomycin and ristocetin was examined directly by the elegant approach of Johnston and Neuhaus (1975). These authors prepared UDP–MurAc–L-Ala–D-isoGlu–L-Lys–D-Ala–D-Ala in which the ϵ-amino group of the lysine residue was spin-labelled by acylation with the 2,2,5,5-tetramethyl-N-oxylpyrroline-3-carbonyl (tempyo) group. Since the electron spin resonance spectrum is a function of the motion that the probe undergoes and also of the polarity of the solvent around it, any complex formation with vancomycin could be directly measured. The method was applied to the nucleotide precursor, and yielded with vancomycin an association constant of 6.2×10^5 M^{-1}, very close to the value of 7.2×10^5 M^{-1} recorded for the nucleotide precursor with diaminopimelic acid in the third position by Nieto and Perkins (1971b). The value for association of the *tempyo* analog with ristocetin was 6.2×10^4 M^{-1} (Johnston and Neuhaus, 1975). For the first time, the use of the *tempyo* derivatives enabled the association constants to be measured for the first lipid intermediate MurAc-pentapeptide–P–P–undecaprenol, and yielded values of 3.0×10^4 and 2.1×10^4 M^{-1} for vancomycin and ristocetin respectively. Thus in each case the association was less strong than for the corresponding nucleotide precursor, although for ristocetin the difference was only three fold, rather than the twenty-fold observed with vancomycin. These results once again support the suggestion of Ward (1974) that the growing glycan chain with its appended peptide units as yet unmodified by D,D-carboxypeptidase or transpeptidase action, may represent the critical intermediate that associates most strongly with these antibiotics and thus brings peptidoglycan polymerization to a halt.

5. RISTOCETIN AND PLATELET AGGREGATION

Howard and Firkin (1971) originally observed that ristocetin, withdrawn from clinical use because of a high incidence of thrombocytopenia in patients receiving the drug, induced the aggregation of platelets from the platelet-rich plasma (PRP; citrated blood centrifuged at low speed to remove the blood corpuscles) of normal people, but not from that of some patients with von Willebrand's disease. Howard *et al.* (1973) later used ristocetin to sub-divide von Willebrand patients into two groups, in one of which the platelets were not aggregated by ristocetin, whereas all responded to ADP. Other work soon showed that factor VIII would correct the deficiency in platelet-aggregation observed in von Willebrand's disease (e.g. Weiss *et al.*, 1973) and gradually an overall picture was built up. It has been proposed (Coller, 1978) that the platelet aggregation induced in normal PRP by ristocetin requires, first, a plasma factor (the von Willebrand factor, vWF) that is lacking or decreased in von Willebrand's disease and secondly, a platelet component that is deficient in the Bernard–Soulier syndrome (Weiss *et al.*, 1974; Howard *et al.*, 1973). The latter component is probably a membrane glycoprotein (Jenkins *et al.*, 1976; Caen *et al.*, 1976) that serves as a receptor both for ristocetin and thence for human vWF, whereby aggregation is caused, and also for bovine vWF except that in this case there is no requirement for ristocetin (Kirby and Mills, 1975). The platelet factor remains unaffected by formalin (Allain *et al.*, 1975) but is decreased by proteolytic enzymes (Jenkins *et al.*, 1976).

Although vancomycin and ristocetin have similar binding sites for peptides (see earlier sections), vancomycin does not itself aggregate platelets (Coller *et al.*, 1975), although there is evidence that it inhibits the action of ristocetin in this respect (Roper *et al.*, 1975; Moake *et al.*, 1977; Coller and Gralnick, 1977) presumably by competing for the same binding sites. One wonders whether the membrane glycoprotein that binds ristocetin has an acyl-D-Ala–D-Ala-like C-terminus; in a normal protein this could only be –Gly–Gly. Indeed, vancomycin did not interfere with vWF or factor VIII coagulant activities in normal platelet-poor plasma and evidence for its role as a competitor of ristocetin was strong (Moake *et al.*, 1977). Attempts were made to characterize these interactions further by making structural modifications of the antibiotics. Coller and Gralnick (1977) treated both ristocetin and vancomycin with the water-soluble carbodi-imide 1-(3-dimethyl-aminopropyl)3-ethyl carbodiimide (EDC) in the presence of glycine methyl ester. This procedure had the effect of converting phenolic groups to *O*-arylisoureas and amidating carboxyl groups to form the neutral glycine methyl ester derivatives. The phenolic groups could be regenerated by the use of hydroxylamine, but not the carboxyl groups. The involvement of a carboxyl function could not be investigated in ristocetin, since only vancomycin has a free carboxyl group.

The EDC-treated ristocetin lost both its ability to aggregate platelets and its antibiotic activity, and each activity was restored when hydroxylamine was used to remove the substituents. Vancomycin prolonged or inhibited the ristocetin-induced agglutination to an extent dependent upon its relative concentration, effects that were enhanced by pre-incubation with platelets but not with plasma. Reaction with EDC in the presence of glycine methyl ester destroyed most of the antibiotic activity of vancomycin, and about half of it could be restored by subsequent reaction with hydroxylamine. At this stage the product was able to cause agglutination of platelets in the presence of normal, but not von Willebrand, plasma. The authors concluded that their results supported the idea that the net positive charge on ristocetin was required to induce agglutination and adduced as evidence the fact that the modified vancomycin, with a net charge of $+2$ at pH 5.5 and uncharged between pH 8 and 9, could also induce agglutination. Later, Coller (1978) performed experiments on the electrical mobility of platelets in the presence of vWF and ristocetin that lent some support to these ideas, but also suggested that vWF bound to the platelets at a site different from that occupied by ristocetin. This led to the idea that reduction in net surface charge, brought about by the ristocetin, permitted the binding of vWF and subsequent agglutination. Bovine vWF, even without ristocetin, agglutinated and reduced the electrical mobility, of normal, but not Bernard–Soulier or trypsinized, platelets.

Modified ristocetin (ristomycin) was also examined by Boda *et al.* (1979). These authors confirmed that although neither vancomycin nor actinoidin would cause human platelets to aggregate in the presence of vWF, both antibiotics inhibited the ristocetin-induced agglutination. When they prepared *bis-N,N*-trifluoroacetylristomycin they found that it would induce agglutination, a result at variance with the conclusions on charge made by Coller (1978). On the other hand carboxyristomycin, in which the ristocetin carboxymethyl group had been hydrolyzed to yield the free acid, apparently neither induced platelet aggregation nor inhibited it when unchanged ristocetin had been used to induce it. Unfortunately, we do not know whether the carboxy-ristomycin was still antibiotically active, a piece of information essential for an interpretation of its lack of inductive or inhibitory effect.

The very large vWF molecule ($\geqslant 4.6 \times 10^6$ daltons) could be reduced by dithiothreitol to a main component of 208 kdal and smaller ones of 197, 174 and 154 kdal (Martin *et al.*, 1980). Trypsin degradation of the non-reduced protein yielded a series of smaller fragments and ristocetin-co-factor activity rapidly disappeared. After 45 min reaction the chief remaining co-factor activity resided in a major fragment of 116 kdal. Although this fragment had a lower specific activity than the intact molecule, its isolation promotes the hope that the specific molecular structures may eventually be characterized.

At present the exact molecular relationship between ristocetin-induced platelet aggregation and the normal processes of blood clotting are not understood, but clearly considerable progress has been made in this relatively novel and rapidly moving line of research.

6. RESURGENCE OF CLINICAL INTEREST IN VANCOMYCIN

In the late seventies came a reversal in the fortunes of vancomycin as a therapeutic agent (Esposito and Gleckman, 1977; Cook and Farrar, 1978). Specific conditions in which its use was considered valuable included severe infections caused by Gram-positive cocci such as staphylococci or streptococci, e.g. in bacterial endocarditis, particularly when the patients were known to be allergic to penicillin, or where their status in this respect was unknown and the gravity of their condition did not allow time for adequate investigation. Vancomycin has also been used to combat staphylococcal infections in patients with restricted venous access who need long-term haemodialysis (Esposito and Gleckman, 1977).

To achieve appropriate serum levels the antibiotic cannot be administered orally, but can be maintained at serum concentrations of $6\text{--}14\,\mu g/ml$ by intravenous dosage of 500 mg every six hours (Geraci, 1977). These concentrations are bactericidal for most strains of staphylococci and streptococci. At the same time, therapeutic levels are found in the pleural, pericardial, ascitic and synovial fluids. Indeed, experimental work with rabbits suggested that the antibiotic could be used to combat pneumococcal meningitis (Beam, 1981). Concentrations of vancomycin equivalent to the MIC were achieved in the CSF and the brain generally and resulted in the death of the bacteria. Vancomycin was found to be superior to penicillin or chloramphenicol for the treatment of penicillin-resistant strains.

The revived clinical interest in vancomycin has resulted in an increased need to measure tissue concentrations. It was originally shown by Perkins and Nieto (1970) that vancomycin could be iodinated (with ^{125}I if desired) and still remain antibiotically active. This reaction formed the basis of a radioimmunoassay that gave very good correlations with microbiological methods (Crossley *et al.*, 1980) and labelling with ^{125}I directly or with ^3H by formation of [^3H] propionylvancomycin permitted radioimmunoassay with limits of 0.04 or 4 ng/ml respectively (Fong *et al.*, 1981).

Because vancomycin is essentially not absorbed from the gastrointestinal tract it reaches high levels there after oral administration, and has therefore been used successfully in the treatment of staphylococcal enterocolitis (Wallace *et al.*, 1965; Kahn and Hall, 1966). Similarly, the drug has more recently been used to treat pseudomembranous colitis that has arisen in response to earlier treatment with other antibiotics. This often fatal condition is caused by the multiplication in the gut of toxigenic *Clostridium difficile*, but the oral administration of vancomycin has proved effective in correcting the diarrhoea, eliminating the toxin from the feces and causing the disappearance of the pseudomembranes from the colonic wall (Tedesco *et al.*, 1978; Keighley *et al.*, 1978) and the drug has also been used successfully in children (Batts *et al.*, 1980). There have been some reports of relapses after cessation of therapy, but Rampling *et al.* (1980) have proposed that in cases where such a risk seems likely prophylactic resumption of oral vancomycin should be used. It seems likely that teicoplanin may play an increasing role in the treatment of similar infections (Williams and Grüneberg, 1984).

Acknowledgements—The author wishes to thank Dr. D. H. Williams for access to unpublished material. During preparation of this review he was in receipt of a Grant from the Medical Research Council.

REFERENCES

ALLAIN, J. P., COOPER, H. A., WAGNER, R. H. and BRINKHOUS, K. M. (1975) Platelets fixed with paraformaldehyde: a new reagent for assay of von Willebrand factor and platelet aggregation factor. *J. Lab. clin. Med.* **85**: 318–328.

ANDERSON, J. S., MATSUHASHI, M., HASKIN, M. A. and STROMINGER, J. L. (1965) Lipid-phosphoacetylmuramyl-pentapeptide and lipid-phosphodisaccharide-pentapeptide: presumed membrane transport intermediates in cell wall synthesis. *Proc. natn. Acad. Sci. U.S.A.* **53**: 881–889.

ANDERSON, J. S., MATSUHASHI, M., HASKIN, M. A. and STROMINGER, J. L. (1967) Biosynthesis of the peptidoglycan of bacterial cell walls. II. Phospholipid carriers in the reaction sequence. *J. biol. Chem.* **242**: 3180–3190.

BARDONE, M. R., PATERNOSTER, M. and CORONELLI, C. (1978) Teichomycins, new antibiotics from *Actinoplanes teichomyceticus* nov. sp. II. Extraction and chemical characterization. *J. Antibiot.* **31**: 170–177.

BATTS, D. H., MARTIN, D., HOLMES, R., SILVA, J. and FEKETY, F. R. (1980) Treatment of antibiotic-associated *Clostridium difficile* diarrhea with oral vancomycin. *J. Pediat.* **97**: 151–153.

BEAM, T. R. (1981) Vancomycin therapy of experimental pneumococcal meningitis caused by penicillin-sensitive and resistant strains. *J. Antimicrob. Chemother.* **7**: 89–99.

BEST, G. K. and DURHAM, N. N. (1965) Vancomycin adsorption to *Bacillus subtilis* cell walls. *Archs Biochem. Biophys.* **111**: 685–691.

BODA, Z., SOLUM, N. O., SZTARICSKAI, F. and RAK, K. (1979) Study of platelet agglutination induced by the antibiotics of the vancomycin group: ristocetin, ristomycin, actinoidin and vancomycin. *Thromb. Diath. haemorrh.* **42**: 1164–1180.

BOGDANOVSKY, D., BRICAS, E. and DEZELÉE, P. (1969) Identity of mucoendopeptidase and carboxypeptidase I of *Escherichia coli*, enzymes hydrolyzing bonds of the D-D-configuration and inhibited by penicillins. *C.R. Acad. Sci., Series D.* **269**: 390–393.

BOGNAR, R., SZTARICSKAI, F., MUNK, M. E. and TAMAS, J. (1974) Structure and stereochemistry of ristosamine. *J. org. Chem.* **39**: 2971–2974.

BONGINI, A., FEENEY, J., WILLIAMSON, M. P. and WILLIAMS, D. H. (1981) Assignment of the carbon-13 spectrum of vancomycin and its derivatives. *J. chem. Soc. Perkin II*. 201–206.

BORDET, C. and PERKINS, H. R. (1970) Iodinated vancomycin and mucopeptide biosynthesis by cell-free preparations from *Micrococcus lysodeikticus*. *Biochem. J.* **119**, 877–883.

BRAZHNIKOVA, M. G., LOMAKINA, N. N., LAVROVA, M. F., TOLSZTYKH, I. V., YURINA, M. SZ. and KLYUEVA, L. M. (1963) Isolation and properties of ristomycin. *Antibiotiki.* **8**: 392–396.

BROWN, J. P., FEENEY, J. and BURGEN, A. S. V. (1975a) A nuclear magnetic resonance study of the interaction between vancomycin and acetyl-D-alanyl-D-alanine in aqueous solution. *Molec. Pharmac.* **11**: 119–125.

BROWN, J. P., TERENIUS, L., FEENEY, J. and BURGEN, A. S. V. (1975b) A structure–activity study by nuclear magnetic resonance of peptide interactions with vancomycin. *Molec. Pharmac.* **11**: 126–132.

CAEN, J. P., NURDEN, A. T., JEANNEAU, C., MICHEL, H., TOBELEM, C., LEVY-TOLEDANO, S., SULTAN, Y., VALENSI, F. and BERNARD, J. (1976) Bernard–Soulier syndrome: a new glycoprotein abnormality. Its relationship with platelet adhesion to subendothelium and with the factor VIII von Willebrand protein. *J. Lab. clin. Med.* **87**: 586–596.

CHATTERJEE, A. N. and PERKINS, H. R. (1966) Compounds formed between nucleotides related to the biosynthesis of bacterial cell wall and vancomycin. *Biochem. biophys. Res. Commun.* **24**: 489–494.

COLLER, B. S. (1978) The effects of ristocetin and von Willebrand factor on platelet electrophoretic mobility. *J. clin. Invest.* **61**: 1168–1175.

COLLER, B. S. and GRALNICK, H. R. (1977) Studies on the mechanism of ristocetin-induced platelet agglutination. Effects of structural modification of ristocetin and vancomycin. *J. clin. Invest.* **60**: 302–312.

COLLER, B. S., LUNDBERG, W. B. and GRALNICK, H. R. (1975) Effects of vancomycin on platelets, plasma proteins and hepatitis B surface antigen. *Thromb. Diath. haemorrh.* **34**: 83–93.

CONVERT, O., BONGINI, A. and FEENEY, J. (1980) A ^{1}H nuclear magnetic resonance study of the interactions of vancomycin with N-acetyl-D-alanyl-D-alanine and related peptides. *J. chem. Soc. Perkin II*. 1262–1270.

COOK, F. V. and FARRAR, W. E. Jr. (1978) Vancomycin revisited. *Ann. intern. Med.* **88**: 813–818.

CROSSLEY, K. B., ROTSCHAFER, J. C., CHERN, M. M., MEAD, K. R. and ZASKE, D. E. (1980) Comparison of a radioimmunoassay and a microbiological assay for measurement of serum vancomycin concentrations. *Antimicrob. Agents Chemother.* **17**: 654–657.

ELLESTAD, G. A., SWENSON W. and McGAHREN, W. J. (1983) Epimerization and stereochemistry of avoparcin. *J. Antibiotics* **36**: 1683–1690.

ESPOSITO, A. L. and GLECKMAN, R. A. (1977) Vancomycin. A second look. *J. Am. Med. Ass.* **238**: 1756–1757.

FESIK, S. W., ARMITAGE, I. M., ELLESTAD, G. A. and McGAHREN, W. J. (1984a) Nuclear magnetic resonance studies on the antibiotic avoparcin. Conformational properties in relation to antibacterial activity. *Mol. Pharmacol.* **25**: 275–280.

FESIK, S. W., ARMITAGE, I. M., ELLESTAD, G. A. and McGAHREN, W. J. (1984b) Nuclear magnetic resonance studies on the interaction of avoparcin with model receptors of bacterial cell walls. *Mol. Pharmacol.* **25**: 281–286.

FONG, K-L. L., HO. D-H. W., BOGERD. L., PAN, T., BROWN, N. S., GENTRY, L. and BODEY, G. P. Jr. (1981). Sensitive radioimmunoassay for vancomycin. *Antimicrob. Ag. Chemother.* **19**: 139–143.

GERACI, J. E. (1977) Vancomycin *Mayo Clin. Proc.* **52**: 631–634.

GRUNDY, W. E., SINCLAIR, A. C., THERIAULT, R. J., GOLDSTEIN, A. W., RICKHER, C. J., WARREN, H. B. Jr., OLIVER, T. J. and SYLVESTER, J. C. (1957) Ristocetin, microbiologic properties. In *Antibiotics Annual 1956–1957* p. 687–692. WELCH, H. & MARTI-IBANEZ, F. (eds.). Medical Encyclopaedia Inc., New York.

GRÜNEBERG, R. N., RIDGWAY, G. L., CREMER, A. W. F. and FELMINGHAM, D. F. (1983) The sensitivity of gram positive pathogens to teichomycin and vancomycin. *Drugs Exp. Clin. Res.* **9**: 139–141.

HAMMES, W. P. and NEUHAUS, F. C. (1974) On the mechanism of action of vancomycin: inhibition of peptidoglycan synthesis in *Gaffkya homari*. *Antimicrob. Ag. Chemother.* **6**: 722–728.

HARRIS, C. M., KOPECKA H. and HARRIS, T. M. (1983) Vancomycin: structure and transformation to CDP-I. *J. Am. Chem. Soc.* **105**: 6915–6922.

HOWARD, M. A. and FIRKIN, B. G. (1971) Ristocetin—a new tool in the investigation of platelet aggregation. *Thromb. Diath. Haemorrh.* **26**: 362–369.

HOWARD, M. A., HUTTON, R. A. and HARDISTY, R. M. (1973) Hereditary giant platelet syndrome: a disorder of a new aspect of platelet function. *Brit. med. J.* **2**: 586–588.

IZAKI, K. and STROMINGER, J. L. (1968) Biosynthesis of the peptidoglycan of bacterial cell walls XIV. Purification and properties of two D-alanine carboxypeptidases from *Escherichia coli*. *J. biol. Chem.* **243**: 3193–3201.

JENKINS, C. S. P., PHILLIPS, D. R., CLEMETSON, K. J., MEYER, D., LARRIEU, M-J. and LUSCHER, E. F. (1976) Platelet membrane glycoprotein implicated in ristocetin-induced aggregation. Studies on the proteins on platelets from patients with Bernard–Soulier syndrome and von Willebrand's disease. *J. clin. Invest.* **57**: 112–124.

JOHNSON, A. W., SMITH, R. M. and GUTHRIE, R. D. (1972) Vancosamine: the structure and configuration of a novel amino-sugar from vancomycin. *J. chem. Soc. Perkin I.* 2153–2159.

JOHNSON, C. R. (1962) Transannular sulfoxide–ketone interaction. A prospectus of the vancomycin structure. Ph.D. Thesis: University of Illinois, Urbana.

JOHNSTON, L. S. and NEUHAUS, F. C. (1975) Initial membrane reaction in the biosynthesis of peptidoglycan. Spin-labelled intermediates as receptors for vancomycin and ristocetin. *Biochemistry* **14**: 2754–2760.

JORDAN, D. C. (1961) Effect of vancomycin on the synthesis of the cell wall mucopeptide of *Staphylococcus aureus*. *Biochem. biophys. Res. Commun.* **6**: 167–170.

JORDAN, D. C. (1965) Effect of vancomycin on the synthesis of the cell wall and cytoplasmic membrane of *Staphylococcus aureus*. *Can. J. Microbiol.* **11**: 390–393.

KAHN, M. Y. and HALL, W. H. (1966) Staphylococcal enterocolitis—treatment with oral vancomycin. *Ann. intern. Med.* **65**: 1–8.

KALMAN, J. R. and WILLIAMS, D. H. (1980a) An NMR study of the structure of the antibiotic ristocetin A. The negative nuclear Overhauser effect in structure elucidation. *J. Am. chem. Soc.* **102**: 897–905.

KALMAN, J. R. and WILLIAMS, D. H. (1980b) An NMR study of the interaction between the antibiotic ristocetin A and a cell wall peptide analogue. Negative nuclear Overhauser effects in the investigation of drug binding sites. *J. Am. Chem. Soc.* **102**: 906–912.

KEIGHLEY, M. R. B., BURDON, D. W., ARABI, Y., ALEXANDER-WILLIAMS, J., THOMPSON, H., YOUNGS, D., JOHNSON, M., BENTLEY, S., GEORGE, R. H. and MOGG, G. A. G. (1978) Randomised controlled trial of vancomycin for pseudomembranous colitis and postoperative diarrhoea. *Brit. med. J.* **2**: 1667–1669.

KIRBY, E. and MILLS, D. C. B. (1975) The interaction of bovine factor VIII with human platelets. *J. clin. Invest.* **56**: 491–502.

KUCERS, A. and BENNETT, N. M. (1975) *The Use of Antibiotics: A Comprehensive Review with Clinical Emphasis* (2nd edn.) pp. 417–423. Lippincott, J. B. Co., Philadelphia.

KUNSTMANN, M. P., MITSCHER, L. A., PORTER, J. M., SHAY, A. J. and DARKEN. M. A. (1969) LL-AV290, a new antibiotic. I. Fermentation, isolation, and characterization. *Antimicrob. Agents Chemother. 1968* 242–245.

LEYH-BOUILLE, M., GHUYSEN, J-M., NIETO, M., PERKINS, H. R. SCHLEIFER, K. H. and KANDLER, O. (1970) On the *Streptomyces albus* G DD-carboxypeptidase. Mechanism of action of penicillin, vancomycin and ristocetin. *Biochemistry*, **9**: 2971–2975.

LIGHTBOWN, J. W. (1964) Antibiotics with specific affinities Part I: Ristocetin and vancomycin *Exp. Chemother.* **3**: 271–289.

LOMAKINA, N. N., YURINA, M. S., SCHEINKER, Yu. N. and TURCHIN, K. F. (1972) Structure of amino acids in the antibiotic ristomycin: Amino acids B and C. *Antibiotiki* **17**: 488–492.

McCORMICK, M. H., STARK, W. M., PITTENGER, G. E., PITTENGER, R. C. and McGUIRE, J. M. (1956) Vancomycin, a new antibiotic I. Chemical and biologic properties. *Antibiotics A.* **1955–1956**: 606–611.

McGAHREN, W. J., MARTIN, J. H., MORTON, G. O., HARGREAVES, R. T., LEESE, R. A., LOVELL, F. M. and ELLESTAD, G. A. (1979) Avoparcin. *J. Am. chem. soc.* **101**: 2237–2239.

McGAHREN, W. J., MARTIN, J. H., MORTON, G. O., HARGREAVES, R. T., LEESE, R. A., LOVELL, F. M., ELLESTAD, G. A., O'BRIEN, E. and HOLKER, J. S. E. (1980) Structure of avoparcin components. *J. Am. chem. Soc.* **102**: 1671–1684.

MARSHALL, F. J. (1965) Structure studies on vancomycin. *J. med. Chem.* **8**: 18–22.

MARTIN, S. E., MARDER, V. J., FRANCIS, C. W., LOFTUS, L. S. and BARLOW, G. H. (1980) Enzymatic degradation of the factor VIII von Willebrand protein: a unique tryptic fragment with ristocetin cofactor activity. *Blood*, **55**: 848–858.

MOAKE, J. L., CIMO, P. L., PETERSON, D. M., ROPER, P. and NATELSON, E. A. (1977) Inhibition of ristocetin-induced platelet agglutination by vancomycin. *Blood*, **50**: 397–406.

NIETO, M. and PERKINS, H. R. (1971a) Physicochemical properties of vancomycin and iodovancomycin and their complexes with diacetyl-L-lysyl-D-alanyl-D-alanine. *Biochem. J.* **123**: 773–787.

NIETO, M. and PERKINS, H. R. (1971b) Modifications of the acyl-D-alanyl–D-alanine terminus affecting complex formation with vancomycin. *Biochem. J.* **123**: 789–803.

NIETO, M. and PERKINS, H. R. (1971c) The specificity of combination between ristocetins and peptides related to bacterial cell wall mucopeptide precursors. *Biochem. J.* **124**: 845–852.

NIETO, M., PERKINS, H. R. and REYNOLDS, P. E. (1972) Reversal by a specific peptide (diacetyl-$\alpha\gamma$-diaminobutyr-yl-D-alanyl–D-alanine) of vancomycin inhibition in intact bacteria and cell-free preparations. *Biochem. J.* **126**: 139–149.

PALLANZA, R., BERTI, M., GOLDSTEIN, B. P., MAPELLI, E., RANDISI, E., SCOTTI, R. and ARIOLI, V. (1983) Teichomycin: in vitro and in vivo evaluation in comparison to other antibiotics. *J. Antimicrob. Chemother.* **11**: 419–425.

PARK, J. T. (1952) Uridine-5'-pyrophosphate derivatives I. Isolation from *Staphylococcus aureus*. II. A structure common to three derivatives III. Amino acid containing derivatives. *J. biol. Chem.* **194**: 877–884, 885–895, 897–904.

PERKINS, H. R. (1969) Specificity of combination between mucopeptide precursors and vancomycin or ristocetin. *Biochem. J.* **11**: 195–205.

PERKINS, H. R. and NIETO, M. (1970) The preparation of iodinated vancomycin and its distribution in bacteria treated with the antibiotic. *Biochem. J.* **116**: 83–92.

PHILLIP, J. E., SCHENCK, J. R., HARGIE, M. P., HOLPER, J. C. and GRUNDY, W. E. (1960) The increased activity of ristocetins A and B following acid hydrolysis. *Antimicrob. Agents A. 1960* 10–16.

RAMPLING, A., WARREN, R. E. and SYKES, H. V. (1980) Relapse of Clostridium colitis after vancomycin therapy. *J. Antimicrob. Chemother.* **6**: 551–552.

REYNOLDS, P. E. (1961) Studies on the mode of action of vancomycin. *Biochim. biophys. Acta* **52**: 403–405.

REYNOLDS, P. E. (1966) Antibiotics affecting cell-wall synthesis. *Symp. Soc. gen. Microbiol.* **16**: 47–69

RILEY, H. D. Jr. (1970) Vancomycin and novobiocin. *Med. Clins N. Am.* **54**: 1277–1289.

ROGERS, H. J., PERKINS, H. R. and WARD, J. B. (1980) *Microbial Cell Walls and Membranes.* Chapman & Hall: London & New York.

ROPER, P., PETERSON, D. M. and MOAKE, J. L. (1975) Vancomycin inhibition of platelet aggregation induced by ristocetin, collagen and ADP. *Abstr. Am. Soc. Hematology.* **201**.

SHELDRICK G. M., JONES, P. G., KENNARD, O., WILLIAMS, D. H. and SMITH, G. A. (1978) Structure of vancomycin and its complex with acetyl-D-alanyl–D-alanine. *Nature (Lond)* **271**: 223–225.

SMITH, G. A., SMITH, K. A. and WILLIAMS, D. H. (1975) Structural studies on the antibiotic vancomycin: evidence for the presence of modified phenylglycine and β-hydroxytyrosine units. *J. chem. Soc Perkin I.* 2108–2115.

SMITH, K. A., WILLIAMS, D. H. and SMITH, G. A. (1974) Structural studies on the antibiotic vancomycin: the nature of the aromatic rings. *J. chem. Soc. Perkin I.* 2369–2376.

SZTARICSKAI, F., HARRIS, C. M., NESZMÉLYI, A. and HARRIS, T. M. (1980) Structural studies of ristocetin A (ristomycin A): carbohydrate-aglycone linkages. *J. Am. chem. Soc.* **102**: 7093–7099.

TEDESCO, F., MARKHAM, R., GURWITH, M., CHRISTIE, D. and BARTLETT, J. G. (1978) Oral vancomycin for antibiotic-associated pseudomembranous colitis *Lancet* **2**: 226–228.

VAN HEIJENOORT, Y., DERRIEN, M. and VAN HEIJENOORT, J. (1978) Polymerization by transglycosylation in the biosynthesis of the peptidoglycan of *Escherichia coli* K12 and its inhibition by antibiotics. *FEBS Lett.* **89**: 141–144.

WALLACE, J. F., SMITH, R. H. and PETERSDORF, R. G. (1965) Oral administration of vancomycin in the treatment of staphylococcal enterocolitis *New Engl. J. Med.* **272**: 1014–1015.

WALLAS, C. H. and STROMINGER, J. L. (1963) Ristocetins, inhibitors of cell wall synthesis in *Stapaylococcus aureus. J. biol. Chem.* **238**: 2264–2266.

WARD, J. B. (1974) The synthesis of peptidoglycan in an autolysin-deficient mutant of *Bacillus licheniformis* N.C.T.C. 6346 and the effect of β-lactam antibiotics, bacitracin and vancomycin. *Biochem. J.* **141**: 227–241.

WEISS, H. J., ROGERS, J and BRAND, H. (1973) Defective ristocetin-induced platelet aggregation in von Wille-brand's disease and its correction by factor VIII. *J. clin. Invest.* **52**: 2697–2707.

WEISS, H. J., TSCHOPP, T. B., BAUMGARTNER, H. R., SUSSMAN, I., JOHNSON, M. M. and EGAN, J. J. (1974) Decreased adhesion of giant (Bernard–Soulier) platelets to subendothelium. *Am. J. Med.* **57**: 920–925.

WERINGA, W. D., WILLIAMS, D. H., FEENEY, J., BROWN, J. P. and KING, R. W. (1972) The structure of an amino-sugar from the antibiotic vancomycin. *J. chem. Soc. Perkin I.* 443–446.

WILLIAMS, A. H. and GRÜNEBERG, R. N. (1984). Teicoplanin. *J. Antimicrob. Chemother.* **14**: 441–445.

WILLIAMS, D. H. and BUTCHER, D. W. (1981) The binding site of the antibiotic vancomycin for a cell wall peptide analogue. *J. Am. chem. Soc.* **103**: 5697–5700.

WILLIAMS, D. H. and KALMAN, J. R. (1977) Structural and mode of action studies on the antibiotic vancomycin. Evidence from 270-MHz proton magnetic resonance. *J. Am. chem. Soc.* **99**: 2768–2774.

WILLIAMS, D. H., RAJANANDA, V. and KALMAN, J. R. (1979) On the structure and mode of action of the antibiotic ristocetin A. *J. chem. Soc. Perkin I.* 787–792.

WILLIAMSON, M. P. and WILLIAMS, D. H. (1980) A ^{13}C-NMR study of the carbohydrate portion of ristocetin A. *Tetrahedron Lett.* **21**: 4187–4188.

WILLIAMSON, M. P. and WILLIAMS, D. H. (1981a) A carbon-13 nuclear-magnetic resonance study of ristocetins A and B and their derivatives. *J. chem. Soc. Perkin I.* 1483–1491.

WILLIAMSON, M. P. and WILLIAMS, D. H. (1981b) Structure revision of the antibiotic vancomycin: the use of nuclear Overhauser effect difference spectroscopy. *J. Am. chem. Soc.* **103**: 6580–6585.

CHAPTER 5

MODE OF ACTION OF β-LACTAM ANTIBIOTICS

DONALD J. TIPPER

Department of Molecular Genetics and Microbiology, University of Massachusetts Medical School, Worcester, MA 01605, U.S.A.

1. INTRODUCTION

The action of β-lactam antibiotics on sensitive bacteria can be regarded as a two-stage process. In the first stage, the antibiotics bind to primary receptors, physically identified as membrane-associated penicillin-binding protein (PBP's). These proteins perform central roles in the cell cycle-related, morphogenetic synthesis of cell wall peptidoglycan. Inactivation of PBP's by bound antibiotic has immediate, biochemically definable effects on their function. The second stage encompasses the physiological effects on the sensitive cell initiated by this primary receptor–ligand interaction.

In a majority of sensitive bacteria, growing in hypotonic media, exposure of growing cells to a sufficient concentration of β-lactam antibiotic will result in cell death. In many cases, this appears to be due to loss of normal control over autolytic enzymes, transient activation of which is a normal part of the cell cycle. Association of death with autolysis has been clearly established in several bacterial species, but the mechanisms involved are poorly understood. Even less well understood are the mechanisms by which β-lactam antibiotics can lead to death without apparent autolysis in certain species, and to reversible inhibition of growth and macromolecular synthesis (a 'tolerant' response: Tomasz, 1979) in other sensitive bacteria. Inevitably, therefore, this review deals mainly with the primary interactions of PBP's with substrates and inhibitors. Lethal consequences are discussed in Section 8. In all of these phenomena, disruption of the normal cell growth cycle is clearly involved. Unfortunately, analysis of the integration of genome replication and expression, cell mass increase, wall synthesis, morphogenesis and cell division within the cell cycle remains one of the least tractable and most complex problems in bacterial physiology. Investigation of the functions of individual PBP's and of the results of selective inhibition of these PBP's by β-lactam antibiotics is probably the most fruitful avenue currently available for investigation of control of wall synthesis in the cell cycle.

Early observations on the mode of action of benzylpenicillin (Penicillin G, penicillin) (Gardner, 1940; Strominger, 1977) implicated the cell wall of sensitive cells as the primary target since the grossly visible effects of cell swelling and lysis suggested a weakening of this structure, whose chemical composition and properties were, at that time completely unknown. A great deal of work on the structure and biosynthesis of bacterial cell walls was necessary before the primary target of inhibition could be identified as the transpeptidation event central to the cross-linking and structural integrity of the bacterial cell wall peptidoglycan. As first postulated (Wise and Park, 1965; Tipper and Strominger, 1965), a single 'transpeptidase' target was envisioned. One purpose of this review is to demonstrate the extent to which this hypothesis has been modified and extended as PBP's have become identified with transpeptidases and enzymes of related function, and as the complexity of β-lactam antibiotic targets and their functions has become more clear. Most progress has been made in *Escherichia coli*, whose PBP's will, therefore, be a major focus of this review.

A second objective of this review is to summarize the evidence supporting the hypothesis (Tipper and Strominger, 1965) that transpeptidation involves an acyl-D-alanyl-Enzyme intermediate and that β-lactam antibiotics are structural analogs of acyl-D-alanyl-D-alanine donor substrates for transpeptidation. It was also suggested (Tipper and Strominger, 1965) that the mechanisms of transpeptidases and β-lactamases could be analogous, having evolved from a common ancestral gene, so that the β-lactamases might also employ an Acyl-Enzyme intermediate mechanism. The data supporting this hypothesis will also be summarized. A third objective is to discuss briefly the potential that current understanding of the mode of action of β-lactam antibiotics has for supplementing the current approach to β-lactam antibiotic development, based on empirical structure–activity analyses, by a rational approach to specifically designed inhibitors of PBP function. Strategies for circumventing bacterially acquired resistance mechanisms will also be touched upon.

The intense interest still generated by this field is reflected in the steady stream of published reviews on β-lactam antibiotics and their bacterial cell wall targets. I shall refer frequently to that by Ward (1984) on peptidoglycan structure and biosynthesis, to those by Spratt (1983) and by Waxman and Strominger (1983) on membrane-bound penicillin binding proteins (PBP's), to those by Ghuysen *et al.* (1980, 1981, 1984) on the soluble penicillin-sensitive D,D-carboxypeptidases of *Streptomyces* and *Actinomadura* species, to those by Tomasz (1979, 1980) on the mechanisms of bactericidal and tolerant responses to β-lactam antibiotics and to that by Boyd (1982) on structure–activity relationships.

The interest in β-lactam antibiotics is generated by the major role this class of antibiotics continues to play in human medicine, a role enhanced by the utility of these potentially bactercidal and relatively nontoxic antibiotics in treatment of the ever-increasing population of patients with severely compromised immune systems. The variety of opportunistic pathogens which may be involved includes species such as *Pseudomonas aeruginosa* which are intrinsically resistant to many antibiotics. This species, in particular, provides a major challenge to the medical chemists who continue to attempt to broaden the spectrum of activity of β-lactam antibiotics to cover such recalcitrant species. A more severe problem is presented by the acquisition of resistance to β-lactam antibiotics by ordinarily sensitive species. These include historically recognized scourges such as the gonococci, pneumococci and staphylococci, as well as opportunistic species such as the pseudomonads. These issues are summarized in Section 2.

2. LIMITATIONS OF β-LACTAM ANTIBIOTICS

It is now well established, as outlined in Section 3, that the primary targets of β-lactam antibiotic action are the PBP's involved in late stages of bacterial cell wall peptidoglycan synthesis. Because peptidoglycan is responsible for maintaining the integrity of bacterial cell walls, disruption of its structure in cells growing in a hypotonic environment leads to lysis and death. The observation that such damaged cells can survive as osmotically fragile spheroplasts or protoplasts in an isotonic medium, provided early insight into the mode of action of penicillin. The potential of spheroplasts for reversion to bacterial form has long been invoked as a mechanism for recrudescence of, for example, upper urinary tract infections, following cessation of β-lactam antibiotic treatment. However, its clinical significance is uncertain.

It is clear that lysis, when it occurs in response to β-lactam antibiotics, is due to inappropriate activation of autolytic peptidoglycan hydrolases (see Section 8). The tolerance of non-growing cells to exposure to normally lethal concentrations of most β-lactam antibiotics is due to the dominance of inhibition of autolysin activity in nongrowing cells. The well-documented antagonism between bacteriostasis and β-lactam antibiotics is a predictable correlate. This has been confirmed, largely through the work of Tomasz and his associates (Tomasz, 1979, 1980; Williamson and Tomasz, 1980), who showed that the autolytic response to β-lactam antibiotic exposure of growing cells of such highly susceptible species as *Streptococcus pneumoniae* could be prevented by mutation (resulting in loss of autolytic activity) or low medium pH (at which the autolysin is inactive). Prevention of autolysis results in a tolerant response: the minimal inhibitory concentration (MIC) is not altered, but the antibiotics become bacteriostatic (see Section 8). Mutations to tolerance of this type are of clinical significance, as reported for *Staphylococci* (Sabath *et al.*, 1977), and more recently for *Listeria* and many strains of *Streptococcus faecium* (Tomasz, 1980). Not surprisingly, endocarditis, whose treatment requires a bactericidal response, acts as a selective niche for tolerant mutants (Horne and Tomasz, 1980).

Recent studies employing chemostat cultures of *E. coli* have shown that the rate of loss of viability and autolysis of a given strain in response to a constant concentration of a given β-lactam antibiotic is constant with respect to the cell generation time (Tuomanen *et al.*, 1986). Thus for strain 205 and Cefonicid at ten times its minimal inhibitory concentration (MIC), the rate of killing was 0.22 logs per generation over a ten-fold range in generation time. The rate of killing varied with strain, antibiotic, and antibiotic concentration.

Just as the obvious potential and early success of penicillin in treating bacterial infectious disease led to intensive investigation of bacterial cell wall structure, the failures in its use led to analysis of the mechanisms of intrinsic and acquired resistance.

The essential requirement for susceptibility is a cell wall peptidoglycan structure of the murein type described in Section 3. Evolution of this structure, containing muramic acid and peptide cross-links synthesized by transpeptidation from acyl-D-Ala-D-Ala donors, is extremely ancient. Appearance of murein coincides with the divergence, several billion years ago, of the precursors of contemporary Archebacteria from those of contemporary Eubacteria and Eukaryotic cells (Fox *et al.*, 1980). The success of the murein structure is such that, through countless subsequent generations, Eubacteria have retained a common glycan structure and cross-linkage mechanism, as well as the basic structure of the murein peptide subunits. The presence of murein is a hallmark of this redefined prokaryotic kingdom (Fox *et al.*, 1980), the best studied class of contemporary prokaryotes. Fortunately, all recognized human bacterial pathogens and normal flora belong to the Eubacteria so that all, with the exception of the Mycoplasmas, which have discarded their cell wall and its biosynthetic machinery, are potentially susceptible to β-lactam antibiotics. The antibiotic susceptibility of normal flora is valuable when they act as opportunistic pathogens, but a potential problem when they are bystander victims of chemotherapy. Massive suppression of gut flora can result from such inadvertent activity, particularly if this suppression includes the predominant Gram negative anaerobic components. Super infection can result, sometimes with severe pathological consequences.

The ultimate determinants of the efficacy of a given β-lactam antibiotic against a Eubacterial infection are the susceptibility of its essential bacterial PBP components, the primary targets, to binding and stable acylation by the drug, and access of the drug to these targets. Analysis of the PBP's in isolated membranes from a wide variety of bacteria, including such intrinsically resistant species as *Pseudomonas aeruginosa*, has failed to show variations in β-lactam susceptibility that could account for the wide variations in sensitivity of the intact bacteria to the effects of equal extracellular concentrations of these antibiotics. This variation is, instead, almost entirely determined by variation in the effective concentrations of these drugs at their site of action.

The first factor determining effective antibiotic concentration is the site of infection. Access of β-lactam antibiotics to obligate intracellular pathogens (*Chamydia* and *Rickettsia*) is prevented by the location of the growing bacterial cells. Resistance of acid-fast bacteria is presumably determined mostly by the impermeability of their lipid-rich cell walls, although the slow growth rate and sequestration of *M. tuberculosis* in tubercles must also play a part. For other extracellular bacterial pathogens, local antibiotic concentration is determined by the site of infection, by various pharmacological factors related to uptake, distribution, secretion, sequestration and inactivation of the drug within host tissues, and by the ability of the patient to tolerate the antibiotic. The latter is limited mostly by allergy and effects on normal flora, since the direct toxicity of almost all β-lactam antibiotics is very low (Brown and Martin, 1981).

The ratio between the extracellular drug concentration and the concentration at the site of the PBP targets of antibiotic action, which lie on the exterior of the cytoplasmic membrane, is primarily determined by the rate of permeation of each drug through the surrounding cell wall and by its susceptibility to β-lactamases produced by the bacterium.

In Gram positive bacteria, the cell wall is, in general, freely permeable to β-lactam antibiotics. This seems to be true even in the relatively resistant group D streptococci, whose resistance seems to be exceptional in being related primarily to a relatively low intrinsic affinity of their PBP's for penicillin (Williamson *et al.*, 1983). The complexity of this issue has been illustrated by the recent studies of Canepari *et al.* (1986). For rapidly growing wild-type *Streptococcus faecium*, PBP3 appears to be essential in that MIC's for β-lactam antibiotics coincide with the relatively low concentrations necessary for its saturation. For slowly growing cells, however, the MIC is many-fold higher and now coincides with the concentration necessary to saturate all of the PBP's, including PBP5, the species with the lowest antibiotic affinity (see section 5.2.2). Thus killing targets and mechanisms may vary with growth conditions in any given bacterial strain.

Gram positive bacteria are generally highly susceptible to penicillin, unless they produce β-lactamase. Beta-lactamase production is only of significance, at present, for staphylococci. For staphylococci, the extracellular antibiotic concentration is determined by bacterial population density and susceptibility to their inducible, secreted class A β-lactamase. Selection of plasmid-bearing staphylococci carrying the gene for this enzyme, conferring resistance to penicillin, was the first major setback suffered in what has become a continuing struggle to adapt β-lactam antibiotics to the treatment of infectious disease. This first challenge was met by the development of methicillin, and later by more effective semisynthetic penicillin derivatives, which retained sufficient affinity for the *S. aureus* PBP's to kill at low concentrations while being resistant to the *S. aureus* β-lactamase. It was not long before mutants of *S. aureus* resistant to the methicillin class of antibiotics began to be recognized in the clinic, further establishing the pattern of reverses that have been encountered with each new advance in β-lactam antibiotic chemotherapy.

In contrast to the simple picture in Gram positive bacteria, Gram negative bacteria have evolved a selectively permeable cell wall component, the outer membrane, which allows them to control, very effectively, the composition of the periplasmic fluid space that lies between this outer membrane and the cytoplasmic membrane. Access to the periplasm, the immediate environment of the PBP's, is determined by the rate of passive diffusion through the outer membrane. This is largely determined, for hydrophilic components such as the β-lactam antibiotics, by the selectivity of the aqueous pores created by the outer membrane porin transmembrane components (Nikaido, 1981; Chapter 7). The periplasm provides a small compartment in which secreted enzymes, such as β-lactamases, can reach high concentrations. These and the other proteins which modify or bind ligands diffusing through the outer membrane, give the cell control over the degradation, import and export of such ligands.

The permeability of the outer membrane varies markedly among Gram negative bacteria, being generally high in *Neisseria*, very low in *Pseudomonads*, and intermediate in *Enterobacteriaceae*. While gonorrhea was (initially) universally treatable with penicillin, further development of semi-synthetic 6-amino penicillanic acid derivatives such as ampicillin, and of cephalosporin derivatives such as cephalothin, was necessary to produce β-lactam antibiotics capable of effectively permeating the walls of *Enterobacteriaceae*. The impressive variety of β-lactamases that Gram negative bacteria are able to produce, capable of hydrolyzing both penicillin and cephalosporin derivatives, and the facility with which plasmids carrying the ubiquitous class A β-lactamases could be transmitted, was the next major barrier to effective β-lactam antibiotic therapy thrown up by bacterial pathogens. Introduction of each new class of β-lactam antibiotics into clinical practice has revealed a new facet of the daunting ability of pathogenic bacteria to meet these challenges to their survival. Indiscriminate use has certainly shortened the period of usefulness of many antibiotic variants, but the innate adaptability of bacteria is primarily responsible for what seems, in retrospect, to be an inevitable series of reverses. For example, β-

lactamase-determined resistance of *Enterobacteriaceae* to ampicillin appeared very early, due to the prevalence and ease of transmission of plasmids carrying transposons expressing class A β-lactamases. This was followed more recently, but inevitably in the face of strong selection, by acquisition of plasmids producing the same β-lactamase by *N. gonorrhea* and *Haemophilus influenzae*. The role played by overproduction of the chromosomal class C β-lactamases in resistance to the next generation of semi synthetic antibiotics became clear more slowly. In *Enterobacter cloacae*, this results from constitutive expression of *ampC* which is normally represented by the *ampR* gene product. In *E. coli*, where expression of *ampC* is constitutive but weak, over-expression results from gene duplication, acquisition of a more efficient promoter, or loss of a growth rate-dependent attenuation system. This resistance is dependent on low rates of permeation of these antibiotics into the periplasmic space and it was suggested that nonhydrolytic 'trapping' of the drug by binding to β-lactamase (Sanders, 1984) is sufficient to give protection. However, it has recently been shown (Vu and Nikaido, 1985; Chapter 7) that in *Enterobacter cloacae*, such resistance is mostly due to the slow but significant rate of hydrolysis of even these β-lactamase resistant third generation β-lactam antibiotics by the high constitutive levels of Class C β-lactamase present. At low, physiologically significant antibiotic levels, this rate, in conjunction with slow permeation of the outer membrane, is sufficient to protect the PBP targets (see Section 7.1).

Mutations leading to small, incremental steps in resistance to penicillin, long recognized in the gonococcus, are primarily due to decreased affinity of PBP's for the drug (see Section 6), though reduction in outer membrane permeability is also involved. This type of mutation, where compatible with viability and pathogenicity, is clearly an ever-present threat to the utility of β-lactam antibiotics. The prevalence of such mutations as causes of treatment failure can be expected to increase as the use of β-lactamase-resistant drugs increases.

3. THE STRUCTURE AND BIOSYNTHESIS OF BACTERIAL CELL WALL PEPTIDOGLYCAN

The structure of *Escherichia coli* cell wall peptidoglycan is illustrated in Fig. 1. The glycan structure, shown in detailed in Fig. 1(a), is universal in murein: it consists of alternating β-1,4 linked residues of *N*-acetyl-D-glucosamine (GlcNAc) and of *N*-acetylmuramic acid (MurNAc), the 3-*O*-D-lactyl ether derivative of GlcNAc. The glycan is a modified form of chitin and is drawn in the flat ribbon conformation (Tipper, 1970), in which chitin is constrained by hydrogen bonds. X-ray scattering data and theoretical analyses of conformation indicate significant helical twist in this structure in peptidoglycan (Labischinski *et al.*, 1979). MurNAc provides the carboxylate group to which the peptide chains are attached. The strict alternation of GlcNAc and MurNAc [represented as G and M in Fig. 1(c)] in the glycan is ensured by synthesis of the disaccharide repeating subunit prior to polymerization.

All peptidoglycans initially carry a peptide subunit on each MurNAc residue. That illustrated in Fig. 1(a) is the L-Ala-D-Glu-mDAP-D-Ala-D-Ala pentapeptide (mDAP is meso-diaminopimelic acid) that constitutes the nascent peptide subunit of the type Alγ peptidoglycan (nomenclature of Schleifer and Kandler, 1972) found, for example, in *E. coli*. This structure is probably common to all Gram negative bacteria and also occurs in many Gram positive bacteria. In the mature peptidoglycan of *E. coli*, transpeptidation and D,D-carboxypeptidase action convert about 66% of the nascent peptide subunits shown in Fig. 1(a) into the cross-linked dimers shown in Fig. 1(b). Most of the rest exist as monomers, lacking one or both of their D-alanine residues due to carboxypeptidase action. The mature peptidoglycan, shown schematically as a two-dimensional net in Fig. 1(c), is cross-linked into a continuous, cell-sized polymer that has the shape of the cell from which it is derived. This is the murein sacculus of Weidel and Pelzer (1964). In Gram negative bacteria, the peptidoglycan layer, located adjacent to the inner layer of the outer membrane, may actually be a two-dimensional monolayer. The Alγ peptidoglycan is the simplest and most

138 D. J. TIPPER

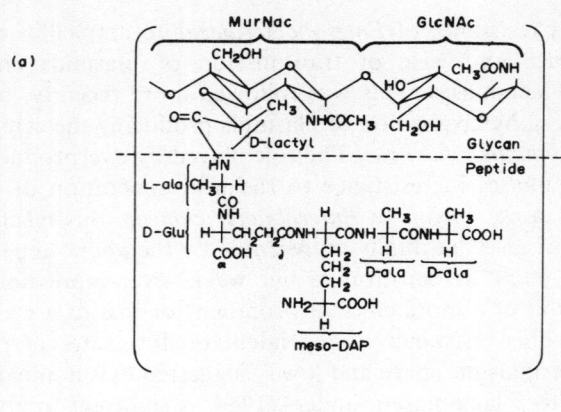

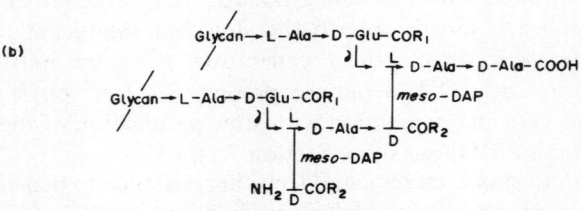

Fig. 1. Structure of the type A1γ peptidoglycan of *Escherichia coli* cell walls. (a) The repeating disaccharide of the glycan consists of β-1,4 linked subunits of *N*-acetylmuramic acid (MurNAc) and *N*-Acetyl-D-glucosamine (GlcNAc). MurNAc is the 3-*O*-D-lactyl derivative of G1cNAc. These disaccharides are themselves linked β-1,4 so that the glycan is a modified form of chitin. The flat ribbon conformation of chitin is illustrated. The pentapeptide L-Ala-D-Glu-meso-DAP-D-Ala-D-Ala is linked to the D-lactyl moiety of MurNAc in each repeating disaccharide subunit in the nascent polymer, but may subsequently be modified by transpeptidation or carboxypeptidase action. Meso DAP is meso-diaminopimelic acid. It is linked at its L center to the γ carboxyl of D-glutamate and to the D-Ala-D-Ala dipeptide. (b) A cross-linked dimer. In the convention employed, an α peptide linkage is represented as a horizontal line, while linkages to or from a non-α-COOH or NH₂ are shown as vertical lines. In *E. coli* (and Gram negative cell walls in general) R1 = R₂ = OH. In *Bacillus subtilis* (Gram positive) R1 = OH and R2 = NH₂ in the vegetative cell wall, but R1 = R2 = OH in the spore cortex. Other variations in amidation of the A1γ structure occur in other Gram positive cell walls. Cross-linkage has eliminated a D-Ala residue from the N-terminal (left-hand, lower) peptide unit, while D,D-carboxypeptidase action would eliminate a D-Ala residue from the C-terminal (right-hand, upper) peptide unit. (c) Schematic representation of a two-dimensional peptidoglycan net giving approximate molecular dimensions. Glycan chains, here represented as chains of M (MurNAc) and G (GlcNAc), in *E. coli* average 50 disaccharide units in length while the peptides in *E. coli* consist mostly of monomers (vertical lines with the lower end representing the free D-Ala carboxy terminus and the short horizontal line representing the free amino terminal group on meso-DAP) and dimers (horizontal cross-linked 'H girders'). Since dimers comprise about two-thirds of the peptide units, the average degree of cross-linkage is 33%. This figure is adapted from the review by Tipper and Wright (1979), in *The Bacteria*, Vol. 7, pp. 291–426 (Academic Press, New York) as modified in *β-Lactam Antibiotics for Clinical Use*, (Queener, Queener and Weber, eds.). Marcel Dekker, New York (1986), with the permission of the publishers and editors.

economical murein and a thin layer is clearly all that is needed for cell viability when it is accompanied and protected against enzymatic attack by the Gram negative outer membrane. As suggested by Schleifer and Kandler (1972), this combination may represent a highly successful and sophisticated variant of the Eubacterial peptidoglycan patterns of relatively recent evolutionary origin. Minor modifications in its structure occur in *E. coli*, including covalent linkage to lipoprotein and rare DAP–DAP cross-links (Glauner and Schwarz, 1983).

The walls of Gram positive bacteria have a much higher peptidoglycan content in a multilayered structure to which other polymers are covalently attached. This produces a wall which is much thicker than in Gram negative bacteria, but also much more permeable, with a sieving limit sufficient to allow easy passage of not only all β-lactam antibiotics, but also larger antibiotics such as bacitracin, vancomycin, moenomycin, etc. which are inactive against Gram negative bacteria. The Gram positive peptidoglycan contains many variants in its peptide structure, but all derive from the pentapeptide (A)-D-Glu-(B)-D-Ala-D-Ala where (A) is usually L-alanine and D-Glu is always γ linked to (B), which is usually a dibasic amino acid (meso-DAP, L-lysine, L-ornithine, etc.). This tripeptide is linked through an Lα linkage to the ubiquitous D-Ala-D-Ala C-terminal dipeptide. In the classification of Schleifer and Kandler (1972), type A1 structures are cross-linked directly between the penultimate D-alanine residue and the ω amino group of (B), as in the A1γ structure of *E. coli* [Fig. 1(b)]. In type A2, A3 and A4 structures, an intervening peptide occurs, but linkage is still to the ω amino group of (B). In type B structures, the amino acceptor for cross-link formation is a dibasic amino acid that forms part of a cross-bridge peptide attached to the α carboxyl group of D-glutamate. It is not necessary that (B) also be dibasic in type B structures, since it is not the peptide branch point.

The 'stem' pentapeptide, lacking cross-bridge amino acids, was first recognized in the nucleotide-peptide peptidoglycan precursor whose discovery in *S. aureus* cells treated with penicillin (Park, 1952) was a pivotal event in the study of peptidoglycan structure and biosynthesis. This nucleotide is a peptidoglycan precursor in all Eubacteria and has the general sequence UDP-MurNAc-(A)-D-Glu-(B)-D-Ala-D-Ala in which MurNAc is activated for transfer by its pyrophosphate linkage.

In the biosynthesis of peptidoglycan (Fig. 2), formation of this nucleotide-pentapeptide, the first phase, is the culmination of a series of cytoplasmic events. A universal aspect of its synthesis is addition of D-Ala-D-Ala as a presynthesized dipeptide, providing the donor substrate for transpeptidation. Formation of this dipeptide by alanine racemase and D-Ala-D-Ala synthetase is a target for antibiotic alanine analogs with broad spectra of antibacterial activities (Neuhaus and Hammes, 1981; Chapter 2). All inhibitors of this phase of peptidoglycan synthesis must cross both cell wall and cytoplasmic membrane permeability barriers to reach their targets.

The second phase of peptidoglycan biosynthesis takes place on the inner surface of the cytoplasmic membrane and is initiated by transfer of phospho-MurNAc-pentapeptide to undecaprenyl-phosphate, (Lipid-P), the membrane-bound anchor for construction of the peptidoglycan subunit. The disaccharide repeating unit of the glycan is produced by addition of GlcNAc (Fig. 2), followed by other species-specific modifications such as addition of cross-bridge amino acids, amidation of free amino groups, etc. (not shown). Following transfer of the lipid-linked completed subunit to the exterior of the cytoplasmic membrane, the third phase is initiated by polymerization of the glycan by transglycosylation, the target of vancomycin action (Perkins, 1982; Chapter 3). The chain grows from its reducing end (Fig. 3), and addition of each disaccharide-peptide subunit releases a molecule of Lipid-PP which must be hydrolyzed by the bacitracin-sensitive pyrophosphorylase (Toscano and Storm, 1982; Chapter 4) before it can be used as a recycled carrier for glycan polymerization (Fig. 2). This extracellular phase continues with formation of mature peptidoglycan by transpeptidation, D,D- and L,D-carboxypeptidase action, covalent attachment of other polymers and limited hydrolysis (controlled autolysin action).

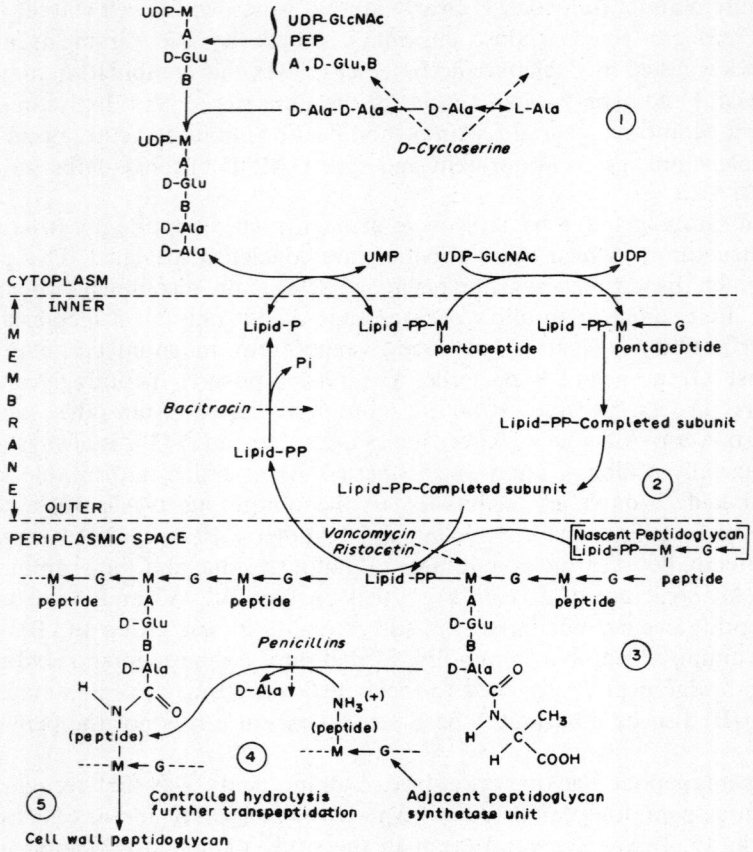

FIG. 2. Biosynthesis of peptidoglycan. Peptidoglycans of all of the types found in *Eubacteria* are synthesized according to this general scheme.(1) The first stage (top) involves cytoplasmic enzymes, substrates and products, and results in synthesis of UDP-MurNAc-pentapeptide [(A)-D-Glu-(B)-D-Ala-D-Ala]. (A) is usually L-alanine and (B) is usually a dibasic amino acid such as meso-DAP or L-lysine. The fourth and fifth amino acids are invariably added as the pre-synthesized dipeptide, D-alanyl-D-alanine, whose synthesis is inhibited by D-cycloserine. (2) The second stage (center) involves both cytoplasmic and membrane-bound substrates. The enzymes and products are bound to the inner surface of the cytoplasmic membrane. The first step in this 'lipid cycle' is transfer of phospho-MurNAc-pentapeptide from UMP to Lipid-P. Lipid-P is undecaprenyl-phosphate, the carrier lipid for bacterial exocellular polysaccharide biosynthesis. Following translocation of phospho-MurNAc-pentapeptide to this carrier, addition of GlcNAc completes the disaccharide. The peptide subunit is completed by species-specific modifications: addition of cross-bridge amino acids, amidation of D-Glu or meso-DAP, and other modifications, none of which are shown. The completed subunit then translocates to the exterior surface of the membrane for polymerization. (3) Polymerization (step 3) occurs by transglycosylation at the reducing end of the glycan, releasing Lipid-pyrophosphate (Lipid-PP). Transglycosylation is inhibited by vancomycin, ristocetin and related antibiotics. The Lipid-PP released is converted back to Lipid-P acceptor by the bacitracin-sensitive membrane-bound pyrophosphatase, completing the lipid cycle. (4) The fourth stage includes cross-link formation by transpeptidation, and also D,D-carboxypeptidase action (not shown), both resulting in loss of the terminal D-alanine residue. These enzymes, like the transglycosylases, are located on the outer surface of the cytoplasmic membrane, and certain PBP's perform both transglycosylase and transpeptidase functions, so that stages (3) and (4) are sometimes tightly coupled events. Other cell wall polymers are covalently attached to nascent-peptidoglycan at this stage by other membrane-associated polymerases and transferases (not shown). (5) In stage 5, controlled hydrolysis and delayed transpeptidation of peptidoglycan modifies the maturing structure to allow cell expansion, morphogenesis and separation.

No peptidoglycan is completely cross-linked. The highest known levels are found in *S. aureus* (75%) and many bacteria, like *E. coli*, have only about 33% cross-links, so that oligomers of peptide subunits average 1.5 units in length [Fig. 1(c)]. The glycan is much more highly polymerized, with an average chain length of 60 to 100 disaccharide units (Tipper and Wright, 1979), presumably controlled by hydrolysis. Autolytic glycan

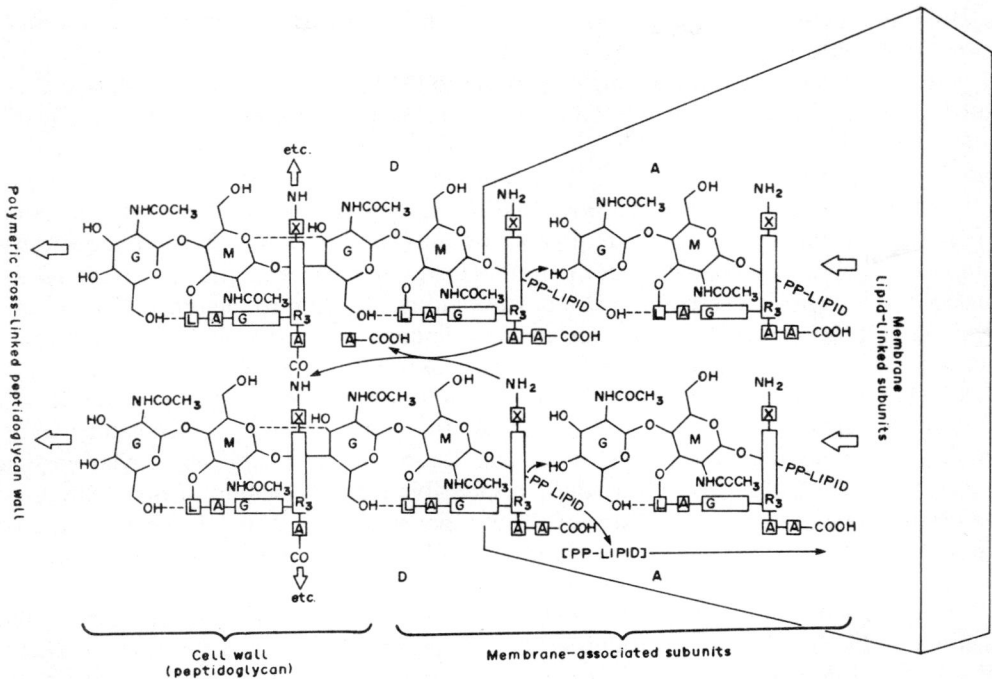

FIG. 3. Polymerization and cross-linking by transpeptidation of a nascent type A2 peptidoglycan. Two parallel peptidoglycan polymerizing sites are shown. Each consists of an Acceptor (A) and Donor (D) site for transglycosylation. A nascent subunit in the A site consists of GlcNAc (G), MurNAc (M), with its 3-O-D-lactyl moiety (L), linked to a pentapeptide A-G-R_3-AA-COOH (A = alanine, G = γ-linked D-glutamate) substituted on the dibasic amino acid (R_3) by a cross-bridge peptide, X-NH_2. This is the acceptor for transglycosylation from nascent glycan in the D site. Both substrates are bound to membrane by Lipid-PP. Transglycosylation releases Lipid-PP from the donor (polymeric) substrate and results in translocation of the newly added subunit to the D site, so that chain growth occurs at the reducing end. Hydrogen bonds defining the chitin-like conformation of the glycan are shown as dashed lines. Transpeptidation between the two nascent peptidoglycan chains is shown as a concomitant event, involving a PBP in close proximity to, or part of, the transglycosylase, resulting in cross-link formation between the amino acceptor (X-NH_2) of the lower chain and the penultimate D-alanine residue of the donor subunit of the upper chain, with release of a terminal D-alanine (A-COOH) residue. Cross-linkage to other adjacent nascent chains, being synthesized by a linear array of polymerizing sites (not shown), could produce a sheet of peptidoglycan. Cross-linkage in which both donor and acceptor substrates are nascent peptidoglycan, as shown, possibly occurs during cross-wall formation (see text).

This figure is adapted from the review by Tipper and Wright (1979), in *The Bacteria* Vol. 7, pp. 291–426 (Academic Press, New York) as modified in *β-Lactam Antibiotics for Clinical Use*, (Queener, Queener and Weber, eds.), Marcel Dekker, New York (1986), with the permission of the publishers and editors.

hydrolases have only been identified in some bacteria, but may have to exist in all in order to control glycan length. The extent of peptide cross-linkage is controlled either by the efficiency of transpeptidation, or by subsequent peptide hydrolysis, for example, by D,D-endopeptidase action. This activity is recognized *in vitro* in PBP 4 of *E. coli* (Section 5.2), but has been identified in only a few other bacteria. The relationship between D,D-transpeptidase, D,D-carboxypeptidase, and D,D-endopeptidase action is illustrated for the *E. coli* A1γ peptidoglycan in Fig. 4. All potentially employ an acyl-D-Ala-D-(X) substrate, and so are potentially inhibited by β-lactam antibiotics (Section 4).

The sequence of events involved in the maturation of the nascent polymer of peptidoglycan during extension of the bacterial cell wall is only partially understood and is a matter of some controversy (Ward, 1984; Chapter 1). The transglycosylases, transpeptidases, D,D- and L,D-carboxypeptidases which are involved in this process, most of which appear to be PBP's, are all membrane proteins presumably anchored on the outer surface of the cytoplasmic membrane. They may be clustered in functionally oriented groups of 'spinnerettes' or 'knitting machines' at annular sites of active longitudinal- or cross-wall extension. The biochemical evidence supports both a functionally integrated assembly line, as schematically shown in Fig. 3, and temporal and presumably physical separation of polymerizing activities.

It has recently become clear, from analysis of the PBP's of *E. coli* (Section 4), that these penicillin-sensitive enzymes include bifunctional transglycosylase/transpeptidase enzymes (PBP's 1A, 1B, and 3 at least) which presumably perform these two functions in a concerted fashion, as shown in Fig. 3. It was originally hypothesized (Tipper and Wright, 1979) that such a concerted mechanism would be essential to ensure efficient juxtaposition of polymeric peptidoglycan donor and acceptor substrates with membrane-bound trans-peptidase, resulting in cross-link formation. However, early experiments in *S. aureus* showed that uncross-linked peptide monomer could be chased into oligomers (Tipper and Strominger, 1968) and a slow increase in cross-linkage of previously polymerized pep-tidoglycan has been shown in *Bacillus megaterium* (Fordham and Gilvarg, 1974), *S. faecalis* (Dezelee and Shockman, 1975), and *E. coli* (DePedro and Schwarz, 1981). It now seems likely, at least in *E. coli* and *S. aureus*, that this represents a secondary trans-peptidation event, while initial transpeptidation occurs coupled to transglycosylation. The delayed transpeptidation may be partially responsible for remodelling of pre-synthesized peptidoglycan to allow cellular expansion. The responsible PBP, PBP 4, has been identified in *E. coli* and *S. aureus* (assignation of the same PBP number is purely coincidental and does not imply similar structures or functions: Section 5).

Although *S. aureus* PBP 4 acts as a D,D-carboxypeptidase *in vitro* (Kozarich and Strominger, 1978), there is no evidence of such activity *in vivo* and deletion of PBP 4 activity, by selective inhibition by cefoxitin or by mutation, leads to a 50% reduction in average cross-linking of the *S. aureus* cell wall peptidoglycan (Wyke *et al.*, 1981). The mutants are viable in the laboratory, but hypersensitive to β-lactam antibiotics. Mutants selected for resistance regain PBP 4 (Ward, 1984; Chapter 1).

In *E. coli* PBP 4 was initially classified as a D,D-carboxypeptidase, although it also functions as a D,D-endopeptidase *in vitro*. Either function should reduce cross-linkage, yet deficiency of PBP 4 activity in *dacB* mutants (Section 5.1.2) has no effect on viability in the laboratory although delayed transpeptidation is abolished (DePedro and Schwartz. (1981). It has recently been suggested (Glauner and Sahwartz, 1983) that PBP 4 catalyzes form-ation of the rare DAP–DAP cross-links in *E. coli* peptidoglycan.

It is generally accepted that glycan polymerization is normally accompanied by immediate linkage to preexisting murein by transpeptidation. It has been suggested (Mirelman *et al.*, 1977; Mirelman, 1979) that, in rod-shaped bacteria such as *E. coli*, cross-linkage to preexisting murein is characteristic of extension of cylindrical peripheral wall, while centripetal growth of cross walls at developing septa involves cross-link formation between strands of nascent 'soluble' peptidoglycan. It is not clear which of these acceptor substrates might be preferred by the bifunctional PBP's: Fig. 3, showing cross-linkage by this mechanism between nascent strands, describes only one possible acceptor. Organization of polymerization sites with respect to each other and preexisting murein, would clearly be important in determining the acceptor used. This may well depend on the PBP involved. While Mirelman's (1979) hypothesis is unproven, it is clear that different high molecular weight, bifunctional PBP's are involved in cylindrical wall extension and cross-wall synthesis, at least in *E. coli* (Section 5).

Besides the essential high molecular weight PBP's, the lower molecular weight D,D-carboxypeptidase components found in most Eubacteria may also play a role in morphogenesis. Since removal of the terminal D-alanine residue by D,D-carboxypeptidase action prevents a peptide unit from acting as a donor in transpeptidation, it was suggested, when these activities were discovered (Izaki *et al.*, 1966), that they function to control the extent of cross-link formation. While the data on mutants lacking these enzymes fails to support this hypothesis (see Section 4), a role in morphogenesis is suggested by the observation that overproduction of *E. coli* PBP-5 results in rounded cell formation (Markiewicz *et al.*, 1982). It may be that the tetra- or tri-peptide products of carboxypeptidase action are preferred or essential acceptor substrates for cross-wall synthesis. This is made more plausible by the intriguing and apparently unusual role this

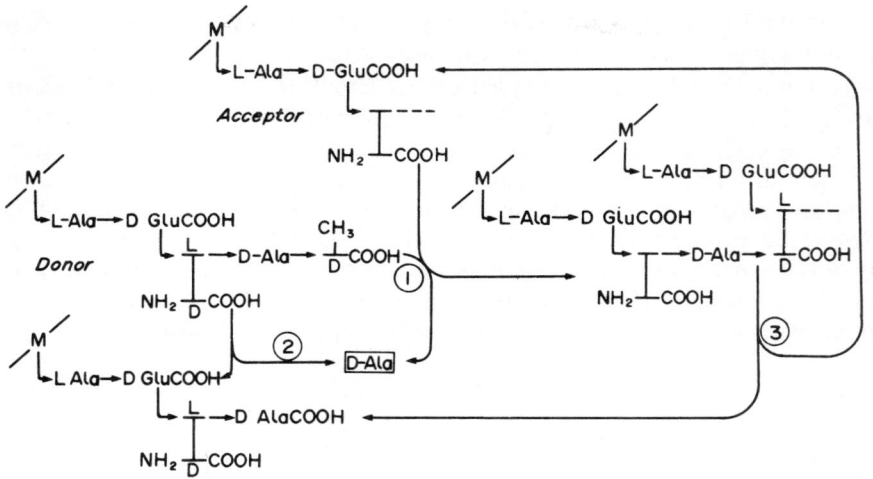

FIG. 4. The relationship between transpeptidase, D,D-carboxypeptidase, and D,D-endopeptidase functions of PBP's. The substrate shown is the Alγ peptidoglycan of *E. coli* cell walls. *Reaction 1:* transpeptidation. A PBP that is primarily a transpeptidase (e.g. *E. coli* PBP 1A, 1Bs) binds a nascent peptidoglycan subunit to its donor site, producing acyl-D-Ala-ENZ (Fig. 5), with release of the terminal D-alanine residue. Binding of a suitable peptidoglycan subunit in the acceptor site leads to transpeptidation. *Reaction 2:* D,D-carboxypeptidase action. The first step, binding of a peptidoglycan subunit to the donor site, enzyme acylation, and release of the terminal D-alanine, occurs as for transpeptidation. However, binding of water to the acceptor site (e.g., of *E. coli* PBP 5 or 6) leads to D,D-carboxypeptidase reaction and release of the peptidoglycan subunit. *Reaction 3:* D,D-endopeptidase action. Binding of previously cross-linked peptidoglycan (e.g., to *E. coli* PBP 4) leads, by a reversal of reaction 1, to release of an amino terminal peptide fragment and acyl-D-Ala-ENZ formation. Hydrolysis of the latter by water (reaction 2) completes the D,D-endopeptidase hydrolysis of the cross-link. The PBP 4 intermediate could alternatively act as a transpeptidation donor (Fig. 5), potentially resulting in a re-orientation of cross-links.

This figure is adapted from the review by Tipper and Wright (1979), in *The Bacteria*, Vol. 7, pp. 291–426 (Academic Press, New York) as modified in *β-Lactam Antibiotics for Clinical Use*, (Queener, Queener and Weber, eds), Marcel Dekker, New York (1986), with the permission of the publishers and editors.

type of mechanism plays in cross-link formation in *Gaffkya homari* (Hammes and Kandler, 1976).

In Gram positive bacilli or *Pseudomonas aeruginosa*, all with type Alγ peptidoglycans, pentapeptides on nascent peptidoglycan chains act as acceptors in transpeptidation (Ward, Chapter 1). In contrast, a penicillin-resistant transpeptidase in *G. homari* uses tripeptides in nascent peptidoglycan as acceptors in wall–membrane preparations (Hammes and Seidel, 1978). The carboxypeptidases involved in tripeptide formation act only on nascent peptidoglycan and are the penicillin-sensitive targets in this organism.

Any role for D,D-carboxypeptidases in controlling transpeptidation, either positive or negative, implies that they have access to their pentapeptide substrate before transpeptidation occurs, suggesting at least partial separation of transglycosylation and transpeptidation events. Possibly the major transpeptidase system detected *in vitro* in preparations from *G. homari* is only one of several systems existing in all cell types, including *G. homari*, and *G. homari* is unusual in that this activity predominates in its disrupted cells. While this seems unlikely, it is probable that multiple transpeptidation systems exist in all bacteria and that those seen *in vitro* represent only the most robust or the most prevalent.

Separation of glycan polymerization from transpeptidation is also suggested by the detection of a rapidly labeled, soluble, uncross-linked peptidoglycan of short chain length purported to be a biosynthetic intermediate in whole cells of *B. megaterium* (Fuchs-Cleveland and Gilvarg, 1976). It has the properties expected of a lipid-linked precursor of cross-linked murein, and a similar material has been detected in *E. coli* (Mett *et al.*, 1980). However, as pointed out by Ward (1984; Chapter 1), the quantities detected are very small, and no chase into cross-linked peptidoglycan has been demonstrated. It has been suggested (Goodell *et al.*, 1983) that they are autolytic artefacts. It remains possible that part of the peptidoglycan, perhaps with specific functions, is made in this way

Investigation of the role of the multiple PBP's in *E. coli* and other bacterial species which afford independent lethal targets for β-lactam antibiotics (see Section 5), leads to the suggestion that each may play a terminal role in a peptidoglycan synthetic pathway of unique function. Different polymerizing systems may be involved, for example, in cylindrical and cross-wall synthesis, in cell expansion, and in cell division. If so, then analysis of total biosynthetic pools may emphasize a component unique to one such pathway at the expense of others. Minor components may be associated with an essential minor synthetic pathway. While they may, therefore, have real significance, they should be regarded with some skepticism until this significance is demonstrated.

4. INHIBITION OF TRANSPEPTIDATION BY PENICILLIN

By 1964, the biosynthetic pathway leading to the polymerization of uncross-linked, soluble peptidoglycan from lipid intermediates (Fig. 2) had been demonstrated *in vitro* without finding any step sensitive to penicillin. The accumulation of nucleotide pentapeptide caused by penicillin (Park, 1952) occurs only in some Gram positive bacteria. While an essential clue to biosynthetic studies, this turned out to be a red herring as far as identifying the primary target for penicillin was concerned. This target turned out to be much further down the pathway, on the other side of the membrane from the cytoplasmic site of nucleotide precursor synthesis. The species-specific accumulation of nucleotide intermediates in response to penicillin apparently reflects variation in the feedback contol of this complex pathway.

Parallel studies of peptidoglycan structure in *S. aureus* (Ghuysen *et al.*, 1965) led to the realization that cross-linkage probably involved the penultimate D-alanine residue of the nucleotide precursor, leading to the hypothesis of cross-link formation by transpeptidation, involving coupled cleavage of the D-alanyl-D-alanine linkage and formation of the D-alanyl-acceptor cross-link. Inhibition of transpeptidation became the prime candidate for penicillin action and this was soon confirmed by *in vivo* studies. In *S. aureus*, it was shown that penicillin caused an increase, in newly synthesized peptidoglycan, of both total alanine content (Wise and Park, 1965) and of uncross-linked peptide monomers retaining both D-alanine residues (Tipper and Strominger, 1965). This observation was extended in later studies (Tipper and Strominger, 1968) to include other β-lactam antibiotics (methicillin, ampicillin and cephalothin), and more detailed analyses of the peptidoglycan structure in inhibited cells. These studies also demonstrated a precursor-product relationship between uncross-linked peptide monomer and cross-linked oligomers in *S. aureus* peptidoglycan. In retrospect, it seems likely that this reflected PBP-4 activity (Wyke *et al.*, 1981).

It was also hypothesized (Tipper and Strominger, 1965) that transpeptidation was a two-step reaction involving an acyl-enzyme intermediate. Interaction of transpeptidase and acyl-D-alanyl-D-alanine donor substrates would form an acyl-D-alanyl-ENZ intermediate, with release of D-alanine, to be followed by transfer of the Acyl-D-alanyl residue to the free amino group of an acceptor substrate (Fig. 5). Penicillin was proposed to act as an analog of the donor substrate, efficiently acylating the transpeptidase because of the relatively high reactivity of its β-lactam bond (Fig. 5). Stable acylation would inhibit transpeptidation, explaining the observed effects on cross-linkage. At that time, the coupling of this primary event to cell death and lysis was predicted to be a direct consequence of weakening of the peptidoglycan. These effects are now known to be indirect (Section 8). The rest of this hypothesis, however, has withstood subsequent detailed analysis, as described in Section 7, and is now accepted as being essentially correct. A natural extension of this hypothesis, predicting a mechanistic and evolutionary relationship between β-lactamases and transpeptidases (Fig. 5) (Tipper and Strominger, 1965), has also been substantiated (Section 7.3).

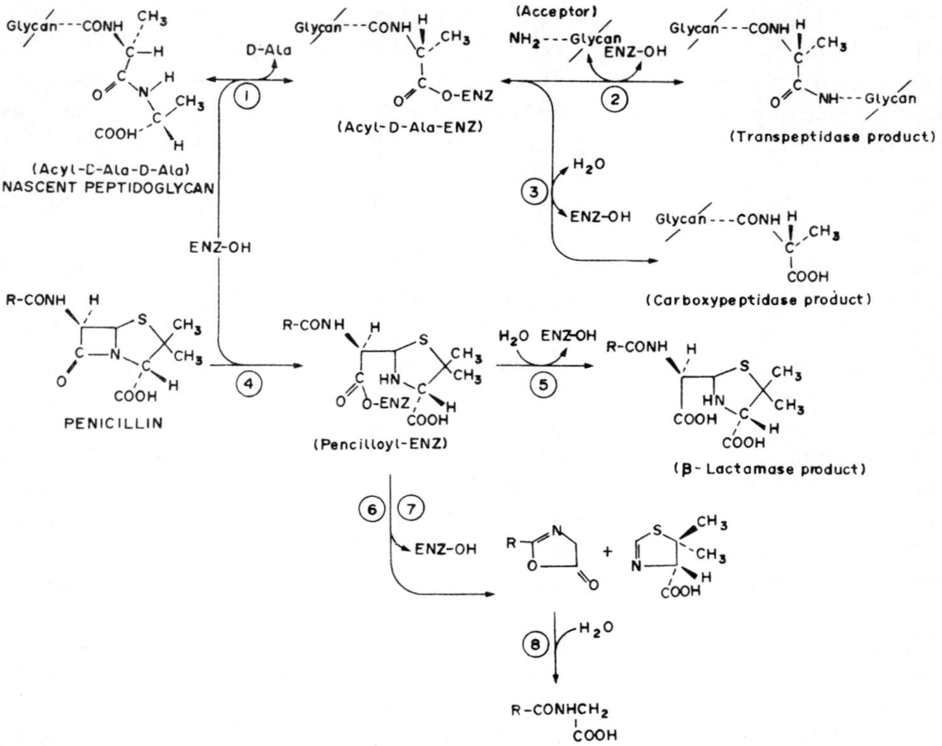

FIG. 5. Transpeptidation and its inhibition by β-lactam antibiotics. A nascent polymerized peptidoglycan subunit (Fig. 1) binds to the transpeptidase PBP (ENZ-OH), leading to acylation of the active site serine residue (acyl-D-ala-ENZ) and release of the terminal D-ala residue (reaction 1). Binding of the N-terminal acceptor group of an adjacent peptidoglycan subunit (NH_2-Glycan) results in peptide cross-link formation and release of PBP (ENZ-OH; reaction 2). If the PBP is a D,D-carboxypeptidase, water acts as the acceptor (reaction 3). Beta-lactam antibiotics, such as the penicillin shown, act as donor substrate analogs, binding to and acylating the L-serine residue in the donor site of the PBP, producing penicilloyl-ENZ (reaction 4). This may be a very stable product, causing inhibition of PBP function. Hydrolysis (reaction 5) will result in β-lactamase action, regenerating active PBP (ENZ-OH). This is the normal mechanism of breakdown of PBP derivatives with relatively short half-lives. Beta-lactamases have evolved to perform this reaction with high efficiency. PBP's inactivated by acylation by β-lactam antibiotics may be reactivated relatively slowly by other breakdown pathways, such as the fragmentation shown (reactions 6, 7 and 8). Other pathways for fragmentation of unstable, acylated PBP derivatives may produce stable, permanently inactivated enzyme derivatives (not shown).

This figure is adapted from the review by Tipper and Wright (1979), in *The Bacteria*, Vol. 7, pp. 291–426 (Academic Press, New York) as modified in *β-Lactam Antibiotics for Clinical Use*, (Queener, Queener and Weber, eds), Marcel Dekker, New York (1986), with the permission of the publishers and editors.

The stably acylated 'transpeptidase' became the obvious candidate for the previously recognized penicillin-binding components whose saturation, in penicillin-sensitive cells, was found to correlate well with minimal inhibitory concentrations (MIC's) (Cooper, 1956). These were soon identified with the penicillin binding proteins (PBP's) of bacterial cytoplasmic membranes (see Section 5).

Transpeptidation and its inhibition by penicillin was soon demonstrated *in vitro* in membrane preparations from *E. coli*, using lipid-linked disaccharide-peptide as substrate (Izaki *et al.*, 1966). In these preparations the acceptor for transpeptidation is either residual fragments of nascent peptidoglycan, or the newly polymerized peptidoglycan itself. This system is inefficient since it is now known that preexisting murein is the major natural acceptor. Activity in such membrane preparations is effectively restricted to the simplest A1 types of peptidoglycan, lacking the additional requirements imposed by the presence of cross-bridge peptide. It was later found that preservation of the natural association of membrane enzymes and cell wall murein transpeptidation substrates in wall–membrane preparations or permeabilized cells produced a much better model system for transpeptidation. Use of these systems has confirmed the inhibition of transpeptidation by β-lactam antibiotics in a wide variety of bacteria (Ward, 1984; Chapter 1).

The initial studies in *E. coli* membranes also led to the discovery of D,D-carboxypeptidases and their sensitivity to penicillin. It was obvious that, just as penicillinases could be variants of transpeptidases in which the penicilloyl-ENZ intermediate was rapidly hydrolyzed, a D,D-carboxypeptidase could be an additional variant in which acyl-D-ananyl-ENZ is rapidly hydrolyzed (Fig. 4). It would thus be inhibited by penicillin by the same mechanism (Fig. 5) (Izaki *et al.*, 1966).

The D,D-carboxypeptidase activity in *E. coli* membranes and in several Gram positive bacilli was subsequently shown to reside in several low molecular weight PBP's (Blumberg and Strominger, 1974). Because these are by far the most abundant PBP's, and because they retain their *in vitro* activity as penicillin-sensitive carboxypeptidases during solubilization and purification, these PBP's have been the principal models for *in vitro* analysis of the interaction between PBP's, acyl-D-alanyl-D-model substrates for hydrolysis and transpeptidation, and β-lactam antibiotics (Blumberg and Strominger, 1974). Major advances in this field have derived from analysis of the unusual soluble secreted D,D-carboxypeptidases of *Streptomyces* R61, *Actinomadura* R39 and *Streptomyces albus* G (Ghuysen, 1984; Ghuysen *et al.*, 1980, 1981, 1984). Members of this group of Gram positive organisms have apparently found it advantageous to evolve genes for secretion of PBP-related soluble enzymes of this type, possibly as a primitive form of protection against β-lactam antibiotics produced by other microorganisms in their soil habitat (Kelley *et al.*, 1986). The *S. albus* G enzyme contains Zn^{2+}, like the *Bacillus cereus* Class B β-lactamase (Joris *et al.*, 1983). Neither appears to involve an acyl-enzyme intermediate or to be related by evolution or mechanism to the PBP transpeptidases, and they will not be discussed further. The R61 and R39 enzymes, however, do involve acyl-enzyme intermediates and are capable of model transpeptidation reactions. Crystals of the R61 enzyme are yielding to X-ray structural analysis (Kelly *et al.*, 1982, 1986) and, in consequence, provide the most incisive data available on interaction of a penicillin-sensitive enzyme with normal substrates and β-lactam inhibitors. These enzymes are discussed again in Section 7. The next section deals exclusively with membrane-bound PBP's.

5. PENICILLIN BINDING PROTEINS (PBP's)

Early studies of the binding of [^{35}S]penicillin to sensitive cells (Cooper, 1956), demonstrated that label bound to a small number of high affinity sites in a form stable to 2% sodium dodecyl sulfate (SDS), aqueous phenol, or boiling in water, and would not exchange with a vast excess of unlabeled drug. Covalent binding as a penicilloyl ester was suggested, but the binding components were not identified. They have now been equated with the cytoplasmic membrane PBP's which, in several instances, have been shown to form stable penicilloyl esters of an active site serine residue (Section 7).

PBP's will bind covalently to affinity columns containing, for example, bound ampicillin derivatives, and can be eluted with hydroxylamine. The release of active PBP is an enzymatic process in which hydroxylamine acts as a transpeptidation receptor for the penicilloyl group. This procedure allows purification of active solubilized PBP's.

PBP's number 10^3 to 10^4 per cell and tend to fall into two classes: the first comprises abundant, relatively low molecular weight PBP's with *in vitro* D,D-carboxypeptidase activity. They are relatively easily purified because of their abundance and retention of activity with simple model substrates during purification. The second class of PBP's comprises the much less abundant high molecular weight components whose purification is correspondingly more difficult and which frequently lack demonstrable *in vitro* activities.

Spratt and Pardee (1975) devised a simple, reproducible technique for PBP visualization, involving saturation of membrane preparations with labeled [^{14}C] penicillin, immediate denaturation with ionic detergent (which stabilizes the penicilloyl-PBP by preventing enzyme-catalyzed hydrolysis or fragmentation), fractionation by SDS-polyacrylamide gel electrophoresis and detection by fluorography. PBP's are numbered in order of decreasing molecular size, that is, in order of increasing mobility on SDS-PAGE. There is no necessary relationship between similarly numbered PBP's from different organisms. When better techniques resolve a previously identified and numbered component into subspecies, they are designated by alphabetical letter: thus *E. coli* PBP 1 has become PBP 1A, 1B and 1C (Section 5).

To be identified in this manner, PBP's must be membrane components forming covalent adducts with penicillin which are stable in boiling 2% SDS. It is also necessary that the PBP's remain active during membrane preparation, since selective penicilloylation of PBP's is an enzymatic process: penicillin concentrations well above those required to saturate active PBP's are required to non-specifically acylate non-PBP membrane proteins. Although penicillin may also be involved in noncovalent protein interactions, transient covalent interactions, or interactions with nonmembrane protein components, studies of PBP function described below have invariably identified one of the covalently labeled membrane PBP's as the significant target. No other interactions need be invoked to explain the action of these antibiotics. Correlative studies have usually identified the lethal targets of *β*-lactam antibiotics among the high molecular weight class of PBP's. Mutant studies (Section 6) also indicate that this class of PBP's performs essential functions.

Binding of other *β*-lactam antibiotics to PBP's has usually been inferred from competition with labeled penicillin, although direct studies have also been performed with several other labeled drugs (mecillinam, cefoxitin, ampicillin, moxalactam, etc; Waxman and Strominger, 1983). Although some of these compounds have very high specificity for certain PBP's, none has been found to bind to a protein that does not also bind penicillin. Thus penicillin is relatively nonselective, and it appears that the targets for all *β*-lactam antibiotics are to be found among PBP's, the proteins that bind penicillin, which are, therefore, aptly named.

The synthesis of [^{3}H]-labeled penicillin of much higher specificity than the commercially available [^{14}C]penicillin used in most studies of PBP's allows direct labeling of cells *in vivo* (e.g. Williamson *et al.*, 1983), so that direct correlations can be made between PBP saturation and physiological effects. In the absence of *β*-lactamase activity, comparison of *in vivo* with *in vitro* binding also provides a measure of cell wall permeability. Limited permeability is generally responsible for *β*-lactamase-independent resistance (Section 2). Beta-lactam resistant mutants with modified PBP's of low affinity also exist (Section 6).

All eubacterial species examined contain at least three PBP's and some as many as eight or nine. The functions of these multiple PBP components may be demonstrated in a variety of ways (Spratt, 1975, 1983). Where *β*-lactam antibiotics are known with highly preferential binding to a single PBP, correlations can be drawn between *in vitro* assays for saturation of this PBP by the antibiotic and physiological and biochemical effects *in vivo*. Studies of mutants which cause permanent or conditional loss of a PBP, and whose phenotype mimics that produced by saturation of the same PBP, can be equally revealing. Such mutants are usually selected for resistance to an antibiotic reacting specifically with this PBP. Co-reversion of resistance and physiological phenotypes is necessary to prove that both result from the same PBP mutation. Where PBP's have been cloned, study of the *in vivo* effect of over-production of these PBP's, and studies of their *in vitro* activities may give the most direct evidence of function. While all PBP's probably do not function as transpeptidases *in vivo*, it seems likely that all are involved in binding to acyl-D-alanyl-D-alanine substrates. The most complete information is available for *E. coli* whose PBP's are described below.

5.1. *E. COLI* PBP's

E. coli contains seven PBP's (Table 1). An eighth PBP, called PBP 1C, has only been detected using an iodinated penicillin derivative (Schwarz *et al.*, 1981). Its significance and properties are not clear, and it will not be discussed further. Following the initial naming of PBP's 1 to 6 (Spratt and Pardee, 1975), PBP 1 was resolved into a slower component,

TABLE 1. *Properties of E. coli PBP's*

PBP	Molecular weight (kd)	Molecules per cell	Gene name(s)		Map position	Selective inhibitors	Consequences of inactivation	Functions
1A	92	200	*pon A*	*mrc A*	73.5	Cephaloridine, cefsulodin		Transglycosylases and primary transpeptidases
1B	~90	250	*pon B*	*mrc B*	3.3		Rapid cell lysis if both inactivated	Essential for cylindrical cell wall synthesis
2	66	20	*pbpA*	*mrd A*	14.4	Mecillinam, clavulanic acid, *N*-formimidoyl thienamycin	Spherical; non growing cells	Transpeptidase required for initiation of cylindrical wall growth at sites of septation
3	60	50	*pbpB*	*ftsI*	1.8	Cephalexin, cefuroxime, azthreonam, furazlocillin	Filamentous, non-septate cells	A transglycosylase/transpeptidase required for septum cross-wall synthesis
4	49	110	*dacB*		68		Delayed transpeptidation absent	A secondary transpeptidase D,D-carboxypeptidase or D,D-endopeptidase acting on maturing peptidoglycan
5	42	1800	*dacA*		13.7		None obvious	A D,D-carboxypeptidase
6	40	600	*dacC*				None obvious	A D,D-carboxypeptidase

The molecular weights given are for the mature forms of the enzymes. As demonstrated for PBP's 1B, 3 and 5, each probably has a leader peptide in its gene which is removed during secretion to the exterior of the cytoplasmic membrane. PBP 1C is not listed since little is known about its properties. Beta-lactam antibiotics which interact with strong preference with individual 'essential' PBP's (PBP's 1B, 2 and 3) are listed. Most of these also react strongly with PBP 1A, but since this is not a lethal event if active PBP 1B remains, this is not usually significant. The *dacC* mutant has not been mapped. The 'molecules per cell' are approximations based on measurement of bound radioactivity and assuming stoichiometric penicillin binding.

PBP 1A, and a faster component, PBP 1B, which itself consists of a cluster of closely related species called PBP 1B's (Spratt *et al.*, 1977; Tamaki *et al.*, 1977; Suzuki *et al.*, 1978). Concomitant loss of all PBP 1B's by a single point mutation (*ponB*⁻), and recovery of all members by reversion (Suzuki *et al.*, 1978), indicate that all derive from a single gene product, presumably by variation in processing (Nakagawa and Matsuhashi, 1982). They will be referred to as PBP 1B. It has recently been reported (J. T. park: quoted in Waxman and Strominger, 1983) that an *iap*-mutation, which affects processing of alkaline phosphatase, results in synthesis of a single PBP 1B. The *iap* gene product is probably involved in nonessential proteolytic processing of several secreted *E. coli* proteins.

5.1.1. *PBP's 1A, 1B, 2 and 3*

E. coli PBP's 1A and 1B both have combined transglycosylase and transpeptidase activities *in vitro* (Nakagawa *et al.*, 1979; Suzuki *et al.*, 1980; Ishino *et al.*, 1980). This was demonstrated utilizing the cloned genes to obtain purified preparations derived from cells overproducing these PBP's. Beta-lactam antibiotics inhibit the cross-linkage but not the polymerization of peptidoglycan catalyzed by these PBP's, indicating selective inhibition of their transpeptidase activity and lack of interdependent function of the two active sites of these enzymes. Similar results have been obtained for PBP 3 (Ishino and Matsuhashi, 1981). Transpeptidase activity is also deduced for PBP 2 since cells carrying the cloned PBP 2 gene and overproducing PBP 2 give membrane preparations having mecillinam-sensitive transpeptidation (Ishino *et al.*, 1982). Transglycosylase activity of PBP 2, the least abundant *E. coli* PBP (Table 1) has not been assessed.

The genes of PBP 1A (*ponA* or *mrcA*), and for PBP 1B (*ponB* or *mrcB*) (Table 1), are widely separated on the *E. coli* chromosome, yet the similarity in the properties and functions of these PBP's suggest a relatively recent derivation from a common ancestral gene. Both gene products exist in low quantities and have similar sizes and functions. DNA sequence analyses would directly test this hypothesis, but have yet to be published.

It has recently been shown (Keck *et al.*, 1985) that the active sites peptides of PBP's 1A, 1B, and 3 all occur near the middle of these proteins and show marked similarity, sharing the consensus sequence Gly (Acylated)-Ser Xaa Xaa Lys Pro around the acylated serine residue (see Section 7.3). PBP's 1A and 1B are reported to share about 30% overall amino acid sequence homology, indicating a relatively close relationship, although neither shows extensive homology to PBP 3 outside of the active site.

Neither loss of detectable PBP 1A due to a *ponA*⁻ mutation, nor loss of detectable PBP 1B due to a *ponB*⁻ mutation is lethal. However, a doubly defective mutant could not be constructed (Suzuki *et al.*, 1980). Availability of a mutant in which penicillin binding to PBP 1A is temperature-sensitive (*ponA*ᵗˢ) allowed construction of a *ponB*⁻ *ponA*ᵗˢ double mutant (Suzuki *et al.*, 1980) which was temperature-sensitive for growth. Thus PBP 1A activity is essential in the absence of PBP 1B function.

Unless mutant construction guarantees inactivation by deletion, it is by no means certain that mutations leading to loss of a detectable PBP causes parallel loss of *in vivo* function. Nor is it clear whether cell viability requires 1, 10 or 100% of the normally available activity of any given PBP. Nevertheless, for the high molecular weight 'essential' PBP's of *E. coli*, which include PBP's 1A, 1B, 2 and 3, the data on mutant phenotypes, allied to those on the effects of selective inhibition by *β*-lactam antibiotics, indicate that apparent loss of a PBP (loss of penicillin binding) equates with functional loss, and that normal growth requires a large fraction of the wild-type activity of each PBP. As will be described below, the latter is not true for PBP's 4, 5 and 6.

The mutant data, therefore, are consistent with the hypothesis that PBP's 1A and 1B perform similar functions and can compensate reciprocally for loss of either gene product. This apparent redundancy of function may only reflect minimal requirements for survival in the laboratory: persistence of both genes and minor variations in known properties of the two PBP's indicate that at least partially discrete *in vivo* functions probably exist for these PBP's and presumably improve survival. As discussed above, it is also possible that retention of a small fraction of the activity of both gene products is necessary for survival.

As discussed in section 5.2.2, the ability of different PBP's to substitute for one another, which determines the number of independently essential PBP's or killing targets, is probably dependent on growth conditions as well as genotype.

Beta-lactam antibiotic binding studies also indicate that PBP 1A function is dispensable in the presence of active PBP 1B. Most β-lactam antibiotics, except for antibiotics highly selective for PBP 2 (such as mecillinam) saturate PBP 1A at concentrations well below their MIC. This has little detectable result, and the MIC for each of these antibiotics correspond to the higher concentration at which they saturate PBP 1B, 2 or 3. An antibiotic such as cephaloridine, which saturates both PBP's 1A and 1B before saturating 2 or 3, causes lysis of morphologically normal cells at its MIC (Table 1). In a $ponB^-$ mutant, the MIC is reduced to that required to saturate PBP 1A, and exposure to this concentration again is accompanied by lysis.

An antibiotic such as penicillin, ampicillin or cephalothin, which saturates PBP3 before it saturates PBP 1B, causes formation of non septate filamentous cells at its MIC. This is a lethal event though a variety of conditional *E. coli* mutations are known leading to reversible inhibition of septation. In a $ponB^-$ mutant, the MIC of each of these antibiotics is reduced to that required to saturate PBP 1A, and lysis without elongation occurs at this concentration. In $ponB^+$ strains, antibiotics such as ampicillin cause swelling and eventual lysis of filamentous *E. coli* cells as the concentration is increased above their MIC, corresponding to the saturation of PBP 1B. Cephalexin, which is much more selective for PBP 3 (Table 1), causes only filamentation over a wide concentration range above its MIC. It is concluded the PBP's 1A and 1B function interchangeable in the extension of cylindrical peripheral cell wall in *E. coli*, at least in laboratory growth conditions, while PBP 3 is required for cross-wall synthesis at septa. Only inhibition of the former process in growing cells results in activation of autolysins and cell lysis. Death due to PBP 3 inhibition must have a different mechanism (Section 8). The slower rate of lysis of $ponA^-$ mutants (Spratt *et al.*, 1977) suggests tighter linkage of autolysin action with PBP 1A than with PBP 1B function. This, and the formation of hyper-cross-linked peptidoglycans by PBP 1A *in vitro* (Tomioka *et al.*, 1982), suggest differential functions for PBP's 1A and 1B.

Mutant phenotypes confirm these conclusions. Thus a mutant with temperature-sensitive PBP 3 also grows as long filamentous cells at the nonpermissive temperature (Spratt, 1977), while the $ponA^{ts}/ponB^-$ double mutant lyses at nonpermissive temperature (Suzuki *et al.*, 1978). The $ponB^-$ mutants lose most of the transglycosylase and trans-peptidase activity detectable in membrane preparations, probably indicating that PBP 1B activities are least sensitive to disruption, a further differentiation of properties of the PBP 1 components. A temperature-sensitive mutant was described, apparently lacking only PBP 1B (Tamaki *et al.*, 1977). This may indicate that PBP 1B functions are not completely redundant in the presence of PBP 1A. However, it was not clearly shown that this phenotype resulted from a single mutation.

Mecillinam, analogs of this amidino-penicillin derivative (Lund and Tybring, 1972), clavulanic acid and thienamycin derivatives (see Fig. 6) all have a high affinity for PBP 2 which is saturated at their MIC (Table 1), causing formation of inviable ovoid cells. For mecillinam, which is most highly selective for PBP 2, these ovoid cells remain osmotically stable even at much higher concentrations. The other antibiotics show less marked preference for PBP 2 and cause lysis at higher concentrations, presumably due to saturation of PBP's 1Aand 1B.

The specificity of mecillinam for PBP 2 means that a mutation in PBP 2 causing it to lose affinity for mecillinam is sufficient to produce a mecillinam-resistant cell. Such mutants reside in *pbpA* (*mrdA*), the structural gene for PBP 2 (Table 1). Conditional or nonconditional mecillinam resistance is associated with disappearance of detectable PBP 2 and formation of viable, round cells (Iwaya *et al.*, 1978). The very small amounts of PBP 2 present in normal cells (Table 1), therefore, apparently control the initiation of new annular zones of cylindrical cell wall synthesis at sites of septation in *E. coli*. It is not clear why inactivation of PBP 2, but not mutational loss, is lethal. Similarly, mutants in *pbpB*

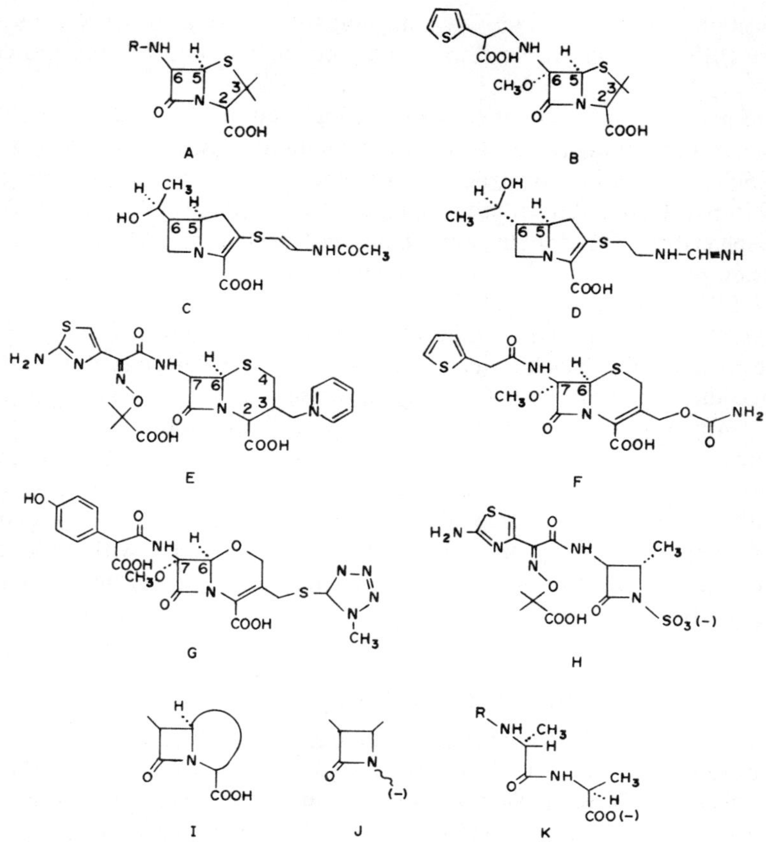

FIG. 6. Structure of representative β-lactam antibiotics. A solid line to a ring substituent indicates a configuration projecting toward the viewer. A dotted line projects away, toward the α face in penams. Thus two adjacent ring substituents indicated with solid lines are *cis* (on the same face). A; The penam bicyclic ring structure of 6-β aminoacyl penicillanic acid derivatives such as penicillin (R = benzyl). B; Temocillin, a 6 α methoxypenam. C; Epithienamycin D, a 5R 6R (*cis*) carbapenam. Note replacement of S by CH_2 and the double bond in the 5-membered ring. D; N-formimidoyl thienamycin (imipenem), a 5R 6S (trans) carbapenem. E; Ceftazidime. A Δ2 cephem in which the acyl group on the 7-β amino group contains the oxime structure found to give resistance to many β-lactamases. F; Cefoxitin. A cephamycin (7-α methoxy Δ2 cephem). G; Moxalactam. A 7-α methoxy oxacephem. Note replacement of S by 0 in the ring structure. H; Aztreonam. An active monobactam with the same oxide side chain as in ceftazidime. I; The common denominator of bicyclic active β-lactams (Boyd, 1982). J; the even simpler structure common to all active β-lactams, including monobactams. Placement of the negative charge in space relative to the β-lactam ring is critical (Cohen, 1983). K; Acyl-D-alanyl-D-alanine.

(ftsI), the gene for PBP 3, can be selected using concentrations of cephalexin at which only PBP 3 is affected. Such mutants have reduced affinity of PBP 3 for β-lactam antibiotics (Spratt, 1977).

In conclusion, inhibition of either PBP 1A plus PBP 1B, PBP 2 or PBP 3 activity is lethal to growing *E. coli* cells. Only for the PBP 1's is lysis associated with lethality. All of these high molecular weight PBP's appear to be transpeptidases *in vitro*, and all but PBP 2 have also been shown to be transglycosylases *in vitro*. It appears that all perform essential functions in the *E. coli* cell cycle, catalyzing or controlling cylindrical or cross-wall synthesis. They are independent, lethal targets for β-lactam antibiotics.

5.1.2. *PBP's 4, 5 and 6*

E. coli mutants apparently lacking PBP 4, 5 and 6 activity (*dacB⁻*, *dacA⁻*, or *dacC⁻*, respectively) are viable, as is the *dac A⁻ dacB⁻* double mutant, even though it retained only 10% of the total *in vitro* D,D-carboxypeptidase activity (Suzuki *et al.*, 1978). It may be that these mutants retain low levels of activity sufficient for viability. However, much of the activity of these PBP's appears to be dispensable and their role in normal growth is not clear.

The increased pentapeptide content of the peptidoglycan in $dacA^-$ and $dacC^-$ mutants does indicate that both function as D,D-carboxypeptidases *in vivo*, as well as *in vitro* (DePedro and Schwarz, 1981). Construction of viable deletion mutants of PBP 5 (Spratt, 1980) and PBP 6 (Broome-Smith and Spratt, 1982) indicate that both PBP's are individually dispensable. The double mutant has not been reported, so that it remains possible that they perform redundant but essential functions.

The gene for PBP 5 (*dacA*) is closely linked to *pbpA* in a cluster also containing *rodA* (*mrdB*). Like $pbpA^-$ mutants, $rodA^-$ mutants are round. Moreover, over-production of PBP 5 produces round cells (Markiewicz *et al.*, 1982), so that this gene cluster appears to share morphogenetic functions. D,D-Carboxypeptidase activity increases *in vivo* at cell division, suggesting a possible role for PBP 5 in cell division. Possibly the tri- or tetrapeptide products of D,D- and L,D-carboxypeptidase action act as acceptors in transpeptidation associated with cross-wall synthesis in cell division (Section 3). However, the low molecular weight and relatively abundant PBP's 4, 5 and 6 of *E. coli* contain no identified lethal targets. Possibly their very abundance, coupled with redundancy of function, protects cells from the potential consequences of total inhibition of these low molecular weight PBP's.

5.2. PBP's OF GRAM POSITIVE BACTERIA

The low molecular weight PBP's of Gram positive species such as *B. subtilis* were among the first PBP's purified, because of their relative abundance. Although some of these PBP's, such as PBP 4 of *S. aureus*, have clear roles in peptidoglycan synthesis, they seem to be largely dispensable, like their counterparts in *E. coli*. The carboxypeptidases of *G. homari* are obviously an exception (Section 3).

The lethal target or essential PBP's of several Gram positive species have been identified among the high molecular weight components by a variety of techniques (e.g. Reynolds *et al.*, 1978). However, in the absence of cloned genes and the opportunity to test the effects of true deletions and the effects of over-production, the available data must be interpreted with caution. These high molecular weight PBP's are also generally more abundant than their *E. coli* counterparts, making purification from normal cells feasible. However, attempts at measuring *in vitro* enzymatic activities have generally been negative, although transglycosylase and low level transpeptidase activities have been reported in PBP mixtures from *Bacillus* species (Waxman and Strominger, 1983) using a depsipeptide substrate. Taku *et al.* (1982) purified a transglycosylase from *B. megaterium* membranes that turned out to be a penicillin-sensitive PBP apparently identical to PBP 4. Examples of assignments of PBP's as lethal targets, and the evidence supporting these assignations, are given below. The list is by no means exhaustive.

5.2.1. B. subtilis

Mutations resulting in stepwise increase in the resistance of *B. subtilis* to cloxacillin were shown to be paralleled by reductions in affinity of PBP 2a for cloxacillin (Buchanan, 1977). No alteration in PBP 2a affinity for penicillin or in penicillin MIC occurred, demonstrating that PBP modifications selected by resistance to a specific β-lactam antibiotic may not affect sensitivity to acylation by a second β-lactam antibiotic. PBP 2a is clearly implicated as the cloxacillin target in *B. subtilis*. This PBP, however, reacts poorly with cephalosporins. The MIC's of cephalosporins correlate with saturation of PBP 2b which is, therefore, implicated as a second lethal target. One of the cloxacillin-resistant mutants had a PBP 2a of modified size, lacked PBP's 1a and 1b and produced cells of larger diameter (Kleppe *et al.*, 1982). Morphogenetic roles similar to those played by *E. coli* PBP's are implied for the different *B. subtilis* high molecular weight PBP's.

5.2.2. *Cocci:* S. aureus, Streptococcus pneumoniae, *and* Streptococcus faecium

Since *S. aureus* mutants lacking PBP 1 or PBP 4 are viable and clinical isolates of Methicillin-resistant strains have modified PBP 2 or 3 (see Section 6), it is likely that the lethal targets for β-lactam antibiotics in *S. aureus* include PBP's 2 and 3, but not PBP's 1 and 4. Similarly, analyses of PBP's of clinically-isolated penicillin-resistant pneumococci implicate several high-molecular weight PBP's as lethal targets (see Section 6). Thus in Gram positive cocci, as in bacilli and *E. coli*, multiple lethal targets apparently occur among PBP's. These PBP's presumably play separate roles in cell wall biosynthesis. A series of recent studies of the response of *Streptococcus faecium* to β-lactam antibiotics (Fontana *et al.*, 1985; Canepari *et al.*, 1986) have shown that the importance of PBP's, and their roles as 'lethal targets', vary with growth conditions. Thus, as mentioned in section 2, PBP 3 is a lethal target in cells growing rapidly at 45°C, and the MIC for penicillin is 0.04 μg/ml, the concentration required for its saturation. By contrast, saturation of PBP 3 is apparently irrelevant for cells growing slowly at 30°C, which are killed only by 8 μg/ml, the concentration necessary to saturate all of the six PBP species, including PBP 5, the species with the lowest affinity for penicillin. A mutant lacking PBP 5 is hypersensitive at 30°C, while a strain overproducing PBP 5 has an MIC of 40 μg/ml at either 30 or 45°C, corresponding to the concentration required for PBP 5 saturation. It appears that all of the PBP functions in this organism, growing at 30°C, can be supplied by PBP 5, making the others redundant under these conditions of slow growth. In contrast, the higher growth rate at 45°C demands PBP 3 functions which can only be supplied by PBP 5 if presnt at abnormally high concentrations. These results imply that a major selective pressure for the maintenance of a variety of PBP genes is not necessarily a set of unique, ubiquitously indispensible functions in cell wall synthesis, but rather a differential ability to perform such essential functions under particular conditions of growth stress. Together with the data of Tuomanen *et al.* (1986) on growth rate effects on β-lactam induced lethality and Vu and Nikaido's data on resistance due to inefficient β-lactamase action, this implies that *in vitro* assessment of the efficacy of a given antibiotic for a particular pathogenic bacterial strain may require mimicking not only the *in vivo* antibiotic concentrations but also its growth rate. Enterococcal endocarditis is an obvious example.

6. PBP MUTATIONS AND RESISTANCE TO β-LACTAM ANTIBIOTICS

As described in Section 5.1.1, the extreme selectivity of mecillinam for *E. coli* PBP 2, and the marked selectivity of cephalexin for PBP 3, allows ready selection of PBP 2 (mrdA) and PBP 3 (pbpB) mutants in the laboratory, since mutations in the genes for these single PBP's is sufficient to confer resistance.

Resistance to an antibiotic which saturates several essential PBP's over a narrow concentration range would presumably require simultaneous mutations in each of the genes for these sensitive PBP's, an improbable event. Nevertheless, such mutants have been seen both in the laboratory and in the clinic. Mutations of this type, and mutations affecting cell wall permeability in Gram negative bacteria, are now recognized as mechanisms of clinically acquired β-lactam resistance. Their prevalence is significant and is bound to increase.

The best known examples of clinically important resistance to β-lactam antibiotics dependent on PBP alterations are methicillin resistance in *S. aureus* and penicillin resistance in the gonococcus. Methicillin resistance appeared not long after the introduction of this β-lactamase-resistant drug into clinical usage. Resistance retains unexplained characteristics, such as expression in only a small fraction of cells in typical strains. Resistance of one highly resistant atypical strain, portraying homogeneous ('constitutive') resistance (strain MR-1) was correlated with a marked drop in affinity of PBP 3 for methicillin and other β-lactams (Hayes *et al.*, 1981). Affinities of PBP's 1, 2 and 4 for methicillin in this strain remained high so that low concentrations of methicillin caused a marked decrease in peptidoglycan cross-linkage, equivalent to that observed in a mutant lacking PBP 4 (Wyke *et al.*, 1981–1982). This had no effect on cellular growth rate or morphology.

In other studies, (Brown and Reynolds, 1980), a reduction in methicillin affinity of PBP 3 was also observed in typical methicillin-resistant strains. Strain 13136 p⁻m⁺ was resistant to all β-lactam antibiotics tested at 30°C, but had normal sensitivity at 40°C. At 30°C, its membranes contained a new PBP, in addition to normal amounts of the four *S. aureus* PBP's with normal affinities for penicillin. This new PBP, which comigrated with PBP 3, was present in large amounts, and was labeled by [^{14}C]penicillin inefficiently and with a short half-life (Brown and Reynolds, 1983). It was absent from membranes of cells grown at 40°C and it was proposed (Brown and Reynolds, 1980) that it may be an inefficient PBP which takes over the function of other essential PBP's when they are inactivated. It has now been demonstrated (P. Reynolds, personal communication) that this new methicillin-resistant PBP band, called PBP 2′, is present in all methicillin-resistant strains examined. It produces a band intermediate between wild-type PBP's 2 and 3. Its existence, and minor differences in electrophoretic band resolution, probably explains the discrepancies between these observations and those of Hayes *et al.* (1981) and Hartman and Tomasz (1981). It appears that, in *S. aureus*, the lethal targets for β-lactam antibiotics include PBP's 1, 2 and possibly 3 (P. Reynolds, personal communication), while PBP 4 appears to be dispensable.

Neisseria gonorrhoea strains, resistant to β-lactam antibiotics due to the presence of β-lactamase producing plasmids, have been known for several years. Prior to their appearance, however, an alarming, progressive increase in resistance to penicillin was observed in the clinic, typical of the type of incremental penicillin resistance first documented by Demerec (1945) in *S. aureus*. This resistance involves both reduction in gonococcal outer membrane permeability, partially circumventable by the use of ampicillin, and reduction in affinity of PBP's, PBP's 1 and 2 are both altered and therefore both are implicated as lethal targets. Reduction in affinity is first seen for PBP 2, the PBP with the highest intrinsic affinity, followed by second-step alterations in PBP 1 (Dougherty *et al.*, 1980; Barbour, 1981).

Resistance due to PBP modification is, of course, not confined to *N. gonorrhoea* and *S. aureus*. It has recently been documented in *Streptococcus pneumoniae*, a species in which β-lactamase production has yet to appear (Hakenbeck *et al.*, 1980; Williamson *et al.*, 1981; Zighelboim and Tomasz, 1980). Increases in the MIC of as much as 1,000-fold above the 0.01 μg/ml typical of earlier isolates have been observed, associated with multiple changes in PBP affinities, indicating the presence of multiple lethal targets (Hakenbeck *et al.*, 1980). Resistance in two serotypes of *Pseudomonas aeruginosa* due to PBP modification was seen to develop in the same cystic fibrosis patient during chemotherapy with piperacilin (Godfrey *et al.*, 1981). Progressive changes in several PBP's occurred.

As pointed out by Spratt (1983), these observations are disquieting in that widespread resistance due to PBP alterations has so far been seen only in circumstance where β-lactamase production plays no part, but can be expected to occur in any pathogen once β-lactamase defenses have been overcome. Thus mutants are already prevalent where β-lactamase is absent, as in the pneumococcus and in the gonococcus, or where the β-lactamase is highly restricted in substrate profile, as in *S. aureus*. In Gram negative bacilli, resistance due to β-lactamase production is a flexible and formidable defense when accompanied by limited outer membrane permeability. Even very low rates of hydrolysis of slowly penetrating antibiotics by class C β-lactamases is sufficient to give resistance (Vu and Nikaido, 1985). Resistance is dependent on low permeation rates and could be enhanced by reduction in permeability due to porin modification. Increased production of a selectively acylated essential PBP can also give resistance. It seems likely, however, that if this level of defence is surmounted by further modifications in β-lactam antibiotic structure, Gram negative bacilli will be just as capable of surviving modifications in essential PBP genes, resulting in reduced antibiotic affinity, as are the cocci listed above. The medical and pharmaceutical professions can resign themselves to a continuation of the prolonged war of attrition between bugs and β-lactam drugs. The clues and characteristics that may be employed in design of future generations of *β*-lactam weapons for use in this struggle are discussed in Section 7.2.

Since interspecific transfer of *β*-lactamase production in Gram positive bacteria is unknown, clinical infections due to Gram positive pathogens provide the most fertile field for inadvertent selection of resistance due to PBP alterations. Most surprising is the continued high sensitivity of Group A streptococci in spite of many years of use of penicillin at extremely low levels in prophylaxis against such infections in individuals with life-threatening allergy to group A streptococcal antigens. As pointed out by Butmann and Tomasz (1982), since resistant group A streptococcal mutants with altered PBP's can be readily selected in the laboratory, it must be supposed that such alterations are incompatible with pathogenicity, if not with viability. Such constraints may be more prevalent in Gram positive bacteria, where polymers covalently attached to peptidoglycan are important determinants of pathogenicity. Attachment of these polymers may be dependent on functional integration of their synthetic enzymes with those of peptidoglycan synthesis, especially with PBP's. It has, for example, been demonstrated that teichoic acid attachment to peptidoglycan is inhibited by penicillin in Gram positive bacilli (Ward, 1984) and pneumococci (Fisher and Tomasz, 1984). Increasingly troublesome PBP mutations can be anticipated in species (*S. aureus*, pneumococcus, gonococcus) where they have already been seen, and can certainly be anticipated in Gram negative bacilli with increased use of derivatives like moxalactam and azthreonam, with resistance to all of their known *β*-lactamases. The next phase in modifying therapeutic regimens in response to the selection of *β*-lactam resistant strains may be taken as a preemptive measure. It may be necessary to design or screen *β*-lactam antibiotics or (more likely) mixtures of such antibiotics which strike at multiple lethal target PBP's, and to tailor such drugs or mixtures to specific pathogens or groups of pathogens. If this becomes necessary, the clinician will, more than ever, be dependent on the microbiological lab for pathogen identification, and on infectious disease services for advice on chemotherapy.

7. *β*-LACTAM ANTIBIOTICS AS SUBSTRATE ANALOGS

7.1. KINETICS OF INTERACTION OF PBP'S WITH SUBSTRATES AND INHIBITORS

The structural mimicry of *β*-lactam antibiotics for the acyl-D-alanyl-D-alanine donor substrates for transpeptidation, postulated as the reason for their ability to acylate and inactivate these enzymes (Tipper and Strominger, 1965), is clearly not exact. The *β*-lactam structural types now known to include highly active antibiotics are very varied (Fig. 6), including both bicyclic compounds (penams, Δ2 cephams, cephamycins, penems, 5R 6S and 5R 6R carbapenems, etc.) and activated monocyclic compounds such as aztreonam (Fig. 6).

The structural requirements for binding to the active sites of PBP's are clearly flexible. An even wider variety of structures is found among effective *β*-lactamase inhibitors. Fortunately, the requirements for interaction with PBP's and *β*-lactamases, while similar, are not identical, allowing developing of *β*-lactamase-resistant antibiotics.

Nevertheless, as previously summarized (Tipper, 1979), it seems likely that the active sites of all PBP's are designed to accommodate optimally a particular acyl-D-Ala-D-Ala conformation and that all PBP inhibitors, in order to have affinity for these sites, have to bear adequate resemblance to the conformation and chemical structure of this natural substrate. As emphasized by Cohen (1983), and Boyd (1982), the common denominator of active inhibitors (Fig. 6), bears only elemental resemblance to a dipeptide. Moreover, it is possible to explain the wide variety of active *β*-lactam structures, or the marked preference for specific PBP's shown by some *β*-lactam antibiotics, in terms of substrate mimicry. Rather it is apparent, from kinetic analyses of interactions of PBP's with both peptide substrates and *β*-lactam inhibitors (see below), the initial binding is not rate-determining. Although this initial interaction does require affinity for the active site, resulting in a K_m for reversible binding commensurate with available substrate concentrations, efficiency of the reaction catalyzed is determined largely by the rate of acylation of the enzyme by the transiently bound substrate. An 'induced fit' model of catalysis is favored (Ghuysen, 1984; see below). Only basic configurational aspects of the critical amide bond of the acyl-D-Ala-D-Ala natural substrates must be reproduced in the β-lactam ring and its surrounding structures. Virudachalam and Rao (1977) were able to rationalize the structure–activity data then available in terms of the possible conformational overlaps of acyl-D-Ala-D-Ala and β-lactam inhibitors. They showed that such overlap was only possible in penams and cephems if they have an L-configuration at the C6 and C7 position, respectively, of their β-lactam rings (Fig. 6), since the β-lactam ring forces the acylamino substituent to adopt positions normally allowed only for D-aminoacyl centers at the equivalent position in an open chain. Moreover, while this overlap is compatible with 6α or 7α methoxy substituents (as in cephamycins, Fig. 6), it is incompatible with a 6α or 7α methyl substituent. It had been postulated (Tipper and Strominger, 1965), in the absence of such analysis, that mimicry of penicillins for the normal substrate would be enhanced by 6α methyl substituents. Conformational analyses (Virudachalam and Rao, 1977) nicely rationalize the inactivity of such derivatives.

In related studies (Virudachalam and Rao, 1978), it was shown that the effects of substituting acyl-D-Ala-D-Ala with other D-amino acids on transpeptidation efficiency, using *G. homari* wall-membrane preparations (Carpenter *et al.*, 1976), and *B. megaterium* preparations (Marquet *et al.*, 1976), could be rationalized in just the same way. Thus, if it is assumed that these enzymes require a substrate conformation that mimics the highly constrained conformation of penicillin in solution, then the ease with which the substituted peptides can adopt this conformation correlates well with the experimentally derived data on their effectiveness as substrates. Once again, structural mimicry between the β-lactam inhibitor and the acyl-D-Ala-D-Ala substrates is supported.

It was also postulated (Tipper and Strominger, 1965), that a penam 6-acyl group resembling, for example, the γ-D-glutamyl-meso-diaminopimelyl acyl substituent of the natural acyl-D-Ala-D-Ala substrate, would also enhance activity. However, such derivatives, while quite active, showed no advantage over the benzoyl group of penicillin. It is quite clear, from the wide variety of complex acyl groups found to enhance β-lactam antibiotic activity, that this enhancement has little to do with substrate mimicry. Recent X-ray structural analyses of the *Streptomyces* R61 D,D-carboxypeptidase (Kelly *et al.*, 1982) have confirmed that these penam C_6 and cephem C_7 aminoacyl side chains and the acyl substituent of natural substrates occupy only partially overlapping space within the active site of this particular atypical PBP. They presumably interact with different parts of the polypeptide with separate requirements for optimization of this interaction.

Kinetic analyses were first applied to the readily purifiable penicillin-sensitive soluble D,D-carboxypeptidases of *Streptomyces* R61 and *Actinomadura* R39 by Ghuysen and his colleagues (1980). These enzymes react with simple model peptide substrates as both carboxypeptidases and transpeptidases with substrate specificity related to the peptidoglycan structures of the parent organisms. Similar analyses have been applied to the easily solubilized, low molecular weight D,D-carboxypeptidases of bacilli (Waxman *et al.*, 1980). Extrapolating from these enzymes to the larger, membrane-bound essential PBP's of these and other bacterial species clearly involves many assumptions. However, the accumulating data on the relatedness of these two groups of PBP's molecules in *E. coli* suggests that the basic findings are probably applicable.

Ghuysen *et al.*, 1980, 1981 formulated simple kinetic models of the form:

$$\mathrm{E+S} \underset{k_{-1}}{\overset{k_1}{\rightleftharpoons}} \mathrm{E.S} \underset{\mathrm{D\text{-}Ala}}{\overset{k_2}{\longrightarrow}} \mathrm{E\text{-}P} \underset{\mathrm{H_2O}}{\overset{k_3}{\longrightarrow}} \mathrm{E.P\text{-}OH} \underset{k_{-4}}{\overset{k_4}{\rightleftharpoons}} \mathrm{E+P\text{-}OH}$$

where k_1/k_{-1} is the dissociation constant (K_M) for reversible binding of substrate (S) to enzyme (E), k_2 is the rate constant for acylation of the active site and k_3 is the rate constant for hydrolysis of the acyl enzyme resulting in D,D-carboxypeptidase action.

For an efficient D,D-carboxypeptidase, the K_m must allow for adequate occupancy at the available substrate concentration and both k_2 and k_3 must be rapid. The dissociation rate of the hydrolyzed product (k_4/k_{-4}) is generally so high that it plays no effective role in the overall kinetics. If H_2O is replaced by an amino acceptor, the kinetic model is for transpeptidation. The initial binding constant (K_M) and rates of acylation (k_2) and transpeptidation (k_3) determine the overall rate of transpeptidation, as for hydrolysis. Reaction with a β-lactam inhibitor (I), by the substrate analog hypothesis, follows similar initial steps, although the reactions involved in dissociation of the acyl-ENZ may differ:

$$E + I \underset{k_{-1}}{\overset{k_1}{\rightleftharpoons}} E.I \xrightarrow{k_2} E\text{-}I \xrightarrow{k_3} E + P$$

The hydrolysis or transpeptidation step (rate k_3) characteristic of the normal substrate is prevented when the enzyme is acylated by a β-lactam because the analog of the C-terminal D-Alanine remains attached to the acyl-ENZ, presumably blocking access to H_2O or amino-acceptor (Fig. 5). For an effective inhibitor, the K_D for initial binding (k_1/k_{-1}) must allow adequate occupancy at therapeutically available drug concentrations, k_2 must be as rapid as possible, but k_3 should be as slow as possible. For a β-lactamase, k_3 is the rate constant for hydrolysis of the acyl enzyme, E-I. β-lactamase inhibitors are designed to acylate the enzymes efficiently (high k_2) but to be highly resistant to hydrolysis (low k_3). The postulated role of β-lactamases in resistance to third generation β-lactam antibiotics in certain Gram negative bacteria is dependent on a K_D for stoichiometric binding which is below the K_m of target PBP's in the same organism for the same antibiotic, so that the drug is initially titrated by the β-lactamase, followed by a rate of hydrolysis (k_2) which exceeds the rate of permeation of the antibiotic through the outer membrane.

Analysis of the R61, R39 and bacillus enzymes shows that their K_M values for substrate binding are in the millimolar range. As suggested by Waxman and Strominger (1983), the juxtaposition of membrane-bound enzyme, membrane-bound donor substrate and nascent cell wall acceptor may yield a high effective *in vivo* substrate concentration such that no evolutionary pressure has been exerted for high substrate affinities. The K_D values for β-lactam inhibitors are in the same range and are essentially unrelated to inhibitory efficiency, which correlates instead with k_2, the acylation efficiency. The results suggest that, once recognition of the substrate D-Ala-D-Ala peptide or of the 'elemental' analogous component of a β-lactam antibiotic (Fig. 6) results in reversible binding to the active site, interaction of other components of substrate or inhibitor with adjacent components of the active site may be involved in an 'induced fit' which, by modifying both substrate and enzyme conformation, enhances the acylation rate (Ghuysen *et al.*, 1980). Thus, while initial β-lactam binding has specific requirements related to substrate mimicry but is relatively nonselective, the effectiveness of secondary interactions of the β-lactam acylamino side chains with adjacent secondary binding sites in the PBP is probably a major determinant of acylation efficiency and of discrimination between PBP targets. Since the components of the active site involved in these secondary interactions differ for normal substrates and inhibitors, structural mimicry cannot be a guide to the design of acyl substituents. Without detailed knowledge of the chemistry of sufficient PBP active sites to allow generalization, the design of β-lactam antibiotics must remain guided by empirical analyses of structure–activity relationships for whole organisms and for specific PBP's. The X-ray crystallographic data on the R61 enzyme (Kelly *et al.*, 1982; 1986) is a major step towards gathering the data required for rational drug design. The catalytically important interactions between enzyme side chains and the side chains of substrates and inhibitors may soon be defined at the atomic level, at least for this serine D,D-peptidase. However, much more needs to be done.

7.2. STRUCTURE–ACTIVITY RELATIONSHIPS

Structure–activity analyses (Boyd, 1982) have demonstrated that a potent β-lactam antibiotic must have sufficient chemical reactivity in its β-lactam bond (too reactive a drug would be unstable in water), defined primarily by the reactivity of its carbonyl to nucleophilic attack, in order to acylate PBP active sites efficiently. This reactivity is enhanced inductively by C6 N-acyl substituents in penams, by C7 N-acyl and by C3′ electrophilic groups in $\Delta 2$ Cephems, by C_6 and C_3 substituents in penams and by the sulfonate group in monobactams (Fig. 6).

While necessary to ensure acylation, such reactivity is insufficient to ensure potency. This depends on 'fit' to the active site itself, as described in Section 7.1, and on resistance to hydrolysis of the acyl-enzyme. The 'fit' depends on relatedness to the normal acyl-D-Ala-D-Ala substrate. The inhibitor–enzyme interactions must also modify these components to facilitate acylation.

It was originally hypothesized (Tipper and Strominger, 1965) that the more nearly single-bonded character of the β-lactam linkage in penicillin, constrained by the nonplanar character of the double ring system, would make it a much stronger acylating agent than the planar peptide bond of acyl-D-Ala-D-Ala, and that the β-lactam would be closer in structure to a transition state in cleavage of the normal substrate than to the substrate itself, possibly leading to high affinity for the active site of a transpeptidase and facile acylation. Analysis of the relatedness between tetrahedral transition states in enzyme acylation by acyl-D-Ala-D-Ala and β-lactams (Boyd, 1979) indicates a good match, although certain conformations of the parent peptide also matched well. This suggests (Boyd, 1982) that the PBP's could readily recognize the β-lactam as substrates, without their having much advantage in initial binding. Their advantage would be in subsequent acylation rate. Kinetic analyses (Section 7.1) do demonstrate that acylating efficiency, rather than binding affinity is paramount. While structure–activity relationships (Boyd, 1982) show that activity increases with the length (single-bonded character) of the β-lactam bond, this may be determined more by adjacent electron withdrawing groups than by configurational distortion of the β-lactam amide bond. Clearly, this must be true for monobactams. In these, the N-sulfonate is essential to activate the adjacent β-lactam carbonyl to nucleophilic attack (Fig. 6).

Resistance to deacylation must depend on steric hindrance to hydrolysis, inherent in the antibiotic structure, or on competing fragmentation or tautomerisation reactions which stabilize the ester linkage (Boyd, 1982). The latter mechanism is illustrated by the loss of the C3′ substituent in cephalosporins and by the inactivation of β-lactamases by agents such as the 6β halo-penicillins, for which the kinetics of inactivation are progressive: several inhibitor molecules may be hydrolyzed before conversion of transiently acylated enzyme to the stable adduct happens to precede hydrolysis.

To be resistant to β-lactamase hydrolysis, β-lactam antibiotics must either lose affinity for the β-lactamase active site, while retaining that for PBP's, lose the ability to activate this site once bound (low k_2), or become resistant to deacylation (low k_3). The relatedness of β-lactamases and PBP's (Section 7.3) makes achievement of differential binding and acylation difficult to achieve. However, stability of an acylated β-lactamase (high k_2, low k_3 for a β-lactamase) is obviously compatible with efficient PBP inactivation (high k_2, low k_3 for PBP's). This is the mechanism of resistance of most of the β-lactamase-resistant antibiotics. Unfortunately, it leaves them susceptible to slow hydrolysis by class C β-lactamases. The simplest solution to this dilemma is to use a mixture of a β-lactamase inhibitor and a potent β-lactam antibiotic, since the components of this mixture can be separately optimized for function (Neu, Chapter 8). To be effective against a particular organism, both drugs must be able to penetrate the cell wall efficiently and the β-lactamase inhibitor must have a considerably lower k_M for the β-lactamase than does the antibiotic. Many combinations have been tested clinically. One difficulty, as summarized in Section 6, is the necessity for tailoring such mixtures to specific pathogens. Nevertheless, this strategy may prolong the useful life of available β-lactam antibiotics.

7.3. Characterization of Acyl Enzyme Intermediates. Relatedness of PBP's and β-Lactamases

The basic validity of the substrate analog theory (Tipper and Stromager, 1965) has been proven by demonstrating that model acyl-D-Ala-D-Ala substrates and β-lactam antibiotics acylate the same serine residue in the PBP 5 D,D-carboxypeptidases of *B. subtilis* (Waxman and Stromager, 1980) and *B. stearothermophilus* (Yocum *et al.*, 1982), in the *Streptomyces* R61 exocellular D,D-carboxypeptidase (Georgopapadakou *et al.*, 1981; Yocum *et al.*, 1982) and the *Actinoma dura* R-39 enzyme (Duez *et al.*, 1981), and in *E. coli* PBP 6 (Yocum *et al.*, 1982).

Isolation of stoichiometric penicilloyl derivatives of PBP's is relatively facile because of the very long half-lives of penicilloyl-enzyme derivatives, but the acyl enzyme formed with model peptide substrates, such as diacetyl-L-lysyl-D-alanyl-D-alanine, can only be trapped if $k_2 > k_3$ (Section 7.1). This requirement is not usually met by such peptide substrates, but was achieved for several PBP's by use of the depsipeptide analog, diacetyl-L-lysyl-D-alanyl-D-lactate, for which k_2 is markedly accelerated (Rasmussen and Stromager, 1978; Yocum *et al.*, 1979). The serine residue acylated by both substrates and inhibitors in the *Bacillus* and *E. coli* PBP's listed, and the sequences surrounding this residue are shown in Table 2. This table also shows the sequences acylated by penicillin in *E. coli* PBP 5 (Yocum *et al.*, 1982) and by inhibitory β-lactam derivatives in the TEM Class A β-lactamase (Knott-Hunzicker *et al.*, 1979).

The active site serine residue is near the *N*-terminus of all of these enzymes, and at residue 36 in both of the Bacillus PBP's. These enzymes are clearly closely related, especially around the active site serine residue and in a region 12–16 residues upstream from this site. The Gly Lys Ile/Val Leu sequence at this location is conserved in all of the sequences shown, suggesting a primary role in the enzyme mechanism.

Structure–activity relationships for β-lactam antibiotics demonstrate a clear requirement for a negative charge strategically placed relative to the β-lactam band (Cohen, 1983), as in all the examples shown in Fig. 6. This is presumably equivalent to the C-terminal carboxylate group of the natural peptide substrate, and indicates that the active site must have an appropriately placed positive charge to interact with this group. The Lys residues in this conserved upstream sequence is a candidate, as is the conserved Lys residue two residues after the acylation site. More extensive comparisons favor the latter (see below). Structural analyses of the R61 enzyme indicate that inhibitors and substrates associate with the N-termini of two adjacent α helices. The positive charges associated with these termini are an alternate candidate for anchoring the negative charge on the substrate (Kelly *et al.*, 1982).

The *E. coli* PBP 5 sequence shows distinct relatedness to the Bacillus sequences at the same regions conserved between these two Gram positive sequences. The available sequence for *E. coli* PBP 6 (Spratt, 1983) can also be aligned by the Gly Lys Val sequence (Table 2). The data on the Streptomyces enzyme sequences is insufficient for comparison (Table 2).

Interestingly, the carboxypeptidases show sequence conservation only in their *N*-terminal regions, that is, in the regions surrounding the acylation sites. The C-terminal regions of these PBP's may be responsible for the unique functions of these PBP's and have evolved to interact with quite distinct cellular components. The PBP's seem to be largely exposed to solvent on the exterior of the cytoplasmic membrane with a hydrophobic domain anchoring them to the membrane. This domain is C-terminal in the Bacillus D,D-carboxypeptidases, so that proteolytic treatment releases a soluble, catalytically active, major N-terminal fragment. This may also be true for higher molecular weight PBP's (Waxman and Stromager, 1983).

Comparison of these low molecular weight carboxypeptidase PBP sequences with the *E. coli* PBP 3 sequence (Table 2) is especially interesting, since possible homology with the Gly Lys Ile/Val Leu upstream segment of the D,D-carboxypeptidases is found, but occurs near the center of PBP 3 (residues 218–234) rather than at the N-terminus (Table 2; Spratt, 1983). This suggests that the bifunctional PBP 3 may have a transpeptidase

TABLE 2. *Homologies Around Active Site Serine Residues in PBP's and β-Lactamases*

E. coli PBP 6
NH₂ AEQTVEAPSVDASAWFLMDYAXGKV---

B. stearothermophilus PBP 5
NH₂-ESAPLDIRADAAILVDAQTGKILYEKNIDTVLGIASMTKM---

B. subtilis PBP 5
NH₂-ASDPIDINASAAIMIEASSGKILYSKNADKRLPIASMTKMMTEYLLEAIDQGKVKWDQTYTPD---

E. coli PBP 5
NH₂-DDLNIKTMIPGVPQIDAESYILIDYNSGKVLAEQNADVRRDPASLTKMMTSYVIGQAMKAGKFKETDLVTIG---

TEM β-lactamase
NH₂-HPETLVKDAEDQLGARVGYIELDLNSGKILESFRPEERFPMMSTFKVLLCGAVLSRVDAGQEQLGRRIHYS---

B. subtilis PBP 5
NH₂-ASDPIDINASAAIMIEASSGKILYSKNADKRLPIASMTKMMTEYLLEAIDQGKVKWDQTYTPD---

S. aureus β-lactamase
RFAYASTSKAIN

Actinomadura R 39
LPASNEV

E. coli PBP 3 (218–234)
SAVLVDVNTGEVLAMAN

Alignment of N-terminal sequences of *E. coli* PBP's 5 and 6 with the PBP 5's of *B. subtilis* and *B. stearothermophilus* and the Tn3 TEM β-lactamase (Gram negative, class A) (Spratt, 1983). The serine residues acylated by substrates or inhibitors are indicated by a filled circle, and are aligned vertically. Exact homologies between adjacent sequences are indicated by * and, from the N-terminus to about 10 residues beyond the acylation site, average 60% between the two bacillus PBP 5's, about 40% between the *E. coli* and *B. subtilis* PBP 5 sequences, and 24% between these and the β-lactamase sequence. Note that many amino acid substitutions in the active site region are conservative (not indicated). Also shown are the sequences around the activation site in the Gram positive class A β-lactamases of *S. aureus*, *B. cereus* and *B. licheniformis*, the sequence of the acylated peptide in the *Actinomadura* R39 soluble D,D-carboxypeptidase, and an alignment (shown above the sequence) suggested by Spratt (1983) between residues 218–234 of *E. coli* PBP 3 and residues 19–35 of *E. coli* PBP 5. Limited homology of this region to the aligned region (residues 11–27) of the Bacillus PBP's is also apparent.

(carboxypeptidase-like) C-terminal domain and a transglycosylase N-terminal domain. Sequence comparisons with other bifunctional PBP's may clarify this relationship. As described in section 5.1.1, the sequences of the active site peptides of *E. coli* PBP's 1A, 1B, and 3 have been determined (Keck *et al.*, 1985). They share only the (Acylated) Ser Xaa Xaa Lys sequence with the low molecular weight PBP's and are centrally located in the sequences predicted from sequence analysis of the cloned genes. This region of PBP 3 (residues 311–314) is considerably removed from the segment (residues 218–234) shown in Table 2, though their proximity in the native protein is unknown.

A clear relationship between the class A β-lactamases and the D,D-carboxypeptidases is revealed by simple linear comparison of the N-terminal sequence (Table 2) (Waxman and Strominger, 1980; Spratt, 1983). The marked difference in size between these low molecular weight PBP's (40 kd) and the class A β-lactamases (29–30 kd) argues against extensive sequence homology, particularly at the C-terminus, and the hypothesis of common ancestry has been questioned. Convergent rather than divergent evolution must obviously be considered. The relationship must be even more obscure for the high molecular weight PBP's (60–90 kd) where sequence homology to the β-lactamases is limited even at the active site, consisting only of the (acylated) Ser Xaa Xaa Lys sequence and other scattered residues. However, limited secondary structural data has previously indicated similarity between β-lactamases and D,D-carboxypeptidases (Moews *et al.*, 1981) and X-ray crystallographic data for the *B. licheniformis* 749/C β-lactamase has finally reached the level of resolution allowing accurate determination of secondary structure (Kelly *et al.*, 1986). This structure has been found to resemble the *Streptomyces* R61 D,D-carboxypeptidase closely, matching all of the α helical and β-sheet components surrounding the active site of this enzyme, so that a close relationship is implied, supporting the validity of the hypothesis (Tipper and Strominger, 1965) of common ancestry for these enzymes. However, chain continuity was not determined for the β-lactamase structure and higher resolution analysis of the similar class A β-lactamase from *S. aureus* PC1 reveals that connections between secondary structure elements differ in important respects from those reported for the R61 D,D-carboxypeptidase. Nevertheless, this analysis reveals that the catalytic arrangements are strikingly similar "strongly suggesting an evolutionary relationship" (Herzberg and Moult, 1987). Presumably β-lactamases evolved from PBP's in response to β-lactam antibiotic production, losing their C-terminal, hydrophobic membrane-binding regions, which are presumably involved in control of carboxypeptidase action, and gaining a facility for hydrolysis of the penicilloyl-enzyme intermediate. Beta-lactamases have N-terminal secretion signal peptides, as is probably true of all of the PBP's, since the functional domains of both enzyme types must be secreted through the cytoplasmic membrane. This has been demonstrated for *E. coli* PBP's 5 and 6 (Pratt *et al.*, 1981).

Similarity between known PBP sequences (Table 2) and sequences of the class C inducible chromosomal β-lactamases, which also employ an acyl enzyme intermediate, is much less distinct and its significance is unclear (Spratt, 1983). A much more distant divergence of ancestral genes is suggested than between PBP's and the class A enzymes. The Zn^{2+}-containing class B enzyme of *B. cereus* is unrelated in mechanism, structure, and presumably in origin, although it may be related to the penicillin-insensitive Zn^{2+}-containing D,D-carboxypeptidase of *Streptomyces albus* (Joris *et al.*, 1983).

Studies of substrate specificity also confirm the mechanistic and structural relationship between Class A β-lactamases and D,D-carboxypeptidases. Thus phenylpropynal, a specific β-lactamase inhibitor, also inactivates *E. coli* PBP's 5 and 6, while the depsipeptide PBP substrate (Section 7.1) is slowly hydrolyzed by the TEM β-lactamase (Waxman and Strominger, 1983).

8. MECHANISMS OF LETHALITY

The bactericidal action of penicillin on pneumococci has been convincingly associated with the activation of their autolytic *N*-acetylmuramyl-L-alanine amidase by the studies of Tomasz *et al.* (Horne and Tomasz, 1980; Tomasz, 1979, 1980; Williamson and Tomasz,

1980). This enzyme only binds to and hydrolyzes the cell wall when its covalently attached wall teichoic acid (C-substance) contains choline. Choline, a growth requirement for pneumococci, can be replaced by ethanolamine, producing cells with autolysin-resistant walls. When exposed to penicillin, these cells remain intact and viable, but are growth-inhibited. The MIC, very low for normal pneumococci, remains unchanged, but the MBC (minimal bactericidal concentration) is greatly increased. This bacteriostatic response to β-lactam antibiotics is called tolerance and is also seen in mutants (grown with choline) lacking most of their autolysin activity. Such mutants can be selected by resistance to deoxycholate, which kills normal pneumococci by nonspecific activation of their autolysin, probably as a consequence of solubilization of their lipoteichoic acid (see below). Normal strains grown at a pH well below that at which the autolysin is optimally active are also tolerant. Thus the lethal effects of autolysin activation can be aborted either by growth conditions unsuitable for autolysin action or by mutation. The tolerant mutants contain the normal complement of PBP's and these are normally susceptible to acylation by penicillin in vivo (Tomasz, 1980).

Lethality of penicillin action in the autolysin-defective mutants can be restored by exogenously supplied pneumococcal autolysin. Autolysin does not lyse cells unexposed to penicillin, indicating that lysis is a consequence of labilization of cell wall substrate or loss of an autolysin inhibitor. Sensitization to exogenous or endogenous autolysin correlates with the secretion of pneumococcal lipoteichoic acid (Forssman antigen) from the cells, occurring after exposure to penicillin. Lipoteichoic acids, known only in Gram positive bacteria, are not covalently bound to peptidoglycan (unlike wall teichoic acids), have a glycolipid terminus anchored in the cytoplasmic membrane, and a poly(glycerophosphate) backbone extending through the cell wall matrix. Inhibition of autolysis can be reimposed (and lethality prevented) in pneumococci exposed to penicillin by relatively high ex-ocellular concentrations of pneumococcal lipoteichoic acid, which also contains choline. Inhibition is specific to this homologous lipoteichoic acid, possibly because of a site on the enzyme for tight binding to choline-containing activator or inhibitor polymers.

The role of choline-containing polymers in autolysin control is unique to pneumococci. However, lipoteichoic acids have also been shown to negatively control autolysins in other streptococci (S. faecium), staphylococci and Bacillus subtilis. A role for autolysin in penicillin lethality is implied in all of these organisms by correlations between the pH dependence of lethality and autolysin action. As inhibitors of autolysis, the lipoteichoic acids of these organisms are interchangeable. The characteristics important to the inhibitory polymer in these other organisms appear to be only amphipathicity and the presence of a polyanionic glycerophosphate backbone, unsubstituted by (cationic) D-alanine ester groups (Fischer et al., 1981). This type of polymer, variably substituted by alanine, is found in most Gram positive bacteria and may play a general role in autolysin control. However, it is absent in Gram negative bacteria, and even in Gram positive bacteria its role is not always clear. Thus, in group A streptococci (see below), death apparently precedes teichoic acid release, suggesting that this release may be a consequence not a cause of cell wall degradation (Kessler and van de Rijn, 1981).

The oral streptococci, S. sanguis and S. mutans, are naturally tolerant to β-lactam antibiotics, even though the MIC's of penicillin for these organisms are below 1 μg/ml. This natural tolerance is broken by addition of exogenous lysin (C-phage associated lysin), exactly as in the autolysin-defective S. pneumoniae mutants. Moreover, as for these S. pneumoniae mutants, deoxycholate is not lethal for S. sanguis or S. mutans. Lipoteichoic acid release does occur in penicillin-treated S. sanguis and in the S. pneumoniae mutants, and presumably renders them sensitive to the exogenous lysin. Not surprisingly, therefore, deoxycholate also causes S. sanguis to become lysin-sensitive (Horne and Tomasz, 1980).

Just as deoxycholate-selected, autolysin-defective S. pneumoniae strains are tolerant, tolerant strains selected with cell wall synthesis inhibitors are frequently (about 75%) autolysin-defective. Nevertheless, some tolerant strains selected in this way retained normal autolysin activity (Williamson and Tomasz, 1980). Two types were found; one type selected with penicillin or a mixture of D-cycloserine plus β-chloro-D-alanine, and the other type selected with bacitracin or vancomycin (see Fig. 3). The first type was tolerant only to penicillin or the alanine analogs. The second was tolerant to all of the antibiotics. It was suggested (Williamson and Tomasz, 1980), on the basis of these findings, that autolysin activation involves at least two sequential steps, only one of which is common to the mechanism of activation triggered by all four inhibitors. Since LTA release occurred in all of the mutants on exposure to penicillin, this may precede, or be necessary but not sufficient for, autolysin activation. As shown schematically below; at least two events may have to occur, in parallel (as shown), or sequentially; (1) is lipoteichoic acid (LTA) release, and (2) and (3) are unknown events, selectively triggered by exposure to certain cell wall synthesis inhibitors and possibly associated with the synthetic components indicated, either of which may complete the requirements for autolysin activation. Activation of events (2) and (3) is affected by the tolerance mutations selected by the same antibiotics which normally trigger these mechanisms. The common denominator of autolysin activation may be perturbation of membrane protein structural organization, particularly at sites actively involved in cell wall biosynthesis (see section 3), where controlled autolysis for remodelling of pre-existing polymer may normally occur.

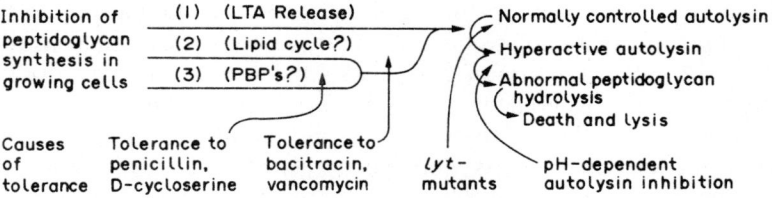

Cells in which macromolecular synthesis is prevented by amino acid starvation, or by exposure to bacteriostatic antibiotics such as chloramphenicol, are usually not killed by exposure to normally lethal concentrations of β-lactam antibiotics. It also seems likely that control of autolysin activation is tied to the cell growth cycle, since transient cell cycle-dependent autolysin activation has been shown to occur in E. coli. Blockage of protein synthesis may block the cell cycle at some quiescent stage, removing some precondition for autolysin activation, resulting in protection from killing by β-lactam antibiotics. Similar reasoning may explain why inhibition of PBP 1A plus 1B's results in lysis in E. coli, while inhibition of E. coli PBP 2 or 3 fails to cause lysis. Perhaps cells in which these PBP's are inactivated accumulate at a different phase in the growth cycle, and only in the case of PBP 1A and 1B's is this phase associated with autolysin activation. The strict correlation found between the generation time of E. coli and the rate of loss of viability and lysis in response to β-lactam antibiotics (Tuomanen et al., 1986) is consistent with this. It has also been observed recently that sub-lethal concentrations of β-lactam antibiotics interrupt the cell division cycle of Streptococcus faecium at two different stages: an early stage prior to the completion of chromosomal replication (e.g., N-formimidoyl thienamycin), and a later stage, probably associated with septation (e.g., cefoxitin) (Pucci et al., 1986). Agents separately affecting these two stages acted syngergistically. However, earlier studies seem to rule out a requirement for completion of a cell cycle for killing by penicillin (Lark, 1958). Implicit in this model and in the phenomenon of tolerance, is a feedback effect of PBP inactivation on cell growth and protein synthesis. The mechanism is not understood, but may be related to the re 1A-controlled stringent response of mRNA synthesis to amino acid starvation (Goodell and Tomasz, 1980).

Suprisingly, studies of cell walls of amino acid-starved E. coli cells suggest a different, more direct mechanism of protection. Amino acid starvation apparently causes rapid production of an autolysin-resistant, chemically modified peptidoglycan. Thus reduced substrate sensitivity, as well as (or rather than) aborted autolysin activation may be the mechanism of the antagonism between bacteriostatic antibiotics and cell wall synthesis inhibitors (Goodell and Tomasz, 1980).

Although autolysin activation in bacteria is widely implicated in death due to exposure to β-lactam antibiotics, by physiological observations and the type of experiments described above, its role is not always obvious or certain. Selective inhibition of *E. coli* PBP's 2 or 3 causes death without immediate lysis (Section 5.2.1). Similarly, group A streptococci, while exquisitely sensitive to penicillin, do not lyse when killed by β-lactam antibiotics, although massive (if delayed) release of LTA results. Penicillin-tolerant, but not penicillin-resistant group A streptococci have been isolated in the clinic.

It is suggested by Tomasz (1980) that the autolysin type responsible for massive penicillin-induced lysis in species such as *S. pneumoniae* is normally responsible for extensive peptidoglycan hydrolysis during cell separation and that, for some unknown reason, the capacity for over-production of this activity has been retained during evolution of a high proportion of eubacteria. The viability of pneumococcal mutants defective in 95–98% of this activity indicates that this super-abundance is not essential for growth in the laboratory. A second type of highly controlled murein hydrolase activity may be required for subtle remodelling of pre-synthesized peptidoglycan to allow cell expansion and morphogenesis, and possibly to allow insertion of new peptidoglycan polymer (Weidel and Pelzer, 1964). It is possible that abnormal activation of this system is responsible for death of group A streptococci exposed to penicillin or of *E. coli* exposed to mecillinam or cephalexin (selective inhibitors of PBP's 2 and 3; Table 1). Alternatively, it may be that the inhibition of protein synthesis, seen in the tolerant response of *S. sanguis* to penicillin, is irreversible in the lethal response of group A streptococci to the same drug. Whatever the explanation of these phenomena, it resides in species-specific aspects of bacterial physiology which are poorly understood. It seems paradoxical that penicillin blocks protein synthesis in tolerant mutants while an unrelated block in protein synthesis can prevent penicillin from killing non-tolerant bacteria. Since penicillin does not induce tolerance to itself, the sequence of autolysin activation and protein synthesis inhibition following exposure to penicillin must be critical. Perhaps only the relative rates of imposition of protein synthesis inhibition (and consequent autolysin-resistant peptidoglycan synthesis?) and autolysin activation determine whether the response is tolerance or lethality.

Persistence, a phenomenon first recognized in the early years of penicillin use (Bigger, 1944) and apparently responsible for the occasional failure of penicillin therapy of staphylococci infections prior to the emergence of β-lactamase producing strains, is a phenomenon probably related to tolerance but with a different phenotype and mechanism. In clinical isolates of β-lactam sensitive strains of many species, such as *S. aureus* and *E. coli*, about 1 in 10^6 of the cell population survives despite prolonged exposure to bactericidal concentrations of the antibiotic under growth conditions. The survivors grow out once antibiotic is removed, but are not mutant: they have the same 10^{-6} persistance rate as the parent. Recently, mutations at the *hipA* locus of *E. coli* have been found to increase persistance up to 10^{-2}. The gene has been cloned (Moyed and Broderick, 1986) and found to lie very near to the terminus of DNA relication. Mutations are recessive, null mutations are cold-sensitive, and *hipA* point mutations also confer a similar persistence in the face of thymine starvation or a conditional block in DNA synthesis. It is suggested that the *hipA* gene product helps to coordinate termination of DNA replication and the start of a new cell cycle, that persisters are in a temporary arrested or "Go" state resembling stationary growth phase, and that while in this state, arrest of peptidoglycan or DNA synthesis prevents the start of a new cell cycle and so is not lethal. The result is, apparently, a general inhibition of macromolecular synthesis. The bacteriostatic effects of inhibitors of peptidoglycan synthesis in tolerant mutants may, therefore, be due to entry in the "persistent" state, that is, to inhibition of the start of the cell cycle when either cell wall or DNA synthesis is arrested. The *hipA* gene product may be a component of a system designed to assess the balance of these processes prior to start.

It seems likely that the failure of treatment of diseases such as bacterial endocarditis, resulting from an incomplete bactericidal response, may be due to the emergence of mutations to tolerance, as has been recently suggested. It is also clear that persistence will remain a problem in the treatment of infections in the severely immuno-compromised host or in a compromising location such as a heart valve or abscess. Possibly the newer quinolone gyrase inhibitors may prove to avoid this problem, although their bactericidal activity probably requires active DNA synthesis. It is also possible that the control pathway inferred from the phenotype of the *hipA* mutations might be a target for the design of a new class of bacteriostatic antibiotics.

9. CONCLUSION

The enormous variety of β-lactam antibiotics, either currently available for clinical use or under testing for such use, demonstrates that no single solution exists to the complex problem of the optimal design β-lactam antibiotics. These antibiotics must have the appropriate pharmacological properties, be able to penetrate outer membranes of the most recalcitrant Gram negative pathogens, retain high activity against essential bacterial PBP's, and be resistant to the wide variety of β-lactamases which bacteria can produce.

Structure/activity analysis of the role played in antibiotics by the highly varied substituents of the β-lactam ring, in binding to and effectively acylating PBP targets, is complicated by this bewildering variety. Observed PBP specificity, and the lack of more than general guidance provided by analogy to the structure of normal substrates (Section 7.3), further complicate this analysis. Mecillinam, for example, was not designed as a selective inhibitor of PBP's similar to *E. coli* PBP-2, and attempts at such specific design, if desirable, may require detailed analysis of the active sites of each class of lethal target PBP in each group of related pathogens. Certainly, design of new inhibitors which are not simple ad hoc variants of known antibiotics will require more specific information on target enzymes than is available in the large volume of existing structure/function data (Boyd, 1982).

Just as important as data on PBP–antibiotic interactions are data pertaining to the ability of β-lactam antibiotics to reach their PBP targets intact and in adequate concentration (Vu and Nikaido, 1985; Chapter 7). Analysis of the relationship between structure and outer membrane permeability for organisms such as *P. aeruginosa* remains a formidable task (Nikaido, 1981).

Since the class A and C β-lactamases employ the same acyl-ENZ intermediate mechanism as PBP's, a reduced rate of β-lactamase deacylation would seem to be the mechanism of resistance to β-lactamases most compatible with persistence of antibiotic activity. It is not surprising, therefore, that while most of the newer β-lactamase-resistant antibiotic derivatives seem to acylate class A β-lactamases poorly, they still react rapidly with class C enzymes, producing relatively stable acyl-β-lactamase derivatives. Unfortunately, while this confers considerable resistance to hydrolysis, a slow rate of outer membrane permeation, coupled with efficient acylation and effective induction or high levels of constitutive production of these periplasmic Gram-negative β-lactamases, results in resistance due to this slow rate of hydrolysis. Clearly, a mutation resulting in overproduction of a non-essential, low molecular weight PBP with high affinity for a given slowly permeating β-lactam antibiotic could protect the producing cell by trapping the antibiotic. If the PBP also had an adequate rate of turnover, it might even act as a functional β-lactamase, producing high level resistance. It is perhaps fortunate that the abundant, smaller PBP's of Gram negative bacteria have low affinities for many non-penam antibiotics.

Use of new β-lactam antibiotic variants has always preceded knowledge of effective resistance mechanisms waiting to be expressed in bacteria. It is to be hoped that our increasingly sophisticated understanding of these mechanisms will allow prospective design of antibiotics with longer useful lifetimes, as well as the use of strategies such as the use of mixtures to extend the usefulness of existing antibiotics.

As summarized inSections 6 and 7, mixtures of β-lactam antibiotics attacking different PBP's may act synergistically, especially if these PBP's play independent, essential roles in cell growth, as illustrated by the studies of Pucci *et al.* (1986). A strategy already in use (Neu, Chapter 8) is the combination of β-lactam antibiotics with β-lactamase inhibitors. In the future, such mixtures may need to be carefully tailored to the strains of major pathogens predominant in a given location at a given time, because of local strain variation in PBP affinities, cell wall permeability, or β-lactamase production. This will always be an empirical process, but it can be guided by information on the acylation efficiencies of candidate antibiotics for essential pathogen PBP's, by their susceptibility to hydrolysis by pathogen β-lactamases, and by the relative affinities of drugs for target PBP's and for β-lactamase sinks. The role of the different porin components of Gram negative pathogen outer membranes in permeation by the antibiotics and β-lactamase inhibitors will also be pertinent, since this will allow prediction of the effects of porin mutations on susceptibility. The only clear prediction is that the role of β-lactam antibiotics in the optimal chemotherapy of infectious disease will continue to undergo change in response to selected changes in their bacterial targets.

Acknowledgements—I would like to thank Drs. J. B. Ward, G. Shockman, R. B. Sykes, and H. Nikaido for reading and commenting on this manuscript. Figures 1, 3, 4 and 5 are modified versions of figures previously published in *The Bacteria*, Vol. VII (J. R. Sokatch and L. N. Ornston, eds; 1979, Academic Press, Inc.) and more recently in *β-Lactam Antibiotics* (Queener, Queener and Weber, eds: 1986, M. Dekker, Inc.).

This work was supported, in part, by grant AI-10806 from the National Institute of Allergy and Infectious Diseases, NIH, Department of Health and Human Services.

REFERENCES

BARBOUR, A. G. (1981) Properties of the penicillin-binding proteins in *Neisseria gonorrhoeae*. *Antimicrob. Ag. Chemother*. **19**: 316–322.

BIGGER, J. W. (1944) Treatment of staphylococcal infections with penicillin. *Lancet* **ii**: 497–500.

BLUMBERG, P. M. and STROMINGER, J. L. (1974) Interaction of penicillin with the bacterial cell: penicillin-binding proteins and penicillin-sensitive enzymes. *Bacteriol. Rev*. **38**: 291–335.

BOYD, D. B. (1979). Conformational analogy between β-lactam antibiotics and the tetrahedral transition states of a dipeptide. *J. Med. Chem*. **22**: 533–537.

BOYD, D. B., (1982) Theoretical and physicochemical studies on β-lactam antibiotics. In: *The Chemistry and Biology of β-Lactam Antibiotics, Vol.* 1, pp. 437–535, MORIN R. B. and GORMAN M. (eds). Academic Press, New York.

BROOME-SMITH, J. K. and SPRATT, B. G. (1982) Deletion of the penicillin-binding protein 6 gene of *Escherichia coli*. *J. Bacteriol*. **152**: 904–906.

BROWN, K. R. and MARTIN, C. M. (1981) Analysis of safety of β-lactam antibiotics. In: *β-Lactam Antibiotics*, pp. 445–459, SALTON, M. and SHOCKMAN, G. D. (eds). Academic Press, New York.

BROWN, D. F. J. and REYNOLDS, P. E. (1980) Intrinsic resistance to β-lactam antibiotics in *Staphylococcus aureus*. *FEBS Lett*. **122**: 275–278.

BROWN, D. F. J. and REYNOLDS, P. E. (1983) The mechanism of methicillin resistance in Staphylococci. In: *The Target of Penicillin*, pp. 537–542. HAGENBECK, R., HOLTJE, J.-V. and LABISCHINSKI H. (eds). W. de Gruyter, Berlin.

BUCHANAN, C. E. (1977) Altered proteins in penicillin-resistant mutants of *Bacillus subtilis*. In: *Microbiology*, pp. 191–194, SCHLESSINGER, D. (ed.). Am. Soc. Microbiol., Washington, D.C.

BUTMANN, L. and TOMASZ, A. (1982) Penicillin-resistant and penicillin-tolerant mutants of Group A Streptococci. *Antimicrob. Ag. Chemother*. **22**: 128–136.

CANEPARI, P., LLEO, M. D. M., CORNAGLIA, G., FONTANA, R. and SATTA, G. (1986) In *Streptococcus faecium* Penicillin-binding Protein 5 Alone is Sufficient for Growth at Sub-maximal But not at Maximal Rate. *J. of General Microbiol*. **132**: 625–631.

CARPENTER, C. V., GOYER, S. and NEUHAUS, F. C. (1976) Steric effects on penicillin-sensitive peptidoglycan synthesis in a membrane–wall system from *Gaffkya homari*. *Biochemistry* **15**: 3146–3152.

COHEN, N. C. (1983) β-lactam antibiotics: Geometrical requirements for antibacterial activities. *J. Med. Chem*. **26**: 259–264.

COOPER, P. D. (1956) Site of action or radiopenicillin. *Bacteriol. Rev*. **70**: 28–48.

DEMEREC, M. (1945) Production of *Staphylococcus* strains resistant to various concentrations of penicillin. *Proc. natn. Acad. Sci. U.S.A*. **31**: 16–24.

DEPEDRO, M. and SCHWARZ, U. (1981) Heterogeneity of newly inserted and preexisting murein in the sacculus of *Escherichia coli*. *Proc. natn. Acad. Sci. U.S.A*. **78**: 5856–5860.

DEZELEE, P. and SHOCKMAN, G. D. (1975) Studies on the formation of peptide cross-links in the cell wall peptidoglycan of *Streptococcus faecalis*. *J. biol. Chem*. **250**: 6806–6816.

DOUGHERTY, T. J., KOLLER, A. E. and TOMASZ, A. (1980) Penicillin-binding proteins of penicillin-susceptible and intrinsically resistant *Neisseria gonorrhoeae*. *Antimicrob. Ag. Chemother*. **18**: 730–737.

DUEZ, C., JORIS, B., FRERE, J.-M. and GHUYSEN, J.-M. (1981) The penicillin-binding site in the exocellular D,D-carboxypeptidase-transpeptidase of *Actinomadura* R39. *Biochem. J*. **193**: 83–86.

FISCHER, H. and TOMASZ, A. (1984) Production and release of peptidoglycan and wall teichoic acid polymers in pneumococci treated with beta-lactam antibiotics. *J. Bacteriol*. **157**: 507–513.

FISCHER, W., ROSEL, P. and KOCH, H. (1981). Effect of alanine ester substitution and other structural features of lipoteichoic acids on their inhibitory activity against autolysins of *Staphylococcus aureus*. *J. Bacteriol*. **146**: 467–475.

FONTANA, R., GROSSATO, A., ROSSIO, L., CHENG, Y. R. and SATTA, G. (1985) Transition from Resistance to Hypersusceptibility to β-Lactam Antibiotics Associated with Loss of a Low-Affinity Penicillin-Binding Protein in a *Streptococcus faecium* Mutant Highly Resistant to Penicillin. *Antimicrob. Agents and Chemotherapy* **28**: 678–683.

FORDHAM, W. D. and GILVARG, C. (1974) Kinetics of cross-linking of peptidoglycan in *Bacillus megaterium. J. biol. Chem.* **249**: 2478–2482.

FOX, G. E., STACKEBRANDT, E., HESPELL, R. B., GIBSON, J., MANILOFF, J., DYER, T. A., WOLFE, R. S., BALCH, W. E., TANNER, R. S., MAGRUM, L. J., ZABLEN, L. B., BLAKEMORE, R., GUPTA, R., BONEN, L., LEWIS, B. J., STAHL, D. A., LUEHRSEN, K. R., CHEN, K. N. and WOESE, C. R. (1980) The phylogeny of Prokaryotes. *Science* **209**: 457–463.

FUCHS-CLEVELAND, E. and GILVARG, C. (1976) Oligomeric intermediate in peptidoglycan biosynthesis in *Bacillus megaterium. Proc. natn. Acad. Sci. U.S.A.* **73**: 4200–4204.

GARDNER, A. D. (1940) Morphological effects of penicillin on bacteria. *Nature, Lond.* **146**: 837–838.

GEORGOPAPADAKOU N. H., LIN, F. Y., RYONO, D. E., NEUBECK R. and ONDETTI, M. (1981) Chemical modifications of the active site of *Streptomyces* R61 D,D-Carboxypeptidase. *Eur. J. Biochem.* **115**: 53.

GHUYSEN, J-M. (1984) Exploration of active sites of DD-peptidases. In: Proceedings, IUPHAR, 9th International Congress of Pharmacology, Vol. 1, pp. 115–123. PATON, W., MITCHELL, J. and TURNER, P. (eds).

GHUYSEN, J-M., FRÈRE, J-M., LEYH-BOUILLE, M., DIDEBERG, O., LAMOTTE-BRASSEUR, J., PERKINS, H. R. and DECOEN, J. L. (1981) Penicillins and Δ³-cephalosporins as inhibitors and mechanism-based inactivators of D-alanyl-D-Ala peptidases. In: *Topics in Molecular Pharmacology*, pp. 63–97, BURGEN A. S. V. and ROBERTS G. C. K. (eds). Elsevier/North-Holland Biomedical Press.

GHUYSEN, J-M., FRERE, J-M., LEYH-BOUILLE, M., NGUYEN-DISTECHE, M., COYETTE, J., DUSART, J., JORIS, B., DUEZ, C., DIDEBERG, O., CHARLIER, P., DIVE, G. and LAMORRE-BRASSEUR, J. (1984) Bacterial Wall Peptidoglycan, DD-Peptidases and Beta-lactam Antibiotics. *Scand. J. Infect. Dis., Suppl.* **42**: 17–37.

GHUYSEN, J-M., FRÈRE, J. M., LEYH-BOUILLE, M., PERKINS, H. R. and NIETO, M. (1980) The active centres in penicillin-sensitive enzymes. *Phil. Trans. R. Soc. Lond. B.* **289**: 285–301.

GHUYSEN, J. M., TIPPER, D. J. BIRGE, C. M. and STROMINGER, J. L. (1965) Structure of the cell wall of *Staphylococcus aureus* strain Copenhagen. VI. The soluble glycopeptide and its sequential degradation by peptidases. *Biochemistry* **4**: 2245–2254.

GLAUNER, B. and SCHWARZ, U. (1983) The analysis of murein composition with high-pressure liquid chromatography. In: *The Target of Penicillin*, pp. 29–34, HAKENBECK, R., HOLTJE, J. V. and LABISCHINSK, H. (eds) Walter de Gruyter and Co., Berlin.

GODFREY, A. J., BRYAN, L. E. and RABIN, H. R. (1981) β-Lactam resistant *Pseudomonas aeruginosa* with modified penicillin-binding proteins emerging during cystic fibrosis treatment. *Antimicrob. Ag. Chemother.* **19**: 705–711.

GOODELL, E. W., MARKIEWICZ, Z. and SCHWARZ, U. (1983) Absence of oligometric murein intermediates in *Escherichia coli. J. Bacteriol.* **156**: 130–135.

GOODELL, W. and TOMASZ A. (1980) Alteration of *Escherichia coli* murein during amino acid starvation. *J. Bacteriol.* **144**: 1009–1016.

HAKENBECK, R., TARPAY, M. and TOMASZ, A. (1980) Multiple changes of penicillin-binding proteins in penicillin-resistant clinical isolates of *Streptococcus pneumoniae. Antimicrob. Ag. Chemother.* **17**: 364–371.

HAMMES, W. P. and KANDLER, O. (1976) Biosynthesis of peptidoglycan in *Gaffkya homari*. The incorporation of peptidoglycan into the cell wall and the direction of transpeptidation. *Eur. J. Biochem.* **70**: 97–106.

HAMMES, W. P. and SEIDEL, H. (1978) The activities *in vitro* of D,D-carboxypeptidase of *Gaffkya homari* during biosynthesis of peptidoglycan. *Eur. J. Biochem.* **84**: 141–147.

HARTMAN, B. and TOMASZ, A. (1981) Altered penicillin-binding proteins in methicillin-resistant strains of *Staphylococcus aureus Antimicrob. Ag. Chemother.* **19**; 726–735.

HAYES, M. V., CURTIS, N. A. C., WYKE, A. W. and WARD, J. B. (1981) Decreased affinity of a penicillin-binding protein for β-lactam antibiotics in a clinical isolate of *Staphylococcus aureus* resistant to methicillin. *FEMS Microbiol. Lett.* **10**: 119–122.

HERZBERG, O. and MOULT, J. M. (1987) Bacterial resistance to β-lactam antibiotics: Crystal structure of β-lactamase from *Staphylococcus aureus* PC1 at 2.5 Å resolution. *Science* **236**: 694–701.

HORNE, D. and TOMASZ, A. (1980) Lethal effect of a heterologous murein hydrolase on penicillin-treated *Streptococcus sanguis. Antimicrob. Ag. Chemother.* **17**: 235–246.

ISHINO, F. and MATSUHASHI, M. (1981) Peptidoglycan synthetic enzyme activities of highly purified penicillin-binding protein 3 in *Escherichia coli*; a septum-forming reaction sequence. *Biochem. biophys. Res. Commun.* **101**: 905–911.

ISHINO, F., MITSUI, S., TAMAKI, S. and MATSUHASHI, M. (1980) Dual enzyme activities of cell wall peptidoglycan synthesis, peptidoglycan transglycosylase and penicillin-sensitive transpeptidase, in purified preparations of *Escherichia coli* penicillin-binding protein IA. *Biochem. biophys. Res. Commun.* **97**: 287–293.

ISHINO, F., TAMAKI, S., SPRATT, B. G. and MATSUHASHI, M. (1982) A mecillinam-sensitive peptidoglycan cross-linking reaction in *Escherichia coli. Biochem. biophys. Res. Commun.* **109**: 689–696.

IWAYA, M., GOLDMAN, R., TIPPER, D. J., FEINGOLD B. and STROMINGER, J. L. (1978) Morphology of an *Escherichia coli* mutant with a temperature-dependent round cell shape. *J. Bacteriol.* **136**: 1143–1158.

IZAKI, K., MATSUHASHI, M. and STROMINGER, J. L. (1966) Glycopeptide transpeptidase and D-alanine carboxypeptidase: penicillin-sensitive enzymatic reactions. *Proc. natn. Acad. Sci. U.S.A.* **55**; 656–663.

JORIS, B., VAN BEEUMEN, J., CASAGRANDE, F., GERDAY, C., FRERE, J-M. and GHUYSEN, J.M. (1983) The complete amino acid sequence of the Zn^{2+}-containing D-Alanyl-D-Alanine-cleaving carboxypeptidase of *Streptomyces albus* G. *Eur. J. Biochem.* **130**: 53–69.

KECK, W., GLAUNER, B., SCHWARZ, U., BROOME-SMITH, J. K. and SPRATT, B. G. (1985) Sequences of the active-site peptides of three of the high-M_r penicillin-binding proteins of *Escherichia coli* K-12. *Proc. Natl. Acad. Sci USA* **82**: 1999–2003.

KELLY, J. A., DIDEBERG, O., CHARLIER, P., WERY, J. P., LIBERT M., MOEWS, P. C., KNOX, J. R., DUEZ, C., FRAIPONT, CL., JORIS, B., DUSART, J., FRERE, J. M. and GHUYSEN, J-M. (1986) On the Origin of Bacterial Resistance to Penicillin: Comparison of a β-Lactamase and a Penicillin Target. *Science* **231**: 1429–1431.

KELLY, J. A., MOEWS, P. C., KNOX, J. R., FRERE, J-M. and GHUYSEN, J. M. (1982) Penicillin target enzymes and the antibiotic binding site. *Science* **218**: 479–481.

KESSLER, R. E. and VAN DE RIJN, I. (1981) Effects of penicillin on group A streptococci: Loss of viability appears to precede stimulation of release of lipoteichoic acid. *Antimicrob. Ag. Chemother.* **19**: 39–43.

KLEPPE, G., YU, W. and STROMINGER, J. L. (1982) Penicillin-binding proteins in *Bacillus subtilis* mutants. *Antimicrob. Ag. Chemother.* **21**: 979–983.

KNOTT-HUNZIKER, V., WALEY, S. G., ORLEK, B. S. and SAMMES, P. G. (1979) Penicillinase active sites: labelling of serine-44 in β-lactamase I by 6β-bromopenicillanic acid. *FEBS Lett.* **99**: 59–61.

KOZARICH, J. W. and STROMINGER, J. L. (1978) A membrane enzyme from *Staphylococcus aureus* which catalyses transpeptidase, carboxypeptidase and penicillinase activities. *J. biol. Chem.* **253**: 1272–1278.

LABISCHINSKI, H., BARNICKEL, G., BRADACZEK, H. and GIESBRECHT, P. (1979) On the secondary and tertiary structure of murein. Low and medium angle X-ray evidence against chitin-based conformations of bacterial peptidoglycan. *Eur. J. Biochem.* **95**: 147–155.

LARK, K. G. (1958) Variation during the cell-division cycle in the penicillin induction of protoplast-like forms of *Alcaligenes faecalis. Canadian Journal of Microbiology* **4**: 179–189.

LUND, F. and TYBRING L. (1972) 6β-Amidinopenicillanic acids—a new group of antibiotics. *Nature New Biol.* **236**: 135–137.

MARKIEWICZ, Z., BROOME-SMITH, J. K., SCHWARZ, U. and SPRATT, B. G. (1982) Spherical *E. coli* due to elevated levels of D-alanine carboxypeptidase. *Nature, Lond.* **297**: 702–704.

MARQUET, A., NIETO, M. and DIAZ-MAURINO, T. (1976) Membrane-bound D,D-carboxypeptidase and transpeptidase activities from *Bacillus megaterium* KM at pH 7. General properties, substrate specificity and inhibition by β-lactam antibiotics. *Eur. J. Biochem.* **68**: 581–589.

METT, H., BRACHA, R. and MIRELMAN, D. (1980) Soluble nascent peptidoglycan in growing *Escherichia coli* cells. *J. biol. Chem.* **255**: 9584–9890.

MIRELMAN, D. (1979) Biosynthesis and assembly of cell wall peptidoglycan. In: *Bacterial Outer Membranes*, pp. 115–166, INOUYE, M. (ed.). John Wiley and Sons, New York.

Mirelman, D., Yashouv-Gan, Y. and SCHWARZ, U. (1977) Regulation of murein biosynthesis and septum formation in filamentous cells of *Escherichia coli PAT 84. J. Bacteriol.* **129**: 1593–1600.

MOEWS, P. C., KNOX, J. R., WAXMAN, D. J. and STROMINGER, J. L. (1981) Secondary structure relations between beta-lactamases and penicillin-sensitive D-alanine carboxypeptidases. *Int. J. Peptide Protein Res.* **17**: 211–218.

MOYED, H. S. and BRODERICK, S. H. (1986). Molecular cloning and expression of *hipA*, a gene of *Escherichia coli* K-12 that affects frequency of persistence after inhibition of murein synthesis. *J. Bacteriol.* **166**: 399–403.

NAKAGAWA, J. and MATSUHASHI, M. (1982). Molecular divergence of a major peptidoglycan synthetase with transpeptidase activities in *Escherichia coli*-penicillin-binding proteins 1Bs. *Biochem. biophys. Res. Commun.* **105**: 1546–1553.

NAKAGAWA, J., TAMAKA, S. and MATSUHASHI, M. (1979) Purified penicillin binding proteins 1Bs from *Escherichia coli* membrane showing activities of both peptidoglycan polymerase and peptidoglycan cross-linking enzyme. *Agric. Biol. Chem.* **43**: 1379–1380.

NEUHAUS, F. C. and HAMMES, W. P. (1981) Inhibition of cell wall biosynthesis by analogues of alanine. *Pharmac. Ther.* **14**: 265–320.

NIKAIDO, H. (1981) Outer membrane permeability of bacteria: resistance and accessibility of targets. In: *β-Lactam Antibiotics*, pp. 249–260, SALTON, M. and SHOCKMAN G. D., (eds). Academic Press, New York.

PARK, J. T. (1952) Uridine 5'-pyrophosphate derivatives. III. Amino acid-containing derivatives. *J. biol. Chem.* **194,** 897–904.

PERKINS, H. R. (1982) Vancomycin and related antibiotics. *Pharmac. Ther.* **16**: 181–197.

PRATT, J. M., HOLLAND, I. B. and SPRATT, B. G. (1981) Precursor forms of penicillin-binding proteins 5 and 6 of *E. coli* cytoplasmic membrane. *Nature, Lond.* **293**: 307–309.

PUCCI, M. J., HINKS, E. T., DICKER, D. T., HIGGINS, M. L. and DANEO-MOORE, L. (1986) Inhibition by β-Lactam Antibiotics at Two Different Times in the Cell Cycle of *Streptococcus faecium* ATCC 9790. *J. of Bacteriology* **165**: 682–688.

RASMUSSEN, J. R. and STROMINGER, J. L. (1978) Utilization of a depsipeptide substrate for trapping acyl-enzyme intermediates of Penicillin-sensitive D-alanine carboxypeptidases. *Proc. natn. Acad. Sci. U.S.A.* **75**: 84–88.

REYNOLDS, P. E., SHEPHERD, S. T. and CHASE, H. A. (1978) Identification of the binding protein which may be the target of penicillin action in *Bacillus megaterium. Nature, Lond.* **271**: 568–570.

SABATH, L. D., LAVERDIERE, M., WHIELER, N., BLAZEVIC, D. and WILKINSON, B. J. (1977) A new type of penicillin resistance of *Staphylococcus aureus. Lancet* **i**: 443–447.

SANDERS, C. C. (1984) Inducible β-lactamases and non-hydrolytic resistance mechanisms. *J. Antimicrob. Chemother.* **13**: 1–2.

SCHLEIFER, K. H. and KANDLER, O. (1972) Peptidoglycan types of bacterial cell walls and their taxonomic implications. *Bacteriol. Rev.* **36**: 407–477.

SCHWARZ, U., SEEGER, K., WENGENMAYER, F. and STRECKER, H. (1981) Penicillin-binding proteins of *Escherichia coli* identified with a ^{125}I-derivative of ampicillin. *FEMS Microbiol. Lett.* **10**: 107–109.

SPRATT, B. G. (1975) Distinct penicillin binding proteins involved in the division, elongation, and shape of *Escherichia coli, Proc. natn. Acad. Sci. U.S.A.* **72**: 2999–3003.

SPRATT, B. G. (1977) Temperature-sensitive cell division mutants of *Escherichia coli* with thermolabile penicillin-binding proteins. *J. Bacteriol.* **131**: 293–305.

SPRATT, B. G. (1980) Deletion of the penicillin-binding protein 5 gene of *Escherichia coli. J. Bacteriol.* **14**: 1190–1192.

SPRATT, B. G. (1983) Penicillin-binding proteins and the future of β-lactam antibiotics. *J. gen. Microbiol.* **129**: 1247–1260.

SPRATT, B. G., JOBANPUTRA, V. and SCHWARZ, U. (1977) Mutants of *Escherichia coli* which lack a component of penicillin-binding protein 1 are viable. *FEBS Lett.* **79**: 374–378.

SPRATT, B. G. and PARDEE, A. B. (1975) Penicillin-binding proteins and cell shape in *E. coli. Nature, Lond.* **254**: 516–517.

STROMINGER, J. L. (1977) How penicillin kills bacteria: a short history. In: *Microbiology*, pp. 177–181, SCHLESSINGER, D. (ed.). American Society for Microbiology, Washington, D.C.

SUZUKI, H., NISHIMURA, Y., and HIROTA, Y. (1978) On the process of cellular division in *Escherichia coli:* a series of mutants of *E. coli* altered in the penicillin-binding proteins. *Proc. natn. Acad. Sci. U.S.A.* **75**: 664–668.

SUZUKI, H., VAN HEIJENOORT, Y., TAMURA, T., MIZOGUCHI, J., HIROTA, Y. and VAN HEIJENOORT, J. (1980) *In vitro* peptidoglycan polymerization catalyzed by binding protein 1B of *Escherichia coli* K12. *FEBS Lett.* **110**: 245–249.

TAKU, A., STUCKEY, M. and FAN D. P. (1982) Purification of the peptidoglycan transglycosylase of *Bacillus megaterium. J. biol Chem.* **257**: 5018–5022.

TAMAKI, S., NAKAJIMA, S. and MATSUHASHI, M. (1977) Thermosensitive mutation in *Escherichia coli* simultaneously causing defects in penicillin-binding protein 1Bs and in enzyme activity for peptidoglycan synthesis *in vitro. Proc. natn. Acad. Sci. U.S.A.* **74**: 5472–5476.

TIPPER, D. J. (1970) The structure of bacterial cell wall peptidoglycans. *Int. J. Syst. Bacteriol.* **26**: 361–377.

TIPPER, D. J. (1979) The mode of action of β-lactam antibiotics. *Rev. Infect. Dis.* **1**: 39–53.

TIPPER, D. J. and STROMINGER, J. L. (1965) Mechanism of action of penicillins: a proposal based on their structural similarity to acyl-D-ananyl-D-alanine. *Proc. natn. Acad. Sci. U.S.A.* **54**: 1133–1141.

TIPPER, D. J. and STROMINGER, J. L. (1968) Biosynthesis of the peptidoglycan of bacterial cell walls. XII. Inhibition of cross-linking by penicillins and cephalosporins: studies in *Staphylococcus aureus in vivo. J. biol. Chem.* **243**: 3169–3179.

TIPPER, D. J. and WRIGHT, A. (1979) The structure and biosynthesis of bacterial cell walls. In: *The Bacteria*, Vol. 7, pp. 291–426, SOKATCH J. R. and ORNSTON, L. N. (eds). Academic Press, New York.

TOMASZ, A. (1979) The mechanism of the irreversible antimicrobial effects of penicillins: How the beta-lactam antibiotics kill and lyse bacteria. *A. Rev. Microbiol.* **33**: 113–137.

TOMASZ, A. (1980) Penicillin tolerance and the control of the murein hydrolases. In: *β-Lactam Antibiotics*, pp. 227–247, SALTON M. and SHOCKMAN, G. D. (eds). Academic Press, New York.

TOMIOKA, S., ISHINO, F., TAMAKI S. and MATSUHASHI, M. (1982) Formation of hyper-cross-linked peptidoglycan with multiple cross-linkages by a penicillin-binding protein, 1A, of *Escherichia coli. Biochem. biophys. Res. Commun.* **106**: 1175–1182.

TOSCANO, W. H. and STORM, D. R. (1982) Bacitracin. *Pharmac. Ther.* **16**: 199–210.

TUOMANEN, E., COZENS, R., TOSCH, W., ZAK, O. and TOMASZ, A. (1986) The Rate of Killing of *Escherichia coli* by β-Lactam Antibiotics is Strictly Proportional to the Rate of Bacterial Growth. *J. Gen. Microbiol.* **132**: 1297–1304.

VIRUDACHALAM, R. and RAO, V. S. R. (1977) Theoretical studies on β-lactam antibiotics. I. Conformational similarity of penicillins and cephalosporins to X-D-alanyl-D-alanine and corrections of their structure with activity. *Int. J. Peptide Protein Res.* **10**: 51–59.

VIRUDACHALAM, R. and RAO, V. S. R. (1978) Theoretical studies of peptidoglycans. I. Effect of L-alanyl, D-butyl, or D-valyl residues at the positions 4 or 5 of the pentapeptide moiety of peptidoglycan on the cross-linking reaction. *Biopolymers* **17**: 2251–2263.

VU, H. and NIKAIDO, H. (1985) Role of β-Lactam Hydrolysis in the Mechanism of Resistance of a β-Lactamase-Constitutive *Enterobacter cloacae* Strain to Expanded-Spectrum β-Lactams. *Antimicrob. Agents and Chemotherapy* **27**: 393–398.

WARD, J. B. (1984) Biosynthesis of peptidoglycan: Points of attack by wall inhibitors. *Pharmac. Ther.* **25**: 327–369.

WAXMAN, D. J. and STROMINGER, J. L. (1980) Sequence of active site peptides from the penicillin-sensitive D-alanine carboxypeptidase of *Bacillus subtilis. J. biol. Chem.* **255**: 3964–3976.

WAXMAN, D. J. and STROMINGER, J. L. (1983) Penicillin-binding proteins and the mechanism of action of β-lactam antibiotics. *A. Rev. Biochem.* **52**: 825–869.

WAXMAN, D. J., YOCUM, R. R. and STROMINGER, J. L. (1980) *Phil. Trans. R. Soc. London Ser. B.* **289**: 257–271.

WEIDEL, W. and PELZER, H. (1964) Bag-shaped macromolecules—a new outlook on bacterial cell walls. *Adv. Enzymol.* **26**: 193–232.

WILLIAMSON, R., CALDERWOOD, S. B., MOELLERING, R. C. JR. and TOMASZ, A. (1983) Studies on the mechanism of intrinsic resistance to β-lactam antibiotics in Group D streptococci. *J. gen. Microbiol.* **129**: 813–822.

WILLIAMSON, R. and TOMASZ, A. (1980) Antibiotic tolerant mutants of *Streptococcus pneumoniae* that are not deficient in autolytic activity. *J. Bacteriol.* **144**: 105–113.

WILLIAMSON, R., ZIGHELBOIM, S. and TOMASZ, A. (1981) Penicillin-binding proteins of penicillin-resistant and penicillin-tolerant *Streptococcus pneumoniae*. In: *β-Lactam Antibiotics*, pp. 215–225, SALTON, M. and SHOCKMAN, G. (eds). Academic Press, New York.

WISE, E. M. and PARK, J. T. (1965) Penicillin: its basic site of action as an inhibitor of a peptide cross-linking reaction in cell wall mucopeptide synthesis. *Proc. natn. Acad. Sci. U.S.A.* **54**: 75–81.

WYKE, A. W., WARD, J. B. and HAYES, M. V. (1982) Synthesis of Peptidoglycan *in vitro* in methicillin-resistant *Staphylococcus aureus. Eur. J. Biochem.* **127**: 553–558.

WYKE, A. W., WARD, J. B., HAYES, M. V. and CURTIS, N. A. C. (1981) A role *in vivo* for penicillin-binding protein 4 of *Staphylococcus aureus. Eur. J. Biochem.* **119**: 389–393.

YOCUM, R. R., AMANUMA, H., O'BRIEN, T. A., WAXMAN, D. J. and STROMINGER, J. L. (1982) Penicillin is an active site inhibitor for four genera of bacteria. *J. Bacteriol.* **149**: 1150–1153.

Yocum, R. R., Waxman, D. J., Rasmussen, J. R. and Strominger, J. L. (1979) Mechanism of penicillin action: Penicillin and substrate bind covalently to the same active site serine in two bacterial D-alinine-carboxypeptidases. *Proc. natn. Acad. Sci. U.S.A.* **76**: 2730–2734.

Zighelboim, S. and Tomasz, A. (1980) Penicillin-binding proteins of multiple antibiotic-resistant South African strains of *Streptococcus pneumoniae*. *Antimicrob. Ag. Chemother.* **17**: 434–442.

CHAPTER 6

MODERN β-LACTAM ANTIBIOTICS

RICHARD B. SYKES

Glaxo Group Research Ltd, Greenford, Middlesex, UK

DANIEL P. BONNER and EDWARD A. SWABB

The Squibb Institute for Medical Research, Post Office Box 4000, Princeton, New Jersey, NJ 08540, USA

1. INTRODUCTION

Over four decades of antibiotic therapy, the causative organisms involved in significant nosocomial infection have continued to evolve and change. Throughout this period, streptococci, staphylococci, enterics, *Pseudomonas*, anaerobes, *Hemophilus* and *Neisseria* have played important roles as the responsible aetiologic agents. Continual changes in β-lactam antibiotics have been necessary to keep pace with these changing patterns of bacterial infection.

With the introduction of penicillin in the early 1940s, staphylococci and streptococci, which represented the nosocomial pathogens of the day, were soon brought under control. *Hemophilus influenzae* and *Neisseria gonorrhoeae* also succumbed to the action of penicillin. Today, we have at our disposal compounds with high and specific activity against Gram-positive and Gram-negative bacteria, compounds active against anaerobes, and broad spectrum compounds exhibiting activity over a broad bacterial range. In addition, β-lactam molecules are available that prevent the hydrolysis of β-lactams susceptible to hydrolysis.

As with other classes of antibiotics, resistance development among bacteria has posed a constant challenge to β-lactam development. Despite this dynamic situation of changing organisms and changing susceptibilities, the β-lactams have held their place as effective and safe therapeutic agents. In 1983, β-lactam antibiotics accounted for approximately 50% of the world antibiotic market valued at over eight billion dollars.

Although many of the early penicillins and cephalosporins are still prescribed in high volume, the last decade has witnessed an avalanche of new β-lactam-containing molecules. Until 1970 all known anti-microbially active β-lactam-containing compounds were divided into the two chemical types represented by penicillins and cephalosporins. The penicillins contain a β-lactam ring fused to a thiazolidine ring, whereas the cephalosporins have the β-lactam fused to a dihydrothiazine ring (Fig. 1). These are referred to as the classic β-lactams.

The discovery of the 7α-methoxy cephalosporins (Nagarajan *et al.*, 1971) provided the first new, naturally occuring β-lactam nucleus following the isolation of cephalosporin C. Although often referred to colloquially as cephamycins, they are fundamentally ceph-3-ems with a methoxy group in place of hydrogen at the 7α-position of the cephalosporin nucleus (Fig. 1).

The first reported non-classical β-lactams were the amidino penicillins (Lund and Tybring, 1972), produced semi-synthetically from 6-APA. A second group of semi-synthetic non-classic β-lactams are represented by the oxacephems (Fig. 1) and carbacephems in which an oxygen or carbon atom substitutes for sulphur in the dihydro-thiazine ring, (Yoshida *et al.*, 1978; Mochida *et al.*, 1984). All other non-classic β-lactams presently in use or under active investigation are based on molecules isolated from natural sources. Nocardicins (Aoki *et al.*, 1976) represent a series of unique azetidin-2-one antibiotics produced by *Nocardia* species which exhibit weak anti-microbial activity (Fig. 1). Clavulanic acid (Howarth *et al.*, 1976) a streptomycete product has oxygen in place

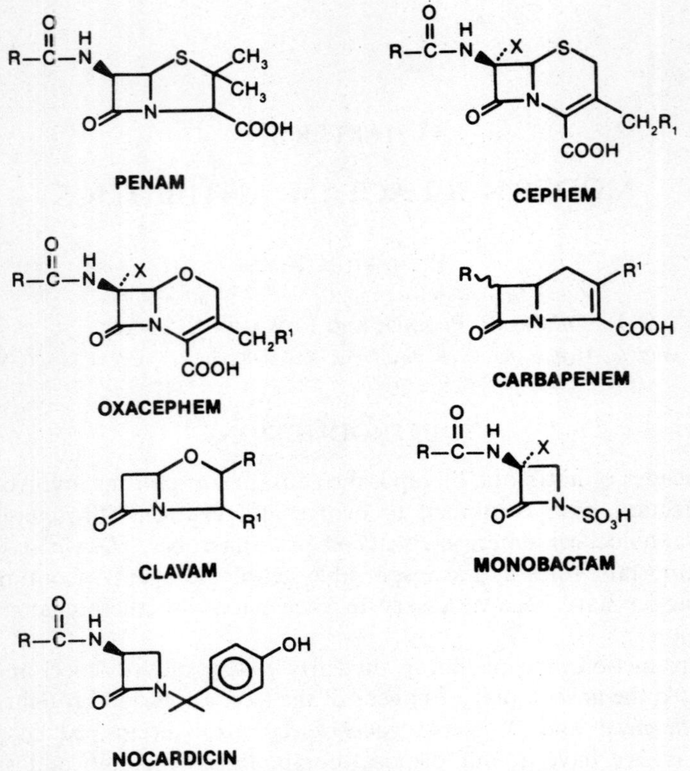

FIG. 1. Basic chemical structures of naturally-occurring β-lactam antibiotics.

of sulfur in the five membered clavam ring (Fig. 1) and represents the first suicide inhibitor of β-lactamases. The carbapenems (Fig. 1) represent a ubiquitous series of molecules produced by streptomycetes and bacteria, and include olivanic acids (Brown *et al.*, 1976), thienamycins (Albers-Schonberg *et al.*, 1978), epithienamycins (Stapley *et al.*, 1977), PS compounds (Okamura *et al.*, 1979), asperenomycins (Tanabe *et al.*, 1982), pluracidomycins (Box *et al.*, 1982), carpetimycins (Nakayama *et al.*, 1981), and SQ 27,860 (Parker *et al.*, 1982). As a family, the carbapenems exhibit potent broad spectrum anti-bacterial activity in addition to their inhibitory activity on the action of β-lactamases.

Following the discovery of β-lactams as products of fungi and actinomycetes, the first reports of β-lactam production by bacteria came in 1981 (Imada *et al.*, 1981; Sykes *et al.*, 1981b). The term monobactam was given to the bacterially-produced monocyclic β-lactam molecules, the first *N*-acyl β-lactam products to be described from bacteria (Sykes *et al.*, 1981b). Subsequently, cephalosporins, carbapenems and β-lactones have been observed as products of bacteria (Sykes *et al.*, 1982b).

As can be seen from the above summary, naturally-occuring β-lactams have been discovered in abundance during the last 10 years. However, during the 'Golden Era' of antibiotic discovery (1955–1965), no such molecules came to light. The rapid growth in the discovery of novel β-lactams over the past 10 years can largely be accounted for by the employment of novel screening techniques. The first β-lactams were discovered by observing zones of inhibition against susceptible wild-type bacteria. The growth in our understanding of the mode of action of β-lactam antibiotics and of their interaction with β-lactamases and the penicillin binding proteins in the cell membrane led to different screening approaches. The majority of β-lactam antibiotics can be monitored by their morphological effects on sensitive test organisms. Clavulanic acid and the carbapenems can be detected in screens devised to look for the effects of β-lactamase inhibition (Brown *et al.*, 1976).

The use of β-lactam supersensitive mutants of *Pseudomonas aeruginosa* derived by successive rounds of mutation was described by Kitano *et al.* (1976), to screen for β-lactams produced by fungi and actinomycetes. Aoki *et al.* (1976) used a β-lactam supersensitive strain of *Escherichia coli* to detect the nocardicins. The use of an *Escherichia coli* mutant-lacking chromosomal β-lactamase and penicillin binding component 1b, led to the discovery by Imada *et al.* (1981) of the monobactams sulfazecin and isosulfazecin in bacterial fermentations.

The screen used by Sykes *et al.* (1981b) which led independently to the discovery of the monobactams was a novel departure from earlier methods that depended on a visible zone of killing. The ability of *Bacillus licheniformis* to produce a β-lactamase in the presence of β-lactams is the basis for this screen (Sykes and Wells, 1985). When *Bacillus licheniformis* is grown in the presence of trace amounts of various β-lactams, β-lactamase is induced and secreted into the surrounding medium. If a chromogenic cephalosporin such as nitrocefin is now added, cleavage of the β-lactam ring occurs leading to a strongly colored product.

This method works only for intact β-lactam rings and is not dependent on intrinsic anti-bacterial activity. All classes of naturally occuring β-lactam antibiotics induce β-lactamase activity in this system, and the only non-β-lactams discovered to date that do so are the β-lactones (Sykes *et al.*, 1982b). Utilizing this technology, β-lactam antibiotics including the monobactams, carbapenems (Parker *et al.*, 1982) and a variety of cephalosporins (Singh *et al.*, 1983, 1984), have been discovered from bacteria.

The constant stream of new penicillins and cephalosporins, and novel β-lactam discoveries has opened innumerable paths for medicinal chemists to explore. From these explorations new and exciting therapeutic agents have begun to emerge (Fig. 2).

In addition to the large number of new compounds being made available for the treatment of infectious diseases, the use of antibiotics in combination has increased. This concept of using antibiotics in combination, although well tested and utilized in practice remains an area for debate in many areas of infectious disease.

Synergy between antibiotics is defined only on the *in vitro* level and is said to be present when the MIC of each drug tested in combination is four-fold or more lower than the MIC of each drug tested individually.

NEW β-LACTAM ANTIBIOTICS

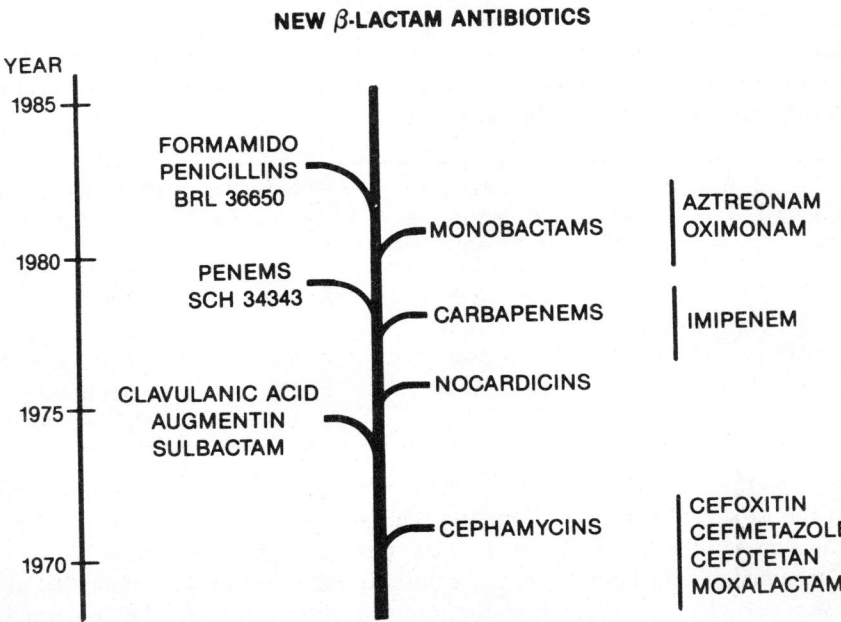

FIG. 2. Significant developments in β-lactam research since 1970.

Among β-lactam antibiotics, synergy can readily be observed with the combination of an enzyme susceptible compound and a β-lactamase inhibitor. For example, in the case of β-lactamase producing staphylococci dramatic changes in MIC values are observed when clavulanic acid is used in combination with ampicillin or amoxicillin. In this particular case, the synergist has little anti-bacterial activity in its own right but acts to protect the β-lactamase susceptible antibiotic against enzymatic inactivation. Such use of β-lactamase inhibitors is discussed in detail.

Antibiotic combinations which contain at least one β-lactam compound in the mix are widely used to achieve either a broader spectrum of activity or increased bactericidal action. Although relatively easy to demonstrate in the laboratory, the clinical significance of synergistic action is not always readily apparent. Perhaps the best and most widely recognised example is the combined use of a penicillin and an aminoglycoside for the treatment of streptococcal endocarditis. In this situation, there is little doubt that the synergistic action observed *in vitro* translates to the *in vivo* situation.

Penicillins and cephalosporins are often administered along with aminoglycosides for the treatment of nosocomial infections in immunosuppressed patients. Many comparative studies have been carried out in an attempt to identify the best pairing of specific β-lactam and specific aminoglycosides. In most instances, combination treatments appear to be similarly efficacious and superior to single drug therapy.

The combined use of β-lactam antibiotics with other β-lactams or with one of the innumerable antibotic classes used in clinical practice, in efforts to broaden the anti-bacterial spectrum of both agents is relatively common in the hospital setting. Whether true synergy is observed between such combinations, is open to question.

This article on modern β-lactam antibiotics is intended to include an in-depth discussion only of compounds that represent new developments in this continually expanding field of research and development. The major groups to be covered are penicillins, cephalosporins, oxacephems, carbapenems, β-lactamase inhibitors and the monobactams.

2. PENICILLINS

2.1. MICROBIOLOGY

The history of the penicillins has until recently, been one of an ever-broadening spectrum of activity. Starting from benzylpenicillin, whose activity is primarily directed against Gram-positive bacteria, we have 40 years later derivatives of 6-aminopenicillanic acid inherently active against most of the common bacterial pathogens of man. Penicillins can be divided into six groups on the basis of their anti-bacterial spectrum, stability to β-lactamases, and activity against *Pseudomonas aeruginosa*. Variation in structural type among these various groups can be seen in Fig. 3.

Group	Anti-bacterial spectrum	Stability to β-lactamases	Activity vs *Pseudomonas*	Representative compound
1	Narrow	No	No	Benzylpenicillin
2	Narrow	Yes	No	Methicillin
3	Broad	No	No	Ampicillin
4	Broad	No	Yes	Piperacillin
5	Narrow	Yes	No	Temocillin
6	Narrow	Yes	Yes	BRL 36650

In answer to the penicillin resistant, β-lactamase producing staphylococci came methicillin and the isoxazoyl penicillins, the first semi-synthetic penicillins. Ampicillin was the first of the semi-synthetic penicillins to show significant activity against Gram-negative bacilli. Carbenicillin and later ticarcillin extended the spectrum of ampicillin to include *Pseudomonas aeruginosa*. Presently, the ureido penicillins, represented by piperacillin (Fig. 3) mezlocillin and azlocillin have extended the spectrum still further to include strains of

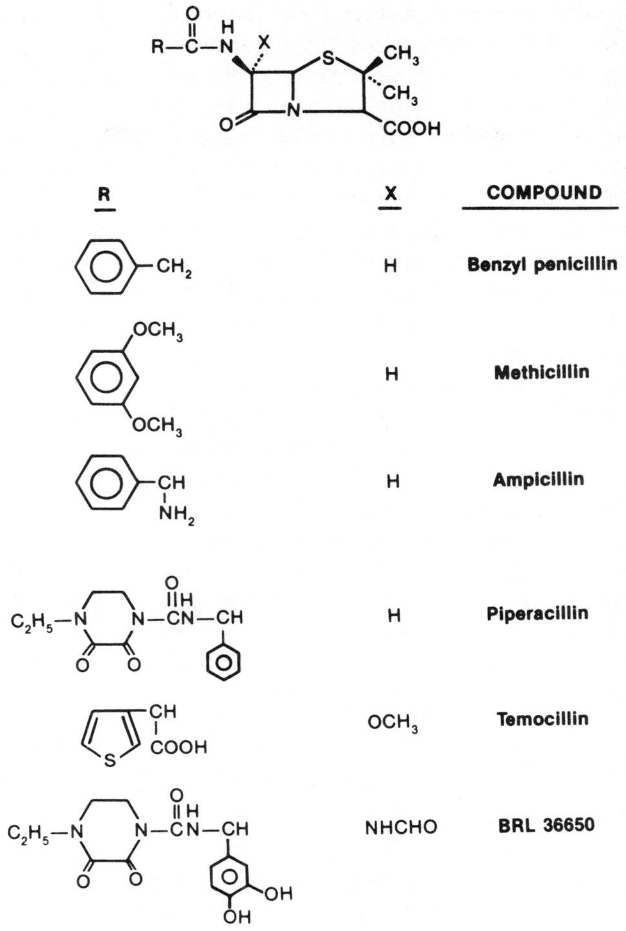

FIG. 3. Structural development among the penicillins.

Klebsiella and *Proteus*. So today, the broad spectrum penicillins claim activity against staphylococci, streptococci, *Hemophilus*, *Neisseria*, members of the *Enterobacteriaceae*, Gram-positive and Gram-negative anaerobes, and non-fermentative bacteria such as *Pseudomonas* and *Acinetobacter*.

Recent developments in the penicillin field have come full circle with a change in direction. Like methicillin, temocillin (6α-methoxy ticarcillin) exhibits a high degree of stability to β-lactamases and has a directed spectrum of activity (Slocombe *et al.*, 1981). In this case, however, the activity is directed not at Gram-positive bacteria but at aerobic Gram-negative bacteria excluding *Pseudomonas*.

The 6α-formamido penicillin, BRL 36650, is a relatively new development in the area of penicillin research (Basker *et al.*, 1984). This compound is reported to exhibit potent activity against Gram-negative bacteria including *Pseudomonas aeruginosa* and *Acinetobacter* sp., while showing little or no activity against Gram-positive organisms.

Among the newer penicillins, piperacillin appears the most potent and broadly active. From a comparative point of view, piperacillin and mezlocillin are more active than azlocillin against *Klebsiella*, whilst piperacillin and azlocillin are the more active against *Pseudomonas aeruginosa*. Piperacillin also appears to have the advantage over the other agents against strains of *Serratia marcescens* (Neu, 1983).

Among the Gram-negative bacteria, the ureido penicillins act through the inhibition of penicillin binding protein 3. As an initial consequence of binding, filamentation results, later followed by cell lysis and death (Metzger, 1982).

While seemingly ideal antibiotics, especially in the situation where empiric therapy may be required, the utility of the ureido penicillins is restricted by their β-lactamase instability. Susceptibility to staphylococcal β-lactamase presents a serious problem due to the high frequency of enzyme producing strains within this group both in and out of the hospital environment. Similarly, for certain groups of Gram-negative bacteria such as *Escherichia coli*, *Klebsiella* and *Hemophilus*, where a significant number of strains produce the plasmid mediated TEM − β-lactamase, the unrestrained use of the ureido penicillins as sole therapy would not augur for high clinical success. Thus, although piperacillin and the other ureido penicillins are active against a broad range of pathogens, they bear the selective yoke of β-lactamase instability which seriously constrains their extended spectrum. The viability of the ureido penicillins as single agents for serious infection of unknown cause will only be known with extended clinical use.

The real potential of the newer penicillins may be realized in combination with aminoglycosides. With such combinations, synergy is frequently observed *in vitro* against the *Enterobacteriaceae*, *Pseudomonas aeruginosa* and *Staphylococcus aureus*. The extent and degree of synergy varies with the particular penicillin and aminoglycoside used, but frequencies of 50–90% have been reported (Drusano *et al.*, 1984).

In an attempt to develop broad spectrum, β-lactamase stable penicillins, a family of compounds known as penems have made their appearance over the last few years (Fig. 4). These compounds exhibit a high degree of activity against Gram-positive and

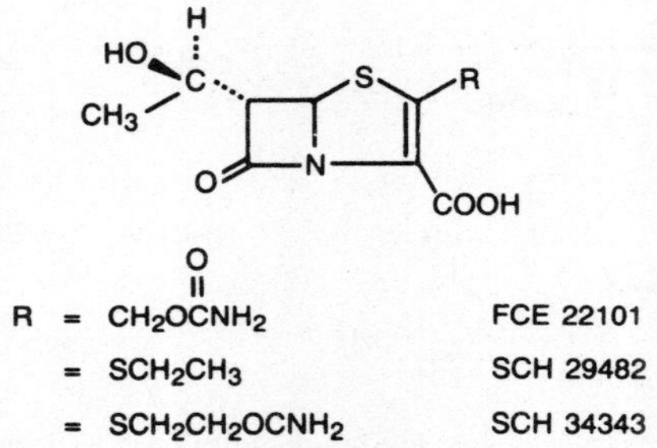

R = CH$_2$OCNH$_2$	FCE 22101
= SCH$_2$CH$_3$	SCH 29482
= SCH$_2$CH$_2$OCNH$_2$	SCH 34343

FIG. 4. Structural relationships among the synthetic penems.

Gram-negative bacteria but lack significant activity against *Pseudomonas aeruginosa* (Hare *et al.*, 1982). Although stable to the action of β-lactamases, like the carbapenems these compounds are susceptible to hydrolysis by mammalian renal dipeptidase (Mikami *et al.*, 1982). SCH 29482 (Fig. 4) (Phillips *et al.*, 1982) was tested extensively in humans and shown to be efficacious following oral administration. However, clinical studies were halted with the discovery that metabolic products excreted into the urine resulted in foul smelling odors. Both FCE 22101 (Sanfilippo *et al.*, 1982) and SCH 34343 (Adam *et al.*, 1984) being progressed by Carlo Erba and Schering, respectively, are injectable antibiotics with properties similar to SCH 29482.

2.2. PHARMACOLOGY

The recently developed ureidopenicillins are not absorbed orally and are therefore administered only parenterally. Pertinent pharmacokinetic properties are shown in Table 1 (Wright and Wilkowske, 1983). These compounds are metabolized only minimally (10%) and are excreted primarily unchanged by the kidney. Biliary excretion also occurs, and tends to compensate for diminished excretion in the presence of renal failure, resulting in only a minimal increase in serum half-life (from 1 to 4 hr), and a minimal need for dosage adjustment. For example, piperacillin administered as a 1-g dose to patients with creatinine clearances in the 0–19 ml/min per 1.73 m^2 range had a half-life of 3.9 hr and a serum clearance of 116 ml/min per 1.73 m^2, compared to corresponding values of 1.0 hr

TABLE 1. *Pharmacokinetic Properties of Ureidopencillins**

	Piperacillin	Mezlocillin	Azlocillin
Protein binding, %	20–40	20–40	20–40
Half-life, hr	1.0	0.8	0.8
Volume of distribution, l	16–19	18–19	18–19
Impaired elimination with renal dysfunction	minimal	minimal	minimal
Urinary excretion in 24 hr, %	70–80	60–70	60–70
Biliary excretion, %	20–30	20–30	20–30

*Adapted from Wright and Wilkowske, 1983.

and 297 ml/min per 1.73 m^2 in patients with creatinine clearances in the 16–102 ml/min per 1.73 m^2 range (Welling *et al.*, 1983). Consequently, patients with severe renal impairment should receive the usual dose at twice the usual dose interval to achieve average serum levels similar to individuals with normal renal function.

These compounds also exhibit non-linear dose-dependent pharmacokinetics, such that increasing the dose results in non-linear increases in antibiotic levels and decreased serum clearance, probably due to saturation of renal and non-renal clearance mechanisms (Bergan, 1981). For example, 1, 2, 4 and 6-gram doses of piperacillin yield peak serum levels of 71, 200, 331 and 452 μg/ml, respectively, half-lives of 0.60, 0.90, 1.02 and 1.05 hr, respectively, and serum clearances of 409, 302, 254 and 210 ml/min per 1.73 m^2 (Tjandramaga *et al.*, 1978).

Piperacillin pharmacokinetics for a 1-g intravenous dose are shown in Fig. 5 along with MIC$_{90}$ values for representative strains of common pathogens. Thus, due to the short half-life, relatively low serum levels and unimpressive activity against the great majority of organisms, large doses of drug are required at frequent intervals to be assured of success. Recommended intravenous doses of ureidopenicillins are 6–18 g/day for mild to moderate infections and 18–24 g/day for severe to life-threatening infections.

Piperacillin decreases the half-life of gentamicin in patients with end-stage renal disease (Thompson *et al.*, 1982), but has no significant effect on the kinetic profile of tobramycin in subjects with normal renal function (Lau *et al.*, 1983).

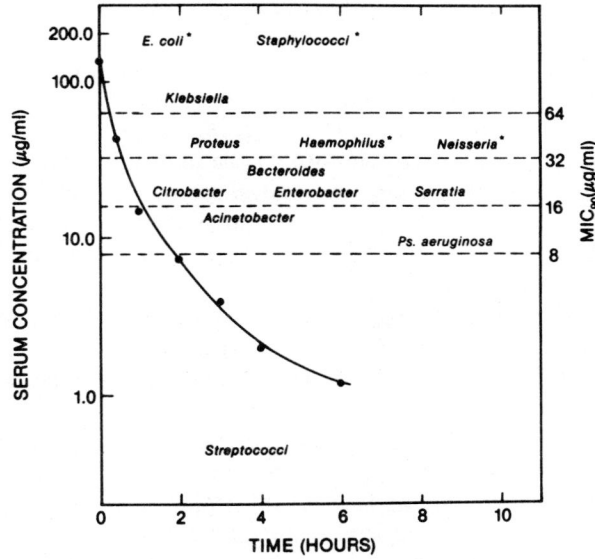

FIG. 5. Interrelationships between serum pharmacokinetics of piperacillin (1 g i.v.) (Evans *et al.*, 1978) and MIC$_{90}$ values (Barry *et al.*, 1985) for a range of clinically important bacteria.
*β-Lactamase producing strains.

3. CEPHALOSPORINS

3.1. Microbiology

Over 20 cephalosporins have become available for clinical use since cephalothin was first introduced in 1965. In addition, a number of new cephalosporins which are currently in various stages of development are expected to make their appearance over the next few years. This plethora of cephalosporins has made it difficult to distinguish one agent from another, particularly among those compounds that lack significant differences in micro-biological or pharmacological properties. Traditionally identified by 'generations' in order of introduction, the cephalosporins can be divided into three groups on the basis of activity spectrum, stability to β-lactamases and significant activity against *Pseudomonas aeruginosa*. The early cephalosporins, such as cephaloridine, cephalothin and cefazolin, display good activity against Gram-positive bacteria and are refractory to staphylococcal β-lactamase. Activity against Gram-negative bacteria such as *Escherichia coli*, *Proteus mirabilis* and *Klebsiella pneumoniae*, is of lesser magnitude and may be further restricted when the organism in question is a β-lactamase producer.

The next wave of cephalosporins, represented by cefuroxime and cefamandole, encom-pass more Gram-negative bacteria in their spectrum, as a result of increases both in inherent activity and β-lactamase stability. Although still resistant to staphylococcal β-lactamase, cefuroxime and cefamandole suffer from incremental decreases in Gram-positive activity.

Recently developed cephalosporins, characterized by the presence of an aminothiazole oxime moiety in the acyl side-chains, are highly active against the enteric bacteria, *Hemophilus* and *Neisseria*, and stable to the inactivating enzymes associated with these organisms. Group 3 compounds represented by ceftazidime, possess notable activity against *Pseudomonas aeruginosa*. As a group, the recently developed cephalosporins exhibit marginal activity against staphylococci and streptococci, despite being stable to Gram-positive β-lactamase.

Group	Anti-bacterial spectrum	Stability to β-lactamases	Activity vs *Pseudomonas*	Representative compound
1	Narrow	Poor	Yes	Cefsulodin
2	Broad	Poor	No	Cefuroxime
3	Broad	Yes	Yes	Ceftazidime

The aminothiazole oxime cephalosporins (Fig. 6), a product of the late 1970s, account for the majority of compounds finding their way to the market place over the last few years. These compounds which continue to dominate cephalosporin research programs fit into the group 3 category. Ceftazidime, an aminothiazole oxime, is representative of the group 3 compounds and is a recent introduction to the cephalosporin armamentarium. Com-pounds in the development stage that are ceftazidime-like include HR-810 and BMY 28142 (Fig. 6). The properties of ceftazidime will be discussed in detail with reference to other cephalosporins where appropriate.

Ceftazidime is distinguished among the new cephalosporins by its good activity against *Pseudomonas aeruginosa* and other *Pseudomonas* species. With MIC_{90} values for *Pseudo-monas* in the single digit range, ceftazidime is 8–16-fold more active than cefotaxime, ceftriaxone and ceftizoxime for this group of non-fermentative bacteria (Harris *et al.*, 1981; Bint *et al.*, 1981). Like cefotaxime and other members of the class, ceftazidime is highly active against the *Enterobacteriaceae*, *Hemophilus* and *Neisseria*, with MIC_{90} values typically at or below 1 μg/ml (Fig. 8). Occasional strains of *Enterobacter* exhibit high level resistance to ceftazidime and related compounds, an event probably mediated principally by permeability difficulties since these compounds are very stable to Class I β-lactamases. When compared to cephaloridine, ceftazidime exhibits at least 100-fold increase in stability against the more common TEM, OXA and SHV plasmid-mediated β-lactamases (Sykes

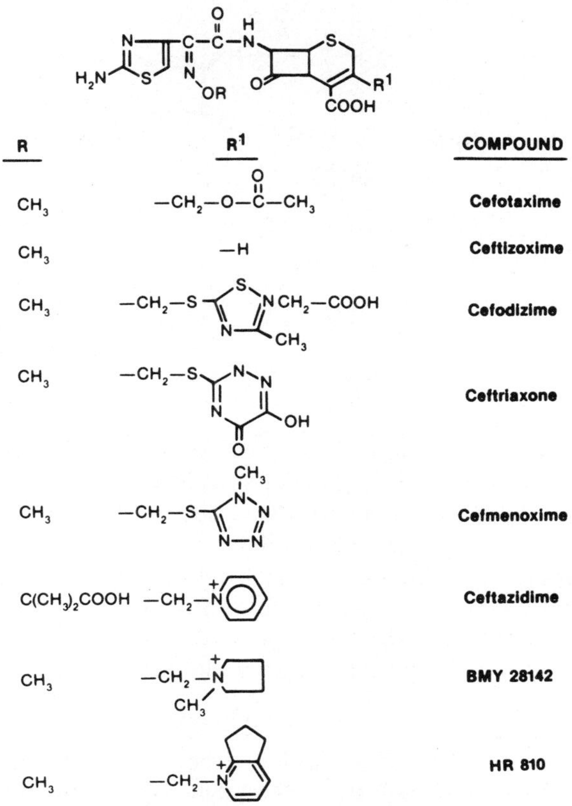

R	R¹	COMPOUND
CH₃	$-CH_2-O-\overset{\overset{O}{\|\|}}{C}-CH_3$	Cefotaxime
CH₃	—H	Ceftizoxime
CH₃	—CH₂—S thiadiazole NCH₂—COOH / CH₃	Cefodizime
CH₃	—CH₂—S triazine OH / O	Ceftriaxone
CH₃	—CH₂—S tetrazole CH₃ / N—N	Cefmenoxime
C(CH₃)₂COOH	—CH₂—N⁺ pyridinium	Ceftazidime
CH₃	—CH₂—N⁺ pyrrolidinium CH₃	BMY 28142
CH₃	—CH₂—N⁺ cyclopenta-fused pyridinium	HR 810

FIG. 6. Structure development among the aminothiazole oxime cephalosporins.

and Bush, 1983). Similarly for the chromosomally determined β-lactamases from *Entero-bacter*, *Proteus*, *Pseudomonas* and *Serratia*, ceftazidime shows a marked improvement in stability over the earlier compounds (Sykes and Bush, 1983). The only β-lactamase showing appreciable hydrolysis of ceftazidime is the relatively uncommon PSE-2 plasmid mediated enzyme encountered in some strains of *Pseudomonas* (Harper, 1981).

Although considered broad spectrum agents, the activity of ceftazidime and related compounds against Gram-positive bacteria is clinically questionable. Against staphylococci and streptococci, ceftazidime is 10–100-fold less active than cephalothin and cephaloridine (Phillips *et al.*, 1981b; Knothe and Dette, 1981). *Streptococcus faecalis* is not susceptible to this class of compounds nor are methicillin-resistant staphylococci. Against anaerobic bacteria a similar situation exists. While some of the Gram-positive anaerobes are marginally susceptible to ceftazidime, Gram-negative anaerobes including the *Bacteroides fragilis* group are poorly inhibited (Phillips *et al.*, 1981b). This is a major distintinguishing factor between the aminothiazole oximes and the cephamycins and oxacephems.

To overcome resistance and provide a broader spectrum of activity, ceftazidime and related compounds have been combined with aminoglycosides and the potential of synergistic interaction studied. *In vitro* synergy has been noted for these combinations against multiply resistant pseudomonads and moderately susceptible members of the *Enterobacteriaceae*. Depending on organism and combination, the extent of synergy varies, but frequencies of 60–90% have been observed (Jones and Packer, 1982; Giamarellou *et al.*, 1984).

In terms of further development, cephalosporin research is once again chasing the goal of broad spectrum antibiotic activity. Two compounds under development, HR-810 (Jones *et al.*, 1984) and BMY 28142 (Neu *et al.*, 1984), both appear to have advantages in this

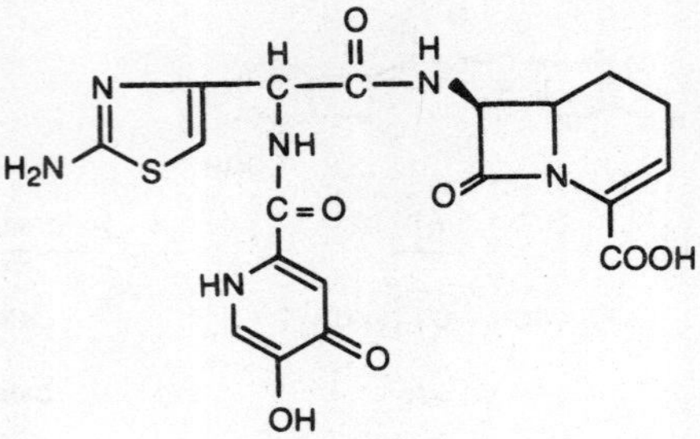

FIG. 7. Carbacephem: KT 4697.

respect. These new molecules retain the activity of ceftazidime against Gram-negative bacteria but in addition, show increased activity against Gram-positive organisms. There is also data to suggest that these compounds may be more effective against cephalosporin resistant *Enterobacter* and *Acinetobacter* strains.

An additional group of compounds closely related to the cephalosporins are the carbacephems. Recently described (Mochida *et al.*, 1984), these molecules exhibit broad spectrum anti-bacterial activity including high activity against *Pseudomonas aeruginosa*. The most potent and metabolically stable compound in this series was KT 4697 (Fig. 7).

3.2. PHARMACOLOGY

The pharmacology of new cephalosporins has recently been reviewed, and is summarized in Table 2. The relatively short half-life of cefotaxime vs the long half-life of ceftriaxone are noteworthy, as this influences greatly the dose interval used in clinical applications. Also, unlike the other new cephalosporins, cefoperazone is eliminated primarily by the biliary route. Ceftazidime has the lowest degree of protein binding.

The serum pharmacokinetic profile of ceftazidime following a 1-g intravenous dose along with MIC_{90} values for commonly encountered bacteria is shown in Fig. 8. Good pharmacokinetic properties and potent activity against the *Enterobacteriaceae*, make ceftazidime a drug of choice for treating such infections. *Pseudomonas aeruginosa* should be covered adequately, but other *Pseudomonas* species, *Acinetobacter* and *Enterobacter* will require high and frequent dosing if good clinical efficacy is to be achieved on a regular basis.

The effects of cefoperazone and ceftazidime on the fecal flora have been studied. Cefoperazone, administered parenterally to patients with various sites of infection, produced a marked reduction in Gram-positive and Gram-negative aerobic bacteria, as well as anaerobes (Alestig *et al.*, 1983). In contrast, in healthy volunteers receiving multiple doses of ceftazidime, there was preservation of fecal anaerobes, with a marked reduction in fecal *Enterobacteriaceae* (Kemmerich *et al.*, 1983).

TABLE 2. *Pharmacokinetic Properties of Cephalosporins**

	Cefotaxime	Ceftizoxime	Ceftriaxone	Cefoperazone	Ceftazidime
Protein binding	40	30	90	90	17
Half-life, hr	1.1	1.9	8	2	1.8
Volume of distribution, l	27	18	9	12	16
Impaired elimination with renal dysfunction	Yes	Yes	Yes	No	Yes
Urinary excretion in 24 hr, %	60	80	80	20	85
Biliary excretion, %	Yes	–	–	Yes	Yes

*Adapted from Neu, 1982, and Barriere and Flaherty, 1984.

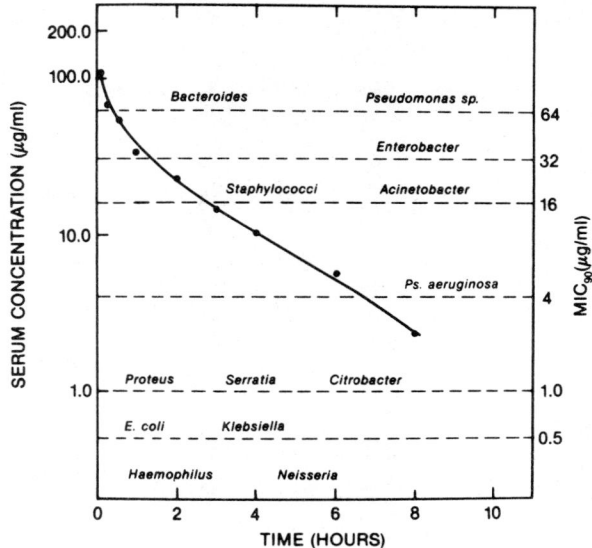

FIG. 8. Interrelationships between serum pharmacokinetics of ceftazidime (1 g i.v.) (Harding *et al.*, 1981b) and MIC$_{90}$ values (Jones *et al.*, 1981) for a range of clinically important bacteria.

Ceftazidime is eliminated primarily in the urine, but also undergoes biliary excretion. The pharmacokinetics are independent of dose over the range 0.25–2.0 g (Harding *et al.*, 1981a). Intravenous doses of 0.5, 1, and 2 g produce serum levels of 39, 83 and 188 μg/ml (Neu, 1982). The pharmacokinetic behavior of ceftazidime is similar in male and female volunteers, with the exception that the peripheral compartment volume of distribution in females was about two-thirds the value for males (attributed to a smaller extracellular fluid volume in females) (Sommers *et al.*, 1983).

Because ceftazidime is primarily eliminated in the urine, it is to be expected that renal insufficiency will delay the elimination of this compound (Welage *et al.*, 1984). The renal excretion of ceftazidime occurs by glomerular filtration only, based upon a ceftazidime/creatinine renal clearance ratio near unity and upon probenecid studies (Harding *et al.*, 1981b). Administration of ceftazidime to patients with normal or moderately impaired renal function can temporarily reduce glomerular filtration by 10 ml/min in patients with bacterial infections (Alestig *et al.*, 1984).

Ceftazidime undergoes hemodialysis, having a serum half-life of 2.8 hr during dialysis compared with 25 hr between dialysis sessions (Fillastre *et al.*, 1983).

In newborn infants, a 50 mg/kg intravenous dose of ceftazidime gave plasma concentrations of 102–124 μg/ml. The elimination half-life ranged from 2.9–6.7 hr and varied inversely with gestational age (McCracken *et al.*, 1984).

4. CEPHAMYCINS AND OXACEPHEMS

4.1. MICROBIOLOGY

Following the discovery of the naturally occuring cephamycins (Nagarajan *et al.*, 1971), clinically useful semi-synthetic derivatives made their appearance (Fig. 9). Cefoxitin, the first of the cephamycins to be used clinically, is now one of the most frequently used antibiotics in the United States. Cefmetazole and cefotetan are marketed in Japan, and cefotetan is being developed for worldwide usage.

Substitution of oxygen for sulfur in the dihydrothiazine ring of the cephamycins led to the development of the oxacephems (Yoshida *et al.*, 1981). Moxalactam was the first oxacephem antibiotic introduced as a broad spectrum agent in 1978. Subsequently, a number of other compounds in the series have been reported (Goto *et al.*, 1984; Komatsu

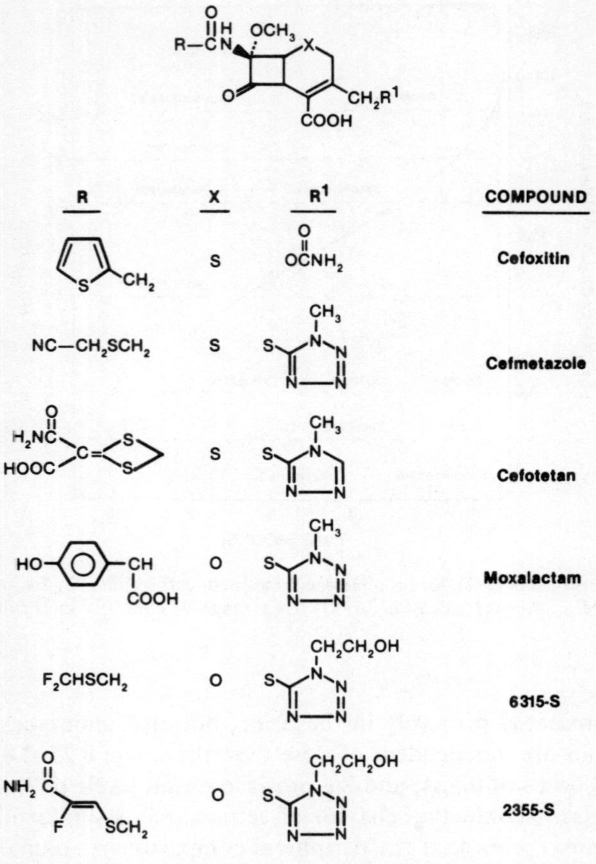

FIG. 9. Structural development among the cephamycins and oxacephems.

et al., 1984). A common feature of all compounds of this type is their remarkable stability to hydrolysis by a wide range of β-lactamases.

The cephamycins and oxacephems can be distinguished on the basis of anti-pseudomonal activity.

Group	Anti-bacterial spectrum	Stability to β-lactamases	Activity vs *Pseudomonas*	Representative compound
Cephamycin	Broad	Yes	No	Cefoxitin
Oxacephem	Broad	Yes	Yes	Moxalactam

Moxalactam exhibits broad spectrum activity against Gram-positive and Gram-negative aerobic and anaerobic bacteria (Carmine *et al.*, 1983). Unlike the cephamycins, moxalactam has moderate activity against *Pseudomonas aeruginosa*. At concentrations of less than 1 μg/ml, it inhibits 90% of strains of *Escherichia coli*, *Klebsiella* species, *Proteus* species, *Morganella morganii*, *Neisseria gonorrhoeae*, *Hemophilus influenzae*, and *Salmonella* species. Ninety per cent of *Enterobacter* and *Serratia* species are inhibited by 8 μg/ml or less. Against *Pseudomonas*, MIC_{90} values are reported to be around 50 μg/ml (Fig. 10).

In contrast to many of the newer β-lactam antibiotics and like cefoxitin, moxalactam exhibits good activity against anaerobes (Phillips *et al.*, 1981b). Anaerobic bacteria, such as *Bacteroides fragilis*, *Fusobacterium nucleatum* and *Clostridium perfingens*, are usually inhibited by 2–16 μg/ml. As a broad spectrum agent, the main weakness of moxalactam lies in its relatively poor activity against staphylococci and streptococci. In most studies,

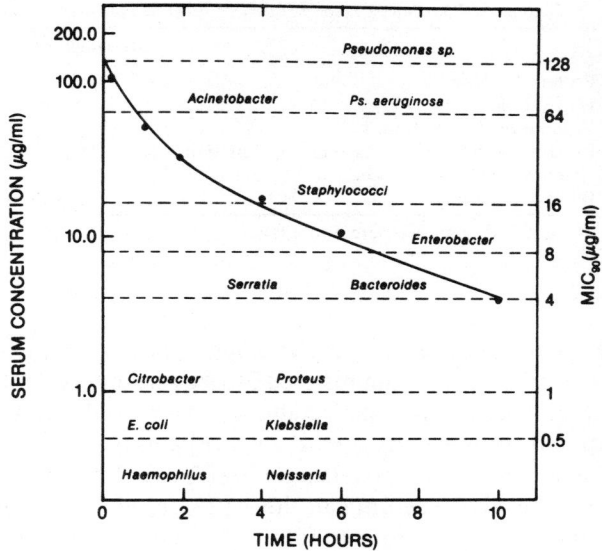

FIG. 10. Interrelationships between serum pharmacokinetics of moxalactam (1 g i.v.) (Luthy et al., 1981) and MIC_{90} values (Jones et al., 1981) for a range of clinically important bacteria.

the level of moxalactam required to inhibit 90% of *Staphylococcus aureus* strains ranges between 6–16 μg/ml; methicillin resistant *Staphylococcus aureus* and *Staphylococcus epidermidis* strains are uniformly resistant. For *Steptococcus pneumoniae*, MIC_{90} values are around 2 μg/ml, whereas the *viridans* group of organisms show values ranging between 2–8 μg/ml. Strains of *Streptococcus faecalis* are resistant to moxalactam (Carmine et al., 1983). Development of the newer oxacephems such as 6315-S and 2355–S (Fig. 9), has been stimulated in part by this deficit of moxalactam.

In vitro, moxalactam shows a high degree of stability to chromosomal and plasmid mediated β-lactamases, including those produced by anaerobes. However, recent reports suggest that moxalactam hydrolysing enzymes are in existence (Warren et al., 1980). Against many of the class 1 chromosomal enzymes, moxalactam has been reported to act as a β-lactamase inactivator (Richmond, 1980). In the case of the *Enterobacter* P99 β-lactamase, moxalactam has a high affinity for the enzyme with an exceptionally low turnover number. The half-life for enzyme release is greater than two hr (Bush et al., 1982). Like the great majority of β-lactam-containing molecules, moxalactam is a potent inducer of certain class 1 β-lactamases. In certain strains of *Enterobacter*, high levels of β-lactamase induced by moxalactam are directly related to drug resistance in the absence of substantial evidence for hydrolysis (Bush et al., 1985).

Moxalactam, like other β-lactam antibiotics, binds to transpeptidase and D-alanine carboxypeptidase, thereby inhibiting the cross-linking reaction in the biosynthesis of the bacterial cell wall peptidoglycan. In *Escherichia coli* moxalactam binds preferentially to PBP 3 but also exhibits high affinity for PBPs 1A, 1B and IV (Komatsu and Nishikawa, 1980).

4.2. PHARMACOLOGY

The first oxacephem available for clinical use is moxalactam, and the pharmacokinetic properties of this compound have been studied extensively (Table 3). Probenecid has no effect on the renal handling of moxalactam. About 30–50% of a dose of moxalactam is removed by hemodialysis (Barriere and Flaherty, 1984), however, peritoneal dialysis does not remove a significant amount of this drug from the body, as indicated by a lack of effect of peritoneal dialysis on the serum half-life of moxalactam (Neu, 1983).

Moxalactam serum pharmacokinetics following a 1 g intravenous dose along with MIC_{90} values for commonly occuring bacterial pathogens are shown in Fig. 10. It is apparent from

TABLE 3. *Pharmacokinetic Properties of Oxacephems**

	Moxalactam
Protein binding, %	50
Half-life, hr	2.3
Volume of distribution, l	20
Impaired elimination with renal dysfunction	Yes
Urinary excretion in 24 hr, %	80
Biliary excretion	Yes

*Adapted from Barriere and Flaherty, 1984.

the figure that adequate coverage for *Pseudomonas*, and *Acinetobacter* will only be obtained if large doses of drug are administered at frequent intervals. Due to the relative insusceptibility of staphylococci to moxalactam, the data would suggest that additional therapy may be required in infections due to such organisms.

The pharmacokinetic profile of moxalactam has been determined in neonates and infants. As might be expected, the serum half-life is prolonged in newborns less than seven days old (5–7.5 hr), and in newborns one to four weeks old (4.4 hr); infants have a half-life of 1.6 hr (Schaad *et al.*, 1981). In elderly volunteers, elimination of moxalactam is mildly impaired due to renal insufficiency (Andritz *et al.*, 1984).

Moxalactam given parenterally to healthy volunteers causes a marked decrease in both anaerobic and aerobic fecal bacteria (Allen *et al.*, 1980). It has been hypothesized that the hypoprothrombinemia and platelet dysfunction caused by moxalactam as well as the cephalosporins, cefamandole and cefoperazone may be related to alterations in gut flora; however, the moxalactam molecule itself or a metabolite may also interfere with the vitamin-K-mediated γ-carboxylation of glutamic acid, a step necessary for prothrombin to bind calcium and exert its biologic effect (Smith and Lipsky, 1983). Moxalactam can also inhibit platelet function, and can lead to a disulfiram-like reaction in subjects ingesting ethanol, an effect also linked to the methyltetrazolethiol side-chain of moxalactam (Buening *et al.*, 1981).

5. CARBAPENEMS

5.1. MICROBIOLOGY

The carbapenems resemble penicillins in having a β-lactam ring fused to a five-membered ring. They differ in that the five-membered ring is unsaturated and does not contain sulfur (Fig. 1). Sulfur is, however, present in all the carbapenems isolated from streptomycetes. Well over 30 examples of carbapenems have been isolated to date and, with the exception of SQ 27,860, which is derived from bacteria (Parker *et al.*, 1982), they are produced by species of *Streptomyces*.

Despite the close chemical similarity between the carbapenems, a wide variety of names are applied to them. *Streptomyces cattleya* produces five thienamycins (Kahan *et al.*, 1979; Rossie *et al.*, 1981). *Streptomyces olivaceus* produces eight olivanic acids (Hood *et al.*, 1979; Box *et al.*, 1982), the PS compounds are produced by *Streptomyces cremeus auratalis* (Okamura *et al.*, 1979), the carpetimycins are from *Streptomyces griseus* (Imada *et al.*, 1980), the asparenomycins are produced by *Streptomyces tokunonensis* (Kawamura *et al.*, 1982) and the pluracidomycins and the epithienamycins by *Streptomyces pluracidomyceticus* (Tsuji *et al.*, 1982) (See Table 4).

Many of the naturally-occuring carbapenems are potent antibiotics, with activity against a broad range of Gram-positive and Gram-negative bacteria (Hoover, 1983). Much of the attraction of this class of compounds lies in their ability to act both as potent antibiotics and as inhibitors of β-lactamase. The configuration of the optically active side-chains (8R, 8S) and whether the C5,6 stereochemistry is *cis* or *trans* are major considerations in the balancing of these activities.

TABLE 4. *Naturally-occurring Carbapenems**

R¹	R²	Stereochemistry (C5,6)	Name	Producing organism
—CH(CH₃)OH	—SCH₂CH₂NH₂	trans	Thienamycin	S. cattleya
—CH(CH₃)OH	—SCH₂CH₂NHCOCH₃	trans	N-acetylthienamycin	S. cattleya
—CH(CH₂)OH	—SCH=CHNHCOCH₃	trans	N-acetyldehydrothienamycin	S. cattleya
—CH₂CH₃	—SCH₂CH₂NH₂	trans	Deshydroxythienamycin	S. cattleya
—CH₂OH	—SCH₂CH₂NH₂	cis	Northienamycin	S. cattleya
—CH(CH₃)OH	—SOCH=CHNHCOCH₃	trans	Epithienamycin B sulfoxide	S. pluracidomyceticus
—CH(CH₃)OH	—SOCH=CHNHCOCH₃	cis	Epithienamycin D sulfoxide	S. pluracidomyceticus
—CH(CH₃)OH	—SCH₂CH₂N:COCH₃	cis	MM22380	S. olivaceus
—CH(CH₃)OH	—SCH₂CH₂NHCOCH₃	trans	MM22381	S. olivaceus
—CH(CH₃)OH	—SCH=CHNHCOCH₃	cis	MM22382	S. olivaceus
—CH(CH₃)OH	—SCH=CHNHCOCH₃	trans	MM22383	S. olivaceus
—CH(CH₃)OSO₃H	—SCH=CHNHCOCH₃	cis	MM13902	S. olivaceus
—CH(CH₃)OSO₃H	—SCH₂CH₂NHCOCH₃	cis	MM17880	S. olivaceus
—CH(CH₃)OSO₃H	—SCH=CHNHCOCH₃	cis	MM4450	S. olivaceus
—CH(CH₃)OSO₃H	—SCH=CHNHCOCH₂CH₃	cis	MM27696	S. olivaceus
—CH₂CH₃	—SCH₂CH₂NHCOCH₃	trans	PS5	S. cremeus auraitilis
—CH(CH₃)CH₃	—SCH₂CH₂NHCOCH₃	trans	PS6	S. cremeus auraitilis
—CH₂CH₃	—SCH=CHNHCOCH₃	trans	PS7	S. cremeus auraitilis
—C(CH₃)CH₃	—SCH=CHNHCOCH₃	trans	PS8	S. cremeus auraitilis
—C(CH₃)CH₂OH	—SOCH=CHNHCOCH₃	cis	Carpetimycin A: C19393H₂	S. griseus (cryophilus)
—C(CH₃)CH₃OSO₃H	—SOCH=CHNHCOCH₃	cis	Carpetimycin B: C19393S₂	S. griseus (cryophilus)
—CH(CH₃)CH₃OSO₃H	—SOCH₂COOH	cis	Pluracidomycin B	S. pluracidomyceticus
—CH(CH₃)CH₃OSO₃H	—SOCH(OH)₂	cis	Pluracidomycin C	S. pluracidomyceticus
=C(CH₃)CH₂OH	—SOCH=CHNHCOCH₃		Asparenomycin A	S. tokunonensis
=C(CH₃)CH₂OH	—SOCH₂CH₂NHCOCH₃		Asparenomycin B	S. argenteolus
=C(CH₃)CH₂OH	—SCH=CHNHCOCH₃		Asparenomycin C	S. argenteolus
—CH(CH₃)OSO₃H	—SO₃H	cis	SF2103A: Pluracidomycin A	S. sulfonofaciens
—CH(CH₃)OSO₃H	—SCH₂CH₂NH₂	cis	8U-2107	S. mojinensis
—CH₂CH₃	—SCH₂CH₂NCOCH₃CH₂NHCO	trans	OA6129A	Streptomyces sp.
—CH(CH₃)OH	HOCH₂C(CH₃)CH(OH)CO	cis	OA6129B₁	Streptomyces sp.
—CH(CH₃)OH	HOCH₂C(CH₃)₂CH(OH)CO	trans	OA6129B₂	Streptomyces sp.
—CH(CH₃)OSO₃H	HOCH₂C(CH₃)₂CH(OH)CO	cis	OA6129C	Streptomyces sp.
—H	—H		SQ 27,860	Serratia: Erwinia

*Reproduced from O'Sullivan and Sykes, 1985.

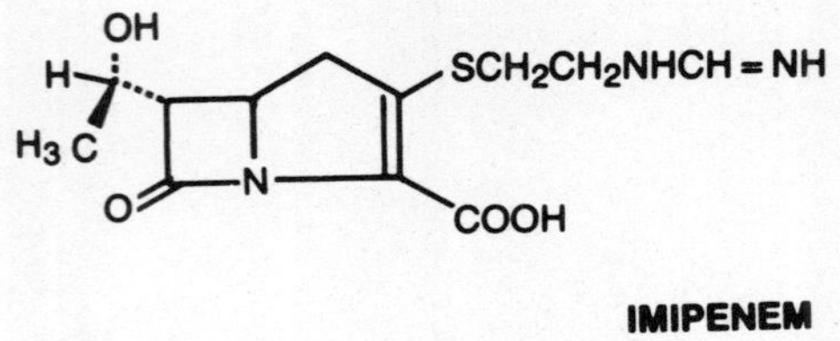

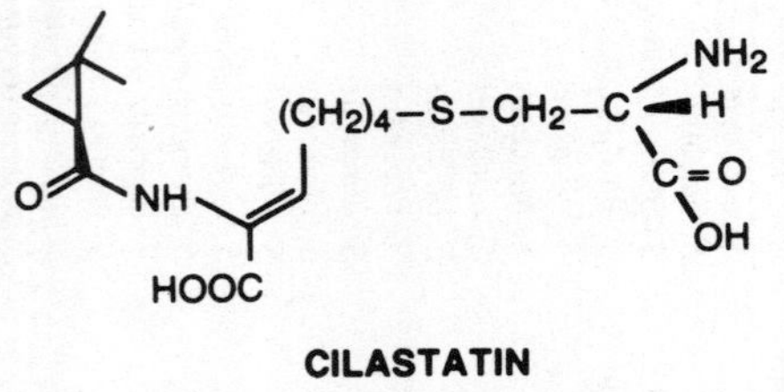

FIG. 11. Imipenem and the dihydropeptidase inhibitor cilastatin.

Although the carbapenems exhibit a high degree of stability to β-lactamases, unlike other β-lactam containing antibiotics (with the exception of penems), they are susceptible to hydrolytic cleavage by mammalian dipeptidase (Kropp *et al.*, 1982).

The first carbapenem to be studied in detail as an anti-microbial agent was thienamycin. Despite the outstanding potency of thienamycin it turned out to be unsuited for clinical development, due to chemical instability (Kahan *et al.*, 1983). Synthesis of the amidine derivative, *N*-formimidoyl thienamycin (imipenem, MK0787) (Fig. 11), resulted in a stable crystalline product with anti-bacterial properties superior to those of thienamycin.

The breadth of spectrum and level of activity of imipenem is unequalled among β-lactam antibiotics. The basis for this activity arises from an ability to interact with multiple PBPs by overcoming the permeation barrier usually afforded by the outer membrane (Vuye, 1982). With *Escherichia coli* imipenem binds preferentially to PBPs 1 and 2, while in *Staphylococcus aureus* the PBPs showing greatest affinity are 1, 3 and 4 (Spratt *et al.*, 1977; Georgopapadakou and Liu, 1980). The morphological consequence for *Escherichia coli* is the conversion to spheres or ellipsoids with death rapidly ensuing, a response typically associated with inhibition of PBP2.

In terms of inherent activity, imipenem resembles the best of the penicillins but has the added advantage of being stable to most of the commonly occuring β-lactamases. In direct enzyme studies imipenem has been found stable to the β-lactamases from *Staphylococcus aureus* and *Bacteriodes fragilis* as well as type 1a, 111a and 1Vc β-lactamases. In addition, against the 1a and *Bacteriodes* enzymes, imipenem was found to be an inhibitor (Richmond, 1981). A larger study involving 28 enzyme preparations representative of plasmid and chromosomally mediated β-lactamases confirmed the stability of imipenem. Only three of the preparations showed detectable hydrolysis of imipenem. Rates were equal to or less than 1 % of that observed for cephaloridine (Hanslo *et al.*, 1981). The only β-lactamase showing appreciable hydrolysis of imipenem is an inducible penicillinase found in strains of *Pseudomonas maltophilia* (Saino *et al.*, 1982). This unusual metal-loenzyme, although having a low affinity for imipenem, exhibits significant hydrolytic activity. However, like the naturally occuring carbapenems, imipenem is susceptible to hydrolysis by mammalian dipeptidase (Mikami *et al.*, 1982).

Imipenem is highly active against Gram-positive bacteria including most staphylococci and streptococci. As with other β-lactam antibiotics the methicillin resistant staphylococci appear non-susceptible to imipenem particularly when the testing is carried out at 30°C. The enterococci vary in their susceptibility to imipenem. In one study, strains of *Streptococcus faecium* were found less susceptible than strains of *Streptococcus faecalis*, with minimal bactericidal concentrations for both species greatly exceeding the minimal

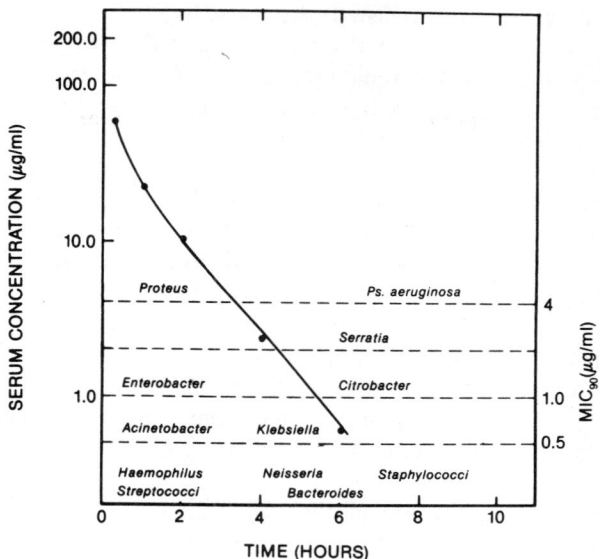

FIG. 12. Interrelationships between serum pharmacokinetics of imipenem (1 g i.v.) (Norrby *et al.*, 1983) and MIC$_{90}$ values (Kahan *et al.*, 1983) for a range of clinically important bacteria.

inhibitory concentrations (Eliopoulos and Mollering, 1981). The activity seen with imipenem against Gram-positive bacteria extends to Gram-negative bacteria as well. Members of the *Enterobacteriaceae* are almost uniformly susceptible to imipenem as are strains of *Neisseria* and *Hemophilus*. Among the non-fermentors, strains of *Pseudomonas aeruginosa* and *Acinetobacter* are generally susceptible. Many other pseudomonads are also susceptible but one group showing marked resistance are strains of *Pseudomonas maltophilia*, perhaps reflecting the lability of imipenem to the β-lactamase produced by this organism. Gram-positive and Gram-negative anaerobic bacteria are usually susceptible to imipenem. The only exceptions in this area are strains of *Clostridium difficile* which are relatively resistant and occasional isolates of *Bacteriodes fragilis* which may be highly resistant (Tally and Jacobus, 1983) (Fig. 12).

When tested in combination with aminoglycosides, imipenem has shown the potential for synergistic interactions. Against strains of *Pseudomonas aeruginosa* and *Staphylococcus aureus* isolated from patients with endocarditis, enhanced killing has been observed with an imipenem-tobramycin combination (Kallick *et al.*, 1982). Synergy against enterococci has also been observed when imipenem was combined with gentamicin, tobramycin or amikacin (Eliopoulos and Moellering, 1981; Gombert *et al.*, 1983).

5.2. PHARMACOLOGY

Imipenem is the first carbapenem antibiotic to undergo clinical pharmacology studies. A recently published review serves as the basis for the following discussion (Norrby *et al.*, 1983). Imipenem undergoes extensive metabolism by a dipeptidase, dehydropeptidase I, located on the brush border of the proximal tubular cells of the kidney. Renal dipeptidase from swine kidney hydrolyzes imipenem, but not aztreonam, penicillin G, or cephaloridine (Mikami *et al.*, 1982).

Intravenous 20 min infusions of 500 or 1000 mg of imipenem in healthy subjects produced peak serum levels of approximately 33 and 61 μg/ml. The serum half-life was 1 hr, while 0–8 hr urinary recovery varied between 6 and 38% of dose. These relatively low urinary recoveries are explained by the hydrolysis of the β-lactam ring of imipenem by the renal dipeptidase. Plasma protein binding is about 25%. Probenecid produced only a small increase in half-life of imipenem.

Concentrations of imipenem in the sera of volunteers receiving a 1-g intravenous dose are shown in Fig. 12 along with MIC$_{90}$ values for a commonly occuring bacteria. Although highly potent against all organisms listed, the short half-life of the drug will necessitate frequent dosing to cope effectively with *Pseudomonas*, *Proteus* and *Serratia* infections.

Because of some concern that the renal metabolism of imipenem in humans might result in sub-optimal levels of antibiotic in the urinary tract (Kropp *et al.*, 1982), the effect of co-administration of dehydropeptidase inhibitors on the disposition of imipenem was studied. Co-administration of a 0.5 or 1 g dose of imipenem with 0.25, 0.5, or 1 g doses of a dihydropeptidase inhibitor, cilastatin (MK0791) (Fig. 11), resulted in the same half-life for imipenem (1 hr) but a markedly increased urinary recovery of imipenem (70% of dose). Increasing doses of cilastatin caused prolonged inhibition of renal metabolism of imipenem, although plasma kinetics were not affected by the degree of renal metabolism of the drug. Nearly 100% of the radioactivity in a radiolabeled dose of imipenem was recovered in the urine, with biliary excretion being <1%, judging from fecal recovery of radioactivity. Even with co-administration of cilastatin, about 30% of a dose of imipenem could not be recovered as active drug in the urine, suggesting that imipenem is metabolized by mechanisms other than the renal dehydropeptidase and that these metabolites are excreted by the kidneys.

Identification and characterization of the metabolites of imipenem, and the effect of renal and hepatic disease on the disposition of imipenem remain unanswered questions. The kinetics of cilastatin action require further study. Additional studies are also needed to fully describe the complex clinical pharmacology of the imipenem–cilastatin drug combination.

6. MONOBACTAMS

6.1. MICROBIOLOGY

Traditional approaches aimed at improving the biological properties of β-lactam antibiotics have, until recently, focused almost entirely on a bicyclic nucleus. The basic assumption that a fused ring system was essential for meaningful anti-bacterial activity was formulated early in the development of penicillin and has held throughout the discovery and development of the cephalosporins, cephamycins and carbapenems. Discovery of the monocyclic nocardicins and subsequent structure–activity studies on these poorly active molecules gave added support to the fused ring theory. Constraints imposed by this doctrine have focused structural alterations of the β-lactam antibiotics to peripheral changes on the bicyclic framework. The discovery of the monobactams and subsequent molecular variation around the central monobactam ring has initiated a radical departure from this precept.

The term monobactam derives from the unique chemical structure and biological origin of these agents: monocyclic β-lactam antibiotics produced by bacteria. Monobactams have been found as products of six bacterial genera (Table 5) and differ in the nature of the acyl substituent and also in the presence or absence of a methoxy group at the 3 α-position of the β-lactam ring (Fig. 1). All naturally-occuring monobactams are *N*-acyl derivatives of 3-amino-2-oxo-1-azetidinesulfonic acid (3-aminomonobactamic acid). In contrast to the penicillins and cephalosporins which derive from the products of fermentation, monobactams can be prepared synthetically from amino acids.

Although none of the naturally-occuring monobactams exhibit impressive anti-bacterial activity (Sykes *et al.*, 1981a) side-chain modification, as with the penicillins and cephalosporins, has led to the development of potently active molecules.

The first monobactam to be tested clinically was aztreonam, an injectable, directed spectrum antibiotic. A second compound of the aztreonam type (AMA 1080/RO 17–2301) has recently been described (Kondo *et al.*, 1983). In addition to these injectable compounds, an orally available monobactam is under development (Tanaka *et al*, 1984) (Fig. 13). The biological properties of aztreonam will be discussed in detail as the prototype member of the monobactam class.

Aztreonam, like all members of the β-lactam family, interferes with the biosynthesis of bacterial cell walls. In aerobic Gram-negative bacteria, aztreonam causes filamentation at its lowest effective concentration, a morphological effect identical to that observed with the majority of cephalosporins (Russell, 1981). The penicillin binding protein (PBP) profile indicates a very high affiinity for PBP3 for a wide range of aerobic Gram-negative bacteria (Georgopapadakou et al., 1982). The relative inactivity of aztreonam against Gram-positive bacteria and anaerobes derives from a poor interaction with the essential PBPs of these organisms (Sykes et al., 1982a).

As would be expected from any recently developed β-lactam antibiotic, aztreonam shows a high degree of stability to β-lactamases (Bush et al., 1982). The broad spectrum plasmid mediated β-lactamases exhibit little or no observable hydrolytic activity against aztreonam. Among the broad spectrum chromosomally mediated enzymes, the K1 lactamase produced by certain strains of Klebsiella oxytoca is one of the few enzymes which have been shown to hydrolyze aztreonam to any significant degree.

The most diverse group of β-lactamases are represented by the chromosomally mediated cephalosporinases. These enzymes, produced by the great majority of Gram-negative bacteria, may be constitutive or inducible and appear to play an important role in the resistance of many bacteria to cephalosporins (Sykes and Matthew, 1976). The behavior of aztreonam towards this diverse group of enzymes, varies from that of a β-lactamase inhibitor to a poor enzyme substrate. The cephalosporinases produced by strains of Enterobacter are strongly inhibited by aztreonam, which has been reported to act as a tight-binding competitive substrate (Bush et al.,1982) and as a β-lactamase inactivator for these enzymes (Labia et al., 1983). The tenacity with which aztreonam and some of the newer cephalosporins bind to Class 1 β-lactamases has been implicated as an antibiotic resistance mechanism. Studies by Bush et al. (1985) have been unable to confirm these observations for aztreonam. Working with multiply resistant strains of Enterobacter, these workers have shown that resistance appears to be a function of cell impermeability to the drug, and that there is little contact between the periplasmically-located β-lactamase and the potential inhibitor. Recent studies by Vu and Nikaido (1985) would also support these observations.

Chromosomal β-lactamases produced by rare strains of Pseudomonas maltophilia, Bacteroides fragilis (Percival et al., 1981; Phillips et al., 1981a) and a strain of Proteus vulgaris (Seigel et al., 1983) have been shown to hydrolyse aztreonam.

An unusual aspect of aztreonam in its interaction with β-lactamases involves the property of inducibility. Unlike the great majority of β-lactam antibiotics, aztreonam fails to induce β-lactamase production in Class I enzyme producing strains (Bush and Sykes, 1982).

The anti-bacterial spectrum of aztreonam is unique among β-lactam antibiotics. Unlike the great majority of β-lactam containing compounds, aztreonam exhibits little or no activity against Gram-positive bacteria, such as staphylococci and streptococci, or against anaerobic bacteria. In contrast, however, aztreonam is a potent inhibitor of aerobic Gram-negative bacteria. The great majority of Enterobacteriaceae strains are inhibited at less than 1 μg/ml. Particularly sensitive are members of the Proteus-Providencia group, Escherichia coli, Serratia marcescens and Klebsiella pneumoniae (Sykes et al., 1981a, 1982a; Paradelis et al., 1983). Similarly, the drug has proved highly active against ampicillin-sensitive and resistant strains of Hemophilus influenzae and Neisseria gonorrhoeae, with the majority of strains inhibited at less than 0.1 μg/ml. For Pseudomonas aeruginosa, the MIC_{50} value is around 4 μg/ml and the MIC_{90} value around 12 μg/ml (Fig. 4).

In anticipation that aztreonam will be used in combination with other antibiotics either to broaden the coverage for initial therapy or to increase potency against infections of the granulocytopenic host, both in vitro and in vivo interaction studies have been carried out. In combination with nafcillin, cloxacillin, erythromycin or vancomycin, aztreonam produced no deleterious effects on the activity of these compounds against Gram-positive organisms. Likewise, the activity of aztreonam against Gram-negative bacteria was unaffected in the presence of these agents (Tanaka et al., 1983a). In combination with aminoglycoside antibiotics, aztreonam has been reported to exhibit a high incidence of synergistic activity against strains of Pseudomonas aeruginosa (Tanaka et al., 1983b; Rehm et al., 1983).

TABLE 5. *Monobactams Isolated from Natural Sources*

R	R^1	SQ No.	Organism
	OCH$_3$	26,180	Chromobacterium violaceum
	OCH$_3$	26,823	Agrobacterium radiobacter
	OCH$_3$	26,857	Agrobacterium radiobacter
	H	26,700	Agrobacterium radiobacter
	OCH$_3$	26,970	Agrobacterium radiobacter
	OCH$_3$	26,812	Agrobacterium radiobacter

R	R^1	SQ No.	Organism
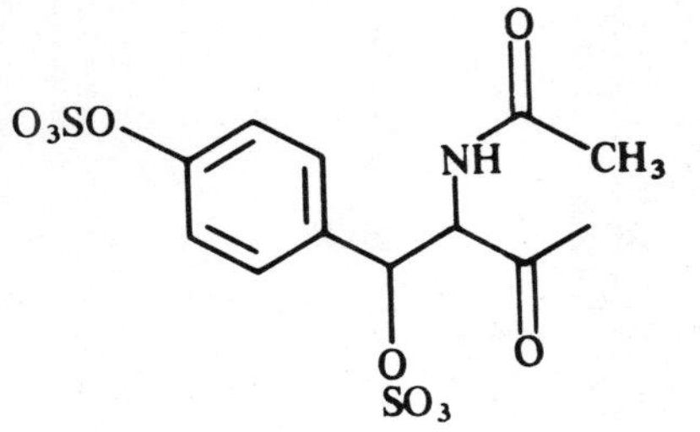	H	28,332	Flexibacter

| 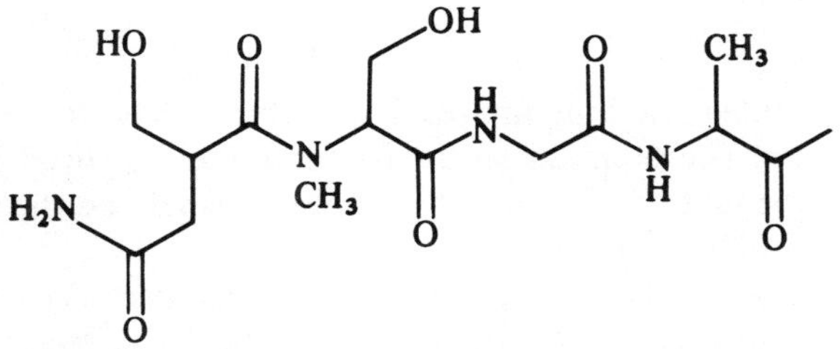 Oligopeptide (MW 1462) | H | 28,502 | Flexibacter |
| Oligopeptide (MW 1446) | H | 28,503 | Flexibacter |

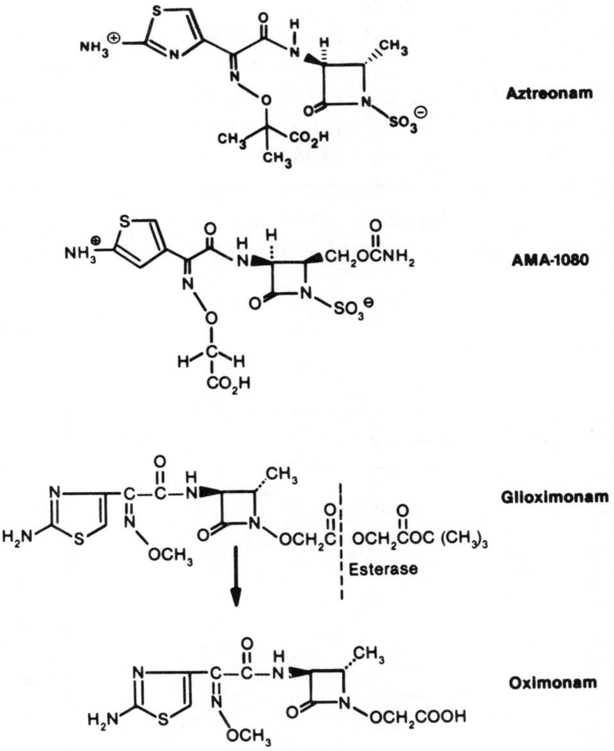

FIG. 13. Monobactams.

6.2. PHARMACOLOGY

The first monobactam antibiotic to undergo clinical development is aztreonam (Swabb *et al.*, 1981). Recently a second monobactam, AMA 1080 or Ro 17-2301, has undergone clinical pharmacology studies (Weidekamm *et al.*, 1984). Key pharmacokinetic properties

TABLE 6. *Pharmacokinetic Properties of Monobactams*

	Aztreonam	AMA1080*
Protein binding, %	56†	18
Half-life, hr	1.7‡, 2.0§	1.8
Volume of distribution, l	11‡, 15§	17
Impaired elimination with renal dysfunction	Yes§	–
Urinary excretion in 24 hr, %	68‡, 74‖	78–89
Biliary excretion, %	15¶	ca. 3

*Weidekam *et al.*, 1984.   §Mihindu *et al.*, 1983.
†Swabb *et al.*, 1983a.   ‖Wise *et al.*, 1982.
‡Swabb *et al.*, 1982.   ¶Swabb *et al.*, 1982b.

of these compounds in healthy volunteers are summarized in Table 6. The two mono-bactams have very similar half-lives. The elimination of aztreonam is impaired in the presence of renal failure, such that the half-life is about three times normal and the serum clearance is one-fourth normal (Mihindu *et al.*, 1983).

Both monobactams are eliminated primarily in the urine in unchanged form. Aztreonam also undergoes biliary excretion, estimated for healthy subjects to be 15%, based upon fecal recovery of radioactivity after a 0.5 g parenteral dose (Swabb *et al.*, 1983b). Aztreonam undergoes metabolism to a minor extent, as indicated by the appearance of 7% of a 0.5 g dose in the urine as the open-β-lactam-ring derivative, SQ 26,992 (analogous to the penicillioate metabolite of penicillin).

These two monobactams display linear pharmacokinetics. Serum concentrations of aztreonam administered as 0.5, 1, and 2-g 30-min intravenous infusions to healthy volunteers were 66, 164 and 225 μg/ml, respectively (Scully *et al.*, 1983), somewhat higher than values for AMA 1080 of 36, 78 and 150 μg/ml after the same intravenous doses infused over 20 min (Weidekamm *et al.*, 1984).

The serum levels of aztreonam following a 1-g intravenous 3-min infusion compared with MIC$_{90}$ values for various Gram-negative and Gram-positive bacteria are shown in Fig. 14. For the *Enterobacteriaceae* as well as *Hemophilus* and *Neisseria*, therapeutic levels

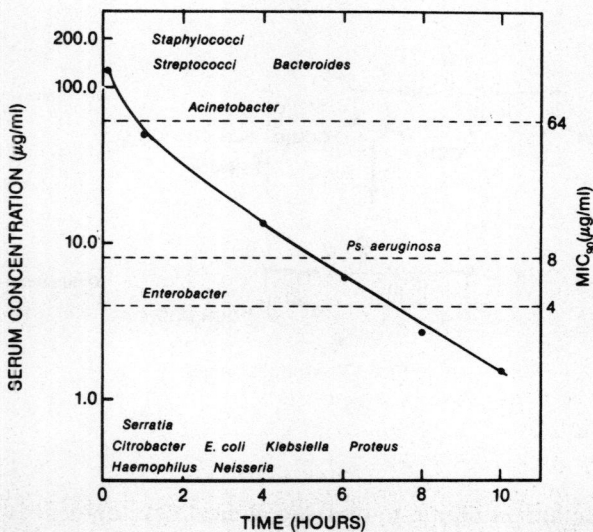

FIG. 14. Interrelationships between serum pharmacokinetics of aztreonam (1 g i.v.) (Swabb *et al.*, 1982) and MIC$_{90}$ values (Jones *et al.*, 1984) for a range of clinically important bacteria.

are achieved for 8–12 hr. Strains of *Enterobacter* and *Pseudomonas*, being less susceptible than the *Enterobacteriaceae*, will be more effectively treated with higher dosage regimens.

Probenecid does not have a major effect on the pharmacokinetic profile of aztreonam, although elimination of aztreonam by net tubular secretion is reduced (Swabb *et al.*, 1983c). No clinically significant drug interaction has been found between aztreonam and cephradine, clindamycin, gentamicin, metronidazole, or nafcillin (Creasey *et al.*, 1984).

Aztreonam undergoes clearance by both hemodialysis and chronic ambulatory peritoneal dialysis (CAPD). Hemodialysis can remove about 50% of a dose in four hr, while CAPD removes only 10% of a dose in 48 hr (Gerig *et al.*, 1984; Fillastre *et al.*, 1985).

The pharmacokinetics of aztreonam in pediatric patients has been reported (Stutman *et al.*, 1984). Newborns <7 days old and <2500 g body weight had impairment of elimination of aztreonam (half-life 5.7 hr). An *in vitro* study showed that, under physiologic conditions, aztreonam (as well as imipenem and azlocillin) did not displace bilirubin bound to albumin, whereas sulfazoxazole, moxalactam and cefoperazone did increase unbound bilirubin (Stutman *et al.*, 1985).

Aztreonam appears to be only poorly immunogenic when given in multiple doses to humans (Adkinson *et al.*, 1984) and to be poorly cross-reactive *in vivo* (Saxon *et al.*, 1984) and *in vitro* (Adkinson *et al.*, 1984) with IgE antibody to penicillin. Also, multiple intravenous doses of aztreonam produce marked reduction in the numbers of fecal aerobic Gram-negative bacilli without notably altering the numbers of fecal anaerobes (Jones *et al.*, 1984).

7. β-LACTAMASE INHIBITORS

7.1. MICROBIOLOGY

The major resistance mechanism to β-lactam antibiotics among bacteria is enzymatic inactivation by β-lactamases. The ability of pathogenic bacteria to produce a diverse array of plasmid or chromosomally-mediated β-lactamases has been a constraining factor on the utility of susceptible β-lactam antibiotics. In recent years, considerable effort has been expended in developing β-lactams refractory to the hydrolytic enzymes, and the appearance of third-generation cephalosporins, oxacephems, carbapenems and the monobactams are the direct result of this approach. However, β-lactamase-stable penicillins exhibiting broad spectrum activity remain elusive. An alternative approach with regard to penicillins, has been to search for molecules capable of inactivating the β-lactamase, thereby protecting the susceptible β-lactam from enzymatic degradation. The ability of alkoxy- (e.g. methicillin) and isoxazolyl- (e.g. cloxacillin) penicillins to inhibit β-lactamases has been known from the early 1960s. These compounds act as competitive inhibitors of some β-lactamases and act synergistically *in vitro* with β-lactamase susceptible β-lactam antibiotics (Cole, 1979). However, the clinical usefulness of such combinations has not been adequately demonstrated.

Since the middle 1970s, several β-lactam compounds have been reported which irreversibly inhibit β-lactamases (Fig. 15). These are the naturally-occuring clavulanic acid and carbapenems and the semi-synthetic penicillanic acid sulfones and halopenicillanic acids. With the exception of the carbapenems, the compounds by themselves are poor antibiotics but act synergistically when combined with β-lactamase-susceptible β-lactams.

Clavulanic acid is a naturally produced compound consisting of a β-lactam ring fused to an oxazolidine ring (Howarth *et al.*, 1976). Clavulanic acid was first isolated from *Streptomyces clavuligerus* in a screening program designed to detect inhibitors of β-lactamases produced by *Klebsiella aerogenes* (Brown *et al.*, 1976). Since the initial report, six other members of the clavam series of β-lactam compounds have been isolated from natural sources (O'Sullivan and Sykes, 1985).

Clavulanic acid, by itself, is a poor anti-bacterial agent with MIC values generally in the range of 25–125 μg/ml for Gram-positive and Gram-negative bacteria. Exceptions have been found with strains of *Neisseria gonorrhoeae* and *Legionella pneumophilia* being inhibited at the level of 1 μg/ml. The importance of clavulanic acid lies in its ability to

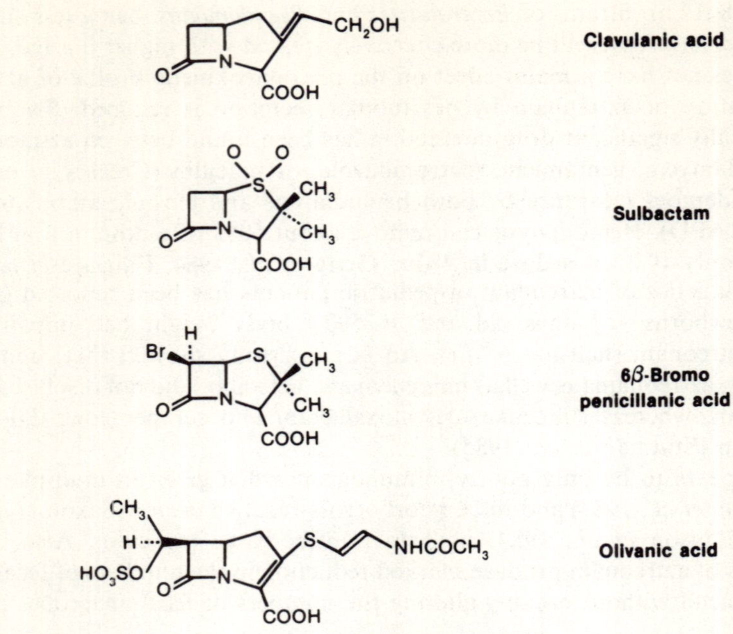

FIG. 15. β-lactamase inhibitors.

inhibit a wide range of β-lactamases of clinical importance, thus potentiating the activity of enzyme susceptible penicillins and cephalosporins against β-lactamase producing resistant bacteria.

The interaction of clavulanic acid with β-lactamase has been studied in three different enzyme systems: the *Escherichia coli* R-TEM enzyme (Charnas *et al.*, 1978; Fisher *et al.*, 1978), the *Staphylococcus aureus* PC1 enzyme (Reading and Hepburn, 1979), and the *Bacillus cereus* 1 enzyme (Durkin and Viswanatha, 1978). All three enzymes are inhibited progressively with the rate and extent of inhibition being different with all three enzymes.

The mechanism of inactivation has been studied extensively with *Escherichia coli* R-TEM β-lactamase. Incubation of the enzyme with clavulanic acid results first in the destruction of the clavulanic acid followed by the formation of a catalytically inactive transient clavulanate–enzyme complex, resulting finally in the formation of a catalytically inactive stable clavulanate–enzyme complex. The transient complex is formed at a faster rate than the irreversibly inactivated complex, but it decomposes to free enzyme and thus eventually all of the enzyme accumulates in the irreversibly inactivated form (Fisher *et al.*, 1978; Fig. 16).

Clavulanic acid shows a broad affinity for penicillin binding proteins of *Escherichia coli*, binding to PBPs 1, 4, 5 and 6 with moderate affinity and poor binding to PBP 3 (Spratt *et al.*, 1977).

The utility of clavulanic acid is seen when combined with a compound such as amoxicillin. Synergistic effects have been noted against amoxicillin-resistant strains of *Staphylococcus aureus*, *Escherichia coli*, *Klebsiella pneumoniae*, *Proteus mirabilis* and *Bacteroides fragilis*. The clavulanic-amoxicillin combination is currently in clinical use

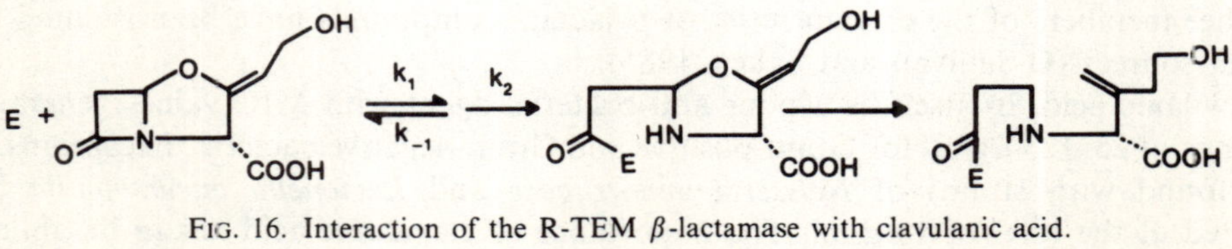

FIG. 16. Interaction of the R-TEM β-lactamase with clavulanic acid.

under the name Augmentin. A combination of clavulanic acid and ticarcillin is also currently undergoing clinical evaluation.

Among the penicillin sulfones, the first such compound to be reported was 6-desaminopenicillanic acid sulfone (CP 45899) (Fig. 15) (English *et al.*, 1978), which resembles clavulanic acid structurally with its lack of substitution at C6 of the β-lactam ring. The compound (sulbactam) is similar to clavulanic acid in profile. Like clavulanic acid, sulbactam is only weakly inhibitory to enzymes exhibiting primarily cephalosporinase activity (Fu and Neu, 1979).

A third group of compounds being developed as β-lactamase inhibitors are the 6-halopenicillanic acids (Fig. 15) (Pratt and Loosemore, 1978). These compounds exhibit weak anti-bacterial activity against most Gram-positive and Gram-negative bacteria (with the exception of *Neisseria*), but are potent inhibitors of various β-lactamases. In this respect, 6α-bromopenicillanic acid and its iodo analogue compare favorably with clavulanic acid whereas the 6-chloropenicillanic acid is less active (Daehne, 1980).

7.2. PHARMACOLOGY

Single oral doses of 250, 500, 750 and 1000 mg of clavulanic acid resulted in dose-proportional mean peak serum levels of 5.8, 10.9, 14.5 and 19.3 μg/ml, respectively (Hoffken *et al.*, 1981; Jackson *et al.*, 1980). Food does not appear to influence the oral absorption of clavulanic acid (Jackson *et al.*, 1980). A 200-mg bolus injection of 1 g amoxicillin and 200 mg clavulanic acid gave peak plasma concentrations of 105 and 28 μg/ml, respectively (Croydon *et al.*, 1981).

TABLE 7. *Pharmacokinetic Properties of β-Lactamase Inhibitors*

	Clavulanic acid (PO)	Sulbactam* (IV)
Protein binding, %	–	–
Half-life, hr	0.97†	0.97
Volume of distribution, l	–	23
Impaired elimination with renal dysfunction	Yes‡	–
Urinary excretion, %	27–39% in 6 hr†	76% in 12 hr
Biliary excretion, %	–	–

*Foulds *et al.*, 1983.
†Jackson *et al.*, 1980.
‡Hoffler and Dalhoff, 1980.

The percentage of a dose absorbed after oral administration of clavulanic acid has not been reported; however, urinary recovery data (Table 7) suggest at least 30% bioavailability after oral administration. It appears to be extensively degraded, and displays 11% degradation/hr in pooled human serum at 37°C (Munch *et al.*, 1981). The serum pharmacokinetic profile and urinary elimination of clavulanic acid is not influenced by co-administration of amoxicillin. Similarly, the pharmacokinetics of amoxicillin are not significantly altered by clavulanic acid (Jackson *et al.*, 1980). Co-administration of probenecid with the combination of amoxicillin and clavulanic acid reduces the renal clearance of amoxicillin and clavulanic acid by 50% and 25%, respectively (Staniforth *et al.*, 1983). While probenecid elevated the serum concentration of amoxicillin, there was no effect on the area under the serum concentration–time curve for clavulanic acid. The pharmacokinetics of a single intravenous dose of clavulanic acid with amoxicillin have been described in pediatric patients (Schaad *et al.*, 1983).

The usual oral dosage in adult patients with moderately severe infections is 250 mg amoxicillin plus 62.5 or 125 mg clavulanic acid every eight hr. Higher doses are suggested in more severe infections (Brogden *et al.*, 1981).

8. CLINICAL ADVANCES AND LIMITATIONS OF
MODERN β-LACTAMS

The newer β-lactams have provided many opportunities to treat serious bacterial infections with lower doses and longer dose intervals, compared with older members of the penicillin and cephalosporin families. Most of these new compounds have been studied in a wide variety of clinical situations: lower respiratory tract infection, urinary tract infections, septicemia, skin and skin structure infections, bone and joint infections, as well as infections in the abdominal and pelvic cavities. There is only limited experience in the therapy of meningitis. However, published clinical experience has not yet led to clear guidelines for the preference of one new β-lactam over another, or the preference of a newer β-lactam over an older, probably cheaper β-lactam. All compounds are widely regarded as having good safety profiles.

The clinical safety of new β-lactam antibiotics has recently been reviewed, and will not be discussed in detail here (Parry, 1984). However, it is important to note that cephalosporin induced coagulopathies are under active investigation, prompted by reports of hypothrombinemia associated with the N-methylthiotetrazole side-chain-containing antibiotics, including moxalactam, cefoperazone and cefamandole (Seeler and Reitan, 1984). These same compounds are also associated with disulfiram-like reactions when ethanol is ingested by patients receiving these agents. Enterococcal superinfections during moxalactam therapy have drawn attention also. In contrast, the new penicillins do not appear to have new or unique toxicities.

Because of the growing concern of rising costs for health care, the pricing of new β-lactam antibiotics is likely to influence their availability on many hospital formularies. There is growing recognition in the field of antibiotic research and development of the importance of demonstrating not only efficacy and safety but also cost effectiveness. The latter factor is likely to play an ever increasing role in antibiotic development over the coming decade.

9. CONCLUDING REMARKS

For almost 45 years β-lactam antibiotics have remained the cornerstone of antibiotic therapy. With the exception of infections caused by mycobacteria and those bacteria which lack peptidoglycan, β-lactam antibiotics have proved safe and efficacious in the treatment of bacterial disease.

The two major resistance mechanisms expressed by bacteria to this group of antibiotics have been apparent from the early days of their clinical usage. Following its introduction, penicillin became progressively less effective against staphylococci due to the production by these organisms of a penicillin hydrolysing enzyme, penicillinase. In addition, penicillin proved to be relatively inactive against the majority of Gram-negative bacteria due to its inability to penetrate the outer membrane layers of these organisms and thus reach the sensitive target proteins located in the cytoplasmic membrane. These two resistance mechanisms, antibiotic exclusion and enzymatic hydrolysis, have continued to plague the β-lactam family up to the present day. The have, in retrospect, been the major driving forces behind the continual development of this antibiotic class. In recent years additional resistance mechanisms have been identified which reside almost exclusively with the Gram-positive bacteria. These include alterations in the target proteins (penicillin binding proteins), and changes that interfere directly with the lytic action of the drug.

From a clinical standpoint, enzymatic hydrolysis of β-lactam molecules has been the cause for greatest concern. Highly efficient enzymes have developed along with the β-lactams such that for every known compound to date there exists a β-lactamase with the capacity to hydrolyse it. The most serious problems have been caused by the plasmid-mediated β-lactamases whose mobile genes have shown little discrimination for bacterial genus or class. Many of the modern β-lactams exhibit little or no susceptibility to these enzymes and thus represent a great stride forward in overcoming the resistance encoded by these ubiquitous genes. Because of their ability to withstand plasmic-determined enzymatic hydrolysis, the new compounds impose no selection for plasmid-carrying strains and are thus to be recommended over enzyme-sensitive molecules. The chromosomally mediated β-lactamases produced in one form or another by the majority of Gram-negative bacteria exhibit weak hydrolytic activity against the new β-lactam compounds and in themselves pose no serious threat.

In terms of intrinsic activity, the new compounds have made important contributions particularly with regard to gram-negative bacteria. In contrast however, the intrinsic activity of Penicillin G against susceptible Gram-positive organisms remains unsurpassed.

With regard to organism selectivity, we have at our disposal compounds directed specifically against Gram-positive and/or Gram-negative bacteria or against a specific genus.

The pharmacokinetic properties of the β-lactams are equally diverse, ranging from the short lived penicillins to cephalosporins with half-lives of up to eight hr.

With the β-lactamase conquered, at least temporarily, the major potential resistance problem for the modern β-lactams is most likely to be penetrability β-lactam-resistant strains of *Enterobacter* producing large amounts of Class I β-lactamase, appear to owe their resistance to antibiotic exclusion rather than antibiotic destruction (Bush *et al.*, 1985). Non-fermenting Gram-negative rods such as pseudomonads and strains of *Acinetobacter* often exhibit high level resistance to β-lactam antibiotics, which again appears to be a function of antibiotic exclusion. Under these circumstances, slow diffusion of the antibiotic into the cell increases the likelihood of becoming prey to an otherwise inefficient β-lactamase (Vu and Nikaido, 1985). Thus, inability of antibiotics to penetrate the outer membrane of these organisms appears to be a major factor contributing to the observed resistance.

These developing trends in antibiotic resistance mechanisms are already shaping the molecules of the future in the constant battle against an ever changing microbial population.

REFERENCES

ADAM, C., NAPLES, L., WEISS, W., SABATELLI, F., HARE, R., LOEBENBERG, D. and MILLER, G. (1984) Evaluation of the *in vitro* antibacterial activity of Sch 34343. 24th Interscience Conference on Antimicrobial Agents and Chemotherapy. Washington DC. Abstract 217.

ADKINSON, N. F., JR., SWABB, E. A. and SUGERMAN, A. A. (1984) Immunology of the monobactam aztreonam. *Antimicrob. Ag. Chemother.* **25**: 93–97.

ALBERS-SCHONBERG, G., ARISON, B. H., HENSENS, O. D., HIRSHIELD, J., HOOGSTEEN, K., KACZKA, E. A., RHODES, R. E., KAHAN, F. M., RATCLIFFE, R. W., WALTON, E., RUSWINKLE, L. J., MORIN, R. B. and CHRISTENSEN, B. G. (1978) Structure and absolute configuration of thienamycin. *J. Am. Chem. Soc.* **100**: 6491–6499.

ALESTIG, K., CARLBERG, H., NORD, C. E. and TROLLFORS, B. (1983) Effect of cefoperazone on faecal flora. *J. Antimicrob. Chemother.* **12**: 163–167.

ALESTIG, K., TROLLFORD, B., ANDERSON, R., OLAISON, L., SUURKULA, M. and NORRBY, S. R. (1984) Ceftazidime and renal function. *J. Antimicrob. Chemother.* **13**: 177–181.

ALLEN, S. D., SIDERS, J. A., CROMER, M. D., FISCHER, J. A., SMITH, J. W. and ISRAEL, K. S. (1980) Effect of LY127935 (6059-S) on human fecal flora. In: *Current Chemotherapy and Infectious Disease*, pp. 101–103, NELSON, J. D. and GRASSI, C. (eds) The American Soc. for Micro., Washington, DC.

ANDRITZ, M. H., SMITH, R. P., BLATCH, A. L., GRIFFIN, P. E., CONROY, J. V., SUTPHEN, N. and HAMMER, M. C. (1984) Pharmacokinetics of moxalactam in elderly subjects. *Antimicrob. Ag. Chemother.* **25**: 33–36.

AOKI, H., SAKAI, H., KOHSAKA, M., KONOMI, T., HOSODA, J., KUBOCHI, Y., IGUCHI, E. and IMANAKA, H. (1976) Nocardicin A, a new monocyclic β-lactam antibiotic. *J. Antibiot.* **29**: 492–500.

BARRIERE, S. L. and FLAHERTY, J. F. (1984) Third-generation cephalosporins: A critical evaluation. *Clin. Pharm.* **3**: 351–369.

BARRY, A. L., THORSBERRY, C., JONES, R. N. and GAVAN, T. L. (1985) Aztreonam: Antibacterial activity. β-lactamase stability and interpretive standards and quality control guidelines for disc diffusion susceptibility test, *Rev. infect. Dis.* (Suppl. 4) **7**: 5594–5604.

BASKER, M. J., EDMONDSON, R. A., KNOTT, S. J., PONSFORD, R. J., SLOCOMBE, B. and WHITE, S. J. (1984) *In vitro* properties of BRL 36650, a novel 6 α-substituted penicillin. *Antimicrob. Ag. Chemother.* **26**: 734–740.

BERGAN, T. (1981) Overview of acylureidopenicillin pharmacokinetics. *Scand. J. infect. Dis* (Suppl.) **29**: 33–48.

BINT, A. J., YOEMAN, P., KILBURN, P., ANDERSON, R. and STANSFIELD, E. (1981) The *in vitro* activity of ceftazidime compared with that of other cephalosporins. *J. Antimicrob. Chemother.* (Suppl. B) **8**: 47–51.

BOX, S. J., CORBETT, D. F., ROBINS, K. G., SPEAR, S. R. and VERRAL, M. S. (1982) A new olivanic acid derivative produced by *Streptomyces olivaceus*. Isolation and structural studies. *J. Antibiot.* **35**: 1394–1396.

BROGDEN, R. N., CARMINE, A., HEEL, R. C., MORLEY, P. A., SPEIGHT, T. M. and AVERY, G. S. (1981)

Amoxycillin/Slavulanic acid: a review of its antibacterial activity, pharmacokinetics and therapeutic use. *Drug* **22**: 337–362.

BROWN, A. G., BUTTERWORTH, D., COLE, M., HANSCOMB, G., HOOD, J. D., READING, C. and ROBINSON, G. N. (1976) Naturally-occurring β-lactamase inhibitors with antibacterial activity. *J. Antibiot.* **29**: 668–669.

BUENING, M. K., WOLD, J. S., ISRAEL, K. S. and KAMMER, R. B. (1981) Disulfiram-like reaction to β-lactams. *J. Am. med. Ass.* **245**: 2027.

BUSH, K. and SYKES, R. B. (1982) Interaction of new β-lactams with β-lactamases and β-lactamase-producing gram-negative rods. In: *New β-Lactam Antibiotics: A Review from Chemistry to Clinical Efficacy of the New Ephalosporins*, pp. 47–63, NEU, H. (ed.) Francis Wood Institute for History of Medicine, Philadelphia.

BUSH, K., FREUDENBERGER, J. S. and SYKES, R. B. (1982) Interaction of aztreonam and related monobactams with β-lactamase for gram negative bacteria. *Antimicrob. Ag. Chemother.* **22**: 414–420.

BUSH, K., TANAKA, S. K., BONNER, D. P. and SYKES, R. B. (1985) Resistance caused by decreased penetration of β-lactam antibiotics into *Enterobacter cloacae*. *Antimicrob. Ag. Chemother.* **27**: 555–560.

CARMINE, A. A., BROGDEN, R. N., HEEL, R. C., ROMANKIEWICZ, J. A., SPEIGHT, T. M. and AVERY, G. S. (1983) Moxalactam (latamoxef) a review of its antibacterial activity, pharmacokinetic properties and therapeutic use. *Drugs* **26**: 279–333.

CHARNAS, R. L., FISHER, J. and KNOWLES, J. R. (1978) Chemical studies on the inactivation of *Escherichia coli* R-TEM β-lactamase by clavulanic acid. *Biochemistry* **17**: 2185–2189.

COLE, M. (1979) Inhibition of β-lactamases. In: *β-Lactamases*, pp. 205–289, HAMILTON-MILLER, J. M. T. and SMITH J. T. (eds) Academic Press, London.

CREASEY, W. A., ADAMOVICS, J., DHRUV, R., PLATT, T. B. and SUGERMAN, A. A. (1984) Pharmacokinetic interaction of aztreonam with other antibiotics. *J. clin. Pharmac.* **24**: 174–180.

CROYDON, E. A. P., JACKSON, D. and STANIFORTH, D. H. (1981) Pharmacokinetics of parenteral "Augmentin". 12th International Congress of Chemotherapy, Florence. Abstract 475.

DAEHNE, W. V. (1980) 6β-Halopenicillanic acids, a group of β-lactamase inhibitors. *J. Antibiot.* **33**: 451–452.

DRUSANO, G. L., SCHIMPFF, S. C. and HEWITT, W. L. (1984) The acylampicillins: mezlocillin, piperacillin and azlocillin. *Rev. infect. Dis.* **6**: 13–32.

DURKIN, J. P. and VISWANATHA, T. (1978) Clavulanic acid inhibition of β-lactamase I from *Bacillus cereus* 569/*HH*. *J. Antibiot.* **31**: 1162–1169.

ELIOPOULOS, G. M. and MOELLERING, R. C., JR. (1981) Susceptibility of enterococcus and *Listeria monocytogenes* to *N*-formimidoyl thienamycin alone and in combination with an aminoglycoside. *Antimicrob. Ag. Chemother.* **19**: 789–793.

ENGLISH, A. R., RETSEMA, J. A., GIRARD, A. E., LYNCH, J. E. and BARTH, W. E. (1978) CP-45,899, a β-lactamase inhibitor that extends the antibacterial spectrum of β-lactams: Initial bacteriological characterization. *Antimicrob. Ag. Chemother.* **14**: 414–419.

EVANS, M. A. L., WILSON, P., LEUNG, T. and WILLIAMS, J. D. (1978) Pharmacokinetics of piperacillin following intravenous administration. *J. Antimicrob. Chemother.* **4**: 255–261.

FILLASTRE, J. P., HUMBERT, G., OLIER, B., LEGUY, F., BORSA, F. and SPENSER, G. R. (1983) Pharmacokinetics of ceftazidime in renal failure. *J. Antimicrob. Chemother.* **11**: 487–488.

FILLASTRE, J. P., LEROY, A., BAUDOIN, C., HUMBERT, G., SWABB, E. A., VERTUCCI, C. and GODIN, M. (1985) Pharmacokinetics of aztreonam in patients with chronic renal failure. *Clin. Pharmac.* **10**: 91–100.

FISHER, J., CHARNAS, R. L. and KNOWLES, J. R. (1978) Kinetic studies on the inactivation of *Escherichia coli* R-TEM β-lactamase by clavulanic acid. *Biochemistry* **17**: 2180–2184.

FOULDS, G., STANKEWICH, J. P., MARSHALL, D. C., O'BRIEN, M. M., HAYES, S. L., WEIDLER, D. J. and MCMAHON, F. G. (1983) Pharmacokinetics of sulbactam in humans. *Antimicrob. Ag. Chemother.* **23**: 692–699.

FU, K. P. and NEU, H. C. (1979) Comparative inhibition of β-lactamases by novel β-lactam compounds. *Antimicrob. Ag. Chemother.* **15**: 171–176.

GEORGOPAPADAKOU, N. and LIU, F. (1980) Binding of β-lactam antibiotics to penicillin-binding proteins of *Staphylococcus aureus* and *Streptococcus faecalis*: relation to antibacterial activity. *Antimicrob. Ag. Chemother.* **18**: 834–836.

GEORGOPAPADAKOU, N., SMITH, S. A. and R. B. (1982) Mode of action of aztreonam. *Antimicrob. Ag. Chemother.* **21**: 950–956.

GERIG, J. S., BOLTON, N. D., SWABB, E. A., SCHELD, W. M. and BOLTON, W. K. (1984) Effect of hemodialysis and CAPD on aztreonam pharmacokinetics in patients with end-stage renal desease. *Kidney Int.* **26**: 308–318.

GIAMARELLOU, H., ZISSIS, N. P., TAGARI, G. and BOUZOS, J. (1984) *In vitro* synergistic activities of aminoglycosides and new β-lactams against multiresistant *Pseudomonas aeruginosa*. *Antimicrob. Ag. Chemother.* **25**: 534–536.

GOMBERT, M. E., BERKOWITZ, L. B. and CUMMINGS, M. C. (1983) Synergistic effect of *N*-formimidoyl thienamycin with gentamicin and amikacin against *Streptococcus faecalis*. *Antimicrob. Ag. Chemother.* **23**: 245–247.

GOTO, S., OGAWA, M., MIYAZPIKI, S., KANEKO, Y. and KAUWAHARA, S. (1984) 6315-S, A novel oxacephem for parenteral: Bacteriological *in vitro* and *in vivo* study. 24th Interscience Conference on Antimicrobial Agents and Chemotherapy. Washington. Abstract 644.

HANSLO, A. K., KING, A., SHANNON, K., WARREN, C. and PHILLIPS, I. (1981) *N*-formimidoyl thienamycin (MK0787): *In vitro* antibacterial activity and susceptibility to β-lactamases compared with that of cefotaxime, moxalactam and other β-lactam antibiotics. *J. Antimicrob. Chemother.* **7**: 607–617.

HARDING, S. M., AYRTON, J., THORNTON, J. E., MUNRO, A. J. and HOGG, M. I. J. (1981a) Pharmacokinetics of ceftazidime in normal subjects. *J. Antimicrob. Chemother.* **8**(Suppl. B): 261.

HARDING, S. M., MUNRO, A. J., THORNTON, J. E., AYRTON, J. and HOGG, M. I. J. (1981b) The comparative pharmacokinetics of ceftazidime and cefotaxime in healthy volunteers. *J. Antimicrob. Chemother.* **8**(Suppl. B): 263–272.

HARE, R. S., MILLER, G. H., NAPLES, L., SABATELLI, F., LOEBENBERG, D. and WAITZ, J. A. (1982) Sch 29482, a new penem antibiotic: evaluation of *in vitro* activity and effect of test conditions. *J. Antimicrob. Chemother.* **9**(Suppl. C): 7–16.

HARPER, P. B. (1981) The *in vitro* properties of ceftazidime. *J. Antimicrob. Chemother.* **8**(Suppl. B): 5–13.

HARRIS, A. M., PLESTED, S. J. and HARPER, P. B. (1981) A comparison of the *in vitro* properties of ceftazidime with those of new broad-spectrum cephalosporins and gentamicin. *J. Antimicrob. Chemother.* **8**(Suppl. B): 43–45.

HOFFKEN, G., WITKOWSKI, G., LODE, H. and KOEPPE, P. (1981) Comparative pharmacokinetics of amoxicillin, clavulanic acid potassium, and their combination. 12th International Congress of Chemotherapy, Florence. Abstract 1043.

HOFFLER, D. and DALHOFF, A. (1980) Pharmacokinetics of clavulanic acid in patients with normal and impaired renal function. In: *Proceedings of the 11th International Congress of Chemotherapy and the 19th Interscience Conference of Antimicrobial Agents and Chemotherapy on Current Chemotherapy and Infectious Deseases*, October 1–5, 1979, pp. 322–323, NELSON, J. D. and GRASSI, C. (eds) Amer. Soc. for Microbiol., Wash., DC.

HOOD, J. D., BOX, S. J. and VERRALL, M. S. (1979) Olivanic acids, a family of β-lactamase inhibitory properties produced by *Streptomyces* species. *J. Antibiot.* **32**: 295–304.

HOOVER, J. R. E. (1983) β-Lactam antibiotics structure activity relationships. In: *Antiobitics Containing the Beta Lactam Structure 2*, pp. 119–145, DEMAIN, A. L. and SOLOMON, N. A. (eds) Springer-Verlag, New York.

HOWARTH, T. T., BROWN, A. G. and KING, T. J. (1976) Clavulanic acid, a novel β-lactam isolated from *Streptomyces clavuligerus. J. chem. Soc. Chem. Commun.* 266–267.

IMADA, A., KITANO, K., KINTAKA, K., MUROI, M. and ASAI, M. (1981) Sulfazecin amd isosulfazecin, novel β-lactam antibiotics of bacterial origin. *Nature* **289**: 590–591.

IMADA, A., NOZAKI, Y., KINTAKA, K., OKONOGI, K., KITANO, K. and HARADA, S. (1980) C-19393 S_2 and H_2, new carbapenem antibiotics 1. Taxonomy of the producing strain, fermentation and antibacterial properties. *J. Antibiot.* **33**: 1417–1424.

JACKSON, D., COOPER, D. L., HARDY, T. L., LANGLEY, P. F., STANIFORTH, D. H. and SUTTON, J. A. (1980) Pharmacokinetic, toxicological and metabolic studies with augmentin. In: *Proceedings of the First Symposium on Augmentin: Clavulanate-Potentiated Amoxycillin*, July 3–4, pp. 87–111, ROLLINSON and WATSON (eds) Excerpta Medica, Amsterdam.

JONES, P. G., BODEY, G. P., SWABB, E. A. and ROSENBAUM, B. (1984) The effect of aztreonam on the throat and stool flora of cancer patients. *Antimicrob. Ag. Chemother.* **26**: 941–943.

JONES, R. N. and PACKER, R. R. (1982) Antimicrobial activity of amikacin combinations against *Enterobacteriaceae* moderately susceptible to third-generation cephalosporins. *Antimicrob. Ag. Chemother.* **22**: 985–989.

JONES, R. N., BARRY, A. L., THORNSBERRY, C., GERLACH, E. H., FUCHS, P. C., GAVAN, T. L. and SOMERS, H. M. (1981) Ceftazidime, a pseudomonas-active cephalosporin: *in vitro* antimicrobial activity evaluation including recommendations for disc diffusion susceptibility tests. *J. Antimicrob. Chemother.* **8**(Suppl. B): 187–211.

JONES, R. N., THORNSBERRY, C. and BARRY A. L. (1984). *In vitro* evaluation of HR810, a new wide spectrum aminothiazoyl α-methoxyimino cephalosporin. *Antimicrob. Ag. Chemother.* **25**: 710–718.

KAHAN, F. M., KROPP, H., SUNDELOF, J. G. and BIRNBAUM, J. (1983) Thienamycin: development of imipenem-cilastatin. *J. Antimicrob. Chemother.* **12**(Suppl. D): 1–35.

KAHAN, J. S., KAHAN, F. M., GEOGELMAN, R., CURRIE, S. A., JACKSON, M., STAPLEY, E. O., MILLER, T. W., MILLER, A. K., HENDLIN, D., MOCHALES, S., HERNADEZ, S., WOODRUFF, H. B. and BIRNBAUM, J. (1979) Thienamycin, a new β-lactam antibiotic 1. Discovery, taxonomy, isolation and physical properties. *J. Antibiot.* **32**: 1–12.

KALLICK, C., RICE, T., NORSEN, J., RAJASHEKARAIAH, K., MARSH, D., MCCULLEY, D. and THADHANI, K. (1982) *In vitro* activity of *N*-formimidoyl thienamycin against *Pseudomonas* and staphylococci associated with endocarditis. Proceedings of the 12th International Congress of Chemotherapy. *Curr. Chemother. Immun.* **1**: 725–726.

KAWAMURA, Y., YASUDA, Y., MAYAMA, M. and TANAKA, K. (1982) Asparenomycins A, B and C, New Carbapenem antibotics. 1. Taxonomic studies on the producing microorganisms. *J. Antibiot.* **35**: 10–14.

KEMMERICH, B., HARTMUT, W., LODE, H., BORNER, K., KOEPPE, P and KNOTHE, H. (1983) Multiple-dose pharmacokinetics of ceftazidime and its influence on fecal flora. *Antimicrob. Ag. Chemother.* **24**: 333–338.

KITANO, K., FUJISAWA, Y., KATAMATO, K., NARA, K. and NAKAO, Y. (1976) Occurrence of 7β-(4 carboxy-butanamido)-cephalosporin compounds in the culture broth of some strains of the genus Cephalosporium. *J. Ferment. Technol.* **54**: 712–719.

KNOTHE, H. and DETTE, G. A. (1981) The *in vitro* activity of ceftazidime against clinically important pathogens. *J. Antimicrob. Chemother.* **8**(Suppl. B): 33–41.

KOMATSU, Y. and NISHIKAWA, J. T. (1980) Moxalactam (6059-S), a new 1-oxa β-lactam: Binding affinity for penicillin-binging proteins of *Escherichia coli* K-12. *Antimicrob. Ag. Chemother.* **17**: 316–321.

KOMATSU, Y., NAGATA, W., MATSUURA, S., HARADA, Y. and YOSHIDA, T. (1984) 2355-S, a new broad spectrum oxacephem for parenteral use: Laboratory evaluation. 24th Interscience Conference on Antimicrobial Agents and Chemotherapy. Washington, DC. Abstract 645.

KONDO, M., KISHINOTO, S., OCHIAI, M., OKONOGI, K. and IMADA, A. (1983) *In vitro* and *in vivo* evaluation of AMA-1080 (Ro 17-2301), Proceedings of the 13th International Congress of Chemotherapy. Vienna, Austria. Paper SE 4.2/15-1.

KROPP, H., SUNDELOF, J. G., HAJDU, R. and KAHAN, F. M. (1982) Metabolism of thienamycin and related carbapenen antibiotics by the renal dipeptidase, dehydropeptidase-I. *Antimicrob. Ag. Chemother.* **22**: 62–70.

LABIA, R., MORAND, A., KAZMIERCZAK, A. and THIAS, C. N. R. S. (1983) Kinetic studies of the interactions of aztreonam with β-lactamases. 23rd Interscience Conference on Antimicrobial Agents and Chemotherapy. Las Vegas. Abstract 329.

LAU, A., LEE, M., FLASCHA, S., PRASAD, R. and SHARIFI, R. (1983) Effect of piperacillin on tobramycin pharmacokinetics in patients with normal renal function. *Antimicrob. Ag. Chemother.* **24**: 533–537.

LUND, F. and TYBRING, L. (1972) 6-β-amidinopenicillanic acids—a new group of antibiotics. *Nature New Biol.* **236**: 135–137.

LUTHY, R., BLASER, J., BONETTI A., SIMMER, H., WISE, R. and SIEGENTHALER, W. (1981) Comparative multiple dose pharmacokinetics of cefotaxime, moxalactam and ceftazidime. *Antimicrob. Ag. Chemother.* **20**: 557–576.

McCRACKEN, G. H., THRELKELD, N. and THOMAS, M. L. (1984) Pharmacokinetics of ceftazidime in newborn infants. *Antimicrob. Ag. Chemother.* **26**: 583–584.

METZGER, K. (1982) Killing of azlocillin- and mezlocillin- induced filamentous forms of *Pseudomonas aeruginosa* by decreasing concentration of penicillin. *J. Antimicrob. Chemother.* **9**(Suppl. A): 11–14.

MIHINDU, J. C. L., SCHELD, W. M., BOLTON, N. D., SPYKER, D. A., SWABB, E. A. and BOLTON, W. K. (1983) Pharmacokinetics of aztreonam in patients with various degrees of renal dysfunction. *Antimicrob. Ag. Chemother.* **24**: 252–261.

MIKAMI, H., OGASHIWA, M., SAINO, Y., INOUE, M. and MITSUHASI S. (1982) Comparative stability of newly introduced β-lactam antibiotics to renal dipeptidase. *Antimicrob. Ag. Chemother.* **22**: 693–695.

MOCHIDA, K., SHIRAKI C., YAMYZAKI, M., HIRATA, T., SATO, K. and OKACHI, R. (1984) Antimicrobial activities of 1-carbacephem compounds and their structure–activity relationships. 24th Interscience Conference on Antimicrobial Agents and Chemotherapy.

MUNCH, R., LUTHY, R., BLASER, J. and SIEGENTHALER, W. (1981) Human pharmacokinetics and CSF penetration of clavulanic acid. *J. Antimicrob. Chemother.* **8**: 29–37.

NAGARAJAN, R., BOECK, L. D., GORMAN, M., HAMILL, R. L., HIGGENS, G. E., HOEHN, M. M., STARK W. M. and WHITNEY, J. G. (1971) β-Lactam antibiotics from *Streptomyces. J. Am. Chem. Soc.* **93**: 2308–2310.

NAKAYAMA, M., KIMURA, S., TANABE, S., MIZOGUCHI, T., WANTANABE, I. and MORI, T. (1981) Structures and absolute configurations of carpetimycins A and B. *J. Antibiot.* **34**: 818–823.

NEU, H. C. (1982) The *in vitro* activity, human pharmacology, and clinical effectiveness of new β-lactam antibiotics. *A. Rev. Pharmac. Toxic.* **22**: 559–642.

NEU, H. C. (1983) Structure–activity relations of new β-lactam compounds and *in vitro* activity against common bacteria. *Rev. infect. Dis.* **5**(Suppl. 2): S319–S337.

NEU H. C., CHIN, N. X. and LABTHAVIKUL, P. (1984) Antibacterial activity of BMY28, 142, an *N*-methyl pyrrolidine aminothiazoyl cephalosporin. 24th Interscience Conference on Antimicrobial Agents and Chemotherapy, Washington, DC. Abstract 660.

NORRBY, S., BJORNEGARD, R. B., FERBER, F. and JONES, K. H. (1983) Pharmacokinetics of imipenem in healthy volunteers. *J. Antimicrob. Chemother.* **12**(Suppl. D): 109–124.

OKAMURA, K., HIRATA, S., KOKI, A., HORI, K., SHIBAMOTO, N., OKMURA, Y., OKABE, M., OKAMOTO, R., KUNONO, K., FUKAGAWA, Y., SHIMAUCHI, Y., ISHIKURA, T. and LEIN, J. (1979) PS-5. A new β-lactam antibiotic. I. Taxonomy of the producing organism, isolation and physico-chemical properties. *J. Antibiot.* **32**: 262–271.

O'SULLIVAN, J. and SYKES, R. B. (1985) β-lactam antibiotics. In: *Biotechnology*, Vol. 4, REHM, H. J. and REED, G. (eds) Verlag Chemie (in press).

PARADELIS, A. G., STATHOPOULOS, G. A., SALPIGIDES, G. N. and CRASSARIS, L. G. (1983) Antibacterial activity of aztreonam: a synthetic monobactam. A comparative study with 13 other antibiotics. *Expl. clin. Pharmac.* **5**: 375–383.

PARKER, W. L., RATHNUM, M. L., WELLS, J. S., TREJO, W. H., PRINCIPE, P. A. and SYKES, R. B. (1982) SQ 27,860, a simple carbapenem produced by species of *Serratia* and *Erwinia. J. Antibiot.* **35**: 653–660.

PARRY, M. F. (1984) Toxic and adverse reactions encountered with new beta-lactam antibiotics. *Bull. N.Y. Acad. Med.* **60**: 358–368.

PERCIVAL, A., THOMAS, E., HART, C. A. and KARAYIANNIS, P. (1981) *In vitro* activity of monobactam, SQ 26,776, against gram-negative bacteria. *J. Antimicrob. Chemother.* **8**(Suppl. E): 49–55.

PHILLIPS, I., KING, A., SHANNON, K. and WARREN, C. (1981a) SQ 26,776: *in vitro* antibacterial activity and susceptibility to β-lactamases (1981) *J. Antimicrob. Chemother.* **8**(Suppl. E): 103–110.

PHILLIPS, I., WISE, R. and NEU, H. C. (1982) An oral penem antibiotic: Sch 29482. *J. Antimicrob. Chemother.* **9**(Suppl. C).

PHILLIPS, I., WARREN, C., SHANNON, K., KING, A. and HANSLO, D. (1981b) Ceftazidime: *in vitro* antibacterial activity and susceptibility to β-lactamases compared with that of cefotaxime, moxalactam and other β-lactam antibiotics. *J. Antimicrob. Chemother.* **8**(Suppl. B): 23–31.

PRATT, R. F. and LOOSEMORE, M. J. (1978) 6β-Bromopenicillanic acid, a potent β-lactamase inhibitor. *Proc. natn. Acad. Sci. U.S.A.* **75**: 4145–4149.

READING, C. and HEPBURN, P. (1979) The inhibition of staphylococcal β-lactamase by clavulanic acid. *Biochem. J.* **179**: 67–76.

REHM, S. J., HALL, C. S., ALANIS, A., WEINSTEIN, A. J. and GAVAN, T. L. (1983). *In vitro* effects of combinations of aztreonam with tobramycin, piperacillin and moxalactam against *Pseudomonas aeruginosa* and *Serratia marcescens*. 23rd Interscience Conference on Antimicrobial Agents and Chemotherapy. Las Vegas. Abstract 30.

RICHMOND, M. H. (1980) The β-lactamase stability of a novel β-lactam antibiotic containing a 7β-methoxycephem nucleus. *J. Antimicrob. Chemother.* **6**: 445–453.

RICHMOND, M. H. (1981) The semi-synthetic thienamycin derivative MK0787 and its properties with respect to a range of β-lactamases from clinically relevant bacterial species. *J. Antimicrob. Chemother.* **7**: 279–285.

ROSSIE, D., DROZD, M. L., KUHRT, M. F., TERMINIELLO, L., CARRE, P. E. and DAWN, S. J. (1981) Mutants of *Streptomyces cattleya* producing *N*-acetyl and deshydroxy carbapenems related to thienamycin. *J. Antibiot.* **34**: 341–343.

RUSSELL, A. D. (1981) *In vitro* studies on SQ 26, 776, a new monobactam antibiotic. *J. Antimicrob. Chemother.* **8**(Suppl. E): 81–88.

SAINO, Y., KOBAYASHI, F., INOUE, M. and MITSUHASHI, S. (1982) Purification and properties of inducible penicillin β-lactamase isolated from *Pseudomonas maltophilia. Antimicrob. Ag. Chemother.* **22**: 564–570.

SANFILIPPO, A., DELLA BRUNA, C., JABES, D., MORVILLO, E. and SCHIOPPACASSI, G. (1982) Biological activity of (5R, 6S, 8R)-6-α-hydroxyethyl-2-acetoxymethyl-2-penem-3-carboxylate. *J. Antibiot.* **35**: 1248–1250.

SAXON, A., HASSNER, A., SWABB, E. A., WHEELER, B. and ADKINSON, N. F., JR. (1984) Lack of cross-reactivity between aztreonam, a monobactam antibiotic and penicillin in penicillin-allergic subjects. *J. infect. Dis.* **149**: 16–22.

SCHAAD, U. B., CASEY, P. A. and COOPER, D. L. (1983) Single-dose pharmacokinetics of intravenous clavulanic acid with amoxicillin in pediatric patients. *Antimicrob. Ag. Chemother.* **23**: 252–255.

SCHAAD, U. B., MCCRACKEN, G. H., JR., THRELKELD, N. and THOMAS, M. L. (1981) Clinical evaluation of a new broad-spectrum oxa-beta-lactam antibiotic, moxalactam, in neonates and infants. *J. Pediatr.* **98**: 129–136.

SCULLY, B. E., SWABB, E. A. and NEU, H. C. (1983) Pharmacology of aztreonam after intravenous infusion. *Antimicrob. Ag. Chemother.* **24**: 18–22.

SEELER, R. A. and REITAN, J. (1984) Cephalosporin induced coagulopathies. *Illinois med. J.* **166**: 351–353.

SIEGEL, J., RYAN, P., APRIL, D. and CHRISTENSON, J. (1983) Unusual β-lactamase stability of RO 17-2301 (AMA-1080), a new monocyclic β-lactam. 23rd Interscience Conference on Antimicrobial Agents and Chemotherapy. Las Vegas. Abstract 189.

Singh, P. D., Johnson, J. H., Ward, P. C., WELLS, J. S., TREJO, W. H. and SYKES, R. B. (1982) A new monobactam produced by a *Flexibacter* sp. Taxonomy, fermentation, isolation, structure determination and biological properties. *J. Antibiot.* **36**: 1246–1251.

SINGH, P. D., YOUNG, M. G., JOHNSON, J. H., CIMARUSTI, C. M. and SYKES, R. B. (1984) Bacterial production of 7-formamidocephalosporins. Isolation and structure determination. *J. Antibiot.* **37**: 773–780.

SLOCOMBE, B., BASKER, M. J., BENTLY, P. H., CLAYTON, J. P., COLE, M., COMBER, K. R., DIXON, R. A., EDMONSON, R. A., JACKSON, D., MERRIKIN, D. J. and SUTHERLAND, R. (1981) BRL 17421 a novel β-lactam antibiotic highly resistant to β-lactamases, giving high and prolonged serum levels in humans. *Antimicrob. Ag. Chemother.* **20**: 38–46.

SMITH, C. R. and LIPSKY, J. J. (1983) Hypoprothrombinemia and platelet dysfunction caused by cephalosporin and oxalactam antibiotics. *J. Antimicrob. Chemother.* **11**: 496–498.

SOMMERS, D. K., WALTERS, L., VAN WYK, M., HARDING, S. M., PATON, A. M. and AYRTON, J. (1983) Pharmacokinetics of ceftazidime in male and female volunteers. *Antimicrob. Ag. Chemother.* **23**: 892–896.

SPRATT, B. G., TOBANPUTRA, V. and ZIMMERMAN, W. (1977) Binding of thienamycin and clavulanic acid to the penicillin-binding proteins of *Escherichia coli*. *Antimicrob. Ag. Chemother.* **12**: 406–409.

STANIFORTH, D. H., JACKSON, D., CLARKE, H. L. and HORTON, R. (1983) Amoxycillin/clavulanic acid: the effect of probenecid. *J. Antimicrob. Chemother.* **12**: 273–275.

STAPLEY, E. O., CASSIDY, P., CURRIE, S. A., DAOUST, D., GEOGELMAN, R., HERNANDEZ, S., JACKSON, M., MATA, J. M., MILLER, A. K., MONAGHAN, R. L., TUNAC, J. B., ZIMMERMAN, S. B. and HENDLIN, D. (1977) Epithienamycins: Biological studies of a new family of β-lactam antibiotics. 17th Interscience Conference on Antimicrobial Agents and Chemotherapy. Abstract 80.

STUTMAN, H. R., MARKS, M. I. and SWABB, E. A. (1984) Single-dose pharmacokinetics of aztreonam in pediatric patients. *Antimicrob. Ag. Chemother.* **26**: 196–199.

STUTMAN, H. R., PARKER, K. M. and MARKS, M. I. (1985) The potential of moxalactam and other new antimicrobials agents for bilirubin-albumin displacement in neonates. *Pediatrics* **75**: 294–298.

SWABB, E. A., LEITZ, M. A., PILKIEWICZ, F. G. and SUGERMAN, A. A. (1981) Pharmacokinetics of the monobactam SQ 26,776 after intravenous doses in healthy subjects. *J. Antimicrob. Chemother.* **8**(Suppl. E): 131–140.

SWABB, E. A., SINGHVI, S. M., LEITZ, M. A., FRANTZ, M. and SUGERMAN, A. A. (1983a) Metabolism and pharmacokinetics of aztreonam in healthy subjects. *Antimicrob. Ag. Chemother.* **24**: 394–400.

SWABB, E. A., SUGERMAN, A. A., FRANTZ, M., PLATT, T. B. and STERN, M. (1983c) Renal handling of the monobactam aztreonam in healthy subjects. *Clin. Pharmac. Ther.* **33**: 609–614.

SWABB, E. A., SUGERMAN, A. A. and McKINSTRY, D. N. (1983b) Multiple-dose pharmacokinetics of the monobactam aztreonam (SQ 26,776) in healthy subjects. *Antimicrob. Ag. Chemother.* **23**: 125–132.

SWABB, E. A., SUGERMAN, A. A., PLATT, T. B., PILKIEWICZ, F. G. and FRANTZ, M. (1982) Single-dose pharmacokinetics of the monobactam aztreonam (SQ 26,776) in healthy subjects. *Antimicrob. Ag. Chemother.* **21**: 944–949.

SYKES, R. B. and BUSH, K. (1983) Interaction of the new cephalosporins with β-lactamase and β-lactamase-producing gram-negative bacilli. *Rev. infect Dis.* **5**(Suppl. 2): 5356–5365.

SYKES, R. B. and MATTHEW, M. (1976) The β-lactamases of gram-negative bacteria and their role in resistance to β-lactam antibiotics. *J. Antimicrob. Chemother.* **2**: 115–157.

SYKES, R. B. and WELLS, J. S. (1985) Screening for β-lactam antibiotics in nature. *J. Antibiot.* **38**: 119–121.

SYKES, R. B., BONNER, D. P., BUSH, K. and GEORGOPAPADAKOU, N. H. (1982a) Aztreonam (SQ 26,776) a synthetic monobactam specifically active against aerobic gram negative bacteria. *Antimicrob. Ag. Chemother.* **21**: 85–92.

SYKES, R. B., BONNER, D. P., BUSH, K., GEORGOPAPADAKOU, N. H. and WELLS, J. S. (1981b) Monobactams–monocyclic β-lactam antibiotics produced by bacteria. *J. Antimicrob. Chemother.* **8**(Suppl. E): 1–16.

SYKES, R. B., CIMARUSTI, C. M., BONNER, D. P., BUSH, K., FLOYD, D. M., GEORGOPAPADAKOU, N. H., KOSTER, W. H., LIU, W. C., PARKER, W. L., PRINCIPE, P. A., RATHNUM, M. L., SLUSARCHYK, W. A., TREJO, W. H. and WELLS, J. S. (1981a) Monocyclic β-lactam antibiotics produced by bacteria. *Nature* **291**: 489–491.

SYKES, R. B., PARKER, L. W. and WELLS, J. S. (1982b) β-lactam antibiotics produced by bacteria. In: *Trends in Antibiotic Research. Genetics, Biosynthesis, Actions and New Substances*, pp. 115–124, UMEZAWA, H., *et al.* (eds) Japan Antibiotics Res. Ass., Tokyo.

TALLEY, F. P. and JACOBUS, N. V. (1983) Susceptibility of anaerobic bacteria to imipenem. *J. Antimicrob. Chemother.* **12**(Suppl. D): 47–51.

TANABE, S., OKUCHI, M., NAKAYAMA, M., KIMURA, S., IWASAKI, A., MIZOGUSHI, T., MURAKAMI, A., ITOH, H. and MORI, T. (1982) A new carbapenem antibiotic, 6643-X. *J. Antibiot.* **35**: 1237–1239.

TANAKA, S. K., BONNER, D. P., SCHWIND, R. A., MINASSIAN, B. F., LALAMA, L. M. and SYKES, R. B. (1984) Oral monobactams: *In vitro* activity of SQ 82,291, 24th Interscience Conference Antimicrobial Agents and Chemotherapy. Washington, DC. Abstract. 137.

TANAKA, S. K., BONNER, D. P. and SYKES, R. B. (1983a) *In vitro* activity of aztreonam in combination with aminoglycosides and other β-lactams against gram positive and gram negative bacteria. In: *13th International Congress of Chemotherapy proceedings*, pp. 27/1–27/5, SPITZY, K. H. and KASLER, K. (eds) Vienna.

TANAKA, S. K., SCHWIND, R. A., MINASSIANS, B. F., LALAMA, L., BONNER, D. P. and SYKES, R. B. (1983b) Synergistic activity of aztreonam–aminoglycoside combinations against antibiotic resistant and susceptible aerobic gram negative bacilli. 23rd Interscience Conference on Antimicrobial Agents and Chemotherapy. Las Vegas. Abstract 31.

THOMPSON, M. I. B., RUSSO, M. E., SAXON, B. J., ATKIN-THOR, E. and MATSEN, J. M. (1982) Gentamicin inactivation by piperacillin or carbenicillin in patients with end-stage renal disease. *Antimicrob. Ag. Chemother.* **21**: 268–273.

TJANDRAMAGA, T. B., MULLIE, A., VERBESSELT, R., DESCHEPPER, P. J. and VERBIST, L. (1978) Piperacillin: Human pharmacokinetics after intravenous and intramuscular administration. *Antimicrob. Ag. Chemother.* **14**: 829–837.

TSUJI, N., NAGASHUMA, K., TERUI, Y., MATSUMOTO, K. and KONDO, E. (1982) The structure of pluracidomycins, new carbapenem antbiotics. *J. Antibiot.* **35**: 536–540.

VU, H. and NIKAIDO, N. (1985) Mechanism of resistance to β-lactamase-constitutive *Enterobacter cloacae* strains to the third generation β-lactams: Trapping or hydolysis. *Antimicrob. Ag. Chemother.* (in press).

VUYE, A. (1982) *In vitro* activity and β-lactamase stability of *N*-formimidoyl thienamycin compared to that of second and third generation cephalosporins. *Chemotherapy* **28**: 267–275.

WARREN, C. A., KING, B. A., SHANNON, K. P., EYKYN, S. J. and PHILLIPS, I. (1980) The *in vitro* antibacterial activity of LY127935 (6059S) a novel 1-oxa-β-lactam antibiotic. *J. Antimicrob. Chemother.* **6**: 607–615.

WEIDEKAMM, E., STOECKEL, K., EGGER, H. J. and ZIEGLER, W. H. (1984) Single-dose pharmocokinetics of Ro 17-2301 (AMA-1080), a monocyclic β-lactam, in humans. *Antimicrob. Ag. Chemother.* **26**: 898–902.

WELAGE, L. S., SCHULTZ, R. W. and SCHENTAG, J. J. (1984) Pharmacokinetics of ceftazidime in patients with renal insufficiency. *Antimicrob. Ag. Chemother.* **25**: 201–204.

WELLING, P. G., CRAIG, W. A., BUNDTZEN, R. W., KWOK, F. W., GERBER, A. U. and MADSEN, P. O. (1983) Pharmacokinetics of piperacillin in subjects with various degrees of renal function. *Antimicrob. Ag. Chemother.* **23**: 881–887.

WISE, R., DYAS, A., HEGARTY, A. and ANDREWS, J. M. (1982) Pharmacokinetics and tissue penetration of aztreonam. *Antimicrob. Ag. Chemother.* **22**: 969–971.

WRIGHT, A. J. and WILKOWSKE, C. J. (1983) The penicillins. *Mayo Clin. Proc.* **58**: 21–32.

YOSHIDA, T. (1981) Structure function relationships of 1-oxacephems and moxalactam. In: *New β-Lactam Antibiotics: A Review from Chemistry to Clinical Efficacy of the New Cephalosporins*, pp. 23–33, NEU, H. (ed.) Pub. Francis Clark Wood Institute for the History of Medicine, Philadelphia.

YOSHIDA, T., NORISADA, M., MATSUULA, S., NAGATA, W. and KUWABARA, S. (1978) 6059–S, A new parenterally active 1-oxacephalosporin: 1. Microbiological studies. 18th Interscience Conference Antimicrobial Agents and Chemotherapy. Atlanta. Abstract. 151.

CHAPTER 7

ROLE OF PERMEABILITY BARRIERS IN RESISTANCE TO β-LACTAM ANTIBIOTICS

HIROSHI NIKAIDO

Department of Microbiology and Immunology, University of California, Berkeley, California 94720, U.S.A.

1. INTRODUCTION

It has been known, since the earliest days (Fleming, 1929), that *penicillin* inhibits Gram-positive bacteria at much lower concentrations than most Gram-negative bacteria, with the exception of such organisms as *Neisseria*. This observation gave rise to the hypothesis that Gram-negative bacteria are covered by an extra barrier layer, which reduces the accessibility of the β-lactams, including penicillin, to the target enzyme. In the early 1960s, there emerged several lines of evidence that strongly supported this hypothesis. First, the 'target' enzymes in isolated *Escherichia coli* membrane preparations were shown to be as sensitive to β-lactams as are the enzymes from Gram-positive bacteria, and the much higher minimum inhibitory concentrations (MICs) observed with intact cells of *E. coli* were interpreted as being due to the failure of β-lactams to penetrate to the target sites (Izaki *et al.*, 1966). Second, the rates of hydrolysis of β-lactams by *β-lactamase*-containing intact cells of Gram-negative bacteria were found to be much slower than those by 'disrupted cell' preparations (Smith, 1963; Hamilton-Miller, 1963). Third, *EDTA treatment* was shown to increase the β-lactam-hydrolyzing activity of intact cells of *Klebsiella aerogenes* and *E. coli*. Since the treatment did not result in the release of the β-lactamase into the medium, the observation strongly suggested that, in untreated cells, the rate of hydrolysis was limited by the rate of substrate penetration through the 'barrier', which became damaged by EDTA (Hamilton-Miller, 1965).

Although the identity of this barrier layer was unclear at the beginning, it was firmly established as the bacterial outer membrane by 1975. Some of the observations that led to this conclusion are as follows:

(i) It became generally recognized that all Gram-negative bacteria are surrounded by an additional membrane layer, the outer membrane, that does not exist in Gram-positive bacterial cells (for example, see Glauert and Thornley, 1969).

(ii) At least some of the Gram-negative β-lactamases were shown to be located in the periplasm, i.e. the space between the outer-membrane-peptidoglycan layer and the underlying cytoplasmic membrane (Neu, 1968).

(iii) The EDTA treatment that damages the barrier was shown to release lipo-polysaccharide, a unique component of the outer membrane (Leive, 1965).

(iv) Isolated outer membrane vesicles were shown to act as a permeability barrier (Nakae and Nikaido, 1975).

Recent studies on the properties of the outer membrane have defined the roles of various outer membrane components in the production of this permeability barrier (Nikaido and Nakae, 1979; Nikaido, 1979a,b; Nikaido and Vaara, 1985). This review will summarize our current knowledge in this area with emphasis on β-lactams.

2. OVERVIEW OF THE POSSIBLE PATHWAYS
OF PENETRATION

2.1. PORIN PATHWAY

Although the Gram-negative bacterial cell is surrounded by the outer membrane, the cell obviously must take up nutrients from, and excrete waste products into, the external medium. Many nutrients and waste products are small, hydrophilic compounds, yet it is common knowledge that the lipid bilayer, which forms the basic continuum of most biological membranes including the outer membrane, usually has very low permeability toward hydrophilic solutes (Stein, 1967). These considerations suggested the presence, in the outer membrane, of a special mechanism that allows the rapid permeation of these small molecules. This mechanism was indeed discovered in the outer membrane of *Escherichia coli* and *Salmonella typhimurium* by a reconstitution approach (Nakae, 1976a,b). When closed lipid vesicles, or *liposomes*, are made without the addition of any membrane protein, their membranes are essentially impermeable to hydrophilic solutes as seen from the retention of radioactive sucrose incorporated into the intravesicular space. However, when the liposomes are made in such a way that fragments of the outer membrane, or an outer membrane protein called *porin*, are incorporated into the bilayer, the intravesicular sucrose was shown to leak out rapidly, and it was suggested that porins are transmembrane proteins with an ability to produce water-filled channels for the diffusion of hydrophilic solutes. The porin channels in *E. coli* or *S. typhimurium* were apparently totally nonspecific, and allowed the diffusion of any hydrophilic solute as long as it was small, i.e. less than about 600 daltons, and hydrophilic (Nakae, 1976a). These properties of the channel, observed in liposomes reconstituted from purified porin, were very similar to the permeability properties of the outer membranes in intact cells (Decad and Nikaido, 1976) or of isolated outer membrane vesicles (Nakae and Nikaido, 1975), although with some special classes of solutes the presence of additional pathways in the outer membrane could be demonstrated (see below).

Porins in most Gram-negative bacteria are proteins with a MW of 35,000–40,000, and are very often one of the most abundant proteins in the cell (Fig. 1). For example, a single *E. coli* cell usually contains 10^5 molecules of porin (Rosenbusch, 1974). Since porin is essential for the uptake of nutrients, mutants lacking the porins completely will not be able to survive, and indeed all 'porinless' mutants isolated so far simply produce diminished amounts of this protein (Bavoil *et al.*, 1977). By using these porin-deficient mutants of *E. coli*, we have shown that at least 90% of cephaloridine (Nikaido *et al.*, 1977b) and of 6-aminopenicillanic acid (Bavoil *et al.*, 1977) cross the outer membrane of wild type cells via the porin channels. Since then, similar observations have been made on many other β-lactam compounds, including ampicillin, cephacetrile, and cefamandole (H. Nikaido and E. Y. Rosenberg, unpublished results). Thus the study of outer membrane permeability for β-lactams essentially means the investigation of the properties of the porin channel, at least in *E. coli* and other enteric bacteria.

Enteric bacteria frequently produce multiple species of porin. Thus *E. coli* K-12 produces OmpF (previously called 1a, Ia, O-9, or b) and OmpC (previously called 1b, Ib, O-8, or c) porins, and *S. typhimurium* produces OmpF ('35K'), OmpC ('36K'), and OmpD ('34K') porins (for details see Osborn and Wu, 1980; Lugtenberg and van Alphen, 1983; Nikaido and Vaara, 1985). *Enterobacter cloacae* was also shown to contain two porin species (Kaneko *et al.*, 1984). All nonenteric species seem to produce a single species of porin characteristic of the strain. The organisms in which porins have been identified so far include *Pseudomonas aeruginosa* (Hancock *et al.*, 1979), *Neisseria gonorrhoeae* (Douglas *et al.*, 1981), *Aeromonas salmonicida* (Darveau *et al.*, 1983), *Brucella* species (Douglas *et al.*, 1984), *Chlamydia trachomatis* (Bavoil *et al.*, 1984), *Campylobacten jejuni* (Huyen *et al.*, 1986), *Haemophilus influenzae* (Vachon *et al.*, 1985), *Rhodopseudomonas capsulata* (Flammann and Weckesser, 1984) and *R. sphaeroides* (Weckesser *et al.*, 1984).

Although the porin channel exhibits no *configurational specificity*, and thus allows the diffusion of any small, hydrophilic solutes, the rates of diffusion of various solutes are

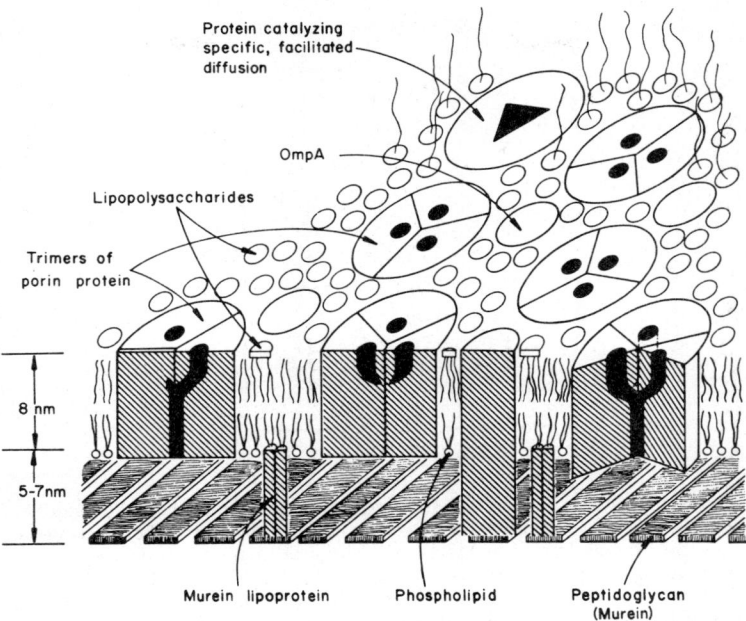

FIG. 1. Schematic representation of the structure of the *E. coli* outer membrane. Note that lipopolysaccharides are found only in the outer leaflet of the bilayer, and that phospholipid molecules are only in the inner leaflet. The polysaccharide chains of lipopolysaccharides, which extend into the medium from the outer surface, are drawn only for some molecules, for clarity. The porins exist as trimers, and according to Dorset *et al.* (1984), the three channels become fused into a single channel at one side (here depicted as the inner side) of the membrane, although more recent study of PhoE porin trimer showed that the channels were not fused together (B. Jap, personal communication). From Nikaido and Vaara (1985) with permission from American Society for Microbiology.

affected greatly by their gross physicochemical properties (Nikaido, 1979b). Since the estimated diameters of the OmpF and OmpC channels of *E. coli* are only 1.16 and 1.04 nm (Nikaido and Rosenberg, 1983), and are very close to the size of the solutes we are interested in, it is obvious that the properties of the solute molecules would profoundly affect their interactions with the rim or the wall of the channels, and thus their rates of diffusion.

Quantitative consideration of the diffusion *rates* is essential for our understanding of the mode of action of β-lactams in Gram-negative bacteria. Since diffusion through the porin channel is a passive process, the periplasmic concentration of any agent will eventually reach the external concentration regardless of the magnitude of the diffusion rates, *if there is no process to inactivate or remove the agent from the periplasmic space* (see Fig. 2a,b). It has often been said in the literature that dilution of the periplasmic concentration by growth might balance the influx of the agent; this argument, however, is not valid, because most β-lactams appear to equilibrate across the outer membrane much more rapidly than the possible rate of dilution by growth (see Section 4.5). Nevertheless it is a well-known fact that β-lactams with high outer membrane permeability tend to be more effective against Gram-negative bacteria (Hamilton-Miller, 1963; Richmond and Sykes, 1973; Zimmermann and Rosselet, 1977). Thus we are led to the conclusion that there must be processes that remove β-lactams from the periplasmic space at a significant rate (see Fig. 2, c and d). The nature of such processes is not completely clear at present. However, many, or even most, Gram-negative bacteria contain low levels of chromosomally determined β-lactamase. Even in strains in which β-lactamase activity cannot be demonstrated by conventional assays, it is nearly impossible to rule out the contribution of enzymatic cleavage, because when external concentrations are in the range of MIC, even very low enzymatic activity may destroy a significant fraction of periplasmic β-lactams. This point is discussed more extensively in Section 4.5 using *E. coli* as an example. There are several other possible pathways for β-lactam removal, including the irreversible binding to penicillin-binding proteins, and possible diffusion into the cytoplasm followed by de-

MEDIUM   PERIPLASM   MEDIUM   PERIPLASM

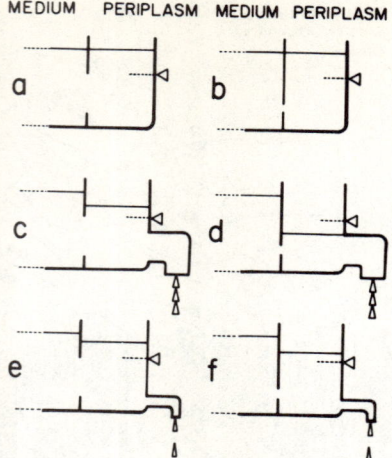

FIG. 2. Relationship between the rates of influx across the outer membrane and the rates of removal from the periplasmic space. The influx rate is represented by the size of the gap between the two compartments; the rate of removal by the size of the faucet. Arrowheads denote the hypothetical concentration necessary to saturate the target enzymes.

In a and b, there is no removal of β-lactams from the periplasmic space, so that the periplasmic concentration will reach the external level regardless of the magnitude of the influx rates; this condition will be approximated by β-lactams that are neither hydrolyzed nor bound tightly by the periplasmic β-lactamase. In c and d, there is a rapid removal, most commonly through hydrolysis by the periplasmic β-lactamase. In this situation, rapid permeation (c) is needed to maintain a high periplasmic concentration. In e and f, there is only a slow removal by the periplasmic enzyme, and even a slow rate of influx would suffice to maintain high periplasmic concentrations (see f).

gradation by cytoplasmic enzymes; however, so far there is little quantitative data for assessing the importance of these pathways.

These considerations lead us to two major sources of confusion and misunderstanding in this field. First, many workers tried to understand the barrier properties of the outer membrane on a qualitative basis. Thus they asked whether the outer membrane is or is not permeable to a given agent, or assumed that the outer membrane should not act as a barrier for any solutes of MW less than 600 daltons, on the basis of experiments in which a near-equilibrium distribution of solutes was measured across the outer membrane (Decad and Nikaido, 1976; Nakae, 1976a,b) (see also Fig. 2a and b). It is clear that this *qualitative* thinking does not correctly reflect the actual situation. The outer membrane, or indeed any physical structure, should and does act as permeability barrier against any solute in the *quantitative* sense, i.e. it slows down the diffusion rate to a certain extent. Thus what is relevant is the *degree* of retardation or restriction of diffusion, not an absolute distinction between 'permeable' and 'impermeable' solutes. Second, when it is admitted that the removal of β-lactams from the periplasm is a significant factor, we realize immediately that the *balance* between the *rate of influx* and the *rate of removal*, rather than the outer membrane permeability alone, determines the periplasmic concentrations of the agent or steady state, and thus its efficacy. Unfortunately this important point is overlooked quite frequently. Thus the observation that a given β-lactam is quite effective in both the wild type strain and a 'hyperpermeable' mutant is often taken as a proof of the high rate of permeation of the agent. Obviously this could alternatively be due to a slow rate of removal (see Fig. 2f) rather than to a high permeability. The significance of removal rates is overlooked, in a similar manner, in many of the methods designed to measure the outer membrane permeability, and thus these methods can produce misleading conclusions (see Section 3). For example, Curtis *et al.* (1985) found that lowering of porin levels due to a regulatory mutation in *E. coli* K-12 did not much affect the MICs of cephalosporins with aminothiazole substituents. Although the authors concluded from this result that these cephalosporins do not use the porin pathway in their passage across the outer membrane, the knowledge that the antibiotic concentration at the target is also dependent on its rate of degradation tells us that such a conclusion is unwarranted, as the experiment involved third-generation cephalosporins with inherently low rates of degradation and wild type *E.*

coli cells with only a very low level of endogenous β-lactamase activity (see Fig. 2, a and b). In fact, in *E. cloacae* the loss (reduction) of porins was shown to increase the MICs of cefotaxime and aztreonam about 30-fold (Werner *et al.*, 1985).

2.2. SPECIFIC PATHWAYS

In the *E. coli* outer membrane, several specific pathways of diffusion are known in addition to the nonspecific porin channel. At present, these specific pathways appear to be divided into two classes. The first group includes those dependent on the presence of 'receptor proteins' for phage lambda and for phage T6. These proteins appear to produce transmembrane channels, which allow the diffusion of very small solutes similarly to the porin channel, but have additional discriminatory mechanisms that favor the diffusion of specific solutes: maltose (and maltodextrins) (Boehler-Kohler *et al.*, 1979; Luckey and Nikaido, 1980a,b) and nucleosides (Hantke, 1976). Since the configurational discrimination of these channels becomes stronger for larger molecules (Luckey and Nikaido, 1980a), one would not expect that β-lactam molecules would diffuse through these channels at significant rates. Indeed, liposomes containing the lambda receptor channel were shown to be essentially impermeable to various β-lactams tested (H. Nikaido, unpublished observation).

The second group of specific pathways transport vitamin B_{12} and iron-chelator complexes (Konisky, 1979; Neilands, 1982). These systems are different from the first group in that the protein component present in the outer membrane can be shown to bind to the solute specifically and with high affinity, and that this transport function requires the wild-type allele of the *tonB* gene. It is not known whether these systems can transport common β-lactams, but this seems highly unlikely in view of the apparently high degree of specificity of these pathways. More recently, however, β-lactam compounds containing iron-chelating structures have been developed, and at least one of them appears to utilize the specific iron-chelator pathway because its action requires the functional *tonB* gene (Watanabe *et al.*, 1987).

Higgins (1984) argues that the high rate of uptake of peptides by *E. coli* and the low apparent K_m values for this process are difficult to explain by the passage of peptides through porin channels alone, and states that he has preliminary evidence suggesting the presence of a peptide-specific channel protein. If such a channel indeed exists, it would be most interesting to study the diffusion of β-lactams through these channels, because β-lactams may be considered to be peptide analogs.

Among nonenteric bacteria, *Pseudomonas aeruginosa* produces proteins that are presumed to be specific channel proteins for phosphate (Hancock *et al.*, 1982) and glucose (Hancock and Carey, 1980). *A priori,* neither of them appeared likely to be involved in the diffusion of β-lactams. However, imipenem-resistant mutants of *P. aeruginosa* were recently found to produce decreased levels of the glucose-channel protein (Quinn *et al.*, 1986; Buscher *et al.*, 1987).

2.3. LIPID BILAYER REGIONS

Lipid bilayer regions of most biological membranes (Stein, 1967) and reconstituted phospholipid bilayer membranes (Cohen and Bangham, 1972) are known to be permeable to lipophilic solutes, which traverse the membrane apparently by first dissolving into the hydrocarbon interior of the membrane. Since some of the β-lactam compounds are rather lipophilic, this pathway might be expected to play a significant role in their penetration through the outer membrane. The rapid exchange of protons and alkali metal cations through the porin channel should dissipate the pH gradient which would otherwise be generated by the diffusion of the lipophilic, uncharged form of the β-lactams through the membrane. However, the Enterobacteriaceae, including *E. coli* and *S. typhimurium* at least, are known to be quite resistant to a number of lipophilic antibiotics and inhibitory agents, including actinomycin D, novobiocin, rifamycin SV, macrolides and various dyes and detergents (Nikaido, 1976). These observations suggest that the outer membrane of *E. coli* and *S. typhimurium*, and its lipid bilayer region, is rather impermeable to lipophilic molecules. This hypothesis was supported strongly by the observation that these organisms become much more sensitive to these agents if the outer membrane structure is altered by

EDTA treatment (Leive, 1974) or by mutational changes in lipopolysaccharide structure (Roantree *et al.*, 1977; Schmidt *et al.*, 1969; Schlecht and Westphal, 1970). Furthermore, the increased sensitivity was indeed shown to be due to increased rates of penetration (Hamilton-Miller, 1965; Nikaido, 1976).

How do these organisms reduce the lipophilic permeability of the lipid bilayer region of the outer membrane? The alterations necessary for increasing its permeability involve either removal or structural alteration of lipopolysaccharides, and therefore it is reasonable to assume that lipopolysaccharides play an important role in this barrier. Practically all lipopolysaccharide molecules are located in the outer half of the outer membrane (Mühlradt and Golecki, 1975; Funahara and Nikaido, 1980). Lipopolysaccharides contain a number of charged groups which must be located close to the membrane surface and at least seven hydrocarbon chains are attached to their backbone structure (Lüderitz *et al.*, 1971; Galanos *et al.*, 1977; Takayama *et al.*, 1983). It is not difficult to imagine that these features would make it difficult for hydrophobic molecules to penetrate through the lipopolysaccharide monolayer into the membrane interior. If this idea is correct, then the outer leaflet of the outer membrane should not only be rich in lipopolysaccharide but should also be essentially devoid of phospholipids. The outer membrane, essentially devoid of regions of phospholipid bilayer, would therefore lack the permeability to hydrophobic solutes characteristic of normal membranes. Indeed covalent labeling and enzyme digestion studies have shown that there are few phospholipid head groups exposed on the surface of *S. typhimurium* cells (Kamio and Nikaido, 1976) (see Fig. 1).

As stated earlier, mutant strains producing lipopolysaccharides of very incomplete structure, i.e. the 'deep rough' mutants, are unusually sensitive to hydrophobic inhibitors (Roantree *et al.*, 1977; Schmidt *et al.*, 1969; Schlecht and Westphal, 1970), and produces outer membranes with high permeability to these agents. Although it is conceivable that these defective lipopolysaccharides themselves served as poor permeability barriers, we found another, even more striking change in the outer membrane of these mutants. These strains could not incorporate normal amounts of proteins into the outer membrane (Ames *et al.*, 1974; Koplow and Goldfine, 1974), and there was a compensatory increase in the amounts of phospholipids (Smit *et al.*, 1975), which were shown to be distributed on both sides of the membrane (Kamio and Nikaido, 1976). Lipophilic agents can traverse this modified outer membrane easily, through the phospholipid bilayer regions, as expected (Nikaido, 1976).

These results indicate that we can safely disregard the possibility of diffusion through lipid bilayer regions, as long as we are concerned only with the penetration of the *usual* type of β-lactam agents into *wild-type* strains of *E. coli* or *S. typhimurium*. However, we should keep in mind that this pathway might become significant under certain conditions. For example, with some nonenteric bacteria, the outer membrane could contain significant numbers of phospholipid molecules in the outer leaflet; in such bacteria the bilayer region would certainly allow the diffusion of some β-lactams. In fact, the phospholipid/protein ratio reported for *Neisseria gonorrhoeae* outer membrane (Lysko and Morse, 1981) is 50–90% higher than that for *S. typhimurium* (Smit *et al.*, 1975), and this observation is consistent with the well-known high sensitivity of the former organism to many hydrophobic antibiotics. As another example, we may consider the penetration of extremely hydrophobic members of the β-lactam family. As will be seen in Section 4, the rate of diffusion through the porin channel becomes very slow for these compounds. On the other hand, the rate of diffusion through the bilayer increases with increased hydrophobicity, and although the rate is low to start with, possibly it could become comparable with the low diffusion rate through the porin channel.

3. METHODS FOR ASSESSING THE PERMEABILITY OF THE OUTER MEMBRANE

As we have emphasized in the preceding section, it is most important to measure permeability in a quantitative manner. However, the rate of diffusion itself is not a reproducible parameter, as it is influenced by a number of other parameters. For passive diffusion processes such as the diffusion through the outer membrane, Fick's first law holds, so that

$$J = P \cdot A \cdot (C_o - C_p) \tag{1}$$

where J is the flux of the solute per unit time per unit mass of cells, P is the permeability coefficient, and A, the area of the membrane per unit mass of cells. C_o and C_p denote the concentration of the solute in the outside medium and periplasmic space, respectively. For a given solute, P is constant for a given strain under constant physiological conditions (growth medium, aeration, temperature, ionic strength, pH, etc.). The rate of diffusion or flux is then dependent on the solute concentration and the value of P. Thus the ultimate aim of the permeability assay should be to determine P or parameters that have direct relationship to P; this will be the criterion used below in order to evaluate the various assay methods proposed.

3.1. 'CRYPTICITY' OR 'PERMEABILITY INDEX'

As we have seen in Section 1, it was noted already by 1963 that the rate of hydrolysis of β-lactams by bacterial extracts is usually significantly higher than the rate of hydrolysis by corresponding amounts of intact cells (Smith, 1963; Hamilton-Miller, 1963). Hamilton-Miller (1963) called the ratio between these two rates the 'permeability index', and used it as an approximate measure of the permeability of the cell surface barrier. This approach was then expanded and applied extensively by Richmond and his associates (Richmond and Sykes, 1973; Richmond and Curtis, 1974), who called this index 'crypticity'. Unfortunately, even with a given β-lactam antibiotic in a given strain in a given set of physiological conditions, it is possible to get almost any value of this index by simply changing the drug concentration in the external medium. This is because the rate of diffusion across the outer membrane can be increased almost infinitely by raising C_o (Eqn 1); thus the crypticity will become lower and lower as C_o is increased. Furthermore, the rate of hydrolysis in intact cells is affected by the V_{max} and K_m of the periplasmic β-lactamase. Thus it is impossible to use this assay to compare the permeability of bacterial strains containing different β-lactamases, or even the same β-lactamase in different amounts. Also one cannot compare crypticity values for different β-lactams and draw conclusions on the relative permeability of these compounds, because the same β-lactamase will exhibit different values of K_m and V_{max} for different compounds.

While some of these limitations were pointed out carefully by pioneering workers (Richmond and Curtis, 1974), it is regrettable that many invalid comparisons have been made and erroneous conclusions drawn through the overinterpretation of crypticity values. The careless use of these indices also tends to give erroneous impressions of the barrier properties of the outer membrane. For example, in *E. coli* cephaloridine usually gives a crypticity value very close to 1, and this has been interpreted often as evidence that "cephaloridine freely diffuses through the cell wall" or "*E. coli* does not possess any permeability barrier against cephaloridine". Actually nothing can be farther from truth. Although cephaloridine is one of the most rapidly penetrating β-lactam compounds (see Section 4), its rate of diffusion across the outer membrane is still at least 10,000 times slower than its rate of free diffusion in bulk water. However, the TEM-type β-lactamase used commonly in crypticity assays has a very high K_m for cephaloridine (Richmond and Sykes, 1973), so that at low C_o, where the crypticity measurement should otherwise become sensitive to the rate of permeation, the overall rate of cephaloridine hydrolysis is determined mostly by the slow reaction rate of the enzyme and is not limited by the outer membrane permeability (see Fig. 2e and f).

There is only one theoretically correct set of conditions where comparisons of crypticity values are valid. When different strains of bacteria are known to contain equal amounts of the identical β-lactamase, then the crypticity values for a given β-lactam (of course tested at the same C_o) should be a valid, semiquantitative index of outer membrane permeability. The data in Table 1, obtained by Richmond and Sykes, are closest to filling

Table 1. *Crypticity Ratios with 'Type IIIa Enzyme' in Different Hosts*

Host strain	Substrate			
	Benzylpenicillin	Ampicillin	Carbenicillin	Cephaloridine
Escherichia coli	30	65	126	1
Pseudomonas aeruginosa	80	60	60	50

Taken from Richmond and Sykes (1973) with the permission of Academic Press. Very large difference in the crypticity ratio with cephaloridine between the two organisms clearly suggest the much lower permeability of the *P. aeruginosa* outer membrane. However, other numbers, such as the higher ratio for ampicillin in comparison with benzylpenicillin in *E. coli*, or similar ratios for ampicillin in both organisms, are misleading and suggest the limitations of this method.

this set of criteria, as the strains presumably contained the same R-factor, although we still cannot rule out the possibility that the expression of the *bla* gene in this R-factor may have been strain dependent. From these data, it seems likely, that the outer membrane of *Pseudomonas aeruginosa* acts as a much more serious barrier for the penetration of cephaloridine than does the outer membrane of *E. coli* (see also Section 4).

There are other sets of conditions in which the comparison of crypticity indices has practical value, although not absolutely justified on theoretical grounds. An example is the situation in which the periplasm contains a very high concentration of β-lactamase. Under these conditions, the β-lactamase activity is far in excess of the rate of influx of substrates through the outer membrane, changes in K_m and V_{max} produced by the use of different β-lactams would be less important, and the rate of permeation becomes the rate-limiting step (Fig. 2c and d). The relative rate of hydrolysis by intact cells or the crypticity index can then give a good indication of the permeability of the outer membrane. This may be the reason why crypticity indices have often led to correct conclusions in comparison between different β-lactams or different strains.

3.2. Sensitivity Comparisons with 'Hyperpermeable' Mutants or Permeabilized Cells

A major problem with the use of crypticity as an indicator of outer membrane permeability is that newer penicillin and cephalosporin derivatives, which tend to be resistant to β-lactamase-catalyzed hydrolysis, cannot be tested. For these compounds, assays based on comparison with 'permeable' cells have been proposed. In a method developed in Richmond's laboratory, the MIC value for an agent with wild-type *E. coli* is compared with that obtained with a hyperpermeable mutant of the same strain (Richmond *et al.*, 1976). This assay is claimed to be less sensitive to the growth condition of the cells, but for each strain one has to isolate at least one hyperpermeable mutant. In contrast, Scudamore *et al.* (1979a) use EDTA-treated cultures as 'permeabilized' cells, i.e. cells in which the barrier properties of the outer membrane have been compromised. Although mutants are not required in this assay, the damage caused by EDTA is gradually repaired in growing cells, so that growth must be followed by turbidimetry only during a short period (usually 35 min) after antibiotic addition. The 50% inhibitory concentration (IC_{50}) for the untreated cells is then divided by the IC_{50} for the EDTA-treated cells, giving a parameter called 'barrier index'.

There is a serious theoretical problem with these methods. Both methods were devised primarily as a way of comparing the penetration rates of different β-lactam compounds. In order for this comparison to be valid, the barrier in permeable cells must either be totally absent, or retard the penetration of all agents to the same extent. It is extremely unlikely that either of these conditions are fulfilled. In the hyperpermeable mutants from Richmond's laboratory, the permeability barrier is still present, because the crypticity values for benzylpenicillin was 2.5, i.e. significantly higher than 1.0, and because the MICs were still much higher than the concentrations needed to saturate some of the presumed targets, i.e. the penicillin-binding proteins in disrupted cell preparations (Richmond *et al.*, 1976; Izaki *et al.*, 1966). A structural alteration of lipopolysaccharide has been reported in one of the mutants (Clark, 1984), but it is not understood how this would alter the permeability of the outer membrane (see also Section 4.6). In any case, neither changes in the porin pathway nor alterations in the bilayer region would produce a uniform, across-the-board increase of permeability to all agents, as the former will primarily affect the penetration of hydrophilic solutes and the latter, that of hydrophobic solutes (see Section 2). In the permeabilized cells used by Scudamore *et al.* (1979a), EDTA treatment is known to remove lipopolysaccharides from the outer membrane (Leive, 1965), and this is most likely to create phospholipid bilayer regions similar to those seen in the 'deep rough' mutants (Section 2.3). This will enhance very strongly the diffusion of hydrophobic agents, but the penetration of hydrophilic agents will be influenced much less. The sensitivity data on EDTA-treated *E. coli* indeed appear to support these predictions (Leive, 1974). This method then will give falsely low values of the barrier index for hydrophilic agents, simply because EDTA treatment does not permeabilize the outer membrane sufficiently for compounds of this class. This prediction is borne out by the low barrier index determined for carbenicillin, far lower than that for benzylpenicillin, indicating a much higher permeability for carbenicillin (Scudamore *et al.*, 1979a). In contrast, it has been shown by more recent methods that β-lactams containing two negatively charged groups, such as carbenicillin, penetrate through the *E. coli* outer membrane much more slowly than the usual, monobasic β-lactams such as benzylpenicillin (see Section 4). Even the crude and semiquantitative crypticity assay shows clearly that carbenicillin penetrates the *E. coli* barrier extremely poorly (Richmond and Sykes, 1973). It appears, therefore, that the barrier index obtained by the method of Scudamore *et al.* (1979a) often leads to misleading conclusions, and does not reflect accurately the barrier properties of the Gram-negative cell surface.

In addition, the outcome of both of these methods depends on the steady state concentration of the agent in the periplasmic space, and, as we have seen in Section 2.1, this parameter is affected by the rate of removal of the agent, principally via enzymatic hydrolysis. This latter rate is variable from one β-lactam compound to another, thus introducing another element of unreliability to these methods. Scudamore *et al.* (1979a) argue that the β-lactamase present could not hydrolyze a significant fraction of the β-lactam molecules in the medium, but this is irrelevant, and what is relevant, i.e. significant hydrolysis of β-lactam molecules within the periplasmic space, requires only a very low total enzyme activity.

3.3. BINDING TO THE PENICILLIN-BINDING PROTEINS

Another proposed assay, applicable only to the diffusion of β-lactamase-resistant agents, is the competitive inhibition of labeling of penicillin-binding proteins (Zimmermann, 1980; Rodriguez-Tebar *et al.*, 1982). Thus intact cells and disrupted cell preparations are treated with a mixture of the β-lactam to be tested and a radiolabeled β-lactam assumed to permeate rapidly through the outer membrane. If the unlabeled β-lactam inhibits the labeling of penicillin-binding proteins in disrupted cells but poorly in intact cells, this is taken as an indication that the tested β-lactam penetrates poorly through the outer membrane.

The major problem with this method is that it is implicitly assumed, if poor inhibition is observed, that this poor inhibition, and therefore the low periplasmic concentration of the tested β-lactam, is due to slow equilibration, or the slow rate of penetration, of the drug across the outer membrane. That is, it assumes that the periplasmic concentration of the β-lactam has not attained the steady state or equilibrium value at the end of the lengthy (usually more than 10 min) labeling period; this is required because the steady state concentration will be equal to the external concentration, regardless of the permeability coefficient, if no degradation occurs (see Fig. 2a and b). However, at least in *E. coli*, the magnitude of the permeability coefficients of β-lactams obtained by the Zimmermann–Rosselet approach (Section 3.4) suggests half-equilibration times in the range of less than 1 sec to 30 sec, and it seems likely that the periplasmic concentration of the β-lactams will have reached its steady-state value early during the labeling period. Thus in order to explain the dependence of the steady state concentrations on outer membrane permeability, we are forced to postulate the presence of a process for removal of β-lactams from the periplasmic space (Fig. 1c–f). The variation in the rates of this removal process and its ill-defined nature undermines the reliability and accuracy of this method. It should be noted, however, that with organisms producing less permeable outer membranes (such as *Pseudomonas aeruginosa*; see Section 4) and with slowly penetrating β-lactams, one may be able to perform the labeling within the non-steady-state portion of the diffusion kinetics. In fact, the results of Zimmermann (1980), obtained with *P. aeruginosa*, appear quite reasonable.

3.4. Exact Methods on Hydrolysis Rates of β-Lactams by Intact Cells

The crypticity index frequently serves as a very rough, qualitative indicator of permeability, but it can be quite misleading when it is used as a quantitative index, as we have seen before. Two laboratories (Sawai *et al.*, 1977; Zimmermann and Rosselet, 1977) attempted to derive a more quantitative index of outer membrane permeability from the rate of hydrolysis of β-lactams by intact cells. Both laboratories recognized that the periplasmic concentration (C_p) of a β-lactam in a cell containing periplasmic β-lactamase molecules is related to its rate of hydrolysis (V) through the Michaelis-Menten relationship

$$V = C_p \cdot V_{max}/(C_p + K_m) \qquad (2)$$

where V_{max} and K_m are the usual kinetic constants of the enzyme. If we assume that the enzyme exhibits the same K_m and V_{max} in the periplasm as in free solution, then we can determine these constants by using sonic extracts of the cells, and thereby calculate C_p by measuring V. This is the extent of analysis by Sawai *et al.* (1977). Although they argued that the ratio between the external concentration (C_o) and periplasmic concentration (C_p) of a β-lactam could be used as an index of barrier property of the outer membrane, this ratio can vary widely for a given β-lactam, depending on the values of C_o and the V_{max} or K_m of the periplasmic β-lactamase, and is not a desirable index of permeability.

Zimmermann and Rosselet (1977), however, developed the theoretical analysis one step further. They made the fundamental and important assumption that, very soon after the addition of β-lactams to cells, a steady state is reached in which the net rate of influx of β-lactam through the outer membrane is balanced by the rate of its hydrolysis in the periplasmic space. Thus the net rate of influx is proportional to the concentration difference of the β-lactam across the outer membrane according to Fick's first law of diffusion, and

$$V = k(C_o - C_p) \qquad (3)$$

where k is a constant directly proportional to the permeability of the outer membrane toward the β-lactam. Since we can determine C_p from Eqn (2), Eqn (3) allows the calculation of k, which is an extremely useful and meaningful measure of outer membrane permeability because, for a given bacterial population and for a given β-lactam, it is independent of C_o, V_{max} or K_m.

Nikaido *et al.* (1977b) have extended this method to permit the calculation of true permeability coefficients of the outer membrane. According to Fick's first law of diffusion,

$$V = P \cdot A \cdot (C_o - C_p) \qquad (4)$$

where P is the permeability coefficient and A is the area of the outer membrane. Comparison with Eqn (3) indicates that $P = k/A$. An example of the calculation is given in Nikaido *et al.* (1983), and the practical aspects of the method have been described in Nikaido (1986).

The Zimmermann–Rosselet assay is one of the very few, theoretically correct methods for assaying outer membrane permeability. However, its practical application obviously requires carefully designed experiments. For example, the precision of the determination of C_p is rapidly lost if assays are done under conditions such that C_p is far above the K_m of the enzyme. For rapidly penetrating compounds, it is best to maximize the value of $(C_o - C_p)$ in order to get the maximum accuracy in the calculation of P according to Eqn (3); this can be achieved by lowering C_o, but at too low concentrations of C_o the precision of the β-lactam assay will suffer. It is also extremely important, especially for slowly penetrating compounds, to prevent cell lysis and damage to the outer membrane, because hydrolysis by enzymes released from, or located in, lysing or damaged cells will make large contributions to the hydrolysis rates by the entire cell population. With *E. coli* and *S. typhimurium*, we have found that addition of Mg^{2+} to growth media, wash buffer, and the assay mixture helps to minimize this problem (Chatterjee *et al.*, 1976; Nikaido *et al.*, 1977a). The contribution from the released enzyme can be estimated by carrying out an assay with the supernatant of the cell suspension (Nikaido *et al.*, 1977a), but that from periplasmic enzyme in 'damaged', leaky cells is impossible to correct for. For this reason, the Zimmermann–Rosselet assay is of somewhat limited value for very poorly penetrating compounds or for bacteria with rather impermeable outer membranes. For example, it has been difficult to measure the very low permeability of *P. aeruginosa* outer membrane with precision (Angus *et al.*, 1982; Yoshimura and Nikaido, 1982).

A major problem with this method is that it requires the enzymatic hydrolysis of β-lactam molecules in the periplasmic space. Thus if the bacterial strain produces an inducible enzyme, it has to be induced. If the strain produces little endogenous β-lactamase, R plasmids coding for a powerful β-lactamase must be introduced. Thus one has to make sure that these procedures do not alter the permeability of the outer membrane. The permeability properties determined in *E. coli* cells containing plasmids R_{TEM} (identical with R6K) (Zimmermann and Rosselet, 1977), R_{471a} (Nikaido *et al.*, 1983) or R_1 (H. Nikaido and E. Y. Rosenberg, unpublished results) are very similar to the properties determined with liposomes containing porins purified from cells not containing R plasmids (Nikaido and Rosenberg, 1983); thus these plasmids, at least in *E. coli*, do not seem to affect outer membrane permeability significantly. Plasmid RP1 has been reported to have pronounced effects on permeability (Curtis and Richmond, 1974). However, a more recent study showed that this conclusion was probably in error (Crowlesmith and Howe, 1980). There are some results, on the other hand, which suggest that group N plasmids alter the outer membrane protein composition (Iyer, 1977; Iyer *et al.*, 1978) of host cells.

Another major problem related to the requirement for β-lactam hydrolysis in this asaay is the difficulty in measuring the permeability of β-lactams that are resistant to enzymatic inactivation. This is an especially serious issue, because most of the recently developed compounds are β-lactamase-resistant. Kojo *et al.* (1980a,b) proposed a solution to this dilemma, applicable to a resistant compound which is slowly hydrolyzed by and is a good inhibitor of the β-lactamase present in a given strain. They first measure the periplasmic concentration of a β-lactam that is easily hydrolyzed by the enzyme, for example cephaloridine, according to the Zimmermann–Rosselet method. They then measure the cephaloridine hydrolysis rates in intact cells in the presence of the test compound. If one knows the K_i value of the test compound for cephaloridine hydrolysis in free solution, this allows one to calculate the periplasmic concentration of this inhibitor. Since the inhibitor is hydrolyzed slowly by the β-lactamase, V_{max} and K_m for this process can be determined, and application of the Zimmermann–Rosselet procedure yields the permeability of the outer membrane to these newer β-lactamase-resistant β-lactams. This method should work if the various implicit assumptions are all correct. Some of them are: (i) the influx of slowly penetrating cephalosporins does not compete with the diffusion of cephaloridine, (ii) exceedingly slow rates of hydrolysis observed when the β-lactamase-stable β-lactams are added to very crude preparations of the enzyme are accurate and are the results of their hydrolysis by the inhibited periplasmic enzyme and (iii) hydrolysis by this enzyme represents the only pathway for the removal of the β-lactamase-resistant β-lactams. Unfortunately, the published data (Kojo *et al.*, 1980b) are internally inconsistent, and it is as yet impossible to evaluate this method critically: experiments were performed at two different β-lactam concentrations, and the C_p values at these two concentrations should produce the same permeability coefficient. Yet calculations based on the data of Table 1 of Kojo et al. (1980b) give values differing by more than an order of magnitude. It is unclear whether the problem lies in the principles of the method or in the actual conditions used. High external concentrations of β-lactams were used, so that the calculated C_p for the inhibitor cephalosporin was up to 400-fold higher than K_i; it is extremely doubtful whether precise measurements of the cephaloridine hydrolytic rates were possible under these conditions, especially in view of the possible contributions of released enzyme molecules and damaged cells, as previously discussed.

Recently Bush et al. (1985) proposed a method for determining the extent of penetration of some β-lactamase-stable compounds across the outer membrane. When these compounds form covalent complexes with periplasmic β-lactamase molecules rapidly, as in the case of aztreonam, one can determine the extent of complex formation from the degree of irreversible inhibition of the enzyme after short exposure of intact cells to the β-lactam. Using this method, it was shown that aztreonam penetrated rather slowly through a wild type E. cloacae outer membrane, and that some mutants, presumably defective in porin(s), had an even lower outer membrane permeability.

3.5. Methods Using Reconstituted Vesicles

It is known that the water-filled channels produced by porins are the major pathway of diffusion for practically all β-lactam antibiotics now in use (Bavoil et al., 1977; Nikaido et al., 1977b). The measurement of the rates of diffusion through these channels in intact, wild-type cells are difficult because there is no easy and rapid way to stop the flux for the termination of assay and because the diffusion rates tend to be too fast for the time resolution of most assay methods. Vesicles of isolated outer membranes do not solve these difficulties and instead create an added problem of poor sealing or 'leakiness' (Nakae and Nikaido, 1975).

It therefore becomes essential to prepare liposomes containing only a few porin channels in order to slow down the diffusion process to an easily measurable rate. This was first accomplished by Nakae (1976a,b) by adding purified porin to a mixture of phospholipids and lipopolysaccharides. However, the method used for measuring the efflux of the labeled solutes from the intravesicular space, i.e. the separation of vesicles from the extravesicular solutes through gel filtration or the use of membrane filters, still lacked the necessary time resolution.

The 'liposome swelling' method, previously used widely for the assay of the permeability of lipid bilayers, has been recently adapted to solve this problem (Luckey and Nikaido, 1980a,b; Nikaido and Rosenberg, 1981, 1983). We make phospholipid liposomes that contain porin molecules within the bilayer membrane and impermeable solutes such as dextran in the intravesicular space. When these liposomes are diluted into an isotonic solution of the test solute, the influx of the test solute through the porin channel is rapidly followed by the influx of water, and the liposomes swell. The swelling decreases the average refractive index of the liposomes and thus their turbidity. The kinetics of swelling can be followed by continuous recording of the optical density of the liposome suspension, with no requirement for stopping the reaction. The diffusion process can be slowed to an easily measurable range by using a porin/lipid ratio of, for example, 1/3600 (w/w) (Nikaido and Rosenberg, 1981), in contrast to the approximately 1/1 (w/w) ratio present in the intact outer membrane (Smit et al., 1975).

In our original procedure (Luckey and Nikaido, 1980a; Nikaido and Rosenberg, 1981) the liposomes were made in dextran in an effort to increase their average refractive index and thus the sensitivity of the assay. These liposomes, however, exhibited anomalous behavior in solutions of electrolytes such as β-lactams, presumably owing to the Donnan effect caused by the presence of charged groups on the dextran molecule; for this reason we now make our liposomes in solutions of stachyose (an uncharged tetrasaccharide)

(Nikaido and Rosenberg, 1983). Briefly, we dry a mixture of 7.2 μmol of egg yolk phosphatidylcholine and 0.4 μmol dicetylphosphate at the bottom of a large test tube, and the film is resuspended by sonication in about 0.2 ml of a solution of purified porin or a suspension of outer membranes in distilled water. The suspension is sonicated until it becomes translucent, and is then dried, under reduced pressure, in a water bath at 45°C. The film is finally resuspended in 0.6 ml of a solution containing 12 mM stachyose, 4 mM Na-NAD, and 1 mM imidazole-NAD buffer, pH 6.0, by a gentle procedure involving hand-shaking, and the liposome suspension is filtered through a Millipore filter (pore diameter: 3 μm) before use.

As we have emphasized elsewhere (Nikaido and Rosenberg, 1983), the flux behavior of electrolytes may become very complex, as the generation of membrane potential accompanying the flux of cation or anion can then produce the movement of counterions. It is theoretically impossible to eliminate this complication completely in a system designed to measure the fluxes of both zwitterionic and anionic compounds, and our system is a compromise that minimizes, but does not completely eliminate, the fluxes induced by gradients of Na^+ and other ions. It is important to ensure that no diffusible anion exists other than the β-lactam, and this is why NAD, which is too large to diffuse easily through E. coli channels, is used as the anionic component of the buffer system. These liposomes behave reproducibly in swelling assays if reconstituted with porins or outer membranes of enteric bacteria. However, with porins producing large channels, such as those of P. aeruginosa (Hancock et al., 1979), this system cannot be used because both stachyose and NAD will diffuse through the channels.

Since we are observing the swelling behavior of multilayered liposomes, only the *initial* rates, which presumably correspond to the swelling of the outermost layer, give us meaningful information; the later part of the swelling curve is difficult to analyze because swelling is then going on simultaneously in many different layers of the multilayered structure.

One assumption in this method is that the swelling rate is limited by the rate of influx of the solute rather than by the rate of diffusion of water. It is, therefore, necessary to measure the latter by diluting the liposomes in water (or dilute buffer), and to use a concentration of porin that will give a much lower rates of swelling upon dilution into isotonic solutions of permeable solutes.

Another assumption of this procedure is that the solutes are crossing the liposome membrane through porin channels. With nonelectrolytes, the validity of this assumption can be easily established by using porin-free vesicles as a control. However, the situation is more complicated with electrolytes such as β-lactams, because it is conceivable that uncharged forms of β-lactams cross the membrane through phospholipid bilayer regions, accompanied by the passage of counterions via the porin channel. This possibility can be checked by using liposomes containing gramicidin A instead of porin; gramicidin will allow the diffusion of positive counterions, but not of β-lactams (Nikaido and Rosenberg, 1983). Use of this control showed that many of the penicillins are indeed too hydrophobic for this assay of porin function. Although it is claimed that this difficulty can be overcome by the use of phospholipids with high melting points (Kobayashi et al., 1982), this conclusion is based on the use of liposomes not containing any carrier for cations, and the authors apparently did not realize the need for the flux of counterions.

In another version of the liposome reconstitution procedure, hydrolytic enzymes are incorporated into intravesicular space, and the rates of hydrolysis of substrates are measured in these proteoliposome suspensions. The difficulty in this method is the production of large, unilamellar vesicles in a reproducible manner. At present the reconstitution with a phospholipid plus large amount of lipopolysaccharide (Barbas et al., 1982; Kobayashi et al., 1982), which tends to widen the interlamellar distance through electrostatic repulsion and eventually produce mostly unilamellar vesicles, seems to be the method of choice. Since one cannot measure the rates of diffusion of nonhydrolyzable agents, and since the size of the vesicles is difficult to control with precision, this method is of limited utility except that one can avoid the leakage of periplasmic enzymes in

Zimmermann–Rosselet assay from cells producing unstable outer membranes, such as *P. aeruginosa*.

4. DIFFUSION OF β-LACTAMS THROUGH THE *E. COLI* OUTER MEMBRANE

Rates of diffusion through porin channels are determined by the gross physicochemical properties of the solutes, and it is desirable, for the purpose of discussion, to separate these properties into independent attributes such as hydrophobicity, size and charge. However, it should be emphasized that these attributes interact with each other. For example, we measure hydrophobicity by taking the octanol/water partition coefficient of uncharged form of the molecule, thereby eliminating, as much as possible, the effects of charge. Yet the real molecule is charged, and charged groups, because of the presence of hydration shell around them, do impart considerable hydrophilicity to the molecule: this is why the zwitterionic compounds show excellent permeability (see Section 4.3), and why their permeation rates seem less influenced by the hydrophobicity of the uncharged skeleton of the molecule—the real molecule is probably well covered by water of hydration. On the other hand, in many cases the effect of charge itself is more important than the general hydration effect, and this is why we generally see the retarding effect of negative charges. It is also conceivable that hydration shell might increase the apparent size of the molecule, but we feel this effect may not be important because the water surrounding the molecule will be exchanged with the water covering the hydrophilic groups on the pore wall.

4.1. EFFECT OF HYDROPHOBICITY

It has frequently been suggested that increased hydrophobicity decreases the efficacy of β-lactam compounds against Gram-negative bacteria, especially *E. coli*. Perhaps this was most clearly stated by Biagi *et al.* (1970), who determined the hydrophobicity of various β-lactams as the R_m values in reverse-phase thin layer chromatography, and found that the efficacy of the cephalosporins, expressed as log $(1/c)$, where c is the molar concentration giving a set degree of inhibition, was correlated by hydrophobicity R_m by the following regression equations.

$$\log (1/c) = 1.928 - 0.527 \, R_m \text{ (for } E. \text{ coli).}$$

$$\log (1/c) = 3.327 + 1.120 \, R_m \text{ (for } Staphylococcus \text{ aureus).}$$

These equations show clearly that there is a positive correlation between hydrophobicity and efficacy in a Gram-positive organism, *S. aureus*, whereas with the Gram-negative organism the higher the hydrophobicity, the less effective was the agent. Since the study used compounds with substituents of diverse nature, the statistical correlation was rather poor, as expected.

Similar analysis with a large number of experimental compounds was performed by Bird and Nayler (1971), who used Hansch's π constants as measures of hydrophobicity. In some cases, a tendency similar to that shown above was noted, but in order to get good correlation coefficients, it was necessary to use equations with terms containing squares of π, as well as other constants such as Hammett and Taft constants. However, this could again be due to the heterogeneity of compounds included in the analysis. Indeed, when the data including only the straight chain aliphatic substituents at the 6-position of penicillins are considered, it becomes very clear (Fig. 3) that the agent becomes more effective with increasing hydrophobicity (or values of π) with *S. aureus* and with decreasing hydrophobicity with *E. coli*. The data for *S. typhi* show a relationship similar to that in *E. coli*, although it is somewhat less clear cut.

That the negative effect of hydrophobicity in Gram-negative organisms was due to the slowing down of diffusion through the outer membrane was first shown by Zimmermann and Rosselet (1977). By using their assay with intact cells (see Section 3.4) with eight

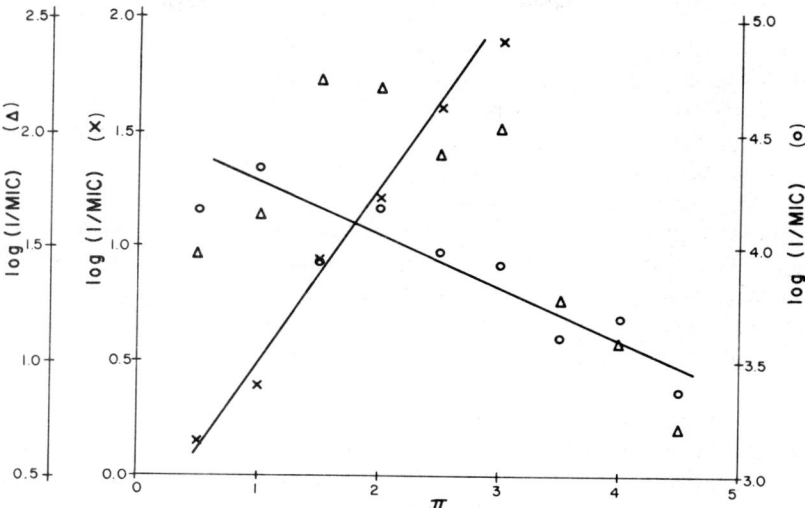

FIG. 3. Efficacy of a homologous series of penicillins in *E. coli*, *Salmonella typhi* and *S. aureus*. Compounds tested were *n*-alkylpenicillins, where the alkyl substituents ranged from CH_3 to C_9H_{19}. log (1/MIC) values against *S. aureus* (×), *E. coli* (○), and *S. typhi* (△) are plotted against the hydrophobicity, or the Hansch π values of the substituent. MIC is expressed in mм. The original data, which formed the basis of correlation equations listed in Bird and Nayler (1971), were kindly supplied by Drs. A. E. Bird and J. H. C. Nayler.

different β-lactams, they found that there was a good correlation between the hydrophilicity and penetration rate, although cephaloridine had an exceptionally high permeability.

This work was extended by Nikaido *et al.* (1983). In the first place, they realized that the *apparent* partition coefficients, used by Zimmermann and Rosselet (1977) as indicators of hydrophobicity, are misleading in an assembly of compounds containing both monoanionic and zwitterionic compounds, because these values are also influenced strongly by the electrical charges on the molecule. Furthermore, they sought to separate the potential effect of charges from the effect of hydrophobicity. They therefore compared only monoanionic cephalosporins of similar size (for structures of β-lactams, see Fig. 4), and expressed the hydrophobicity of the drugs by the octanol/water partition coefficient of the *uncharged form* of the molecule. Finally, they used mutants producing only one porin species. This analysis produced a very good correlation between the hydrophobicity and the outer membrane penetration rate (Fig. 5), showing that a ten-fold increase in the partition coefficient produced approximately five-fold decrease in permeability. In this analysis, the β-lactam compounds were clearly penetrating through porin channels, because the lipid domains of the *E. coli* outer membrane have an unusually low permeability (Section 2.3). This was also corroborated by proteoliposome swelling studies performed with purified porins (Nikaido and Rosenberg, 1983; Yoshimura and Nikaido, 1985), the results of which are shown in Table 2. There was a similar relationship between permeability and hydrophilicity, but in this system the diffusion through the phospholipid bilayer became predominant with the more hydrophobic compounds, confirming that lipid bilayers of the real outer membrane does have an unusually low contribution to the permeation of hydrophobic compounds.

A similar effect of hydrophobicity was observed by Murakami and Yoshida (1982), who compared the penetration rates of various cephalosporins in intact cells by using the Zimmermann–Rosselet method. They found the relative penetration rates of cephaloridine, cefazolin and cephalothin to be 100:23:3, ratios close to the 100:13:2 values found by Nikaido *et al.* (1983). Furthermore, they found that the replacement of the ring sulfur atom at the 1-position with oxygen in cephalothin and cephamandole increased the hydrophilicity and also the penetration rates through both *E. coli* and *Proteus morganii* outer membrane approximately by a factor of two.

As mentioned in Section 2.1, *E. coli* K-12 produces two porins, OmpF and OmpC, in ordinary laboratory media. The apparent size of the OmpF channel is slightly larger than that of the OmpC channel (Nikaido and Rosenberg, 1983). In studies with intact cells of mutants producing only one channel type (Nikaido *et al.*, 1983), it was reported that hydrophobicity had similar effects on penetration through OmpF and OmpC channels. On the other hand, the proteoliposome study with a series of peptides (Nikaido and Rosenberg, 1983) showed that hydrophobicity affected the penetration through the OmpC channel more severely than that through the OmpF channel. We believe that the results of the intact cell assays with the OmpC-porin-containing strains were in error, because the rates of penetration were slow and the accuracy of assays was very poor. Since the OmpC channel is narrower than the OmpF channel, it seems reasonable that the diffusion through the former would be influenced more by the hydrophobicity of the solute.

Because most of the penicillins are too hydrophobic to be tested with the proteoliposome system, direct comparison between penicillins and cephalosporins is difficult. One comparison we can make is between ampicillin and its cephalosporin analogs, cephaloglycin and cephalexin (Table 2); here we see that cephalosporins permeate about two- to three-fold faster. This is to be expected from the difference in hydrophobicity, as penicillins have about four times higher partition coefficients in octanol/water than the corresponding cephalosporins (Yoshimura and Nikaido, 1985). It is interesting that, among these zwitterionic compounds, the calculated hydrophobicity of the uncharged form does not

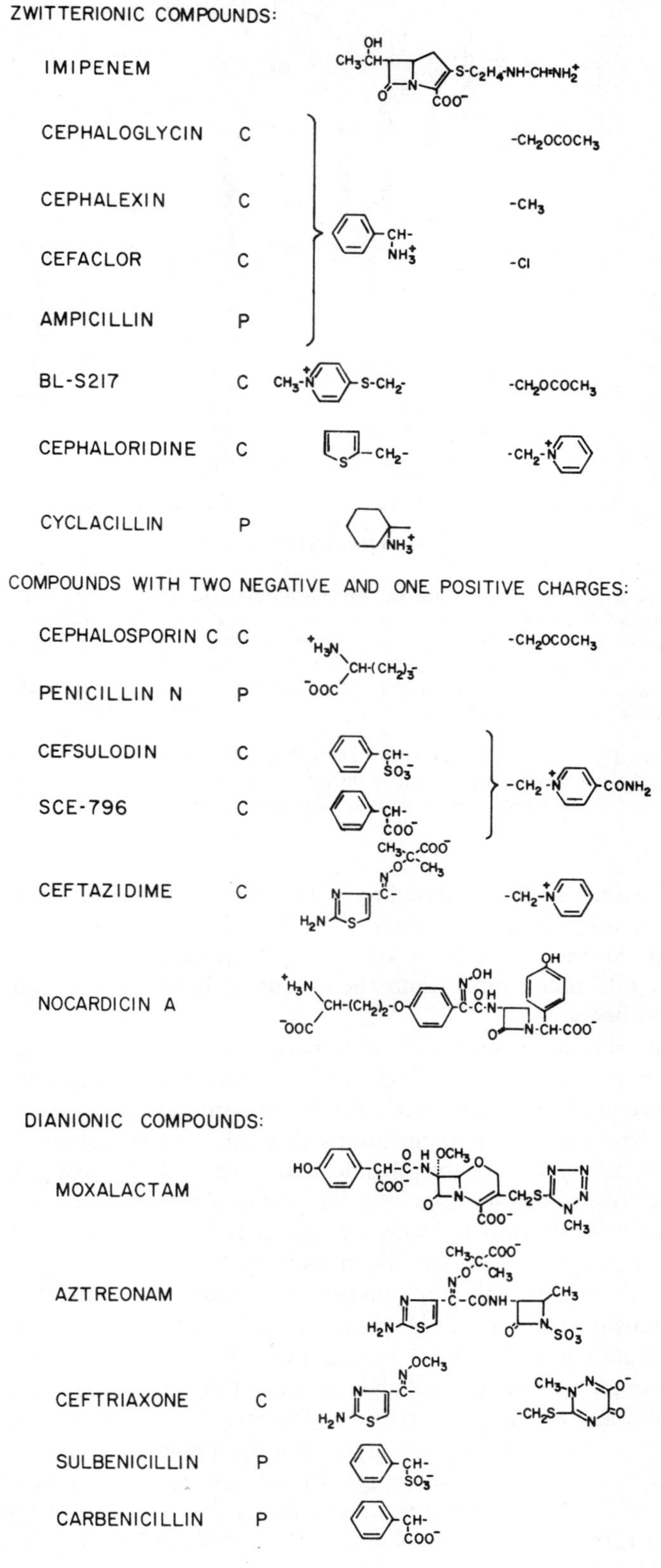

ZWITTERIONIC COMPOUNDS:

IMIPENEM

CEPHALOGLYCIN   C   -CH₂OCOCH₃

CEPHALEXIN   C   -CH₃

CEFACLOR   C   -Cl

AMPICILLIN   P

BL-S217   C

CEPHALORIDINE   C

CYCLACILLIN   P

COMPOUNDS WITH TWO NEGATIVE AND ONE POSITIVE CHARGES:

CEPHALOSPORIN C   C   -CH₂OCOCH₃

PENICILLIN N   P

CEFSULODIN   C

SCE-796   C

CEFTAZIDIME   C

NOCARDICIN A

DIANIONIC COMPOUNDS:

MOXALACTAM

AZTREONAM

CEFTRIAXONE   C

SULBENICILLIN   P

CARBENICILLIN   P

FIG. 4. Struture of β-lactam compounds tested. For compounds based on the traditional cephem (cephalosporin) or penam (penicillin) nucleus, only the substituents are shown. The substituent Z is —OCH₃ in cefmetazole and cefoxitin, and —H in all other compounds with the traditional cephem nucleus.

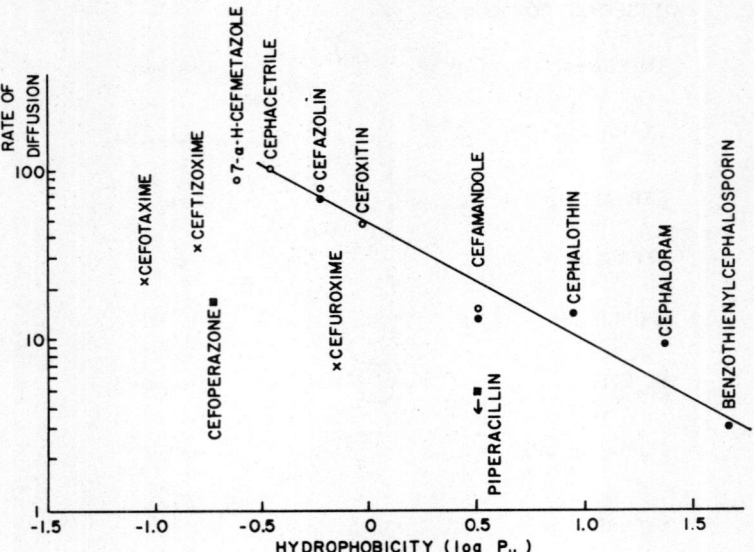

FIG. 5. The permeability of monoanionic cephalosporins. The rate of penetration through the OmpF channel of *E. coli* K12 is expressed as percentages of the rate for cephacetrile. The rates for the 'conventional' cephalosporins determined by the liposome swelling assay (○) are complemented by those determined by the use of whole cells (●) (Nikaido *et al.*, 1983), because the former assay was not usable for more hydrophobic compounds (see Section 3.5). The rates determined by the liposome swelling assay for compounds containing methoxime substituents and for compounds with exceptionally bulky side chains (see Fig. 4) are shown with symbols × and ■, respectively. Hydrophobicity is expressed as the logarithm of P_u, the 1-octanol/water partition coefficient of the uncharged form of the molecule. (From Yoshimura and Nikaido (1985) with permission from American Society for Microbiology.)

have much influence on the permeability within the cephalosporin series, or within the penicillin series (compare cephaloglycin with BL-S217 or ampicillin with cyclacillin in Table 2 and Fig. 6) (see also Section 4.3). Thus the nature of the nucleus seems to affect the penetration rate much more than the extent of hydrophobicity determined by the peripheral substituents.

It has been claimed that penicillins tend to penetrate through nonporin pathways (Sawai *et al.*, 1982), and the relatively high rate of penetration of ampicillin through a phospholipid bilayer (Yamaguchi *et al.*, 1982) has been correlated with this notion. Since many penicillins have very poor permeability through the porin channel due to their high degree of hydrophobicity, it is conceivable that even a slow leakage through nonporin pathways (e.g. diffusion through the lipid bilayer) could come to represent a major share in the overall penetration process. However, this does not necessarily indicate the presence of any specific penetration process for penicillins. In fact the higher permeability of ampicillin through the phospholipid bilayer in comparison with cefazolin and cephaloridine (Yamaguchi *et al.*, 1982) is quite expected. Cefazolin cannot cross the bilayer without the simultaneous influx of counterion, Na^+, which has an exceedingly low permeability through lipid bilayers (Bangham *et al.*, 1967); the situation is entirely different in the outer membrane where Na^+ can easily go through the porin channel (see also Section 3.5). Cephaloridine penetrates lipid bilayers poorly, presumably because its pyridinium moiety carries a permanent positive charge. In contrast, a small but significant portion of ampicillin can exist in the uncharged form that can cross the bilayer without much difficulty. In short, the results of Yamaguchi *et al.* (1982) are irrelevant to the mechanism of penetration of penicillins across the outer membrane.

Thus much of the current data on the permeability of β-lactams can be explained on the basis of gross physico-chemical properties of the compounds and their influence on permeation through the porin channels. Sometimes, however, there appear to be data that

TABLE 2. *Relative Permeation Rates of β-Lactam Antibiotics** *

β-Lactam	Mol. wt.*	Hydrophobicity ($\log P_u$)†	Rel. Diffusion Rate‡ Through OmpF Channel	Rel. Diffusion Rate‡ Through OmpC Channel
Monoanionic compounds:				
Cephacetrile	338	−0.45	100	100
7-α-H-cefmetazole	440	−0.62	82	
Cefazolin	453	−0.24	77	
Cefmetazole	470	−0.60	65	
Cefoxitin	426	−0.02	46	
Ceftizoxime	382	(−0.80)	35	19
Cefotaxime	454	(−1.05)	22	8
Cefoperazone	644	−0.74	16	
Cefamandole	461	0.50	14	
Cefuroxime	410	−0.16	7	
Piperacillin	516	0.50	<5	
Zwitterionic compounds:				
Imipenem	299	(−1.94)	216	280
Cephaloridine	415	(2.04)	167	
Cephalexin	347	(1.28)	129	
Cefaclor	368	(1.10)	123	
Cephaloglycin	405	(0.53)	87	
BL-S217	437	(1.50)	84	
Ampicillin	333	(0.95)	46	
Cyclacillin	341	(1.96)	40	
Dianionic compounds:				
Moxalactam	518	(−2.86)	34	10
Aztreonam	433		22	12
Ceftriaxone	552		20	<4
Sulbenicillin	412	(0.42)	5	
Carbenicillin	376	(1.38)	5	
Compounds with one positive and two negative charges:				
Cephalosporin C	414	(−0.88)	72	
Penicillin N	358	(−0.46)	56	
Cefsulodin	531	(−0.07)	37	
SCE-796	495	(0.89)	34	
Ceftazidime	545	(0.75)	12	<4

The data show the rate of diffusion of β-lactam molecules through the OmpF and OmpC porin channels in reconstituted proteoliposomes in the presence of an identical driving force. For the structure of the compounds, see Fig. 4. Taken from Yoshimura and Nikaido (1985) with the permission of American Society for Microbiology.

*The molecular weights of compounds with net anionic charge(s) are those of free anions.

†Those without parentheses were experimentally determined. Those in parentheses were calculated.

‡The rates were normalized to the swelling rate in cephacetrile. The actual swelling rate of OmpC-containing proteoliposomes in cephacetrile was 25–30% of the rate obtained in proteoliposomes containing the same amount of OmpF porin.

defy rationalization. For example, in the study shown in Fig. 3, Bird and Nayler (1971) obtained sensitivity data with *Salmonella typhi*, which look very different from those for *E. coli*. This is unexpected, because *S. typhimurium* porins are similar to those of *E. coli* (Tokunaga *et al.*, 1979). However, the plotting of the data (Fig. 3) shows the existence of a very similar negative effect of hydrophobicity, except for the prominent peak of activity at $\pi = 1.5$, which could have been caused for example by the peculiarity of the binding site of one of the penicillin-binding proteins in this species.

4.2. EFFECT OF SIZE (of β-lactams)

Proteoliposome swelling experiments showed clearly that the rates of diffusion through the porin channel are affected strongly by the size of the solute molecules, and that disaccharides with the MW of 342, for example, diffuse at rates about two orders of magnitude lower than that of arabinose with the MW of 150 (Nikaido and Rosenberg, 1981, 1983). β-Lactams frequently have MWs in the range of 350–450, and their size significantly retards their diffusion through the *E. coli* porin channels. Furthermore, the

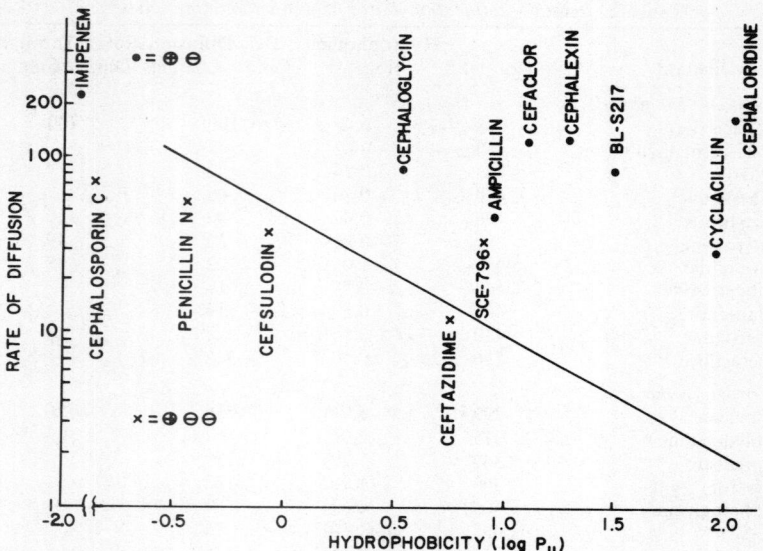

FIG. 6. Rates of penetration of zwitterionic compounds (●) and compounds with one positive and two negative charges (×). Penetration rates through the OmpF channel of *E. coli* in the reconstituted liposomes are shown as percentages of the penetration rate of cephacetrile. The solid line shows the behavior of 'conventional' monoanionic cephalosporins (see Fig. 5). From Yoshimura and Nikaido (1985) with permission of American Society for Microbiology.

permeability through the narrower OmpC channel is at least several times lower than that through the OmpF channel, presumably because the β-lactam molecules tend to get excluded more often from entering the OmpC channel owing to the collision with the rims of the pore (Nikaido and Rosenberg, 1983). Similarly, the OmpF porin channel of *S. typhimurium* shows higher permeability to cephaloridine than the OmpC or OmpD channel (Kobayashi *et al.*, 1982). Although the authors claim that Nikaido *et al.* (1977b) concluded that OmpC and OmpD were the most efficient pores for cephaloridine, no such conclusion was drawn in this work, performed by using strains all of which were deficient in the OmpF protein. In fact the permeability coefficient for OmpC⁺, OmpD⁺, OmpF⁻ strain was only one fifth of that found for OmpF-containing *E. coli* (Nikaido *et al.*, 1983), and this result is consistent with the conclusion that OmpF is the most efficient pore also in *S. typhimurium*.

In spite of their size, the influx rates of some β-lactams through the porin channel are rather impressive. For example, cephaloridine (MW = 415) penetrated nearly twice as rapidly as lactose (MW = 342) (Nikaido and Rosenberg, 1983). Perhaps the compactness of the ring structure and the added hydrophilicity brought about by the presence of zwitterionic charges speed up the diffusion process.

Small differences in size did not produce striking changes in penetration rates (Fig. 5). However, the flux became limited with compounds with unusually large size. This is seen for example with piperacillin and cefoperazone, which diffuse much more slowly than expected from their hydrophobicity values, most probably due to the very large side chain at the 6- (or 7-) position (Fig. 5).

Another case in which the effect of steric hindrance is clearly seen involves those compounds that have substituted oxime groups on the alpha carbon of the 7-substituents (Fig. 5). These compounds, which have dramatically high efficacy for most Gram-negative bacteria, paradoxically penetrate much more slowly, by almost an order of magnitude, than expected from their hydrophobicity values. The basis for this surprising phenomenon was suggested by the nuclear magnetic resonance data (Hashimoto *et al.*, 1976) that in the *syn* isomers these oxime substituents protrude out of the main plane of the cephalosporin nucleus. These substituents thus will produce a significant steric hindrance in the passage of these molecules through the narrow pore. This idea was tested by comparing the *syn* (or *Z*) compounds with their *anti* (or *E*) analogs, in which the substituents will not produce much steric hindrance (Yoshimura and Nikaido, 1985). As shown in Fig. 7, the compounds with the *anti* substituents diffused much more rapidly than their corresponding *syn* analogs, confirming our prediction (Yoshimura and Nikaido, 1985).

Methoxy substituent on the C-7, present in cephamycin derivatives, also had a retardation effect, but this effect was very small, and the penetration rate of cefmetazole, with the methoxy substituent, was decreased only by 20% in comparison with its 7-H analog (Yoshimura and Nikaido, 1985).

Among zwitterionic compounds, hydrophobicity seems to have less effect on the penetration rate than among the monoanionic compounds (see below). Here the size apparently becomes a major influence, and cephalexin with CH_3- substituent at the 3 position diffused consistently faster than cephaloglycin with the bulkier, albeit much more hydrophilic, $CH_3-CO-O-CH_2$- substituent (Table 2). The exceptionally high permeability of imipenem (Table 2) is probably due also to a large extent to the small size of this compound (MW = 299).

Even for average-sized β-lactams, the wider OmpF channel was several times more effective in allowing their influx than the OmpC channel, as described above. Because of this difference in channel diameter, it is expected that the latter will become even more restrictive toward unusually large β-lactams, and the ratio of penetration rates between the two channels would become much higher. This indeed turned out to be the case: it appears that compounds with molecular weights higher than 500 or those with protruding bulky side chains have real difficulty in passing through the OmpC channel. Thus such compounds as *cefoperazone* (MW = 644), *ceftriaxone* (MW = 552), and *ceftazidime* (MW = 545), which penetrate through the OmpF channel with significant rates, cannot pass through the OmpC channel with measurable rates (Table 2). This is a potentially important observation in view of the physiological regulation of the production of OmpF and OmpC proteins, to be discussed below in Section 4.6.

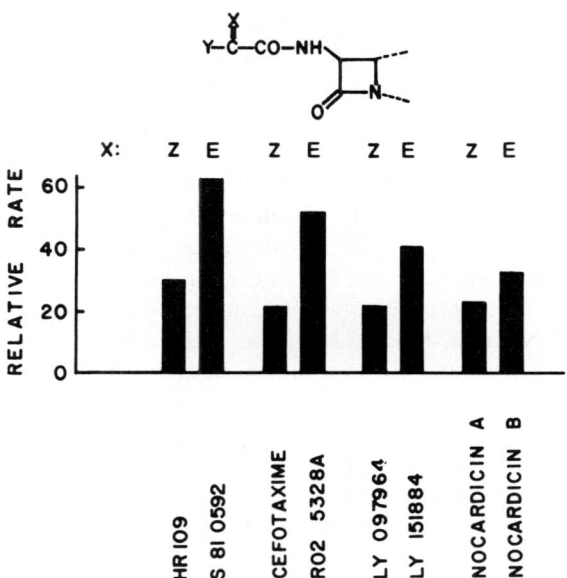

Fig. 7. Comparison of compounds bearing oxime substituents in *Z* and *E* configurations. The relative rates of penetration through the OmpF channel of *E. coli* K12 in reconstituted proteoliposomes are shown as percentages of the penetration rates of cephacetrile. HR109 is an analog of cefotaxime, in which a sulfoxide group replaces the ring sulfur at the 1-position of cefotaxime. S81 0592, R02 5328A, LY151884 and nocardicin B are *E* isomers of HR109, cefotaxime, LY097964, and nocardicin A, respectively. From Yoshimura and Nikaido (1985) with permission of American Society for Microbiology.

4.3. EFFECT OF CHARGES (on β-lactams)

As has already been shown in isolated cases, zwitterionic compounds seem to penetrate through porin channels much more rapidly than compounds carrying a net negative charge (Fig. 6 and Table 2). As stated above, among zwitterionic compounds, the hydrophobicity of the uncharged form does not seem to have a strong influence on the rate of flux. A similar independence from hydrophobicity also seems to exist among compounds carrying two negative and one positive charges, so that SCE-796, a rather hydrophobic compound, seems to diffuse more rapidly than the monoanionic compound of the same hydrophobicity (Fig. 6). As described at the beginning of Section 4, these observations probably reflect the dual effects of charged groups: in addition to the electrical effect, charged groups tend to increase the hydrophilicity of the surface of the molecule through the presence of hydration shells, and this latter effect could accelerate the permeation through the pore.

In contrast to zwitterionic compounds and compounds with two negative charges plus one positive charge, compounds with two negative and no positive charges diffuse into proteoliposomes rather poorly (Table 2). Among them, moxalactam and ceftriaxone showed reasonably high permeability values, presumably due to the very hydrophilic nature of the rest of the molecule. The presence of multiple negative charges appears to retard the penetration through the OmpC channel slightly more than it does that through the OmpF channel, as seen in the proteoliposome experiments with sugars and sugar acids (Fig. 1 of Nikaido and Rosenberg, 1983). It is therefore expected that dianionic β-lactams also will be more severely retarded in their penetration through the OmpC channel, and the experimental data seem to bear this out (Table 2).

A net negative charge seems to be an even more serious detriment to the passage of solutes through the outer membrane of intact cells than to their penetration into proteoliposomes. Thus in cells containing OmpF porin, cephacetrile and cefsulodin, each with one net negative charge, has rates of influx corresponding to 23% and 3% of that of zwitterionic cephaloridine (Nikaido et al., 1983). In contrast, cephacetrile and cefsulodin diffused into proteoliposome vesicles at 60% and 22%, respectively, of the rate of cephaloridine (Yoshimura and Nikaido, 1985). Similarly, the rates of diffusion of the dianionic SCE-20 were 4% and 19% of the rates of flux of the monoanionic cephacetrile, in intact cells and vesicles, respectively (Nikaido et al., 1983; Nikaido and Rosenberg, 1983). This more severe retardation of the negatively charged molecules in intact cells may be related to the presence of a Donnan potential, inside negative, across the outer membrane (Stock et al., 1977).

4.4. PROPERTIES OF PORIN CHANNELS FROM OTHER BACTERIA

In a qualitative sense, porin channels from other bacteria are expected to share the properties of the OmpF channel of E. coli described above. Thus the rate of influx of various compounds is influenced by the size of the solute, as shown in several cases (Bavoil et al., 1984; Douglas et al., 1981, 1984; Flammann and Weckesser, 1984; Weckesser et al., 1984; Yoshimura and Nikaido, 1983). The results with various porin channels are different only in the slope of the permeability vs solute size curve, and the fitting of the curve with theoretically predicted values provided the values of diameter for these channels. Similarly, in most cases bacterial porin channel appeared to favor cations over anions (Benz and Hancock, 1981), except for the Neisseria gonorrhoeae channel (Young et al., 1983). It is also expected that hydrophobicity will slow down the penetration through the channel. However, larger channels will be affected less by size, charge, or hydrophobicity of the solute (see also Section 5).

4.5. RATES OF PENETRATION AND ANTIBACTERIAL ACTIVITY

Among the β-lactam compounds of earlier generations, there was a clear relationship between the activity against Gram-negative organisms, especially E. coli, and their diffusion rates through the porin channel. Thus among penicillins, the earliest compounds with anti-Gram-negative activity, penicillin N and ampicillin, both show good permeability through the OmpF channel (Table 2). Among cephalosporins, the outstanding permeability of cephaloridine is paralleled by its strong activity. Furthermore, we have seen that the correlation between activity and hydrophobicity, seen among β-lactams carrying simple substituents (Fig. 4), can be explained by the rates of diffusion of these compounds.

The correlation, however, is not so simple with the more recent compounds. Certainly there are cases in which increased permeation rates apparently resulted in an increase in activity: for example when the aminothiazole substituent, which increases hydrophilicity and penetration rates (see Table 2 and Fig. 5), was introduced into cefuroxime-type structures bearing the substituted oxime side chain, it produced ceftizoxime and cefotaxime with much lower MIC values than cefuroxime. On the other hand, there are cases in which very high activity is accompanied by a rather low value of permeability. To begin with, the compounds with substituted oxime side chains usually have rather low permeability (Table 2), yet show spectacularly low MIC values (around 0.06 μg/ml) with E. coli; on the other hand, such compounds as cephaloridine or cephacetrile, which penetrate outer membranes perhaps ten times more rapidly, have MIC values nearly two orders of magnitude higher. Similarly, there are compounds such as piperacillin and cefoperazone that show low permeability yet are quite active.

This apparent paradox can be understood by considering the rates of hydrolysis of the drug in the periplasmic space. Even E. coli strains not containing any R plasmid will produce chromosomal β-lactamase. The activity of this constitutive enzyme, in a K-12 strain in which the structural gene has not undergone amplification, is about 0.005 μmol benzylpenicillin hydrolyzed per min per mg cells (Lindström et al., 1970). This rate is very low, and is less than 1% of the rate observed with extracts of cells containing some of the R plasmids coding for TEM-type β-lactamases (Hedges et al., 1974). Such low levels of activity often escape detection, and erroneous statements have been made about the 'absence' of β-lactamases in certain strains. Yet even this level of activity plays a predominant role in determining the MIC, and in producing the apparent correlation between permeability and efficacy of the agents. Using this value and using the permeability coefficient predicted for benzylpenicillin from its hydrophobicity (see Fig. 5), one can calculate that the expected periplasmic concentration of this drug from the equation given by Zimmermann and Rosselet (1977). As seen in Table 3, at external concentrations equal to MIC, the periplasmic concentration reaches levels that would inhibit the penicillin-binding proteins 1 through 3, the main targets of action of most of β-lactams. Similarly, improved permeability of ampicillin and cephaloridine is seen to produce periplasmic concentrations much closer to the external concentration, and to lower the MICs of these agents. We emphasize these conclusions, as the effect of the presence of very weak β-lactamase activity has not been stressed enough in the past.

The notion that the periplasmic concentration is determined by the balance between the influx rate and the hydrolysis rate, first enunciated in a quantitative manner by Zimmermann and Rosselet (1977), leads to the corollary that, if the rate of hydrolysis is negligibly slow, periplasmic concentrations of the drug of even very low permeability will approach its external concentrations (see Fig. 2b). We believe that this is the reason why some of the new compounds are active despite their unimpressive rates of penetration, as most of these compounds, especially those carrying the substituted oxime chain, or the 7-α-methoxy substituent, are usually quite resistant to hydrolysis. Calculation shows that with hydrolysis rates around 1% of cephaloridine, a periplasmic concentration close to 95% of the extracellular level can be maintained even when the permeability is only 1% of cephaloridine (Table 3). Even lower rates of penetration can be tolerated as long as the hydrolysis rate is slower. Thus low permeability is not a problem with β-lactamase-resistant compounds.

It should be emphasized here that we were able to predict the MICs in Table 3 quite accurately by combining the diffusion equation with the Michaelis-Menten equation. This not only shows that enzymatic hydrolysis is the main mechanism of removal, but also allows us to treat the antibiotic–bacteria interaction in a quantitative and predictive manner; it will be seen in section 6 that this approach allows us to determine the relative

Table 3. *Predicted Periplasmic Concentrations of β-Lactams in* E. coli *K12 Wild Type Strain Not Containing any R Plasmids*

	MIC* (μg/ml)	P† (nm/sec)	β-Lactamase‡		Periplasmic conc expected at MIC μg/ml	I_{50} for PBP1-3* μg/ml
			K_m (μM)	V_{max} (nmol/mg/sec)		
Benzylpenicillin	16	20	12	0.1	5.6	0.5–3.0
Ampicillin	3.2	345	6	0.003	3.0	1.4–3.9
Cephaloridine	2.0	1300	2000	0.11	2.0	0.3–2.5
Hypothetical cpd 1	0.1	13	10	0.001	0.095	
Hypothetical cpd 2	0.1	1.3	10	0.0001	0.095	

*From the data of Curtis *et al.* (1979). I_{50} indicates concentrations needed to inhibit, by 50%, the labeling of PBPs 1a, 1b, 2 and 3 by radioactive benzylpenicillin.

†Permeability coefficient of the *E. coli* outer membrane obtained from Yoshimura and Nikaido (1985). The value for benzylpenicillin was read from the curve for 'conventional' monoanionic β-lactams in Fig. 3 of Nikaido *et al.* (1983).

‡Kinetic constants for the chromosomally coded β-lactamase of *E. coli* K12, from Lindström *et al.* (1970).

contribution of hydrolytic and binding processes to the β-lactam resistance in β-lactamase-depressed mutants of *E. cloacae*. Recently Waley (1987) significantly extended this theoretical model. An important conclusion from Waley's analysis is that the balance between the rate of influx and the rate of enzymatic removal can be approximated quantitatively by a parameter called permeability number or P_n, which is obtained by dividing $P \cdot A$ (equation 4) by the 'physiological efficiency' (Pollock, 1965), i.e. V_{max}/K_m, of the periplasmic β-lactamase. If $P_n \ll 1$, the outer membrane barrier is significant and the MIC will be far higher than the β-lactam concentration required to inhibit the PBPs. If $P_n \gg 1$, the outer membrane does not act as a significant barrier and the MIC is close to the concentration needed to inhibit PBPs. Thus P_n is a very useful parameter in considering the function of the outer membrane; one should emphasize that it is inversely proportional to the physiological efficiency, V_{max}/K_m. The importance of the V_{max}/K_m parameter will be emphasized again in section 6.

It is difficult, however, to do precise calculations for wild-type *E. coli* K12 cells, because the hydrolytic activity of the chromosomally determined β-lactamase of *E. coli* K12 toward the more recent compounds has not been described. The interaction between the permeability barrier and β-Lactamase-catalyzed degradation in *E. coli* was analyzed recently in detail, and the results showed that the theoretical analysis can predict the values of MIC quite accurately (Nikaido and Normark, 1987). One can assume that the enzyme would behave similarly to other Gram-negative chromosomal, cephalosporinases, but even here we are hampered by the irrational habit of some workers of carrying out enzyme assays at only one, usually quite high, substrate concentration, rather than determining the K_m and V_{max} values. Thus there are numerous reports that cefuroxime, cefotaxime, ceftazidime, etc. are hydrolyzed with less than 0.1% (or 0.01%) of the rate of cephaloridine, at the substrate concentration of 100 to 500 μM. However, these superficially impressive numbers can be quite misleading. For example, a report from one of the few laboratories which understand this problem reports that *E. cloacae* P99 enzyme has K_m of 580 and 0.32 μM for cephaloridine and cefotaxime, with the relative V_{max} of 100 and 0.003 (Bush *et al.*, 1982). When assayed in the 'conventional' manner, at 500 μM substrate concentration, we would be led to believe that cefotaxime is hydrolyzed at less than 0.01% of the rate of cephaloridine. But at concentrations that matter, that is, at concentrations necessary to inhibit the target penicillin-binding proteins, the situation is very different. At 0.1 μM (0.04–0.05 μg/ml), cefotaxime is hydrolyzed at 0.4% of the rate of cephaloridine, a rate that could be significant in some situations. Furthermore, our recent work (Vu and Nikaido, 1985) showed that the chromosomally mediated β-lactamase of *E. cloacae* 55 M hydrolyzed cefoxitin and cefotaxime at 38 and 16% of the rate of cefazolin, when 0.1 μM substrates were used (see Section 6). These considerations emphasize the importance of reporting meaningful kinetic data when dealing with the substrate profiles of β-lactamases.

Another way to consider the role of permeability is to calculate the half-equilibration time, i.e. the time needed for the periplasmic concentration to reach one-half of the external concentration when the cells are suddenly exposed to β-lactams. This is a hypothetical number calculated from the permeability coefficient (see Nikaido *et al.*, 1983), assuming the total absence of degrading enzymes. This calculation shows that the half-equilibration time is of the order of 0.1 sec or less for the fastest penetrating drugs such as cephaloridine and imipenem, and only 20 sec even for the drugs with the slowest penetration rate we could measure, such as sulbenicillin or carbenicillin (Fig. 8). Thus the penetration of drugs across the outer membrane is quite fast in comparison with the growth rate of cells under normal growth conditions, and this suggests that drugs with even lower permeability could be effective as long as they are resistant to degradation or other mechanisms of removal from the periplasmic space (see Section 6).

4.6. PHYSIOLOGICAL AND GENETIC REGULATION OF PORIN CHANNELS

As stated earlier, *E. coli* K12 produces two porins, OmpF and OmpC, with estimated pore diameters of 1.16 and 1.04 nm, respectively (Nikaido and Rosenberg, 1983). We have seen that the diffusion of larger, dianionic, or more hydrophobic β-lactams becomes more strongly restricted in the narrower OmpC channel. Indeed culturing of *E. coli* K12 cells in the presence of low concentrations of dianionic β-lactams such as sulbenicillin, or of large and dianionic compounds such as moxalactam, selects for mutants lacking the OmpF porin (Harder *et al.*, 1981; Komatsu *et al.*, 1981). These mutants showed higher MICs than the wild type with hydrophobic or dianionic compounds, which obviously have difficulty in penetrating through the remaining, narrower, OmpC channel (see above). However, the MICs for compounds that easily go through the porin channel, including zwitterionic agents and monobasic, hydrophilic agents, were essentially unaltered (Harder *et al.*, 1981). These observations show clearly that, at least under laboratory conditions, *E. coli* cells can use the presence of the two porins to their advantage, and become resistant to certain agents by switching off expression of the wider pore. Genetic analysis of similar mutants, isolated by using cefoxitin, revealed that some were *ompF* mutants and showed a phenotype similar to that described above, i.e. unaltered sensitivity to rapidly penetrating cefazolin and cephaloridine, and increased resistance to agents with low intrinsic rates of penetration, e.g. cefoperazone, moxalactam, cefuroxime, cefotaxime and azthreonam (Jaffé *et al.*, 1982, 1983). Cefoxitin also selected for mutants that were deficient in both porins: these had mutations in the regulatory locus *ompB*, and showed higher MICs than

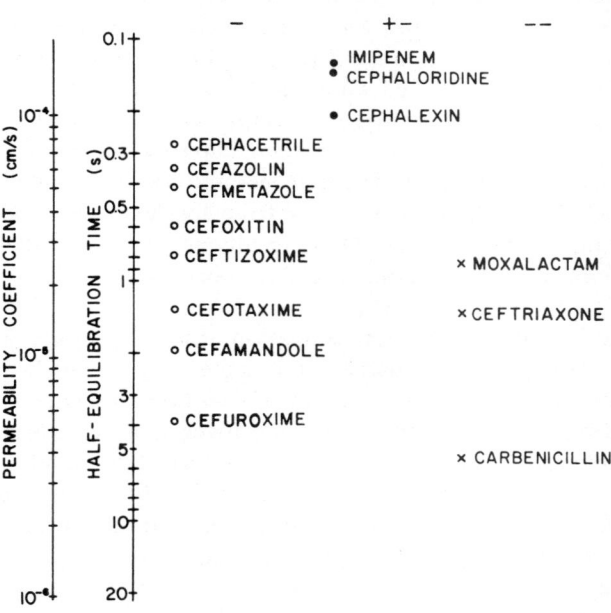

FIG. 8. Calculated half-equilibration times for various β-lactams across *E. coli* outer membrane. Calculation is performed as described by Nikaido *et al.* (1983). + and − signs at the top show the nature of charged groups present at the neutral pH.

the wild type for all β-lactams tested, as expected for such mutants (Jaffé *et al.*, 1982). Even these mutants, however, remained sensitive to imipenem and mecillinam. Although the authors suggest that imipenem uses a non-porin pathway, it seems possible that the extremely high intrinsic permeability of this agent, together with its resistance to hydrolysis by β-lactamases, results in periplasmic concentrations high enough to be inhibitory even when very small numbers of porin channels remain. Mecillinam, a positively charged compound, is also likely to have an exceptionally high permeability through the porin channel (although we could not measure its permeability in proteoliposomes because of its positive charge).

Mutants of a possibly similar type were reported in *Serratia marcescens* (Goldstein *et al.*, 1983). These mutants could be isolated both from clinical cases and in the laboratory, and were characterized by an increase in resistance to a variety of cephalosporins and also to aminoglycosides. The protein pattern of the outer membrane is altered, and a predominant band that could correspond to one of the porins disappears or becomes decreased in the mutants.

The synthesis of OmpF porin is known to be repressed in media of high osmolarity both in *E. coli* (Hasegawa *et al.*, 1976; van Alphen and Lugtenberg, 1977) and in *S. typhimurium* (Smit and Nikaido, 1978). The ecological advantage of this physiological regulation has remained a puzzle until recently, but our recent collaborative work with A. A. Medeiros throws some light on this question. Dr. Medeiros' group isolated an *S. typhimurium* 'parent' strain, harboring an R factor coding for a TEM-type β-lactamase, from a patient suffering from a renal abscess. After a few days of cephalexin therapy, they isolated a 'mutant' strain, which was more resistant to various β-lactams. Analysis of the outer membrane proteins of these strains, grown in Difco nutrient broth, a low osmolarity medium, showed that the parent contained two porins whereas the mutant contained only one. Thus the situation was superficially similar to the mutants isolated *in vitro*, described above. Yet further analysis showed that the mutant was lacking the OmpC porin, rather than the expected OmpF porin. Loss of the narrower OmpC channel is not expected to alter permeability to β-lactams significantly, and this was indeed our observation with the nutrient-broth-grown cells. However, when the cells were grown in the presence of 0.9% NaCl, the parent repressed the production of OmpF porin completely, and contained only the OmpC porin. The mutant contained no detectable amounts of porin under these conditions, and were indeed less permeable to several antibiotics (Medeiros *et al.*, 1987; see also Nikaido, 1984). Taken together with the observation that the production of OmpF porin is repressed at 37°C (Lundrigan and Earhart, 1984), the results strongly suggest that not much OmpF protein is produced while the bacteria are in the bodies of host animals, and that they use the more restrictive OmpC channel nearly exclusively in this environment, which is likely to contain many inhibitory substances. The OmpF porin, then, might be used when the bacteria are in natural bodies of water, an environment in which the most efficient uptake of nutrients from low external concentrations must be carried out by using wider channels. These results also illustrate that precise control of osmolarity of the medium is necessary when assessing the sensitivity of enteric organisms to antibiotics.

Another mechanism of physiological regulation of porin production was discovered by Argast and Boos (1980) and Tommassen and Lugtenberg (1980), who found that a new porin, PhoE, begins to be produced whenever *E. coli* becomes starved for phosphate. The PhoE channel does not retard the diffusion of negatively charged molecules, and sometimes favors anionic molecules over their uncharged analogs (Korteland *et al.*, 1982; Nikaido and Rosenberg, 1983), a feature obviously suited for the efficient uptake of inorganic phosphate and phosphorylated compounds from the medium. Although PhoE channel is of potential interest in accelerating the uptake of negatively charged β-lactams, we are not aware of any specific milieu that would produce the phosphate starvation and depression of PhoE within a host animal.

Several types of mutants altered in outer membrane permeability are known in *E. coli*. As described in Section 2.3, 'deep rough' mutants with lipopolysaccharides of very incomplete structure produce outer membrane permeable to various hydrophobic compounds, including hydrophobic β-lactams (Nikaido, 1976). Mutation in *envA* gene makes the cells more susceptible to both hydrophobic agents such as rifampicin and rather hydrophilic β-lactams. Grundström *et al.* (1980) showed that the lipopolysaccharide content of the outer membrane was decreased by 25% in the mutant. Thus the increased permeability to lipophilic agents can be explained as the consequence of the creation of phospholipid bilayer regions, but the increased penetration rate reported for cephalosporin C is difficult to explain.

Richmond's group have isolated mutants of *E. coli* K-12 that were hypersensitive to a wide range of antibiotics, for use in the study of permeability barrier of the wild type organism (Richmond *et al.*, 1976) (see Section 3.2). The mutants are hypersensitive to hydrophobic agents (the MIC for novobiocin is reduced 40-fold) and also to moderately hydrophilic β-lactams so that the MIC for ampicillin is reduced from six (Curtis *et al.*, 1979) to sixteen (Richmond *et al.*, 1976) fold. It has been reported that the mutant lipopolysaccharide has an altered amino group/phosphate ratio (Clark, 1984). Although it is tempting to assume that the altered lipopolysaccharide changes the permeability of channels by interaction with the porins, no direct measurement of β-lactam penetration rates has been reported, and proteoliposomes containing fragments of outer membrane of the mutant showed identical swelling rates with those containing fragments of the wild type membrane, in solutions of hydrophilic compounds (H. Nikaido, unpublished results). Furthermore, since the periplasmic concentration of ampicillin in the wild type cell should be very close to the external concentration when the latter is near its MIC (Table 3), it is rather unexpected that the MIC would be lowered significantly by further increasing the permeability of porin channel.

5. DIFFUSION OF β-LACTAMS THROUGH THE *P. AERUGINOSA* OUTER MEMBRANE

P. aeruginosa is resistant to a wide range of antibiotics and other deleterious agents (Brown, 1975; Bryan, 1979), and it has been inferred that this property is related to the poor permeability of its outer membrane. However, it was only in 1982 that direct measurements of outer membrane permeability was performed in this species. Angus *et al.* (1982) found that the permeability for nitrocefin, measured by the Zimmermann–Rosselet method (see Section 3.5), was about two orders of magnitude lower than the permeability reported for most other β-lactams in *E. coli*. More direct comparison using cephacetrile and cephaloridine showed permeability coefficients of about 10^{-6} cm/sec (Yoshimura and Nikaido, 1982), 100 to 500-fold lower than the values obtained for *E. coli* using these compounds (Nikaido *et al.*, 1983). Permeability to glucose 6-phosphate and *p*-nitrophenylphosphate was also at least 100-fold lower than that shown by *E. coli* (Yoshimura and Nikaido, 1982).

Since the *P. aeruginosa* porin produces a large channel, allowing the diffusion of polysaccharides of several thousand daltons (Hancock *et al.*, 1979), these results appear paradoxical at first sight. However, reconstitution with purified porin showed that only a very small fraction of the porin molecules produce open channels (Benz and Hancock, 1981; Yoshimura and Nikaido, 1983).

Recently two laboratories reported that most of the *P. aeruginosa* porin channels are far smaller than previously reported, even smaller than those of *E. coli* (Caulcott *et al.*, 1984; Yoneyama and Nakae, 1986). However, this conclusion is not convincing because of the following. (a) These results are in conflict with a large body of internally consistent data suggesting a large diameter for the pores, including radioisotope efflux data (Hancock *et al.*, 1979), liposome swelling results (Yoshimura and Nikaido, 1983), black lipid film experiments (Benz and Hancock, 1981), and the relative insensitivity of the rates of diffusion of β-lactams to their structural modifications (see below). (b) Much of the new results are compatible with the large pore model, if one remembers that smaller sugars diffuse through the porin channel more rapidly than do the larger sugars.

It appears that the high degree of resistance of *P. aeruginosa* to a number of β-lactams can be adequately explained on the basis of this exceptionally low permeability of the outer membrane, combined with the rapid hydrolysis catalyzed by the inducible, chromosomally determined β-lactamase. The β-lactams that show increased antipseudomonad activity probably do so because of their high resistance to the *P. aeruginosa* β-lactamase, their inability to induce the β-lactamase, and/or their high affinity toward the target penicillin-binding proteins.

It is difficult to study the diffusion of β-lactams through the *P. aeruginosa* porin channel. Proteoliposome swelling assay cannot be used except for zwitterionic compounds, as the 'impermeable' anion used in our study of the *E. coli* porin, NAD, will easily pass through the *P. aeruginosa* channel. We cannot use dextran-containing proteoliposomes because of complex and unpredictable behavior of these liposomes in electrolyte solutions (Nikaido and Rosenberg, 1983). The intact cell studies using the Zimmermann–Rosselet method are plagued by the fact that large amounts of enzyme tend to leak out of the cells because of the unstable structure of the *P. aeruginosa* outer membrane, and that they contribute heavily to the total activity measured because of the very low rate of hydrolysis by intact cells. Yet the existing, albeit fragmentary data suggest that diffusion through this channel is affected much less by the properties of the solutes than is diffusion through the narrower *E. coli* channel. For example, in *E. coli*, very hydrophobic nitrocefin molecules penetrate four times more slowly than cephacetrile molecules, yet in *P. aeruginosa* the difference in rates was less than 30% (J. Hellman and H. Nikaido, unpublished results). This relative indifference of the *P. aeruginosa* porin to the physicochemical properties of the solute suggests that it would be difficult to invent an agent showing an exceptional permeability through the general porin channel of this organism. On the other hand, antipseudomonadal agents should be able to tolerate a wide variety of structural alterations, which may create large bulk, high hydrophobicity or multiple negative charges. Indeed efforts to increase the antipseudomonadal activity of β-lactam agents have sometimes resulted in compounds of large size, with sharply decreased activity against *E. coli*. Cefsulodin (MW = 531) may be a good example of this class, and the much higher activity of its penicillin analog, sulbenicillin, toward *E. coli* may in part be due to its smaller size.

Consideration of the interplay between the outer membrane permeation rate and the rate of removal in the periplasm (Section 4.5) predicts that those compounds that are completely resistant to β-lactamase hydrolysis should be very effective against *P. aeruginosa*, in spite of the poor permeability of the outer membrane of this organism. However, there are compounds that do not fit this prediction. Cefuroxime, for example, shows poor activity in spite of its excellent affinity for penicillin-binding proteins and its resistance to β-lactamases. A possible explanation of this phenomenon will be presented in Section 6.

Meadow (1975) showed that mutants of strain PAC1, producing incomplete lipo-polysaccharides, sometimes become hypersensitive to carbenicillin. These mutants showed even more striking hypersensitivity to novobiocin and to other lipophilic agents, and therefore they seemed to be similar to the deep rough mutants of enteric bacteria (see Section 2.3). However, a later study (Koval and Meadow, 1977) suggested that the hypersensitivity and lipopolysaccharide defect were due to two independent mutations. In contrast, one of the rough mutants isolated by Kropinski *et al.* (1978) by phage selection had higher sensitivity to erythromycin, benzylpenicillin and deoxycholate apparently owing to its defective LPS structure.

Zimmermann (1980) isolated a hypersensitive mutant of *P. aeruginosa*, which was useful in demonstrating the presence of barrier properties in the outer membrane of this organism. The mutant was shown to have several alterations in the structure of its lipopolysaccharide, but it was not of the deep rough type (Angus *et al.*, 1982). Although it would be tempting to assume that the altered lipopolysaccharide affects the functions of the pore, evidence for such an idea is still lacking, and the molecular basis for the increased sensitivity of this mutant is unclear.

6. ARE β-LACTAMS 'TRAPPED' NON-HYDROLYTICALLY BY β-LACTAMASES?

In recent years, a number of β-lactam-resistant strains of *Enterobacter cloacae, P. aeruginosa* and *Serratia marcescens* have been isolated from clinical cases as well as in the laboratory. These strains seem to share the following characteristics (Sanders, 1983): (1) they produce the normally inducible, chromosomally coded β-*lactamase* in a constitutive manner, (2) they become resistant to a wide variety of third generation β-lactams, which the β-lactamase does not appear to hydrolyze at significant rates (see Section 4.5). These compounds include cefuroxime, cefotaxime, ceftizoxime, ceftazidime, moxalactam, cefoperazone and azthreonam, and the strains remain sensitive only to imipenem and mecillinam. This puzzling observation was explained by the assumption that the periplasmic β-lactamase, although incapable of hydrolyzing these agents, binds tightly to them, and thereby prevents them from reaching their target sites (Takahashi *et al.*, 1980; Yokota and Azuma, 1980; Then and Angehrn, 1982; Sanders, 1983).

This idea of 'trapping' was challenged on the ground that, for this mechanism to work, the total number of β-lactamase molecules per ml of culture must be larger than the number of β-lactam molecules (Seeberg *et al.*, 1983). However, this argument fails to take into account the presence of the outer membrane barrier. Thus if (1) the outer membrane shows poor permeability to the drug so that only small quantities of the drug crosses the membrane per unit time and (2) the number of β-lactamase molecules in the periplasmic space is very large, then the β-lactamase molecules lost by the irreversible binding process can be replaced by the synthesis of new enzyme molecules as a part of cellular growth, and the cells will be protected.

We have recently tested the two conditions listed above, using an *E. cloaceae* strain producing β-lactamase constitutively. First, we found that the permeability of its outer membrane to cephazolin was only 7% of that of *E. coli* K12. Furthermore, according to Kaneko *et al.* (1984), the major porin of this species seems to produce a rather narrow channel comparable to the OmpC channel of *E. coli*, and therefore the diffusion of most third-generation compounds is expected to be quite slow (see Section 4.2). Secondly, we found that the β-lactamase exists in a very large number of copies, estimated to be 2×10^5 copies per cell (Vu and Nikaido, 1985).

If we assume that one of the third generation agents would penetrate through outer membranes at a rate corresponding to 13% of that of cephacetrile (see Table 2), and that the latter compound has a permeability coefficient of $0.07 \times 7.5 \times 10^{-5}$ cm/sec (i.e. 7% of that in *E. coli*; see Nikaido *et al.*, 1983), then the maximal rate of diffusion of this compound (with an assumed MW of 500) from an external concentration of 2 μg/ml can be calculated as follows.

$$V = P \times A \times C_o$$

where P, A, and C_o denote permeability coefficient, area of the membrane and the external concentration of the solute. Using the value of 132 cm²/mg (Smit *et al.*, 1975) for A,

$$V = 0.13 \times 0.07 \times 7.5 \times 10^{-5} \text{ (cm/sec)} \times 132 \text{ (cm}^2\text{/mg)} \times 0.4 \times 10^{-8} \text{ (mol/cm}^3\text{)}$$

$$\times 6.023 \times 10^{23} \text{ (molecules/mol)}/(2 \times 10^9 \text{ (cells/mg))}$$

$$= 109 \text{ molecules/cell/sec.}$$

Since a cell will produce 2×10^5 molecules of β-lactamase per generation, it will make roughly $2 \times 10^5/30/60 = 111$ molecules of the new enzyme per second, if a doubling time of 30 min is assumed. Thus at least under the condition of rapid growth in the laboratory, the trapping should work effectively, and produce a weak level of resistance to concentrations of the order of 2 μg/ml (but see also below).

These considerations also suggest one explanation for the continued effectiveness of imipenem and mecillinam in these mutants. Imipenem has an exceptionally high permeability (Table 2), and this is likely to be true of mecillinam also because of its positive charge. It is also possible that their strong affinity to penicillin-binding protein-2 also contributes to their efficacy (Sanders, 1983).

The level of resistance observed in mutants isolated from clinical sources or in laboratory, however, is usually much higher, in the range of more than 100 μg/ml. One way to explain this difference is that the *E. cloacae* pores are much more restrictive than the *E. coli* OmpF porin, and that the permeability coefficients for some of the third-generation β-lactams may be much lower than the value assumed above. For example, if the permeability for a third generation drug is 0.5%, rather than 13%, of that for cephacetrile , it is possible to build up a resistance level of up to 50 μg/ml by trapping alone.

This hypothesis, however, does not fit with the result of Seeberg *et al.* (1983) who could transfer the genetic determinant for the β-lactamase into *E. coli* K12, the porin channels of which are not unusually restrictive for the third generation agents, and still could produce a fairly high level of resistance. An obvious alternative explanation is that the β-lactamase makes the cell resistant because it hydrolyzes even the third-generation compounds at a significant rate. As described in Section 4.5, much of the published data on the activity profiles of β-lactamases tend to underestimate the rates of hydrolysis of the new compounds, and a more careful study of this slow hydrolytic degradation should be performed. Our recent study of the chromosomally mediated β-lactamase of *E. cloacae* indeed showed that at 0.1 μM concentration, i.e. the concentration at which the penicillin-binding proteins begin to become inhibited, cefoxitin and cefotaxime are hydrolyzed at 38 and 16% of the rate of cefazolin, respectively (Vu and Nikaido, 1985). These are unexpectedly high rates when one considers that the V_{max} values for these compounds are only 0.002 and 0.001% of that for cefazolin. These data again emphasize the importance of considering the action of β-lactamases at physiologically relevant, very low substrate concentrations, not at the high, physiologically irrelevant concentrations normally employed for such assays, such as 0.1–1 mM. Our data (Vu and Nikaido, 1985) suggest that the high resistance level of this strain of *E. cloacae* can be explained by the hydrolytic activity of the enzyme at least for cefoxitin, cefotaxime and cefoperazone. However, it is clear that the calculated rates of hydrolysis would be unable to lower the periplasmic concentrations of the drugs effectively without the slow rates of their influx through the outer membrane. As emphasized earlier in sections 2.1 and 4.5, the all-important parameter is the *balance* between the rate of influx and the rate of hydrolysis.

The importance of enzyme activity at low substrate concentrations has been emphasized by other workers, and indeed the clearest formulation comes from Pollock (1965) who stated that the 'physiological efficiency', V_{max}/K_m, rather than V_{max}, reflected much better the activity of β-lactamase in real-life situations. Livermore (1983, 1985) noted the high affinities of *P. aeruginosa* β-lactamase toward the third-generation cephalosporins, and predicted that these compounds would be hydrolyzed at significant rates. Such hydrolysis has indeed been observed in a model system with dialysis membrane substituting for the outer membrane in limiting the influx of β-lactams (Livermore *et al.*, 1986b). It is also noteworthy that the resistance of *E. coli* to ampicillin, azlocillin, and mezlocillin were correlated more with the physiological efficiency of the β-lactamase toward these agents than to the V_{max} values (Livermore *et al.*, 1986a), as predicted from the observations above, as well as by the mathematical analysis of Waley (1987) (see also section 4.5).

In conclusion, quantitative studies of β-lactamase-depressed *E. cloacae* suggest that the high resistance level toward third-generation cephalosporins can be explained only by the significant rates of hydrolysis of these compounds, combined with low outer membrane permeability, not by 'trapping'. Although trapping could produce significant resistance levels in organisms with even lower membrane permeability, such a situation has not been documented so far (see also Livermore, 1985).

Bryan *et al.* (1984) found that a *P. aeruginosa* PAO mutant, which produced the β-lactamase constitutively, did not become more resistant to ceftazidime, which the enzyme could not hydrolyze at a significant rate. However, this enzyme has an exceptionally low affinity for ceftazidime ($K_m = 1250\,\mu\text{M}$), and trapping cannot be expected to work with such an enzyme. This study, therefore, does not disprove the trapping hypothesis.

7. GRAM-NEGATIVE BACTERIA WITH VERY HIGH SENSITIVITY TO β-LACTAMS

Some Gram-negative bacteria show exceptionally high sensitivity to β-lactams. For example, *Rhodopseudomonas capsulata* strains are reported to have MICs of 0.006 to 0.06 μg/ml for benzylpenicillin (Weaver *et al.*, 1975). Although it is tempting to attribute this to the large (1.6 nm diameter) size of the porin channels of this organism (Flammann and Weckesser, 1984), we note that a related species, *R. sphaeroides*, is quite resistant to benzylpenicillin with an MIC of 60 μg/ml (Weaver *et al.*, 1975), yet its porin channel is of only slightly smaller size, estimated as 1.3 nm in diameter (Weckesser *et al.*, 1984). Possibly the activity of β-lactamase in these organisms plays an even more important role than the permeability of their outer membranes.

Another well-studied example is *Neisseria gonorrhoeae*. When penicillin was first introduced, the MICs for benzylpenicillin were between 0.002 and 0.02 μg/ml, although currently in some parts of the world up to 50% of strains isolated have a resistance level higher than 0.5 μg/ml (Sparling, 1977). The anion preference of the porin channel (Young *et al.*, 1983) and the generally high permeability of the outer membrane in this species would contribute to the sensitivity, but the low level of chromosomal β-lactamase, which could be detected by analytical isoelectric focusing (Sykes and Matthew, 1976), but not by conventional assays (see Sparling, 1977), may be also very important.

Maness and Sparling (1973) analyzed the resistance pattern of clinical gonococcal isolates to seven agents, and found good correlations among resistance to benzylpenicillin, doxycycline, chloramphenicol and erythromycin. Particularly strong correlations were found between the resistance to a hydrophobic dye, acridine orange, and resistance to doxycycline, chloramphenicol and erythromycin, all rather hydrophobic agents (Nikaido, 1976), but no correlation was found between acridine orange resistance and resistance to streptomycin, a very hydrophilic agent. By genetic analysis through transformation, Sparling and his associates then found that the multiple resistance to hydrophobic agents was coded for by a series of mutations, including *mtr* and *penB*, and that there was another mutation, *env*, which made the strain hypersensitive to these agents (Sparling, 1977). They then hypothesized that the mutations affected the permeability of the outer membrane, and tested this hypothesis by measuring the penetration of a hydrophobic dye, crystal violet, into the cells (Guymon and Sparling, 1975). The results were beautifully clear. There was no uptake in the resistant *mtr* mutant (above the level that is due to the adsorption to the negatively charged cell surface), uptake was extensive in the hypersensitive *env* mutant, and it was at an intermediate level with the wild type. Although Scudamore *et al.* (1979b) claim that *mtr* and *penB* mutants are not much altered in their outer membrane permeability, this conclusion is not convincing in view of the theoretical problems with their methodology (see Section 3.2).

There have been extensive efforts to understand the biochemical basis of this alteration in permeability. The *mtr* mutants were found to contain an extra protein of 52,000 daltons (Guymon *et al.*, 1978). Although *penB* strains were initially thought to have an altered 'principal outer membrane protein' (Guymon *et al.*, 1978), which later was identified as porin (Douglas *et al.*, 1981), more recent study showed that this was due to the cotransformation of the linked *nmp*-1 gene (Cannon *et al.*, 1980). There was no change in the composition of lipopolysaccharides in either *mtr* or *penB* (Guymon *et al.*, 1978), although primary amino groups, which could play an important role in the interaction between lipopolysaccharide molecules, have not been quantitated. In *env* mutants, Lysko and Morse (1981) showed an increase of phospholipid/protein ratio, and thus it seems likely that the increase in permeability here is mediated by the creation of phospholipid bilayer regions, as in the deep rough mutants of enteric bacteria (see Section 2.3).

8. CONCLUSIONS

When the first β-lactam antibiotic, benzylpenicillin, was characterized, it was found to be practically inactive against most Gram-negative bacteria with the exception of a few species such as *N. gonorrhoeae*. In the succeeding decades, very many β-lactam compounds with excellent Gram-negative activity have been produced. We now know that the lack of activity of benzylpenicillin was due to two problems, a poor penetration through the outer membrane and hydrolysis by the periplasmic β-lactamase. In fact we can see that the historical development of broad spectrum β-lactams involved the development of high permeability agents during the earlier phase, but more recently emphasized resistance to β-lactamases, a strategy necessitated by the spread of R factors producing large amounts of these enzymes.

Yet we can see that bacteria have found ways to escape even the most recently developed agents. First, there are organisms that are deficient in porins, so that their outer membrane permeability can be greatly reduced (see Section 4.6). The presence of drugs can select for these strains, although they are expected to be at a significant disadvantage once in a drug-free environment. Secondly, the production of very large numbers of β-lactamase molecules with high affinity to some of the new agents leads to considerable resistance. There is still no general agreement on whether this is due to binding of the ligand alone, or to slow but significant hydrolysis, but as we have seen in Section 6, the outcome, i.e. the resistant phenotype, will be very similar in either case. Finally, R-factors producing new types of β-lactamases capable of hydrolyzing new β-lactams are constantly making their appearance (see Medeiros, 1984). As pointed out by Richmond and Curtis (1974) ten years ago, the Gram-negative bacteria have developed an ingenious strategy by having β-lactamase molecules located in the periplasmic space so that they hydrolyze just a small number of β-lactam molecules trickling across the outer membrane permeability barrier, and it may be a long time before we completely 'win' our battle against these organisms.

Acknowledgement—The work in my laboratory has been supported by Public Health Service Grant AI-09644 from the National Institute of Allergy and Infectious Diseases. I thank many colleagues in the pharmaceutical industry for their advice and interest, and sometimes for their efforts in finding or synthesizing experimental compounds; although I cannot name all, I am particularly indebted to P. H. Bentley, D. Boyd, B. Christensen, L. Ellis, T. Kamiya, R. Morin, J. H. C. Nayler, E. Schrinner, S. Sugawara, R. B. Sykes and T. Yoshida.

REFERENCES

AMES, G. F.-L., SPUDICH, E. N. and NIKAIDO, H. (1974) Protein comparison of the outer membrane of *Salmonella typhimurium*: Effect of lipopolysaccharide mutations. *J. Bacteriol.* **117**: 406–416.

ANGUS, B. L., CAREY, A. M., CANON, D. A., KROPINSKI, A. M. B. and HANCOCK, R. E. W. (1982) Outer membrane permeability in *Pseudomonas aeruginosa*: Comparison of a wild-type with an antibiotic-supersusceptible mutant. *Antimicrob. Ag. Chemother.* **21**: 299–308.

ARGAST, M. and BOOS, W. (1980) Co-regulation in *Escherichia coli* of a novel transport system for *sn*-glycerol-3-phosphate and outer membrane protein Ic (e,E) with alkaline phosphatase and phosphate-binding protein. *J. Bacteriol.* **143**: 142–150.

BANGHAM, A. D., DE GIER, J. and GREVILLE, G. D. (1967) Osmotic properties and water permeability of phospholipid liquid crystals. *Chem. Phys. Lipids* **1**: 225–246.

BARBAS, J. A., RODRIGUEZ-TÉBAR, A. and VÁSQUEZ, D. (1982) A new method to study permeation of β-lactam antibiotics into reconstituted vesicles from the outer membrane of *Pseudomonas aeruginosa* NCTC 10662. *FEBS Lett.* **146**: 381–384.

BAVOIL, P., NIKAIDO, H. and VON MEYENBURG, K. (1977) Pleiotropic transport mutants of *Escherichia coli* lack porin, a major outer membrane protein. *Molec. Gen. Genet.* **158**: 23–33.

BAVOIL, P., OHLIN, A. and SCHAECHTER, J. (1984) Role of disulfide bonding in outer membrane structure and permeability in *Chlamydia trachomatis*. *Infect. Immun.* **44**: 479–485.

BENZ, R. and HANCOCK, R. E. W. (1981) Properties of large ion-permeable pores formed from protein F of *Pseudomonas aeruginosa* in lipid bilayer membranes. *Biochim. biophys. Acta* **646**: 298–308.

BIAGI, G. L., GUERRA, M. C., BARBARO, A. M. and GAMBA, M. F. (1970) Influence of lipophilic character on the antibacterial activity of cephalosporins and penicillins. *J. med. Chem.* **13**: 511–515.

BIRD, A. E. and NAYLER, J. H. C. (1971) Design of penicillins. In: *Drug Design*, Vol. 2, pp. 277–318, ARIENS, E. J. (ed.) Academic Press, New York.

BOEHLER-KOHLER, B. A., BOOS, W., DIETERLE, R. and BENZ, R. (1979) Receptor for bacteriophage lambda of *Escherichia coli* forms larger pores in black lipid membranes than the matrix protein (porin). *J. Bacteriol.* **138**: 33–39.

BROWN, M. R. W. (1975) The role of the cell envelope in resistance. In: *Resistance of Pseudomonas aeruginosa*, pp. 71–107, BROWN, M. R. W. (ed.) John Wiley & Sons, New York.

BRYAN, L. E. (1979) Resistance to antimicrobial agents: The general nature of the problem and the basis of resistance. *Pseudomonas aeruginosa: Clinical manifestations of infection and current therapy*, pp. 219–270, DOGGETT, R. G. (ed.) Academic Press, New York.

BRYAN, L. E., KWAN, S. and GODFREY, A. J. (1984) Resistance of *Pseudomonas aeruginosa* mutants with altered control of chromosomal β-lactamase to piperacillin, ceftazidime, and cefsulodin. *Antimicrob. Ag. Chemother.* **25**: 382–384.

BÜSCHER, K.-H., CULLMANN, W., DICK, W. and OPFERKUCH, W. (1987) Imipenem resistance in *Pseudomonas aeruginosa* resulting from diminished expression of an outer membrane protein. *Antimicrob. Ag. Chemother.* **31**: 703–708.

BUSH, K., FREUDENBERGER, J. S. and SYKES, R. B. (1982) Interaction of azthreonam and related monobactams with β-lactamases from Gram-negative bacteria. *Antimicrob. Ag. Chemother.* **22**: 414–420.

BUSH, K., TANAKA, S. K., BONNER, D. P. and SYKES, R. B. (1985) Resistance caused by decreased penetration of β-lactam antibiotics into *Enterobacter cloacae*. *Antimicrob. Agents Chemother.* **27**: 555–560.

CANNON, J. G., KLAPPER, D. G., BLACKMAN, E. Y. and SPARLING, P. F. (1980) Genetic locus (*nmp*-1) affecting the principal outer membrane protein of *Neisseria gonorrhoeae*. *J. Bacteriol.* **143**: 847–851.

CAULCOTT, C. A., BROWN, M. R. W. and GONDA, I. (1984) Evidence for small pores in theouter membrane of *Pseudomonas aeruginosa*. *FEMS Microbiol. Lett.* **21**: 119–123.

CHATTERJEE, A. K., ROSS, H. and SANDERSON, K. E. (1976) Leakage of periplasmic enzymes from lipopolysaccharide-defective mutants of *Salmonella typhimurium*. *Can. J. Microb.* **22**: 1549–1560.

CLARK, D. (1984) Novel antibiotic hypersensitive mutants of *Escherichia coli*. Genetic mapping and chemical characterization. *FEMS Microbiol. Lett.* **21**: 189–195.

COHEN, B. G. and BANGHAM, A. D. (1972) Diffusion of small non-electrolytes across liposome membranes. *Nature (London)* **236**: 173–174.

CROWLESMITH, I. and HOWE, T. G. B. (1980) Characterization of β-lactamate-deficient (*bla*) mutants of the R plasmid R1 in *Escherichia coli* K-12 and comparison with similar mutants of RP1. *Antimicrob. Ag. Chemother.* **18**: 667–674.

CURTIS, N. A. C. and RICHMOND, M. H. (1974) Effect of R factor-mediated genes on some surface properties of *Escherichia coli*. *Antimicrob. Ag. Chemother.* **6**: 666–671.

CURTIS, N. A. C., ORR, D., ROSS, G. W. and BOULTON, M. G. (1979) Affinities of penicillins and cephalosporins for the penicillin-binding proteins of *Escherichia coli* K-12 and their anti-bacterial activity. *Antimicrob. Ag. Chemother.* **16**: 533–539.

CURTIS, N. A. C., EISENSTADT, R. L., TURNER, K. A. and WHITE, J. A. (1985) Porin-mediated cephalosporin resistance in *Escherichia coli* K-12. *J. Antimicrob. Chemother.* **15**: 642–644.

DARVEAU, R. P., MacINTYRE, S., BUCKLEY, J. T. and HANCOCK, R. E. W. (1983) Purification and reconstitution in lipid bilayer membranes on an outer membrane, pore-forming protein of *Aeromonas salmonicida*. *J. Bacteriol.* **156**: 1006–1011.

DECAD, G. M. and NIKAIDO, H. (1976) Outer membrane of Gram-negative bacteria. XII. Molecular-sieving function of cell wall. *J. Bacteriol.* **128**: 325–336.

DORSET, D. L., ENGEL, A., MASSALSKI, A. and ROSENBUSCH, J. P. (1984) Three dimensional structure of a membrane pore: Electron microscopical analysis of *Escherichia coli* outer membrane matrix porin. *Biophys. J.* **45**: 128–129.

DOUGLAS, J. T., LEE, M. D. and NIKAIDO, H. (1981) Protein I of *Neisseria gonorrhoeae* outer membrane is a porin. *FEMS Microbiol. Lett.* **12**: 305–309.

DOUGLAS, J. T., ROSENBERG, E. Y., NIKAIDO, H., VERSTREATE, D. R. and WINTER, A. J. (1984) Porins of *Brucella* species. *Infect. Immun.* **44**: 16–21.

FLAMMANN, H. T. and WECKESSER, J. (1984) Porin isolated from the cell envelope of *Rhodopsedomonas capsulata*. *J. Bacteriol.* **159**: 410–412.

FLEMING, A. (1929) On the antibacterial action of cultures of a *Penicillium*, with special reference to their use in the isolation of *B. influenzae*. *Br. J. exp. Path.* **10**: 226–236.

FUNAHARA, Y. and NIKAIDO, H. (1980) Asymmetric localization of lipopolysaccharide on the outer membrane of *Salmonella typhimurium*. *J. Bacteriol.* **141**: 1463–1465.

GALANOS, C., LÜDERITZ, O., RIETSCHEL, E. T. and WESTPHAL, O. (1977) Newer aspects of the chemistry and biology of bacterial lipopolysaccharides, with special reference to their lipid A component. In: *Biochemistry of Lipids II*, pp. 239–335, GOODWIN, T. W. (ed.) International Review of Biochemistry, Vol. 14, University Park Press, Baltimore.

GLAUERT, A. M. and THORNLEY, M. J. (1969) The topography of the bacterial cell wall. *A. Rev. Microbiol.* **23**: 159–198.

GOLDSTEIN, F. W., GUTMAN, L., WILLIAMSON, R., COLLATZ, E. and ACAR, J. F. (1983) *In vivo* and *in vitro* emergence of simultaneous resistance to both β-lactam and aminoglycoside antibiotics in a strain of *Serratia marcescens*. *A. Microbiol. Paris* **134A**: 329–337.

GRUNDSTRÖM, T., NORMARK, S. and MAGNUSSON, K.-E. (1980) Over-production of outer membrane protein suppresses *envA*-induced hyperpermeability. *J. Bacteriol.* **144**: 884–890.

GUYMON, L. F. and SPARLING, P. F. (1975) Altered crystal violet permeability and lytic behavior in antibiotic-resistant and -sensitive mutants of *Neisseria gonorrhoeae*. *J. Bacteriol.* **124**: 757–763.

GUYMON, L. F., WALSTAD, D. L. and SPARLING, P. F. (1978) Cell envelope alterations in antibiotic-sensitive and -resistant strains of *Neisseria gonorrhoeae*. *J. Bacteriol.* **136**: 391–401.

HAMILTON-MILLER, J. M. T. (1963) Penicillinase from *Klebsiella aerogenes*. A comparison with penicillinase from Gram-positive species. *Biochem. J.* **87**: 207–214.

HAMILTON-MILLER, J. M. T. (1965) Effect of EDTA upon bacteriol permeability to benzylpenicillin. *Biochem. biophys. Res. Commun.* **20**: 688–691.

HANCOCK, R. E. W. and CAREY, A. M. (1980) protein D1—A glucose-inducible, pore-forming protein from the outer membrane of *Pseudomonas aeruginosa*. *FEMS Microbiol. Lett.* **8**: 105–109.

HANCOCK, R. E. W., DECAD, G. M. and NIKAIDO, H. (1979) Identification of the protein producing transmembrane diffusion pores in the outer membrane of *Pseudomonas aeruginosa* PAO1. *Biochim. biophys. Acta* **554**: 323–331.

HANCOCK, R. E. W., POOL, K. and BENZ, R. (1982) Outer membrane protein P of *Pseudomonas aeruginosa*: Regulation by phosphate deficiency and formation of small anion-specific channels in lipid bilayer membranes. *J. Bacteriol.* **150**: 730–738.

HANTKE, K. (1976) Phage T6-colicin K receptor and nucleoside transport in *Escherichia coli*. *FEBS Lett.* **70**: 109–112.

HARDER, K. J., NIKAIDO H. and MATSUHASHI, M. (1981) Mutants of *Escherichia coli* that are resistant to certain beta-lactam compounds lack of the OmpF porin. *Antimicrob. Ag. Chemother.* **20**: 549–552.

HASEGAWA, Y., YAMADA, H. and MIZUSHIMA, S. (1976) Interaction of outer membrane proteins O-8 and O-9 with peptidoglycan sacculus of *Escherichia coli* K-12. *J. Biochem., Tokyo* **80**: 1401–1409.

HASHIMOTO, M., KOMORI. T. and KAMIYA, T. (1976) Nocardicin A. and B, novel monocylic β-lactam antibiotics from a *Nocardia* species. *J. Am. Chem. Soc.* **98**: 3023–3025.

HEDGES, R. W., DATTA, N., KONTOMICHALOU, P. and SMITH, J. T. (1974) Molecular specificities of R-factor-determined beta-lactamases: Correlation with plasmid compatibility. *J. Bacteriol.* **117**: 56–62.

HIGGINS, C. F. (1984) Peptide transport systems of *Salmonella typhimurium* and *Escherichia coli*. In: *Microbiology—1984*. pp. 17–20, LEIVE, L. and SCHLESSINGER, D. (eds) American Society for Microbiology, Washington, D. C.

HUYER, M., PARR, T. R. Jr., HANCOCK, R. E. W. and PAGE, W. J. (1986) Outer membrane porin protein of *Campylobacter jejeuri*. *FEMS Microbiol. Lett.* **37**: 247–250.

IYER, R. (1977) Plasmid mediated alterations in composition and structure of envelopes of *Escherichia coli* B/r. *Biochim. biophys. Acta* **470**: 258–272.

IYER, R., DARBY, V. and HOLLAND, I. B. (1978) Alterations in the outer membrane proteins of *Escherichia coli* B/r associated with the presence of the R plasmid rRM98. *FEBS Lett.* **85**: 127–132.

IZAKI, K., MATSUHASHI, M. and STROMINGER, J. L. (1966) Glycopeptide transpeptidase and D-alanine carboxypeptidase: Penicillin-sensitive enzymatic reactions. *Proc. natn. Acad. Sci. U.S.A.* **55**: 656–666.

JAFFÉ, A., CHABBERT, Y. A. and SEMONIN, O. (1982) Role of porin proteins OmpF and OmpC in the permeation of β-lactams. *Antimicrob. Ag. Chemother.* **22**: 942–948.

JAFFÉ, A., CHABBERT, Y. A. and DERLOT, E. (1983) Selection and charactrization of β-lactam-resistant *Escherichia coli* K-12 mutants. *Antimicrob. Ag. Chemother.* **23**: 622–625.

KAMIO, Y. and NIKAIDO, H. (1976) Outer membrane of *Salmonella typhimurium*: accessibility of phospholipid head groups to phospholipase C and cyanogen bromide activated dextran. *Biochemistry* **15**: 2561–2570.

KANEKO, M., YAMAGUCHI, A. and SAWAI, T. (1984) Purification and characterization of two kinds of porins from the *Enterobacter cloacae* outer membrane. *J. Bacteriol.* **158**: 1179–1181.

KOBAYASHI, Y., TAKAHASHI, I. and NAKAE, T. (1982) Diffusion of β-lactam antibiotics through liposome membranes containing purified porins. *Antimicrob. Ag. Chemother.* **2**: 775–780.

KOJO, H., SHIGI, Y. and NISHIDA, M. (1980a) A novel method for evaluating the outer membrane permeability to β-lactamase-stable β-lactam antibiotics. *J. Antibiot.* **33**: 310–316.

KOJO, H., SHIGI, Y. and NISHIDA, M. (1980b) *Enterobacter cloacae* outer membrane permeability to ceftizoxime (FK749) and five other new cephalosporin derivatives. *J. Antibiot.* **33**: 317–321.

KOMATSU, Y., MURAKAMI, K. and NISHIKAWA, T. (1981) Penetration of moxalactam into its target proteins in *Escherichia coli* K-12: Comparison of a highly moxalactam-resistant mutant with its parent strain. *Antimicrob. Ag. Chemother.* **20**: 613–619.

KONISKY, J. (1979) Specific transport systems and receptors for colicins and phages. In: *Bacterial Outer Membranes*, pp. 319–359, INOUYE, M. (ed.) John Wiley and Sons, New York.

KOPLOW, J. and GOLDFINE, H. (1974) Alterations in the outer membrane of the cell envelope of heptose-deficient mutants of *Escherichia coli*. *J. Bacteriol.* **117**: 527–543.

KORTELAND, J., TOMMASSEN, J. and LUGTENBERG, B. (1982) PhoE protein pore of the outer membrane of *Escherichia coli* K12 is a particularly efficient channel for organic and inorganic phosphate. *Biochim. biophys. Acta* **690**: 282–289.

KOVAL, S. F. and MEADOW, P. M. (1977) The isolation and characterization of lipopolysaccharide-defective mutants of *Pseudomonas aeruginosa* PAC1. *J. gen. Microbiol.* **98**: 387–398.

KROPINSKI, A. M. B., CHAN, L. and MILAZZO, F. H. (1978) Susceptibility of lipopolysaccharide-defective mutants of *Pseudomonas aeruginosa* strain PAO to dyes, detergents, and antibiotics. *Antimicrob. Ag. Chemother.* **13**: 494–499.

LEIVE, L. (1965) Release of lipopolysaccharide by EDTA treatment of *Escherichia coli*. *Biochem. biophys. Res. Commun.* **21**: 290–296.

LEIVE, L. (1974) The barrier function of the Gram-negative envelope. *Ann. N.Y. Acad. Sci.* **235**: 109–127.

LINDSTRÖM, E. B., BOMAN, H. G. and STEELE, B. B. (1970) Resistance of *Escherichia coli* to penicillins. VI. Purification and characterization of the chromosomally mediated penicillinase present in *ampA*-containing strains. *J. Bacteriol.* **101**: 218–231.

LIVERMORE, D. (1983) Kinetics and significance of the activity of the Sabath and Abrahams' beta-lactamase of *Pseudomonas aeruginosa* against cefotaxime and cefsulodin. *J. Antimicrob. Chemother.* **11**: 169–179.

LIVERMORE, D. (1985) Do β-lactamases 'trap' cephalosporins? *J. Antimicrob. Chemother.* **15**: 511–514.

LIVERMORE, D., MOOSDEEN, F., LINDRIDGE, M. A., KHO, P. and WILLIAMS, J. D. (1986a) Behaviour of TEM-1 β-lactamase as a resistance mechanism to ampicillin, mezlocillin and azlocillin in *Escherichia coli*. *J. Antimicrob. Chemother.* **17**: 139–146.

LIVERMORE, D., RIDDLE, S. J. and DAVY, K. W. M. (1986b) Hydrolytic model for cefotaxime and ceftriaxone resistance in β-lactamase-derepressed *Enterobacter cloacae*. *J. Inf. Dis.* **153**: 619–622.

LUCKEY, M. and NIKAIDO, H. (1980a) Specificity of diffusion channels produced by λ phage receptor protein of *Escherichia coli*. *Proc. natn. Acad. Sci. U.S.A.* **77**: 167–171.

λ LUCKEY, M. and NIKAIDO, H. (1980b) Diffusion of solutes through channels produced by phage lambda receptor protein of *Escherichia coli*: Inhibition by higher oligosaccharides of maltose series. *Biochem. biophys. Res. Commun.* **93**: 166–171.

LÜDERITZ, O., WESTPHAL, O., STAUB, A.-M. and NIKAIDO, H. (1971) Isolation and chemical and immunological characterization of bacterial lipopolysaccharides. In: *Bacterial endotoxins*, pp. 145–233, WEINBAUM, G., KADIS, S. and AJL, S. J. (eds) Microbial Toxins, Vol. 4, Academic Press, New York.

LUGTENBERG, B. and VAN ALPHEN, L. (1983) Molecular architecture and functioning of the outer membrane of *Escherichia coli* and other Gram-negative bacteria. *Biochim. biophys. Acta* **737**: 51–115.

LUNDRIGAN, M. D. and EARHART, C. F. (1984) Gene *envY* of *Escherichia coli* K-12 affects thermoregulation of major porin expression. *J. Bacteriol.* **157**: 262–268.

LYSKO, P. G. and MORSE, S. A. (1981) *Neisseria gonorrhoeae* cell envelope: Permeability to hydrophobic-molecules. *J. Bacteriol.* **145**: 946–952.

MANESS, M. J. and SPARLING, P. F. (1973) Multiple antibiotic resistance due to a single mutation in *Neisseria gonorrhoeae*. *J. Infect. Dis.* **128**: 321–330.

MEADOW, P. M. (1975) Wall and membrane structures in the genes *Pseudomonas*. In: *Genetics and Biochemistry of Pseudomonas*, pp. 67–98, CLARKE, P. H. and RICHMOND, M. H. (eds) John Wiley & Sons, New York.

MEDEIROS, A. A. (1984) Classification and distribution of beta-lactamases 390. In: *Microbiology—1984*, pp. 385–390, LEIVE, L. and SCHLESSINGER, D. (eds) American Society for Microbiology, Washington, D.C.

MEDEIROS, A. A., O'BRIEN, T. F., ROSENBERG, E. Y. and NIKAIDO, H. (1987) A strain of *Salmonella typhimurium* became more resistant to cephalosporins during therapy because it lost its OmpC porin. *J. Inf. Dis.* (in press).

MÜHLRADT, P. F. and GOLECKI, J. R. (1975) Asymmetric distribution and artificial reorientation of lipopolysaccharides in the outer membrane bilayer of *Salmonella typhimurium*. *Eur. J. Biochem.* **51**: 343–352.

MURAKAMI, K. and YOSHIDA, T. (1982) Penetration of cephalosporins and corresponding 1-oxacephalosporins through the outer layer of Gram-negative bacteria and its contribution to antibacterial activity. *Antimicrob. Ag. Chemother.* **21**: 254–258.

NAKAE, T. (1976a) Outer membrane of *Salmonella*. Isolation of protein complex that produces transmembrane channels. *J. biol. Chem.* **251**: 2176–2178.

NAKAE, T. (1976b) Identification of the outer membrane protein of *E. coli* that produces transmembrane channels in reconstituted vesicle membranes. *Biochem. biophys. Res. Commun.* **71**: 877–884.

NAKAE, T. and NIKAIDO, H. (1975) Outer membrane as a diffusion barrier in *Salmonella typhimurium*. Penetration of oligo- and polysaccharides into isolated outer membrane vesicles and cells with degraded peptidoglycan layer. *J. biol. Chem.* **250**: 7359–7365.

NEILANDS, J. B. (1982) Microbial envelope proteins related to iron. *A. Rev. Microbiol.* **36**: 285–309.

NEU, H. C. (1968) The surface localization of penicillinases in *Escherichia coli* and *Salmonella typhimurium*. *Biochem. biophys. Res. Commun.* **32**: 258–263.

NIKAIDO, H. (1976) Outer membrane of *Salmonella typhimurium*. Transmembrane diffusion of some hydrophobic compounds. *Biochim. biophys. Acta* **433**: 118–132.

NIKAIDO, H. (1979a) Permeability of the outer membrane of bacteria. *Angew. Chem. (Internat. Ed.)*, **18**: 337–350.

NIKAIDO, H. (1979b) Non-specific transport through the outer membrane. In: *Bacterial Outer Membranes*, pp. 361–407, INOUYE, M. (ed.) John Wiley & Sons, New York.

NIKAIDO, H. (1984) Outer membrane permeability and beta-lactam resistance, In: *Microbiology—1984*, pp. 381–384, LEIVE, L. and SCHLESSINGER, D. (eds) American Society for Microbiology, Washington, D.C.

NIKAIDO, H. (1986) Transport through the outer membrane of bacteria. *Meth. Enzymol.* **125**: 265–278.

NIKAIDO, H. and NAKAE, T. (1979) The outer membrane of Gram-negative bacteria. *Adv. Microb. Physiol.* **20**: 163–250.

NIKAIDO, H. and NORMARK, S. (1987) Sensitivity of *Escherichia coli* to various β-lactams is determined by the interplay of outer membrane permeability and degradation by periplasmic β-Lactamases: a quantitative predictive treatment. *Mol. Microbiol.* (in press).

NIKAIDO, H. and ROSENBERG, E. Y. (1981) Effect of solute size on diffusion rates through the transmembrane pores of the outer membrane of *Escherichia coli*. *J. gen. Physiol.* **77**: 121–135.

NIKAIDO, H. and ROSENBERG, E. Y. (1983) Porin channels in *Escherichia coli*: Studies with liposomes reconstituted from purified proteins. *J. Bacteriol.* **153**: 241–252.

NIKAIDO, H. and VAARA, M. (1985) Molecular basis of the permeability of bacterial outer membrane. *Microbiol. Rev.* **49**: 1–31.

NIKAIDO, H., BAVOIL, P. and HIROTA, Y. (1977a) Outer membranes of Gram-negative bacteria. XV. Transmembrane diffusion rates in lipoprotein-deficient mutants of *Escherichia coli*. *J. Bacteriol.* **132**: 1045–1047.

NIKAIDO, H., SONG, S. A., SHALTIEL, L. and NURMINEN, M. (1977b) Outer membrane of *Salmonella*. XIV. Reduced transmembrane diffusion rates in porin-deficient mutants. *Biochem biophys. Res. Commun.* **76**: 324–330.

NIKAIDO, H., ROSENBERG, E. Y. and FOULDS, J. (1983) Porin channels in *Escherichia coli*: Studies with β-lactams in intact cells. *J. Bacteriol.* **153**: 232–240.

OSBORN, M. J. and WU, H. C. P. (1980) Proteins of the outer membrane of Gram-negative bacteria. *A. Rev. Microbiol.* **34**: 369–422.

POLLOCK, M. R. (1965) Purification and properties of penicillinases from two strains of *Bacillus licheniformis*. *Biochem. J.* **94**: 666–675.

QUINN, J. P., DUDEK, E. J., DIVINCENZO, C. A., LUCKS, D. A. and LERNER, S. A. (1986) Emergence of resistance to imipenem during therapy for *Pseudomonas aeruginosa* infections. *J. Inf. Dis.* **154**: 289–294.

RICHMOND, M. H. and CURTIS, N. A. C. (1974) The interplay of beta-lactamase and intrinsic factors in the resistance of Gram-negative bacteria to penicillins and cephalosporins. *Ann. N.Y. Acad. Sci.* **235**: 553–567.

RICHMOND, M. H. and SYKES, R. B. (1973) The β-lactamases of Gram-negative bacteria and their possible physiological role. *Adv. Microb. Physiol.* **9**: 31–85.

RICHMOND, M. H., CLARK, D. C. and WOTTON, S. (1976) Indirect method for assessing the penetration of beta-lactamase-nonsusceptible penicillins and cephalosporins in *Escherichia coli* strains. *Antimicrob. Ag. Chemother.* **10**: 215–218.

ROANTREE, R. J., KUO, T.-T. and MACPHEE, D. G. (1977) The effect of defined lipopolysaccharide core defects upon antibiotic resistance of *Salmonella typhimurium*. *J. gen. Microbiol.* **103**: 223–234.

RODRIGUEZ-TÉBAR, A., ROJO, F., MONTILLA, J. C. and VAZQUEZ, D. (1982) Interaction of β-lactam antibiotics with penicillin-binding proteins from *Pseudomonas aeruginosa*. *FEMS Microbiol. Lett.* **14**: 295–298.

ROSENBUSCH, J. P. (1974) Characterization of the major envelope protein from *Escherichia coli*. Regular arrangement on the peptidoglycan and unusual dodecyl sulfate binding. *J. biol. Chem.* **249**: 8019–8029.

SANDERS, C. C. (1983) Novel resistance selected by the new expanded-spectrum cephalosporins: A concern. *J. Infect. Dis.* **147**: 585–589.

SAWAI, T., HIRUMA, R., KAWANA, N., KANEKO, M., TANIYASU, F. and INAMI, A. (1982) Outer membrane permeation of β-lactam antibiotics in *Escherichia coli*, *Proteus mirabilis*, and *Enterobacter cloacae*. *Antimicrob. Ag. Chemother.* **22**: 585–592.

SAWAI, T., MATSUBA, K. and YAMAGISHI, S. (1977) A method for measuring the outer membrane permeability of β-lactama antibiotics in Gram-negative bacteria. *j. Antibiot.* **30**: 1134–1136.

SCHLECHT, S. and WESTPHAL, O. (1970) Untersuchungen zur Typisierung von Salmonella-R-Formen. 4. Typisierung von *S. minnesota*-R-Mutanten mittels Antibiotica. *Zentr. Bakteriol. Parasitenk.* I Orig. **213**: 356–381.

SCHMIDT, G., SCHLECHT, S. and WESTPHAL, O. (1969) Untersuchungen zur Typisierung von Salmonella-R-Formen. 3. Typisierung von *S. minnesota*-Mutanten mittels chemischer Agenzien. *Zentr. Bakteriol. Parasitenk.* I Orig. **212**: 88–96.

SCUDAMORE, R. A., BEVERIDGE, T. J. and GOLDNER, M. (1979a) Outer-membrane penetration barriers as components of intrinsic resistance to beta-lactam and other antibiotics in *Escherichia coli* K-12. *Antimicrob. Ag. Chemother.* **15**: 182–189.

SCUDAMORE, R. A., BEVERIDGE, T. J. and GOLDNER, M. (1979b) Penetrability of the outer membrane of *Neisseria gonorrhoeae* in relation to acquired resistance to penicillin and other antibiotics. *Antimicrob. Ag. Chemother.* **15**: 820–827.

SEEBERG, A. H., TOLXDORFF-NEUTZLING, R. M. and WIEDEMANN, B. (1983) Chromosomal β-lactamases of *Enterobacter cloacae* are responsible for resistance to third generation cephalosporins. *Antimicrob. Ag. Chemother.* **23**: 918–925.

SMIT, J. and NIKAIDO, H. (1978) Outer membrane of Gram-negative bacteria. XVIII. Electron microscopic studies on proin insertion sites and growth of cell surface of *Salmonella typhimurium*. *J. Bacteriol.* **135**: 687–702.

SMIT, J., KAMIO, Y. and NIKAIDO, H. (1975) Outer membrane of *Salmonella typhimurium*: Chemical analysis and freeze-fracture studies with lipopolysaccharide mutants. *J. Bacteriol.* **124**: 942–958.

SMITH, J. T. (1963) Penicillinase and ampicillin resistance in a strain of *Escherichia coli*. *J. gen. Microbiol.* **30**: 299–306.

SPARLING, P. F. (1977) Antibiotic resistance in the Gonococcus, In: *The Gonococcus*, pp. 111–135, ROBERTS, R. B. (ed.) John Wiley & Sons, New York.

STEIN, W. D. (1967) *The Movement of Molecules Across Cell Membranes*, Academic Press, New York.

STOCK, J. B., RAUCH, B. and ROSEMAN, S. (1977) Periplasmic space in *Salmonella typhimurium* and *Escherichia coli*. *J. biol. Chem.* **252**: 7850–7861.

SYKES, R. B. and MATTHEW, M. (1976) The β-lactamases of Gram-negative bacteria and their role in resistance to β-lactam antibiotics. *J. Antimicrob. Chemother.* **2**: 115–157.

TAKAHASHI, I., SAWAI, T., ANDO, T. and YAMAGISHI, S. (1980) Cefoxitin resistance by a chromosomal cephalosporinase in *Escherichia coli*. *J. Antibiot.* **33**: 1037–1042.

TAKAYAMA, K., QURESHI, N. and MASCAGNI, F. (1983) Complete structure of lipid A obtained from the lipopolysaccharides of the heptoseless mutant of *Salmonella typhimurium*. *J. biol. Chem.* **258**: 12801–12802.

THEN, R. L. and ANGEHRN, P. (1982) Trapping of non-hydrolyzable cephalosporins by cephalosporinases in *Enterobacter cloacae* and *Pseudomonas aeruginosa* as possible resistance mechanism. *Antimicrob. Ag. Chemother.* **21**: 771–717.

TOKUNAGA, M., TOKUNAGA, H., OKAJIMA, Y. and NAKAE, T. (1979) Characterization of porins from the outer membrane of *Salmonella typhimurium*. *Eur. J. Biochem.* **95**: 441–448.

TOMMASSEN, J. and LUGTENBERG, B. (1980) Outer membrane protein e of *Escherichia coli* K-12 is coregulated with alkaline phosphatase. *J. Bacteriol.* **143**: 151–157.

VACHON, V., LYEW, D. J. and COULTON, J. W. (1985). Transmembrane permeability channels across the outer membrane of *Haemophilus influenzae* type b. *J. Bacteriol.* **162**: 918–924.

VAN ALPHEN, W. and LUGTENBERG, B. (1977) Influence of osmolarity of the growth medium on the outer membrane protein pattern of *Escherichia coli*. *J. Bacteriol.* **131**: 623–630.

VU, H. V. and NIKAIDO, H. (1985) Role of β-lactum hydrolysis in the mechanism of resistance of a β-lactamase-constitutive *Enterobacter cloacae* strain to the expanded-spectrum β-lactums. *Antimicrob. Ag. Chemother* **27**: 393–398.

WALEY, S. G. (1980) An explicit model for bacterial resistance: application to β-lactam antibiotics. *Microbiol. Sci.* **4**: 143–146.

WATANABE, N., NACASU, T., KATSU, K. and KITOH, K. (1987) E-0702, a new cephalosporin, is incorporated into *Escherichia coli* cells via the *tonB*-dependent system. *Antimicrob. Ag. Chemother.* **31**: 497–504.

WEAVER, P. F., WALL, J. D. and GEST, H. (1975) Characterization of *Rhodopseudomonas capsulata*. *Arch. Microbiol.* **105**: 207–216.

WECKESSER, J., ZALMAN L. S. and NIKAIDO, H. (1984) Porin from *Rhodopseudomonas sphaeroides*. *J. Bacteriol.* **159**: 199–205.

WERNER, V., SANDERS, C. C., SANDERS, W. E., Jr. and GOERING, R. V. (1985) Role of β-lactamase and outer membrane proteins in multiple β-lactam resistance of *Enterobacter cloacae*. *Antimicrob. Agents Chemother.* **27**: 455–459.

YAMAGUCHI, A., HIRUMA, R. and SAWAI, T. (1982) Phospholipid bilayer permeability of beta-lactam antibiotics. *J. Antibiot.* **35**: 1692–1699.

YOKOTA, T. and AZUMA, E. (1980) Biochemical aspects of bacterial resistance to new β-lactam drugs non-hydrolysable by β-lactomases, pp. 333–337. In: *Antiobiotic Resistance*, MITSUHASHI, S., ROSIVAL, L. and KREMERY, V. (eds) Springer Verlag, Berlin.

YONEYAMA, H. and NAKAE, T. (1986) A small diffusion pore in the outer membrane of *Pseudomonas aeruginosa*. *Eur. J. Biochem.* **157**: 33–38.

YOSHIMURA, F. and NIKAIDO, H. (1982) Permeability of *Pseudomonas aeruginosa* outer membrane to hydrophilic solutes. *J. Bacteriol.* **152**: 636–642.

YOSHIMURA, F. and NIKAIDO, H. (1983) Purification and properties of *Pseudomonas aeruginosa* porin. *J. biol. Chem.* **258**: 2308–2314.

YOSHIMURA, F. and NIKAIDO, H. (1985) Diffusion of β-lactam antibiotics through the porin channels of *Escherichia coli* K12. *Antimicrob. Ag. Chemother.* **27**: 84–92.

YOUNG, J. D.-E., BLAKE, M., MAURO, A. and COHN, Z. A. (1983) Properties of the major outer membrane protein from *Neisseria gonorrhoeae* incorporated into model lipid membranes. *Proc. natn. Acad. Sci. U.S.A.* **80**: 3831–3835.

ZIMMERMANN, W. (1980) Penetration of β-lactam antibiotics into their target enzymes in *Pseudomonas aeruginosa*: Comparison of a highly sensitive mutant with its parent strain. *Antimicrob. Ag. Chemother.* **18**: 94–100.

ZIMMERMANN, W. and ROSSELET, A. (1977) The function of the outer membrane of *Escherichia coli* as a permeability barrier to β-lactam antibiotics. *Antimicrob. Ag. Chemother.* **12**: 368–372.

CHAPTER 8

THE ROLE OF β-LACTAMASE INHIBITORS IN CHEMOTHERAPY

HAROLD C. NEU

Departments of Medicine and Pharmacology, College of Physicians and Surgeons, Columbia University, 630 West 168 Street, New York, NY 10032, U.S.A.

1. INTRODUCTION

Resistance to β-lactam antibiotics was known before penicillin G became a clinically useful agent. In 1940 Abraham and Chain reported in a note in *Nature* that they had found a *Bacillus coli* that produced an enzyme which destroyed penicillin. In 1944 Kirby reported in *Science* that an extract of *Staphylococcus* was able to destroy penicillin G. In the past several decades resistance to β-lactams has become an increasingly serious problem. Virtually all *Staphylococcus aureus*, 25% of *Haemophilus influenzae*, *Branhamella catarrhalis*, many *Enterobacteriaceae*, *Bacteroides*, and Pseudomonads possess β-lactamases which hydrolyze the penicillins and cephalosporins currently in clinical use.

There have been several different approaches to the problem of β-lactamase resistance. The most successful have been the synthesis of new β-lactams with increased stability to enzymatic hydrolysis, and the development of inhibitors that bind or inactivate β-lactamases. Although the concept of combining a useful but β-lactamase-sensitive antibiotic with a β-lactamase inhibitor was employed as early as the 1960s, when semi-synthetic anti-staphylococcal β-lactams such as cloxacillin or oxacillin were combined with ampicillin to treat urinary tract infections, this approach in general was not useful because of inadequate inhibition, and rapidly fell into disuse with the availability of the cephalosporin antibiotics. Developing awareness of the variety and increasing prevalence of β-lactamases able to destroy, with varying efficiency, all of the available semi-synthetic cephalosporins, rekindled interest in the search for efficient inhibitors of such β-lactamases and the discovery of clavulanic acid in 1976 (Howarth *et al.*, 1976) made this a reality. Semi-synthetic penicillin derivatives such as the halopenicillanic acids (Pratt and Loosemore, 1978) and the penicillanic sulfones (English *et al.*, 1978) were developed as the mechanism of enzyme inactivation observed with clavulanic acid became understood. This review will examine the β-lactamases of clinical importance and discuss the β-lactamase inhibitors currently available with particular reference to their clinical utility.

2. β-LACTAMASE REACTIONS

β-Lactamases hydrolyze the β-lactam ring of different β-lactam compounds. These include penicillins, cephalosporins, penems, carbapenems, and monobactams. While the mechanisms by which the hydrolysis of these molecules occur are basically identical, they differ in detail depending upon the particular substrate. In general the reaction involves the initial formation of a non-covalent enzyme–substrate complex. This complex undergoes subsequent modification with the formation of an acyl–enzyme intermediate that is probably important in all β-lactamase reactions (Fisher *et al.*, 1980; Knott-Hunzinger *et al.*, 1980). It has been postulated that for β-lactamase enzymes lacking a rigid tertiary structure, the formation of the enzyme–substrate complex induces a conformational change in the enzyme providing an alignment of the active amino acids causing catalysis. Studies with several different β-lactamases have implicated a serine residue as the acylation site (Cartwright and Coulson, 1980; Fisher *et al.*, 1981). The serine is aligned in the occupied active site such that acylation by the carbonyl of the β-lactam ring is favored. Deacylation is followed by release of the hydrolyzed β-lactam molecule and resumption of the normal β-lactamase conformation. In general, β-lactamases are highly efficient catalysts of hydrolysis of suitable substrates. For example, the TEM-2 β-lactamase can hydrolyze 2000 molecules of benzyl penicillin per sec per molecule of enzyme (Fisher *et al.*, 1980).

3. CLASSIFICATION OF β-LACTAMASES

β-Lactamases have been classified in recent years on the basis of the amino acid sequence of the enzymes. Three broad classes, called A, B and C, are recognized (Ambler, 1980; Jaurin and Grundstrom, 1981). Class A is represented by four β-lactamases: the *Staphylococcus aureus* PC1 enzyme; *Bacillus licheniformis* β-lactamase; *B. cereus* β-lactamase I; and *Escherichia coli* R-TEM present in several related gram-negative transposons. The key amino acid in these enzymes is serine, and the proposed mechanism of action of these β-lactamases involves the formation and subsequent hydrolysis of an acyl–enzyme complex in which serine-70 is the amino acid residue which is acylated. In Class A enzymes there is a lysine at position 73 which is important in the interaction of β-lactamase inhibitors with the enzyme.

Class B enzymes are metaloenzymes quite distinct from Class A enzymes. These enzymes possess a thiol group which acts as a ligand to bind zinc which is required for β-lactamase activity. β-Lactamase II, a Class B enzyme, is produced by *B. cereus*. Similar enzymes have been found in some *Bacteroides* and also in *Pseudomonas maltophilia* (Saino *et al.*, 1982; Yotsujii *et al.*, 1983). This enzyme is capable of hydrolyzing substrates which are otherwise β-lactamase stable such as cefoxitin, imipenem, and moxalactam. It is not known whether this enzyme functions via an acyl–enzyme mechanism. There are no known inhibitors of β-lactamases of this type with the exception of agents which chelate the metal ions necessary for β-lactamase activity (Cartwright and Waley, 1983).

Class C β-lactamases are encoded by chromosomal genes producing enzymes such as those present in *Pseudomonas aeruginosa* and the enzyme specified by the amp C gene of *E. coli* K12 (Jaurin and Grundstrom, 1981). In the Class C β-lactamases the amino acid involved in the enzymatic reaction has also been identified as serine which forms an acyl–enzyme complex (Knott-Hunziger *et al.*, 1982).

There has been no attempt to exhaustive classification of the β-lactamases of gram-positive bacteria. Among the gram-positive organisms which contain β-lactamases, only staphylococci are of clinical significance. *S. aureus* β-lactamases can be divided sero-logically into four types (Richmond, 1965). All are predominantly active against penicillins, but penicillins such as methicillin and the isoxazolyl penicillins and nafcillin are not destroyed by these β-lactamases. Most cephalosporins with the exception of cephaloridine are not readily inactivated by *S. aureus* β-lactamases. These enzymes are plasmid-mediated and transfer from one organism to another is by transduction.

The β-lactamases of coagulase-negative staphylococci such as *S. epidermidis* appear to be similar to the β-lactamases of *S. aureus*. These enzymes have been less well studied. In general, staphylococcal β-lactamases are inhibited by β-lactams such as cloxacillin and by β-lactamase inhibitors such as clavulanic acid, sulbactam and halopenicillinates.

A number of alternative classification schemes have been proposed, most antedating amino acid sequence data leading to the ABC classification (Jack and Richmond, 1970; Richmond and Sykes, 1973; Sawai *et al.*, 1968). These classifications of β-lactamases are based primarily upon substrate and inhibition profiles although in recent years additional attention has been paid to isoelectric points. New enzymes are continually being discovered which do not readily fit into the established classifications. Thus new enzymes are best characterized by substrate profile, inhibition profile and isoelectric points. The Richmond–Sykes classification has proved to be of persistent utility, and it is the one

TABLE 1. *Classification of β-Lactamases*

Ambler classification	Richmond–Sykes classification	Bacterial source	Trivial names	Preferred substrate	Genome	Inhibitor susceptibility
A	—	S. aureus / B. licheniformis	PC	Penicillins	Plasmid / Chromosomal	Cloxacillin, clavulanate
	IIIa	Enterobacteriacaea, Haemophilus, Neisseria / Klebsiella	TEM-1, TEM-2 / SHV-1	Penicillins, some cephalosporins	Plasmid	Cloxacillin, clavulanate, not PCMB* clavulanate
	V	E. coli / P. aeruginosa	OXA / PSE	Penicillins, some cephalosporins	Plasmid	Some clavulanate
B	—	B. cereus / B. fragilis / P. maltophilia	II (Zn^{2+} stimulated)	Penicillin + cephalosporins carbapemems	Chromosomal	Chelators of Zn^{2+}
C	Ia	Enterobacter, Morganella, Serratia	P99	Cephalosporins	Chromosomal	Cloxacillin, PCMB, not clavulanate
	Ic	P. vulgaris	S-A	Cephalosporins	Chromosomal	Clavulanate
	Id	P. aeruginosa		Cephalosporins	Chromosomal	Cloxacillin, not clavulanate
	IV	Klebsiella	K-1	Penicillins	Chromosomal	Clavulanate, not cloxacillin

*PCMB = 1

generally recognized by most workers. Table 1 provides a schema relating the various classifications of β-lactamases.

In the Richmond–Sykes classification of gram-negative β-lactamases, Class I β-lactamases are considered primarily to be cephalosporinases. Class I is an extremely large class which includes chromosomally determined β-lactamases present in most of the members of the *Enterobacteriacae* and in *Pseudomonas* species. Class II β-lactamases are primarily active against penicillins, and are found primarily in *Proteus* species. Class III β-lactamases are plasmid determined enzymes. Class IV are chromosomal enzymes which are not inhibited by cloxacillin; whereas Class III enzymes are inhibited by cloxacillin but not by *p*-chloromercuribenzoate. Class V enzymes preferentially attack penicillins, but unlike Class II enzymes, are plasmid-mediated and can frequently hydrolyze the anti-staphylococcal β-lactams such as oxacillin. One of the most useful methods for identifying β-lactamases has been isoelectric focusing as developed by Matthew and Harris (1976). Use of a chromogenic cephalosporin, nitrocefin, has made it possible to assay β-lactamases in crude extracts of microbial organisms.

4. PLASMID-MEDIATED β-LACTAMASES OF GRAM-NEGATIVE BACTERIA

Anderson and Datta in 1965 found that ampicillin resistance in *Salmonella typhimurium* in Great Britain could be transferred to *E. coli*. Subsequently Datta and Kontomichalou (1965) reported the isolation of an ampicillin-resistant *E. coli* from a little girl in Athens whose first name was Temoniera. Both ampicillin resistance and β-lactamase production could be transferred to a recipient *E. coli* indicating that a resistance factor was involved. This first plasmid β-lactamase was called TEM and the name has persisted. Similar trivial names have been given to apparently unique plasmid-mediated β-lactamases as they have been discovered. Plasmid-mediated β-lactamases are constitutive. They can be divided into three classes. The first is a broad spectrum penicillinase which hydrolyzes penicillin and cephaloridine at similar rates. These are the Richmond–Sykes Class IIIa enzymes. The second hydrolyzes the anti-staphylococcal penicillins such as oxacillin, and the third are carbenicillin hydrolyzing enzymes. These are Richmond–Sykes Class V enzymes. Each of these β-lactamases have different isoelectric points.

In the late 1970s plasmid β-lactamases which were inhibited by sulfhydro reagents were discovered. The first, SHV-1, was described by Pitton (1972) and by Petrocheilou *et al.* (1977). This enzyme is found primarily in *Klebsiella pneumoniae*. Matthew (1979) described a second enzyme called HMS-1, in clinical isolates. The HMS refers to Hedges, Matthew and Smith. In 1979 Hedges and Matthew also described a series of *Pseudomonas* β-lactamases, called PSE-1, PSE-2, PSE-3 and PSE-4, which hydrolyzed carbenicillin. These were originally thought to be restricted to *P. aeruginosa*, but it is now known that they are found in many other gram-negative organisms as well. Hence they are more properly called carbenicillinases.

A number of novel, plasmid-mediated β-lactamases have been described in the last several years (Medeiros *et al.*, 1985). They reported new OXA enzymes, OXA-4, 5, 6 and 7, which differed from OXA-1, 2 and 3, in substrate profiles, isoelectric points and inhibition reactions. OXA-4 and OXA-6 are inhibited by cloxacillin.

A β-lactamase has been found in *Haemophilus influenzae*, ROB-1 which may be membrane bound (Medeiros, 1984). Levesque *et al.* (1982) reported a plasmid-determined β-lactamase from a *Chromobacter* which had a pI of 8.1 and preferentially hydrolyzed cephalosporins. Hedges *et al.* (1985) reported a novel carbenicillin hydrolyzing β-lactamase in *Aeromonas hydrophila*, AER-1.

5. DISTRIBUTION OF PLASMID β-LACTAMASES IN CLINICAL ISOLATES

The TEM β-lactamase, Richmond–Sykes Class IIIa enzyme, appears to be the most widely distributed β-lactamase in clinical isolates of gram-negative pathogens. It accounts for 70–80% of isolates of β-lactamase producers throughout the world. Simpson *et al.* (1980) found that the TEM β-lactamase was the most common β-lactamase in bacteria causing urinary tract infections. Matthew (1979) and Roy *et al.* (1983) also noted TEM to be the most common plasmid-mediated enzyme. Medeiros (1984) reported that TEM-1 was found in 72% of *E. coli* isolates obtained from different parts of the world, with the frequency of TEM-1 in different locations ranging from 66% to 93%. In some situations *E. coli* and *P. aeruginosa* may contain several different plasmid-mediated β-lactamases simultaneously. Furthermore, most members of the *Enterobacteriaceae* and many *Pseudomonas* species will contain chromosomally mediated β-lactamases independent of the presence of plasmid-mediated forms. Hence they frequently contain several different enzymes simultaneously with different affinities for β-lactams and different reactions to β-lactamase inhibitors.

β-Lactamase producing *Branhamella catarrhalis* were recognized in 1977 (Malmvall *et al.*, 1977; Percival *et al.*, 1977). It had been believed that this β-lactamase was chromosomally-mediated, but Kamme *et al.* (1983) showed that it was a plasmid-mediated enzyme and could be transferred to other species. The β-lactamases of *Branhamella* have been shown to hydrolyze ampicillin, carbenicillin, mecillinam, and cefaclor with a higher rate than does TEM-1 (Eliasson and Kamme, 1985). Farmer and Reading (1982) showed that *Branhamella* β-lactamases were inhibited by clavulanic acid, and Alvarez *et al.* (1985) showed that 87% of *B. catarrhalis* contained β-lactamases inhibited by a mixture of amoxicillin and clavulanate.

6. CHROMOSOMALLY-MEDIATED β-LACTAMASES

Chromosomally-mediated β-lactamases may be either constitutive or inducible enzymes. Most chromosomally-mediated β-lactamases are in the category of Class I enzymes (Richmond and Sykes, 1973). The enzymes of this type hydrolyze cephalosporins in preference to the penicillins. In general, β-lactamases of this type hydrolyze cephalosporins five to 100 times as readily as benzyl penicillin, and a number of semi-synthetic penicillins and iminomethoxy cephalosporins inhibit these enzymes. The amount of enzyme produced by an individual species is extremely variable. It can range from barely detectable amounts to as much as 10% of the cell protein.

Inducible β-lactamases have been found in many genera. These include: *Acinetobacter*, *Citrobacter*, *Enterobacter*, *Morganella*, *Providencia*, *Pseudomonas* (both *aeruginosa* and other species), *Serratia*, and *Yersinia*. Inducible β-lactamases have recently been found in *Alcaligenes faecalis* (Fujii *et al.*, 1985). Wild-type strains of *P. aeruginosa* invariably produce a chromosomally-mediated inducible β-lactamase which has been referred to as the Sabath–Abraham enzyme (Sabath *et al.*, 1965). Induction of β-lactamases can occur as the result of exposure to substrates or to some of the β-lactamase inhibitors. Seven α-methoxy cephalosporins such as cefoxitin, and also clavulanate and the carbapenems and penems are extremely efficient inducers of β-lactamases in *E. cloacae*, *M. morganii*, *C. freundii*, and *P. aeruginosa*.

E. coli, *Salmonella* species and *Shigella* species produce chromosomally-mediated β-lactamases at a low level. Some *Enterobacter cloacae*, *E. aerogenes*, and *C. freundii* can produce large amounts of constitutive β-lactamases of a cephalosporinase type which will hydrolyze even relatively stable cephalosporins (Vu and Nikaido, 1985).

Klebsiella species produce several extremely important β-lactamases. All *Klebsiella* produce a β-lactamase which hydrolyzes amino- and carboxy-penicillins such as ampicillin and carbenicillin. *Klebsiella oxytoca*, an indole-positive *Klebsiella* species, produces a β-lactamase (called K-1) which is different in properties from that present in *K. pneumoniae* (Hart and Percival, 1982). This enzyme can hydrolyze iminomethoxy cephalosporins and monobactams such as aztreonam.

Most *Bacteroides* species isolated from clinical specimens produce β-lactamases. Olsson *et al.* (1977) found 93% of *B. fragilis* to be β-lactamase producers. The enzymes are constitutive and closely related to each other in terms of substrate profile, inhibition pattern and isoelectric point. Other *Bacteroides* species also produce β-lactamases. Murray and Rosenblatt (1977) reported that 56% of *B. melaninogenicus* produce β-lactamases and Leung and Williams (1978) reported that *B. thetaiotaomicron* and *B. assachrolyticus* produced β-lactamases. Yotsujii *et al.* (1983) reported a novel β-lactamase produced by *B. fragilis* which was capable of hydrolyzing β-lactamase stable compounds such as imipenem and cefoxitin. Saino *et al.* (1982) reported a similar type β-lactamase from *P. maltophilia* which could hydrolyze imipenem.

Most of the sero groups of *Legionella* produce β-lactam inactivating enzymes (Marre *et al.*, 1982; Fu and Neu, 1979a). These enzymes hydrolyze penicillins and cephalosporins but not methoxy or iminomethoxy cephalosporins. Induction has not been detected.

7. β-LACTAMASE ENZYME LOCATION

Gram-positive bacteria produce β-lactamases that are both extracellular and intracellular. In organisms such as *B. cereus*, 80 to 90% of the β-lactamase is found outside the cell. Pathogenic gram-positive bacteria such as staphylococci excrete the majority of their β-lactamase as an extracellular enzyme. High levels of enzyme released into the external environment may result in low concentrations around an individual microorganism. Gram-positive organisms also contain some intracellular enzyme that appears to be membrane bound to lipoprotein. This enzyme has a lower activity than the extracellular enzyme, but may provide a further defense against the residual antibiotic not hydrolyzed by the secreted enzyme, since only small amounts of strategically located enzyme may be needed to protect the β-lactam binding proteins.

β-Lactamases of gram-negative bacteria exist as soluble enzymes in the periplasmic space of the microorganisms reaching high concentrations. In some organisms a periplasmic β-lactamase that has a high affinity (low K_m value) for substrates is highly effective in protecting the microorganism against destruction by an antibiotic whose access to the periplasm is limited by outer membrane permeability.

Nikaido (1984, 1985) has reviewed the role of outer membrane permeability in β-lactamase resistance. The ability of a β-lactam antibiotic to enter a gram-negative bacteria contributes significantly to the efficiency of β-lactamases in protecting the microorganism. This is not true in gram-positive species which contain no significant barrier to the access of small β-lactam antibiotics to the cytoplasmic membrane.

8. CLASSES OF INHIBITORS

β-Lactamase inhibitors may be described using classical enzyme terminology. Although many of the β-lactam compounds are referred to as competitive inhibitors, there are very few true competitive inhibitor substances. Penicilloates and peniollates behave as pure competitive inhibitors of a β-lactamase such as the *B. cereus* β-lactamase I (Kiener and Waley, 1978). Compounds such as cloxacillin or methicillin have been referred to as competitive inhibitors of β-lactamases. However studies by Furth (1975) and Labia *et al.* (1979) have shown that the compounds actually are slowly hydrolyzed. Such inhibitors have been called competitive substrates and include many of the new β-lactam antibiotics such as cefotaxime or the monobactam aztreonam. Competitive substrates have a high affinity for the enzyme but are poor enzyme substrates with a relatively long time required for product formation. A reversible complex forms as with competitive inhibitors, but there is a slow acylation and ultimately a slow deacylation step. Unless careful studies are performed, the initial kinetics would appear to be that of competitive inhibition. Fisher *et al.* (1980) and Bush *et al.* (1982) showed that cefoxitin and aztreonam were excellent competitive substrates, and functionally resemble competitive inhibitors.

There are no clinically useful non-competitive inhibitors of β-lactamases, although several compounds have been shown to function in this type of mechanism. It is assumed that a non-competitive inhibitor binds at a site other than the enzymatic active site. This interaction alters the enzymatic conformation so that substrates can no longer induce a catalytically active form of the enzyme. The compound izumenolide, a sulphated non-β-lactam macrolide, acts as a non-competitive inhibitor of TEM-2 β-lactamase at low concentrations (Bush et al., 1980). Unfortunately this compound does not enter the periplasmic space of gram-negative bacteria except at very high concentrations. Thus it is not a useful β-lactamase inhibitor.

Irreversible inactivators may be of several types. Some may modify the enzyme making it incapable of catalyzing the conversion of a substrate to an eventual product. A reversible enzyme–inhibitor complex forms initially, but this complex proceeds to a product in which the inhibitor is covalently and irreversibly bound to the enzyme. Suicide inactivators are poorly reactive but bind at an enzyme's active site. Interaction of the inhibitor and enzyme results in a species which subsequently may form a covalent linkage with a critical residue in the enzyme. The suicide inhibitor is changed by the enzyme into an inactivating species. The activated species binds at the same site as a substrate and undergoes fragmentation as a result of the normal catalytic reaction of the enzyme. The important β-lactamase inhibitors that have been used clinically such as clavulanic acid and the penicillanic acid sulfone, sulbactam, are suicide inhibitors.

9. MEASUREMENT AND EXPRESSION OF INHIBITOR EFFECTIVENESS

Studies of β-lactamase inhibitors are performed by incubating enzyme and inhibitor together for 10 to 15 min and assaying the activity of enzyme by adding substrate and measuring the rate of hydrolysis. Alternatively substrate and inhibitor are added to the enzyme together and the rate of hydrolysis is measured. The rates are compared with those of controlled reactions, and the concentration of inhibitor that produces 50% inhibition (I_{50}) is found from the equation:

$$I_{50} = I\left(\frac{V_1}{V_0 - V_1}\right)$$

where I is the concentration of inhibitor that gives a rate V_1 and V_0 is the rate of the control lacking the inhibitor.

In determining this type of inhibition, it is necessary to test for reversibility. A standard assay for reversibility has been to dilute the enzyme solution. This may not be an adequate technique for β-lactamases. In general, extensive dialysis or gel filtration is necessary to determine the irreversibility of β-lactamase inactivators. Gel filtration also may be useful in identifying inactive enzyme, and isoelectric focusing of enzyme–inhibitor complex may provide information regarding the types and numbers of complexes formed during the reaction.

10. SPECIFIC β-LACTAMASE INHIBITORS

10.1. CLAVULANIC ACID

Clavulanic acid was isolated from *Streptomyces clavuligerus* and characterized by the group at Beecham Pharmaceuticals in 1976 (Howarth et al., 1976). Clavulanic acid differs from penicillins in that it has an oxazolidine rather than a thiazolidine ring and it lacks an acylamino side chain (Fig. 1). Furthermore, it has an unusual substituent at C2 rather than the two methyl groups normally found in penams. Clavulanic acid has minimal anti-bacterial activity, although it does inhibit some species such as *Neisseria* and some *Bacteroides* at clinically achievable concentrations. It is a potent inhibitor of a number of different β-lactamases of gram-positive and gram-negative bacteria.

The basic mechanisms of clavulanic acid interaction with β-lactamases have been worked out for a number of different enzymes (Cartwright and Coulson, 1979; Charnas et al., 1978; Fisher et al., 1978; Labia and Peduzzi, 1978). The E. coli TEM β-lactamases, S. aureus enzyme and the B. cereus β-lactamase I are all inactivated in a time-dependent process. There appears to be a stoichiometry of about 1:1 for inactivation of the S. aureus

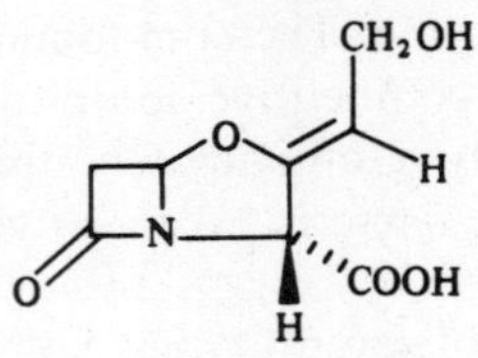

FIG. 1. Structure of clavulanic acid.

β-lactamase. The *E. coli* R TEM-2 enzyme has required 115 turnovers of clavulanic acid before the enzyme is fully inactivated, and the *B. cereus* β-lactamase is not fully inhibited even in the presence of 16,000-fold excess of inhibitor (Table 2). Clavulanic acid interacts with the R-TEM β-lactamase of *E. coli* in three ways (Charnas *et al.*, 1978; Fisher *et al.*, 1978). Clavulanic acid initially acts as a substrate for the enzyme and undergoes hydrolytic reaction. Following that, there is a transient intermediate that slowly regenerates free enzyme, Fig. 2. The ultimate reaction involves the irreversible inactivation of the enzyme. It takes a large number of turnovers of enzyme reaction to achieve ultimate irreversible inactivation. Utilizing isoelectric focusing it has been possible to determine several different protein bands that are distinct from normal enzyme. The inactivated enzyme and the transient complexes have chromophores at 280 nm whose appearance correlates with the loss of enzymatic activity. When clavulanic acid has been labeled with ^{14}C at position C5, C6 and C7, all three inactive enzyme species are labeled indicating that the molecule has attached covalently. O'Hara *et al.* (1983) using nuclear magnetic resonance spectrometry showed that clavulanate bound to TEM β-lactamases with an I_{50} of 0.0001 mg compared to 0.4 mg for imipenem, 0.6 mg for dicloxacillin and 20 mg for cefotaxime.

Clavulanic acid differs in its action on different enzymes. The interaction of clavulanic acid with the *S. aureus* β-lactamase, which is also a Class A enzyme, is different in that the enzyme is inactivated without turnover of inhibitor to form transiently inhibited species. It has been suggested that the inactive species is an enamine, and in this situation irreversible inactivation will not occur. The interaction with different β-lactamases have been studied by Reading and Farmer (1981). The Richmond–Sykes Class IV β-lactamase from *K. pneumoniae* is both transiently and irreversibly inactivated. In contrast, β-lactamases of the Class I types are transiently inhibited.

Overall it appears that clavulanic must undergo the initial steps in a hydrolytic pathway of acyl–enzyme formation, followed by β elimination with proton loss at C6 to give an enamine which is transiently stable. A good leaving group at C5, and an acidic proton at C6 promote the reaction. Although a large number of other clavam derivatives have been produced, the potency of the derivatives is generally of the same order or less than that of clavulanate (Cherry and Newall, 1982).

Clavulanate inhibits β-lactamases of *S. aureus*, the gram-negative plasmid β-lactamases TEM-1, TEM-2, HMS-1, SHV-1, and the PSE enzymes (Table 3). It has relatively good activity against OXA-1 and OXA-2, but is not an effective inhibitor of OXA-3 and does not inhibit the recently described OXA-4, 5, and 6 enzymes (Medeiros *et al.*, 1985). Marked differences are seen for the inhibition of chromosomally determined β-lactamases. For example, the *K. pneumoniae* β-lactamases are inhibited with I_{50}s similar to that required for the TEM enzyme. The same is true for the *P. vulgaris* Type Ic β-lactamase. Most of the Ia type enzymes found in *E. cloacae*, *C. freundii* and the amp C *E. coli* β-lactamase

TABLE 2. *Chemical Characteristics of Inactivation of β-Lactamase Inhibitors*

Agent	Enzyme	Irreversible inactivation	$t_{1/2}$ Transient inactivation	K intact	Hydrolytic turnovers
Clavulanate	TEM-1	Yes	4 min	$5 \times 10^{-4}\,\mathrm{sec}^{-1}$	115
Clavulanate	*K. pneumoniae*	Yes	4 min	$7.2 \times 10^{-5}\,\mathrm{sec}^{-1}$	Yes
Clavulanate	*S. aurenus*	No	160 min	—	No
Clavulanate	*E. cloacae*	No	180 min	—	No
Sulbactam	TEM-1, *E. coli*	Yes		$2.8 \times 10^{-4}\,\mathrm{sec}^{-1}$	5000

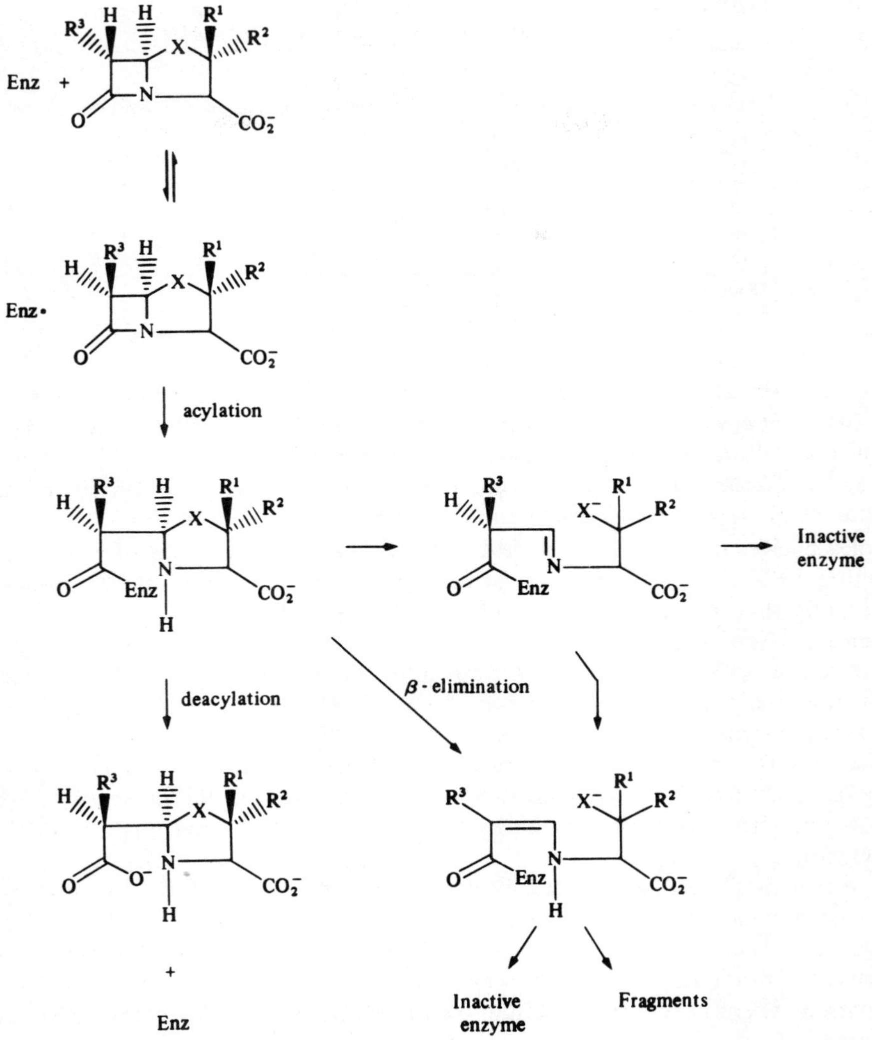

FIG. 2. Scheme for β-lactamase inactivation.

TABLE 3. *Inhibition of Plasmid-mediated β-Lactamases by Clavulanate and Sulfones*

β-Lactamase name	Source	I_{50} (μM)		
		Clavulanate	Sulbactam	6AMPA*
TEM-1	*E. coli*	0.04	1	0.0007
TEM-2	*E. coli*	0.08	1.3	0.001
SHV-1	*E. coli*	0.04	2.7	0.002
HMS-1	*E. coli*	0.2	3.6	0.1
OXA-1	*E. coli*	1.5	4.7	0.004
OXA-2	*E. coli*	1.3	0.3	0.02
OXA-3	*E. coli*	55	12	4.6
PSE-1	*P. aeruginosa*	1.0	3.0	0.04
PSE-2	*P. aeruginosa*	0.04	3.4	0.01
PSE-3	*P. aeruginosa*	0.02	5.5	0.06
PSE-4	*P. aeruginosa*	0.07	3.0	0.02
PC-1	*S. aureus*	0.1	3.6	0.006

*6-aminomethylene penicillanic acid.
Modified from Arisawa and Then, 1982.

TABLE 4. *Inhibition of Chromosomally-mediated β-Lactamases by Clavulanate,*
Sulbactam and 6-Acetyl-methylene Penicillanic Acid (6AMPA)

β-Lactamase type*	Source	I_{50} (μM)		
		Clavulanate	Sulbactam	6AMPA
Ia, P99	E. cloacae	140	7.2	4.7
I	C. freundii	235	7.5	0.1
Ic	P. vulgaris	0.03	0.1	0.004
Id	P. aeruginosa	650	6.5	2.2
II	K. pneumoniae	0.01	0.8	0.008
IV	K. oxytoca	0.08	4.6	0.006

*Richmond-Sykes classification.
Modified from Arisawa and Then, 1982.

are not inhibited at readily achievable concentrations (Table 4). β-Lactamases in *Bacte-*
roides species, *Legionella*, and *Branhamella* are also inhibited by clavulanate. Clavulanate
did not inhibit inducible β-lactamases of organisms such as *Alcaligenes faecalis* (Fujii *et*
al., 1985) or *Flavobacterium* (Sato *et al.*, 1985). But clavulanate did inhibit the inducible
β-lactamase of *Aeromonas* (Zemelman *et al.*, 1984).

Studies by Reading and Farmer (1984) on the penetration of clavulanate into *E. coli*
containing TEM β-lactamases have shown that clavulanate enters the periplasmic space
more readily than do sulbactam or iodopenicillanates (Table 5).

When clavulanate has been combined with β-lactamase unstable compounds, it has
been shown to protect penicillin G, ampicillin, amoxicillin, piperacillin, cefoperazone,
cephalothin, and ticarcillin (Fu and Neu, 1979a, 1981; Hunter *et al.*, 1980; Neu and Fu,
1978, 1980). Slocombe *et al.* (1984) evaluated the efficacy of clavulanate combined with
amoxicillin in the therapy of animal infections produced by *K. pneumoniae*, *S. aureus* and
B. fragilis. They were able to demonstrate that amoxicillin in the presence of clavulanic
acid was protected from inactivation by the bacterial β-lactamases present at the site of
the infection.

One factor that must be considered in the evaluation of clavulanic acid is its potential
as a β-lactamase inducer. Clavulanate is an effective inducer of β-lactamases in *P.*
aeruginosa, *E. cloacae*, and *C. freundii*. Thus the potential exists for clavulanate to decrease
the activity of a compound with which it is combined when these organisms are
encountered. There have been no situations reported in which this potential problem has
been noted. Currently clavulanate is combined with amoxicillin for use as an oral
compound and in selected settings as a parenteral agent. Clavulanate is also combined with
ticarcillin for use as a parenteral agent.

10.2. SULFONES

Sulbactam, CP 45899, is a penicillanic acid sulfone produced by Pfizer (Fig. 3).
Sulbactam itself has only weak anti-bacterial activity against most gram-positive cocci,
Enterobacteriaceae and *Pseudomonas*. It does inhibit *Neisseria* and *Acinetobacter*, and it
has weak activity against *Bacteroides* species (Aswapokee and Neu, 1978; English *et al.*,
1978). The initial studies by English *et al.* (1978) indicated that sulbactam produced
β-lactamase inhibition with cell-free enzymes from *S. aureus* and many *Enterobacteriaceae*.

TABLE 5. *Comparison of the Inhibitory Activity of β-Lactamase*
*Inhibitors with Cell Extracts and Intact Bacterial Cells**

Inhibition	I_{50}, μg/ml		
	Cell-free extract	Intact cells	Permeability index
Clavulanate	0.056	0.69	123
Sulbactam	0.3	23	77
β-bromopenicillanate	0.45	34	76

**E. coli* containing TEM-1 β-lactamases.

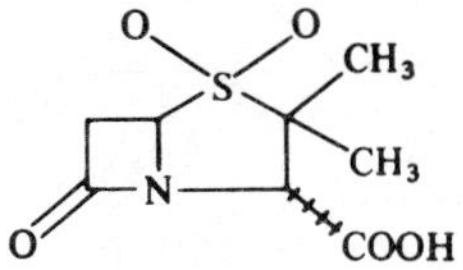

FIG. 3. Structure of sulbactam.

Fu and Neu (1979b) demonstrated similar findings and noted that enzymes exhibiting primary cephalosporinase activity were only weakly inhibited. Jones *et al.* (1985) showed that sulfones combined with ampicillin inhibited *Legionella* species.

Fisher *et al.* (1981) evaluated the interaction of sulbactam with the R-TEM β-lactamase. There are differences between the interaction of clavulanate and sulbactam with this enzyme. For example, clavulanate inactivated R-TEM with a half-time of eight min compared to an inactivation half-time of 44 min for sulbactam and 30-fold more turnovers were required for inactivation with sulbactam compared to clavulanic acid (Table 2). An enzyme-bound chromophore at 280 nm is formed with sulbactam, as with clavulanic acid. Hydroxylamine treatment of inactivated enzyme produces a 25% recovery of catalytic activity in comparison to a 33% return of the activity of the enzyme treated with clavulanate. It has been suggested that loss of a proton at C6 and cleavage of C5–SO_2 leads to a stable β-amino acylic ester derivative of the enzyme and subsequent transamination at C5 leads to permanent inactivation of the enzyme. Brenner and Knowles (1981), using dideuterated sulbactam, have shown that there is a transient stable intermediate and that enzyme is further available for hydrolysis and inactivation. Using the sulbactam dideuterated at C6 they have shown that the 6 β proton is removed during the formation of the transiently inhibited species.

10.3. HALOGENATED SULFONES

A number of other sulfones have been synthesized and evaluated as potential β-lactamase inactivators. Halogenated sulfones have proved to be effective inactivators. Cartwright and Coulson (1979) synthesized a 6-chloro penicillanic acid sulfone and showed that it acted as a progressive inhibitor of staphylococcal β-lactamase producing a characteristic α-chloro, β-aminoacrylic ester. Brenner and Knowles (1984a), in further studies of penicillanic acid sulfones, showed that sulbactam produced a cross-linking of the enzyme by a β-aminoacrylate fragment from C5, C6 and C7.

Knight and Waley (1985) using a penicillanic acid dioxide showed that it was possible to inhibit β-lactamases of the Class C type irreversibly at an alkaline pH (pH 8), but that at lower pHs the inhibition was a transitory affair.

Yamaguchi *et al.* (1985) showed that sulfonation of cloxacillin converted it into an excellent β-lactamase inhibitor of isolated enzymes, but not of intact bacteria.

Another penicillanic acid compound which has been studied extensively *in vitro* is 6-acetyl-methylene penicillanic acid (Ro 15-1903), 6-AMPA (Angehrn and Arisawa, 1982; Arisawa and Then, 1982, 1983). 6-AMPA is chemically characterized by a 6-methylene double-bond connected directly to the β-lactam ring as well as a reactive keto group on the 6-substituent (Fig. 4). It inhibited the R-TEM β-lactamase in a second-order fashion

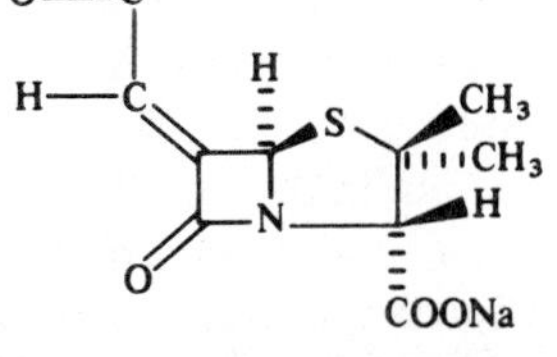

FIG. 4. Structure of 6-acetyl-methylene penicillanic acid.

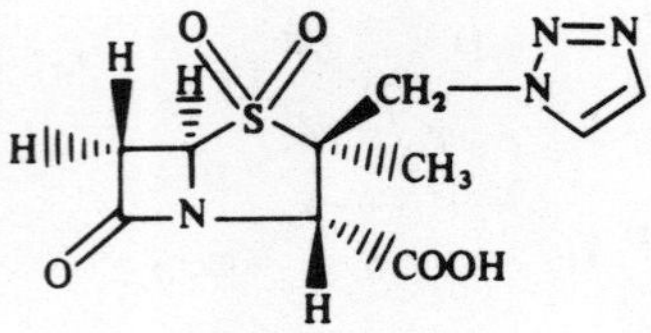

Fig. 5. Structure of YTR-H.

with a rate constant of $0.6\,\mu m^{-1}\cdot sec^{-1}$ (Ariasawa and Then, 1983). The normal enzyme is converted into two inactive forms, and the data suggests that the compound functions as an irreversible active site inhibitor similar to sulbactam and clavulanate (Brenner and Knowles, 1984b).

6-AMPA is an effective inhibitor of *S. aureus* β-lactamase, the TEM β-lactamase and the OXA, SHV, HMS and PSE β-lactamases (Table 3). It is more effective with isolated enzymes than are clavulanic acid or sulbactam. With chromosomal β-lactamases, 6-AMPA is an effective inhibitor of the *P. vulgaris* β-lactamase and to some extent of the Richmond–Sykes Type Ia and Id enzymes present in *P. aeruginosa*, *E. cloacae* and *C. freundii* (Table 4). 6-AMPA is effective as a β-lactamase inhibitor combined with ampicillin or ceftriaxone against *B. fragilis* organisms. Although 6-AMPA is an effective inhibitor of isolated enzymes, Chin and Neu (unpublished) have not found the compound to be useful as a potentiator of the activity of penicillins or cephalosporins against *Enterobacter*, *Citrobacter* or *Pseudomanas* species.

10.4. YTR-H

YTR-H is another sulfone derivative (Fig. 5) which has been shown to inhibit various β-lactamases (Aronoff *et al.*, 1984). YTR-H will produce irreversible inhibition of TEM-1, TEM-2, SHV, *P. vulgaris* Ic enzyme and PSE β-lactamases. It is also highly active against *Branhamella* and *Bacteroides* β-lactamases. YTR-H will allow ampicillin, amoxicillin, piperacillin, and cefazolin to inhibit strains of *E. coli*, *K. pneumoniae*, *S. aureus*, and *B. fragilis* that are resistant to these agents (Chin and Neu, unpublished observations). Similar to the other sulfones, however, it is only poorly active against most of the Richmond–Sykes Type I β-lactamases found in *E. cloacae*, *C. freundii*, and *P. aeruginosa*. Chin and Neu (unpublished observations) have shown that YTR-H has greater penetrability to the periplasmic space than does sulbactam or iodopenicillanates but is, however, not as permeable as clavulanate.

10.5. 6-β-Bromopenicillanic Acid

6-β-bromopenicillanic acid (Fig. 6) has been studied as an inhibitor of β-lactamases of *S. aureus*, *B. careus*, *E. coli* R-TEM, and *P. aeruginosa* (Pratt and Loosemore, 1978). It has been studied in combination with other agents by Wise *et al.* (1981) and by Neu (1983b). 6-β-bromopenicillinate was shown to be an active-site directed irreversible inhibitor of *E. coli* R-TEM and *B. cereus* β-lactamase. Knott-Hunziger *et al.* (1980) showed that labeled bromopenicillanic acid was bound to serine at the active site of the *B. cereus* enzyme. An inactive enzyme derivative is rapidly formed and there is no turnover of inhibitor. A new chromophore forms at 326 nm due to an enzyme-bound dihydro-thiazine (Loosemore *et al.*, 1980). The rapid inactivation of β-lactamase suggests that there is a unique process with the halogenated penicillanic acid derivatives which is different from that seen with sulfones and clavulanate.

Joris *et al.* (1985) showed that 6-bromo and 6-iodo penicillanic acids interact with *Enterobacter* P99 β-lactamase at the active site at rates lower than those for their interaction with Class A β-lactamases.

Neu (1983b) showed that iodopenicillinate and bromopenicillinate inhibited TEM-2, PSE-1, PSE-3, PSE-4 and the *B. cereus* and *S. aureus* β-lactamase. As with other agents, the halo penicillinates were not effective inhibitors of *E. cloacae*, *P. aeruginosa* or of methicillin-resistant *S. aureus*.

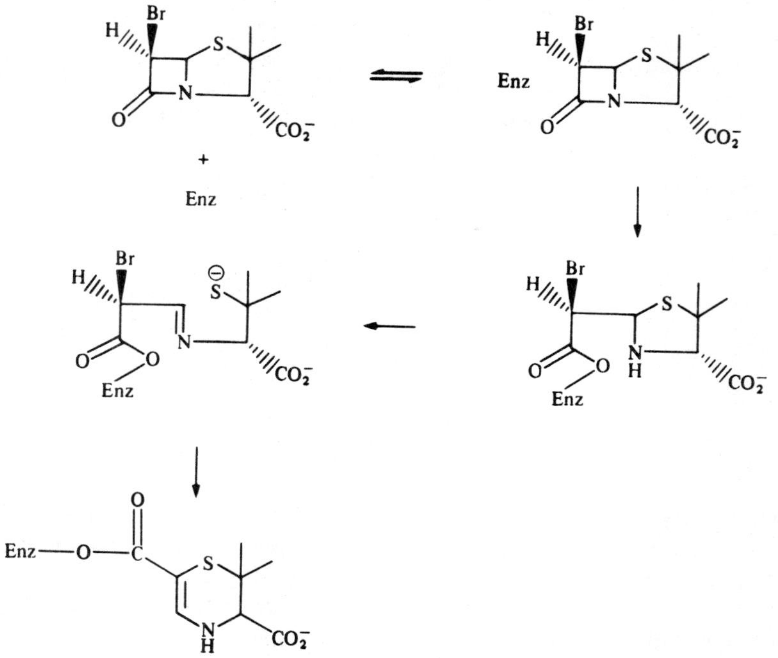

FIG. 6. Structure of 6-bromopenicillanic acid and scheme for β-lactamase inactivation.

Halogenated penicillanates and the penicillanic acid sulfones do not penetrate gram-negative outer membranes as efficiently as clavulanate, and with intact microorganisms, produce less protection for the more permeable unstable β-lactams with which they are combined. This explains the difference between their excellent activity with isolated enzymes and the relatively modest potentiation of the activity of β-lactamase labile compounds seen against intact microorganisms.

Calverley and Beatrup (1983) prepared N-alkyl aminopenicillanic acids which inhibited the E. cloacae P99 β-lactamase with an I_{50} <4 mg/L. Studies in our laboratory with these alkyl aminopenicillanic acids (Chin and Neu, unpublished observations) has indicated that these compounds can be effective inhibitors of some of the cephalosporinases in contrast to clavulanic acid. However, these compounds have no activity when combined with ampicillin and tested with intact microorganisms.

11. OTHER β-LACTAMASE INACTIVATORS

11.1. OLIVANIC ACID AND RELATED COMPOUNDS

The olivanic acids are natural products of *Streptomyces olivaceus* which were isolated by workers at Beecham Pharmaceuticals (Butterworth *et al.*, 1979). Compounds of very similar activity are the thienamycins isolated by workers at Merck. These compounds are carbapenems that have a substitution of carbon for the heterocyclic sulfur of penams and an endocyclic double bond. In the olivanates there is a sulfated side chain and in the thienamycins a hydroxyleythyl group. The side chain on these compounds is either α or β. The C6 substituent is in a transconfiguration while the configuration at C8 is S. Some of these compounds, particularly the thienamycins, are highly active against many bacteria.

β-Lactamases of plasmid and chromosomal origin are inhibited by olivanic acids with penicillinases being more readily inhibited than cephalosporinases. The olivanic acid I_{50} concentrations are in the ng/nl range. In addition, inhibition appears to be progressive and irreversible (Easton and Knowles, 1982) (Fig. 7).

Thienamycin derivatives inhibit TEM Type III and Type IV β-lactamases, but it is not established that this inhibition is of an irreversible type. In view of the extensive

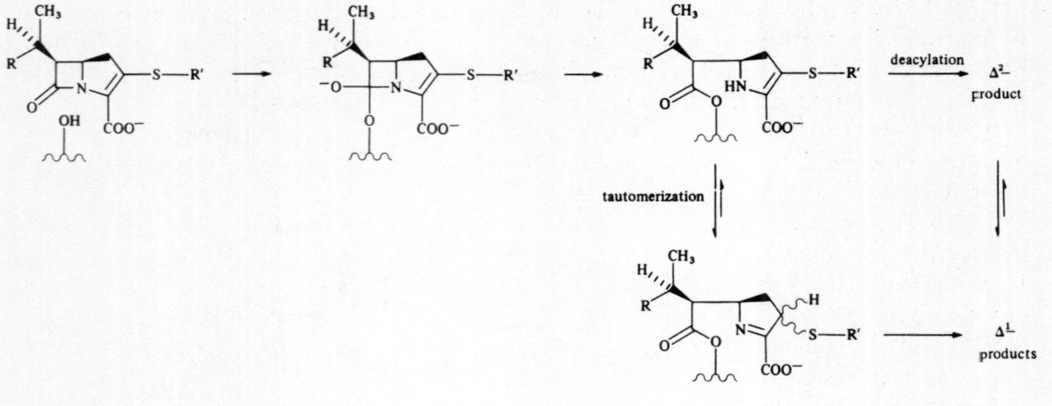

FIG. 7. Proposed sequence of olivanic acid interaction with β-lactamase.

anti-bacterial activity of thienamycin compounds, their use as β-lactamase inhibitors is of secondary importance. The commercially available thienamycin semi-synthetic derivative imipenem has such excellent inhibitory activity inhibiting broad spectrum aerobic and anaerobic bacteria, that its β-lactamase inhibitory properties are difficult to evaluate. Carbapenems are highly effective inducers of β-lactamases in *E. cloacae*, *C. freundii*, *S. marcescens* and *P. aeruginosa*. Although compounds such as imipenem induce β-lactamase activity in these species, the organisms generally remain susceptible to the compounds.

Easton and Knowles (1982) proposed that the interaction of olivanic acid derivatives with the R-TEM β-lactamase was by formation of an acyl–enzyme, the 2-pyrroline, which either deacylates or tautomerizes to the 1-pyrroline. Thus the ability of the agents to inhibit the enzyme is dependent on the partitioning of the acyl–enzyme to the 1-pyrroline and the rate of regeneration of free enzyme from the complex.

Yamaguchi *et al.* (1984) found a novel carbepenem SF 2103A, that inhibited plasmid β-lactamases and the *P. vulgaris* cephalosporinase as substrate inhibitors but irreversibly inhibited the *C. freundii* cephalosporinase.

Nozaki *et al.* (1984) reported the inhibitory activity of cephabacin compounds that contained a 7-formyl amino substituent which would inhibit the cephalosporinase of *P. vulgaris*. It is probable that the cephabacins are substrate inhibitors rather than true suicide inhibitors.

12. CLINICAL USE OF β-LACTAMASE INHIBITORS

There are two β-lactamase inhibitors currently in clinical use or under study. Clavulanate has been combined with amoxicillin at a 2:1 or 4:1 ratio in oral form and in a 2:1 preparation for parenteral use. The oral formulation is licenced for use in the United States, the United Kingdom and a number of other countries. Clavulanate has also been combined with ticarcillin at a concentration of 100 or 200 mg with 3 g of ticarcillin for i.v. use. These preparations are available in the United States, Europe and Great Britain.

Clavulanic acid is moderately well absorbed from the gastrointestinal tract with peak serum levels occurring 40 to 120 min after ingestion. Mean peak serum levels following a dose of 125 mg are 4 μg/ml and approximately 6 μg/ml for a 250 mg dose (Adam *et al.*, 1982; Jackson *et al.*, 1984). The combination of clavulanate with amoxicillin does not significantly alter the pharmacological parameters of either drug. After i.v. infusion of clavulanate combined either with amoxicillin or ticarcillin, peak concentrations of approximately 11 μg/ml after a 250 mg i.v. dose are achieved with levels of 0.2 μg/ml at 6 hr (Scully *et al.*, 1984). In general the administration of food does not impair the absorption of clavulanate.

Clavulanate is well distributed in the body following oral ingestion or i.v. administration, producing therapeutic concentrations in sputum, peritoneal fluid, interstitial fluid, bile, middle ear fluid, and tonsil tissue. In the presence of inflammation, concentrations of 1 μg/ml have been found in cerebrospinal fluid. Urinary concentrations of clavulanate have been well in excess of that required to provide adequate β-lactamase inhibitory activity. The combination of clavulanate and amoxicillin have been shown to be effective in respiratory tract infections, skin infections, sinusitis and urinary tract infections, whether these infections have been due to amoxicillin susceptible or resistant micro-organisms.

Currently the amoxicillin–clavulanate combination provides an alternative form of therapy for infections due to β-lactamase producing staphylococci, β-lactamase producing *H. influenzae* as a cause of otitis media, and urinary infections due to β-lactamase producing *E. coli* and *Klebsiella*. As a parenteral agent the combination may have utility against some mixed infections in which *B. fragilis*, *E. coli*, *Klebsiella*, enterococci and *S. aureus* are present.

The combination of ticarcillin and clavulanate has also been used to treat respiratory infection, cutaneous infections, urinary tract infections, and intraabdominal infections. In general, the results of clinical trials have been favorable with cure rates comparable to those found with comparative agents. Neu (1985) has summarized the studies of ticarcillin–clavulanate in a fixed combination that have been conducted in the United States. Ticarcillin plus clavulanate proved as effective as cefoxitin in treatment of pelvic infections, and it was useful as a prophylactic agent in preventing infection following penetrating abdominal trauma, comparable to the combination of clindamycin and gentamicin. In the treatment of urinary tract infections, ticarcillin–clavulanate compared with piperacillin showed comparable responses.

Sulbactam was combined with ampicillin as an oral preparation, and initial studies of its effectiveness were performed in a number of centers. However, the poor oral absorption of the sulbactam led to a significant amount of diarrhea, and this preparation is no longer in use. Sulbactam has also been combined at a 1:1 ratio with ampicillin, penicillin and with cefoperazone, and studies are currently in progress to evaluate the utility of these combinations.

Sulbactam's pharmacokinetics in humans are similar to those of ampicillin and amoxicillin (Foulds *et al.*, 1983). It is excreted by the kidney producing urinary concentrations comparable to those achieved with ampicillin with which it has been combined. Sulbactam has been used to great gynecological and urinary tract infections (Houang *et al.*, 1984; Nichols *et al.*, 1985). The response rates with *E. coli*, *Klebsiella* species and *Bacteroides* species were comparable to those found with other β-lactamase stable agents. Administered as an i.v. compound, sulbactam has not produced an appreciable degree of diarrhea.

13. CONCLUSIONS

β-Lactamase production will continue to be an extremely important mechanism of resistance to β-lactam antibiotics. The emergence of bacterial resistance has had a marked influence on anti-microbial therapy within the past decade (Neu, 1983a). Many β-lactamase stable cephalosporins have been developed. β-Lactamase inhibition through the use of suicide inhibitors such as clavulanate and sulbactam has proved to be a feasible mechanism to overcome β-lactamase inactivation of labile β-lactam compounds. The data to date from clinical studies do not provide an adequate number of treated patients or sufficient comparative studies to properly evaluate whether the concept of β-lactamase inhibition is as successful as has been the synthesis of new antibiotics. As the clinical experience with clavulanate–amoxicillin and clavulanate–ticarcillin increases, it should be possible to find areas in which these combinations would be preferred to other agents.

Further research into β-lactamase inhibitors may yield agents which will be effective inhibitors of the cephalosporinases, but such agents must be able to penetrate into the periplasm of bacteria at adequate concentrations to be effective. The story of β-lactamase inhibition is an intriguing one since it demonstrates that an understanding of the mechanisms of β-lactamase action and the distribution of the enzymes in nature can be used to find and to synthesize agents that ultimately have clinical utility.

REFERENCES

ABRAHAM, E. P. and CHAIN, E. (1940) An enzyme from bacteria able to destroy penicillin. *Nature* **146**: 837.

ADAM, D., VISER, I. and KOEPPE, P. (1982) Pharmacokinetics of amoxicillin and clavulanic acid administered alone and in combination. *Antimicrob. Ag. Chemother.* **22**: 353–357.

ALVAREZ, S., JONES, M., HOLTSCLAW-BERK, S., GUARDERASS, J. and BERK, S. L. (1985) *In vitro* susceptibility and beta-lactamase production of 53 clinical isolates of *Branhamella catarrhalis. Antimicrob. Ag. Chemother.* **27**: 646–647.

AMBLER, R. P. (1980) The structure of beta-lactamases. *Phil. Trans. R. Soc. (Biol).* **289**: 321–331.

ANDERSON, E. S. and DATTA, N. (1965) Resistance to penicillin and its transfer in *Enterobacteriaceae. Lancet* i: 407–409.

ANGEHRN, P. and ARISAWA, M. (1982) 6-Acetylmethylene penicillanic acid (Ro 15-1903), a potent beta-lactamase inhibitor. *J. Antibiot.* **35**: 1584–1589.

ARISAWA, M. and THEN, R. L. (1982) 6-Acetylmethylene penicillanic acid (Ro 15-1903), a potent β-lactamase inhibitor. *J. Antibiot.* **35**: 1578–1583.

ARISAWA, M. and THEN, R. L. (1983) Inactivation of TEM-1 beta-lactamase by 6-acetylmethylene penicillanic acid. *Biochem. J.* **209**: 609–615.

ARONOFF, S. C., JACOBS, M. R., JOHENNING, S. and YAMATE, S. (1984) Comparative activities of the beta-lactamase inhibitors YTR 830, sodium clavulanate, and sulbactam combined with amoxicillin or ampicillin. *Antimicrob. Ag. Chemother.* **26**: 580–582.

ASWAPOKEE, N. and NEU, H. C. (1978) A sulfonate beta-lactam compound which acts as a beta-lactamase inhibitor. *J. Antibiot.* **31**: 1238–1244.

BRENNER, D. G. and KNOWLES, J. R. (1981) Penicillanic acid sulfone: an unexpected isotope effect in the interaction of 6α and 6β-monodeuterio and 6,6 dideuterio derivatives with RTEM beta-lactamase from *Escherichia coli. Biochemistry* **20**: 3680–3687.

BRENNER, D. G. and KNOWLES, J. R. (1984a) Penicillanic acid sulfone: nature of irreversible inactivation of RTEM beta-lactamase of *Escherichia coli. Biochemistry* **23**: 5833–5839.

BRENNER, D. G. and KNOWLES, J. R. (1984b) 6-(methoxymethylene) penicillanic acid: inactivator of RTEM beta-lactamases from *Escherichia coli. Biochemistry* **23**: 5839–5846.

BUSH, K., BONNER, D. P. and SYKES, R. P. (1980) Izumenolide—a novel beta-lactamase inhibitor produced by micromonospora. *J. Antibiot.* **33**: 1262–1269.

BUSH, K., FREUDENBERGER, J. S. and SYKES, R. B. (1982) Interaction of aztreonam and related monobactams with beta-lactamases from gram-negative bacteria. *Antimicrob. Ag. Chemother.* **22**: 414–421.

BUTTERWORTH, D., COLE, M., HANSCOMB, G. and ROLINSON, G. N. (1979) Olivanic acids, a family of beta-lactam antibiotics with beta-lactamase inhibitory properties produced by streptomyces species. I: Detection, properties and fermentation studies. *J. Antibiot.* **32**: 287–294.

CALVERLEY, M. J. and BEATRUP, M. (1983) *N*-(functionalized alkyl) derivatives of 6-aminopenicillanic acid: a new series of specific inhibitors of beta-lactamase from *Enterobacter cloacae* P99. *J. Antibiot.* **36**: 1507–1515.

CARTWRIGHT, S. J. and COULSON, A. F. (1979) A semisynthetic penicillinase inactivator. *Nature* **278**: 360–361.

CARTWRIGHT, S. J. and COULSON, A. F. W. (1980) Active site of staphylococcal beta-lactamase. *Phil. Trans. Roy. Soc. Ser. B* **289**: 270–272.

CARTWRIGHT, S. J. and WALEY, S. G. (1983) Beta-lactamase inhibitors. *Med. Res. Rev.* **33**: 341–382.

CHARNAS, R. L., FISHER, J. and KNOWLES, J. R. (1978) Chemical studies on the inactivation of *Escherichia coli* RTEM beta-lactamase by clavulanic acid. *Biochemistry* **17**: 2185–2189.

CHERRY, P. C. and NEWALL, C. E. (1982) Clavulanic acid. In: *Chemistry and Biology of Beta-lactam Antibiotics*, Vol. 2, pp. 361–402, MORIN, R. B. and GORMAN, M. (eds) Academic Press, New York.

DATTA, N. and KONTOMICHALOU, P. (1965) Penicillinase resistance controlled by infectious R-factors in *Enterobacteriacae. Nature* **208**: 239–241.

EASTON, C. J. and KNOWLES, J. R. (1982) Inhibition of RTEM beta-lactamase from *Escherichia coli*. Interaction of the enzyme with derivatives of olivanic acid. *Biochemistry* **4**: 2857–2862.

ELIASSON, I. and KAMME, C. (1985) Characterization of the plasmid-mediated beta-lactamase in *Branhamella catarrhalis*, with special reference to its substrate affinity. *J. Antimicrob. Chemother.* **15**: 139–149.

ENGLISH, A. R., RETSEMA, J. A., GIRARD, A. E., LYNCH, J. E. and BARTH, W. E. (1978) CP-45,899, a beta-lactamase inhibitor that extends the antibacterial spectrum of beta-lactams: initial bacteriological characterization. *Antimicrob. Ag. Chemother.* **14**: 414–419.

FARMER, T. and READING, C. (1982) Beta-lactamases of *Branhamella catarrhalis* and their inhibition by clavulanic acid. *Antimicrob. Ag. Chemother.* **21**: 506–508.

FISHER, J., BELASCO, J. G., KHOSLA, S. and KNOWLES, J. R. (1980) Beta-lactamase proceeds via an acyl-enzyme intermediate. Interaction of the *Escherichia coli* R-TEM enzymes with cefoxitin. *Biochemistry* **19**: 2895–2901.

FISHER, J., CHARNAS, R. L., BRADLEY, S. M. and KNOWLES, J. R. (1981) Inactivation of the R-TEM beta-lactamase from *Escherichia coli*. Interaction of penam sulfones with enzyme. *Biochemistry* **20**: 2726–2731.

FISHER, J., CHARNAS, R. L. and KNOWLES, J. R. (1978) Kinetic studies on the inactivation of *Escherichia coli* beta-lactamases by clavulanic acid. *Biochemistry* **17**: 2180–2184.

FOULDS, G., STANKEWICH, J. P., MARSHALL, D. C., O'BRIEN, M. M., HAYES, S. L., WEIDLER, D. J. and MCMAHON, G. (1983) Pharmacokinetics of sulbactam in humans. *Antimicrob. Ag. Chemother.* **23**: 692–599.

FU, K. P. and NEU, H. C. (1979a) Inactivation of beta-lactam antibiotics by *Legionella pneumophila. Antimicrob. Ag. Chemother.* **16**: 561–564.

Fu, K. P. and Neu, H. C. (1979b) Comparative inhibition of beta-lactamases by novel beta-lactam compounds. *Antimicrob. Ag. Chemother.* **15**: 209–212.

Fu, K. P. and Neu, H. C. (1981) Synergistic activity of cefoperazone in combination with beta-lactamase inhibitors. *J. Antimicrob. Chemother.* **7**: 287–292.

Fujii, T., Sato, K., Inoue, M. and Mitsuhashi, S. (1985) Purification and properties of inducible penicillin beta-lactamase isolated from *Alcaligenes faecalis*. *Antimicrob. Ag. Chemother.* **27**: 608–611.

Furth, A. (1975) Purification and properties of a constitutive beta-lactamase from *Pseudomonas aeruginosa* strain Dalgleish. *Biochim. biophys. Acta* **377**: 431–443.

Hart, C. A. and Percival, A. (1982) Resistance to cephalosporins among gentamicin-resistant *Klebsiellae*. *J. Antimicrob. Chemother.* **9**: 275–286.

Hedges, R. W. and Matthew, M. (1979) Acquisition by *Escherichia coli* of plasmid-borne beta-lactamases normally confined to *Pseudomonas* spp. *Plasmid* **2**: 169–178.

Hedges, R. W., Medeiros, A. A., Cohenford, M. and Jacoby, G. A. (1985) Genetic and biochemical properties of AER-1, a novel carbenicillin-hydrolyzing beta-lactamase from *Aeromonas hydrophila*. *Antimicrob. Ag. Chemother.* **27**: 479–484.

Houang, E. T., Watson, C., Howell, R. and Chapman, M. (1984) Ampicillin combined with sulbactam or metronidazole for single-dose chemoprophylaxis in major gynaecological surgery. *J. Antimicrob. Chemother.* **14**: 529–535.

Howarth, T. T., Brown, A. G. and King, T. J. (1976) Clavulanic acid, a novel beta-lactam antibiotic isolated from *Streptomyces clavuligerus*. *J. chem. Soc. Chem. Commun.* 266–267.

Hunter, P. A., Coleman, K., Fisher, J. and Taylor, D. (1980) *In vitro* synergistic properties of clavulanic acid with ampicillin, amoxicillin and ticarcillin. *J. Antimicrob. Chemother.* **6**: 455–470.

Jack, G. W. and Richmond, M. H. (1970) A comparative study of eight distinct beta-lactamases synthesized by gram-negative bacteria. *J. gen. Microbiol.* **61**: 43–61.

Jackson, D., Cooper, D. L., Filer, C. W. and Langley, P. F. (1984) Augmentin: absorption, excretion and pharmacokinetic studies in man. *Post-grad. Med.* Sept–Oct 1984, 51–70.

Jaurin, B. and Grundstrom, T. (1981) AmpC cephalosporinase of *Escherichia coli* K12 has a different evolutionary origin from the beta-lactamases of the penicillinase type. *Proc. natn. Acad. Sci. U.S.A.* **78**: 4897–4901.

Jones, R. N., Thornsberry, C., Wilson, H. W. and McDougal, L. K. (1985) The *in vitro* activity of sulphones alone and in combination with ampicillin or amoxicillin against *Legionella pneumophila* and other *Legionella* spp. including beta-lactamase studies. *Diag. Microbiol. infect. Dis.* **3**: 179–183.

Joris, B., DeMeester, F., Galleni, M., Reckinger, G., Coyetter, J., Frere, J. M. and VanBeeumen, J. (1985) The beta-lactamase of *Enterobacter cloacae* P99. Chemical properties, *N*-terminal sequence and interaction with beta-halogen-penicillanates. *Biochem. J.* **228**: 241–248.

Kamme, C., Vang, M. and Stahl, S. (1983) Transfer of beta-lactamase production in *Branhamella catarrhalis*. *Scand. J. infect. Dis.* **15**: 225–226.

Kiener, P. A. and Waley, S. G. (1978) Reversible inhibitors of penicillinases. *Biochem. J.* **169**: 197–204.

Kirby, W. M. M. (1944) Extraction of a highly potent penicillin inactivator from penicillin-resistant staphylococci. *Science* **99**: 452–453.

Knight, G. G. and Waley, S. G. (1985) Inhibition of Class C beta-lactamases by (1′R,6R)-6-(1′hydroxy) benzyl penicillanic SS-dioxide. *Biochem. J.* **225**: 435–439.

Knott-Hunziger, V., Petursson, C., Jayatilake, G. S., Waley, S. G., Jaurin, B. and Grundstrom, T. (1982) Active sites of beta-lactamases. The chromosomal beta-lactamases of *Pseudomonas aeruginosa* and *Escherichia coli*. *Biochem. J.* **201**: 621–627.

Knott-Hunziger, V., Redhead, K., Petursson, S. and Waley, S. G. (1980) Beta-lactamase action: isolation of an active-site serine peptide from the *Pseudomonas* enzyme and a penicillin. *FEBS Lett.* **121**: 8–10.

Labia, R. and Peduzzi, J. (1978) Cinetique de l'inhibition de beta-lactamases per l'acide clavulanique. *Biochim. biophys. Acta* **526**: 572–579.

Labia, R., Barthelemy, M., Fabre, C., Guionie, M. and Peduzzi, J. (1979) Kinetic studies of three R-factor mediated beta-lactamases. In: *Beta-lactamases*, pp. 429–442, Hamilton-Miller, J. M. T. and Smith, J. T. (eds) Academic Press, London.

Leung, T. and Williams, J. D. (1978) Beta-lactamases of subspecies of *Bacteroides fragilis*. *J. Antimicrob. Chemother.* **4**: 47–54.

Levesque, R., Roy, P. H., Letarte, R. and Pechere, P. (1982) Plasmid-mediated cephalosporinase from *Achromobacter* species. *J. infect. Dis.* **145**: 753–761.

Loosemore, M. J., Cohen, S. A. and Pratt, R. F. (1980) Inactivation of *Bacillus cereus* beta-lactamase 1 by 6-β-bromopenicillanic acid: kinetics. *Biochemistry* **19**: 3990–3995.

Malmvall, B. E., Brorsson, J. E. and Johnsson, J. (1977) *In vitro* sensitivity to penicillin V and beta-lactamase production of *Branhamella catarrhalis*. *J. Antimicrob. Chemother.* **3**: 374–375.

Marre, R., Medeiros, A. A. and Pascule, A. W. (1982) Characterization of the beta-lactamase of six species of *Legionella*. *J. Bacteriol.* **151**: 216–221.

Matthew, M. (1979) Plasmid-mediated beta-lactamases of gram-negative bacteria: properties and distribution. *J. Antimicrob. Chemother.* **5**: 349–358.

Matthew, M. and Harris, A. M. (1976) Identification of beta-lactamases by analytical isoelectric focusing correlation with bacterial taxonomy. *J. gen. Microbiol.* **94**: 55–67.

Medeiros, A. A. (1984) Beta-lactamases. *Br. med. Bull.* **40**: 18–27.

Medeiros, A. A., Cohenford, M. and Jacob, G. A. (1985) Five novel plasmid-determined beta-lactamases. *Antimicrob. Ag. Chemother.* **27**: 715–719.

Murray, P. R. and Rosenblatt, J. E. (1977) Penicillin resistance and penicillinase production in clinical isolates of *Bacteroides melaninogenicus*. *Antimicrob. Ag. Chemother.* **11**: 605–608.

Neu, H. C. (1983a) The emergence of bacterial resistance and its influence on empiric therapy. *Rev. infect. Dis.* **5**: 9–20.

NEU, H. C. (1983b) Beta-lactamase inhibitory activity of iodopenicillanate and bromopenicillanate. *Antimicrob. Ag. Chemother.* **23**: 63–66.

NEU, H. C. (1985) Beta-lactamase inhibition: therapeutic advances. *Am. J. Med.* **79** (Suppl.) (in press).

NEU, H. C. and FU, K. P. (1978) Clavulanic acid, a novel inhibitor of beta-lactamases. *Antimicrob. Ag. Chemother.* **14**: 650–655.

NEU, H. C. and FU, K. P. (1980) Synergistic activity of piperacillin in combination with beta-lactamase inhibitors. *Antimicrob. Ag. Chemother.* **18**: 582–585.

NICHOLS, R. L., SMITH, J. W., ADINOLFI, M. F., GALLI, R. and VIVODA, L. M. (1985) Inhibition of beta-lactamase-induced resistance in soft tissue infections. *Archs Surg.* **120**: 36–42.

NIKAIDO, H. (1984) Outer membrane permeability and beta-lactam resistance. In: *Microbiology 1984*, LEIVE, L. and SCHLESSINGER, D. (eds) Am. Soc. Microbiol., Washington, DC.

NIKAIDO, H. (1985) Role of permeability barriers in resistance to β-lactam antibiotics. *Pharmac. Ther.* **27**: 197–231.

NOZAKI, K., OKONOGI, K., KATAYAMA, N., ONO, H., HARADA, S., KONDO, M. and OKAZAKI, H. (1984) Cephabacins, new cephem antibiotics of bacterial origin. IV. Antibacterial activities, stability to beta-lactamases and mode of action. *J. Antibiot.* **37**: 1555–1565.

O'HARA, K., SHIOMI, Y. and KUNO, M. (1983) Comparative study of the activities of beta-lactamase inhibitors by nuclear magnetic resonance spectrometry. *Jap. J. Antibiot.* **36**: 2763–2768.

OLSSON, B., DORNBUSH, K. and NORD, C. E. (1977) Susceptibility to beta-lactam antibiotics and production of beta-lactamase in *Bacteroides fragilis. Med. Microbiol. Immunol.* **163**: 183–194.

PERCIVAL, A., CORKILL, J. E., ROWLANDS, J. and SYKES, R. B. (1977) Pathogenicity of and beta-lactamase production by *Branhamella* (*Neisseria*) *catarrhalis. Lancet* **ii**: 1175.

PETROCHEILOU, V., SYKES, R. B. and RICHMOND, M. H. (1977) Novel R-plasmid-mediated beta-lactamase from *Klebsiella aerogenes. Antimicrob. Ag. Chemother.* **12**: 126–128.

PITTON, J. S. (1982) Mechanisms of bacterial resistance to antibiotics. In: *Review of Physiology*, Vol. 65, pp. 15–93, ADIRNA, R. H. (ed.) Springer-Verlag, Berlin.

PRATT, R. F. and LOOSEMORE, M. J. (1978) 6-β-bromopenicillanic acid, a potent beta-lactamase inhibitor. *Proc. natn. Acad. Sci. U.S.A.* **75**: 4145–4149.

READING, C. and FARMER, T. (1981) The inhibition of beta-lactamases from gram-negative bacteria by clavulanic acid. *Biochem. J.* **199**: 779–787.

READING, C. and FARMER, T. (1984) The inhibition of periplasmic beta-lactamase in *E. coli* by clavulanic acid and other beta-lactamase inhibitors. *Post-grad. Med.* Sept–Oct 1984, 163–168.

RICHMOND, M. H. (1965) Wild-type variants of exopenicillinase from *Staphylococcus aureus. Biochem. J.* **88**: 452–549.

RICHMOND, M. H. and SYKES, R. B. (1973) The beta-lactamases of gram-negative bacteria and their possible physiological role. *Adv. Microbiol. Phys.* **9**: 31–88.

ROY, C., FOZ, A., SEGURA, C., TIRADO, M., FUSTER, C. and REIG, R. (1983) Plasmid-mediated beta-lactamases identified in a group of 204 ampicillin-resistant *Enterobacteriacae. J. Antimicrob. Chemother.* **12**: 507–510.

SABATH, L. D., JAGO, M. and ABRAHAM, E. P. (1965) Cephalosporinase and penicillinase activities of a beta-lactamase from *Pseudomonas pyocyanae. Biochem. J.* **96**: 739–752.

SAINO, Y., KOBAYASHI, F., INOUE, M. and MITSUHASHI, S. (1982) Purification and properties of an inducible penicillin beta-lactamase from *Pseudomonas maltophilia. Antimicrob. Ag. Chemother.* **22**: 564–570.

SATO, K., FUJII, T., OKAMOTO, R., INOUE, M. and MITSUHASHI, S. (1985) Biochemical properties of a β-lactamase produced by *Flavobacterium adoratum. Antimicrob. Ag. Chemother.* **27**: 612–614.

SAWAI, T., MITSUHASHI, S. and YAMAGISHI, S. (1968) Drug resistance of enterobacteria. Comparison of beta-lactamases in gram-negative and bacteria resistance to alpha-aminobenzyl-penicillin. *Jap. J. Microbiol.* **12**: 423–434.

SCULLY, B. E., STEINMAN, R., CHIN, N. X. and NEU, H. C. (1984) The pharmacology of clavulanic acid and ticarcillin combined. *Chemioterapia* **3**: 385–389.

SIMPSON, I. N., HARPER, P. B. and O'CALLAGHAN, C. H. (1980) Principal beta-lactamase responsible for resistance to beta-lactam antibiotics in urinary tract infections. *Antimicrob. Ag. Chemother.* **17**: 929–936.

SLOCOMBE, B., BEALE, A. S., BOON, R. J., GRIFFIN, K. E., MASTERS, P. J., SUTHERLAND, R. and WHITE, A. R. (1984) Antibacterial activity *in vitro* and *in vivo* of amoxicillin in the presence of clavulanic acid. *Post-grad. Med.* Sept–Oct 1984, 29–49.

VU, H. and NIKAIDO, H. (1985) Role of beta-lactamase hydrolysis in the mechanism of resistance of a beta-lactamase constitutive *Enterobacter cloacae* strain to expanded-spectrum beta-lactams. *Antimicrob. Ag. Chemother.* **27**: 393–398.

WISE, R., ANDREWS, J. M. and PATEL, N. (1981) 6-β-bromo and 6-β-iodo penicillanic acids, two novel beta-lactamase inhibitors. *J. Antimicrob. Chemother.* **7**: 531–536.

YAMAGUCHI, A., ADACHI, A., HIRATA, T., ADACHI, H. and SAWAI, T. (1985) Conversion of cloxacillin into a progressive inhibitor of beta-lactamases by sulfonation and its activity against various types of these enzymes. *J. Antibiot.* **38**: 83–93.

YAMAGUCHI, A., HIRATA, T. and SAWAI, T. (1984) Novel carbapenem derivative SF 2103A: studies on the mode of beta-lactamase inactivation. *Antimicrob. Ag. Chemother.* **25**: 348–353.

YOTSUJII, A., MIAMI, S., INOUE, M. and MITSUHASHI, S. (1983) Properties of a novel beta-lactamase produced by *Bacteroides fragilis. Antimicrob. Ag. Chemother.* **24**: 925–929.

ZEMELMAN, R., GONZALEZ, C., MONDACA, M. A., SILVA, J., MERINO, G. and DOMINGUEZ, M. (1984) Resistance of *Aeromonas hydrophilia* to beta-lactam antibiotics. *J. Antimicrob. Chemother.* **14**: 575–579.